# Pediatric Oncology

For further volumes:
http://www.springer.com/series/5421

Each volume of the series "Pediatric Oncology" covers the whole spectrum of the disease concerned, from research issues to clinical management, and is edited by internationally highly respected experts in a comprehensive and clearly structured way. The user-friendly layout allows quick reference to in-depth information. The series is designed for all health-care personnel interested in high-level education in pediatric oncology.

Cindy L. Schwartz • Wendy L. Hobbie
Louis S. Constine • Kathleen S. Ruccione
Editors

# Survivors of Childhood and Adolescent Cancer

## A Multidisciplinary Approach

**Third Edition**

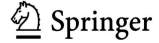

*Editors*

Cindy L. Schwartz
Department of Pediatrics
MD Anderson Cancer Center
Houston, TX
USA

Wendy L. Hobbie
Division of Oncology
Children's Hospital of Philadelphia
Philadelphia, PA
USA

Louis S. Constine
Departments of Radiation Oncology
and Pediatrics
University of Rochester Medical Center
James P. Wilmot Cancer Ctr.
Rochester, NY
USA

Kathleen S. Ruccione
Center for Cancer And Blood Diseases
Children's Hospital Los Angeles
Los Angeles, CA
USA

ISSN 1613-5318          ISSN 2191-0812    (electronic)
Pediatric Oncology
ISBN 978-3-319-16434-2          ISBN 978-3-319-16435-9    (eBook)
DOI 10.1007/978-3-319-16435-9

Library of Congress Control Number: 2015947443

Springer Cham Heidelberg New York Dordrecht London

Printed on acid-free paper

Springer International Publishing AG Switzerland is part of Springer Science+Business Media
(www.springer.com)

# Foreword

About two decades ago, when the first volume in this series was being prepared, most pediatric oncologists recognized that successful treatment would lead to cure for the majority of children with cancer. This 3rd edition continues to bring to clinicians useful advice regarding the management of children who have completed treatment and who are destined to live for decades. Some of the children will bear the brunt of late complications and their lives will be shorter than those of their peers; but many will have benefited greatly from the alterations in therapy designed to limit long-term toxicity, a therapy that was proven to be effective using the clinical trials approach that pediatric oncologists have embraced for almost half a century.

Efforts to improve the care of adult survivors of childhood cancer depend very much on understanding the relations between earlier therapy and future health. Quality of life is affected by problems real or anticipated resulting from medical complications, such as cardiac, pulmonary, gastrointestinal, neurologic, and endocrine late effects. Cognitive function and fertility are also major problems recognized in long-term survivors. However, with longer follow-up of more individuals, it is now possible to attempt to relate early treatment to the extent of these effects. It then makes possible the creation of therapeutic protocols that continue to test whether the most intensive therapy and that which results in the most serious late complications are truly necessary for successful tumor eradication in all children with a specific diagnosis.

Some readers may ask: "Why was this 3rd edition needed?" Since the preparation of the 2nd edition, there has been a proliferation of studies concerning longer-term complications in survivors of cancer in childhood, and their results have been reported in numerous publications, hence, this new edition. No other publication offers the wealth of information that clinicians need to care for children, adolescents, and adults who have survived cancer in childhood.

During my professional lifetime, a dramatic improvement in the survival rates for children with cancer has taken place. But this is old news. Even before the first edition of this extraordinary resource for pediatricians and other care givers first appeared in 1994, we began to recognize that "cure" would be possible for at least three of every four children and adolescents diagnosed with cancer. But since the publication of the 2nd edition in 2006, the emphasis has changed. The focus is now on two important issues: can pediatric oncology care providers devise treatment that maintains these excellent survival rates while avoiding therapy that we know is or suspect could be harmful in the long term, and how can we educate and empower survivors to understand their medical histories and enable them to take charge of their health?

Specialists in pediatric cancer share the responsibility for the care of survivors with general practitioners, during both pediatric and adult years, the specialists providing data derived from the study of large cohorts of long-term survivors and the generalists instituting health-promoting and early detection practices intended to prevent more serious disease. General practitioners can educate survivors to follow good health practices and avoid risk-taking behaviors, such as smoking, excess food and alcohol consumption, and unsafe sex. Counseling the long-term survivor in ways that will ensure early detection and prevention without raising unnecessary concerns requires sensitivity as well as the knowledge of specific long-term complications that could be associated with earlier disease and treatment. Although most of the effects of surgical procedures, radiation therapy, and drug combinations offered now are well known to pediatric oncologists, newer, perhaps more aggressive, treatments for children with resistant disease are currently under clinical investigation and, should they prove successful and enable more children to survive, their effects will not become known for many years. The combined efforts of pediatric oncology care providers and general practitioners will be required to observe, catalog, and report the consequences of newer approaches to cure.

One of the most salutary improvements during the last decade in treatment for children with cancer has been the emphasis on the so-called prognostic factors in selecting treatment appropriate to the risk of recurrence and sparing those children who derive no added benefit from more aggressive programs. This process needs to continue, and concern for long-term deleterious effects should enter into consideration of future regimens.

At present, the overall balance between the risks and benefits of therapy for childhood cancer lies clearly in the direction of benefit, even for the most aggressive treatment programs currently in clinical trials. As new treatments become widely accepted, follow-up designed to keep track of late-occurring toxicities should be incorporated into the clinical care of patients receiving therapy so that future generations are able to assess the impact of these treatments on long-term quality of life. It is important to learn more about the lifelong effects on specific age, disease, and treatment modality cohorts for the purpose of evaluating long-term risk-benefit ratios, as well as to increase our knowledge of the mechanism of the disease we produce.

Future young adult childhood cancer patients will benefit from changes in therapy that reduced or eliminated some of the agents responsible for many of the medical problems experienced by patients treated during the decades of the 1970s and 1980s. Nevertheless, possible long-term effects of childhood cancer and its treatment may become evident as survivors age. Several questions remain regarding the long-term complications of therapy. Clinicians need more data regarding the effects of aging to guide them in managing former patients.

Caregivers and pediatric cancer survivors who are now adults seek the optimal venue in which to receive care as independent adults. In addition, oncology care providers need to determine whether the models for research and clinical care of survivors created in pediatric oncology can be applied to survivors of adult-onset cancer. Providing a smooth transition for these patients to age-appropriate risk-based health care is a priority, and this can only occur by actively addressing the barriers faced by survivors, providers, and the health-care system. Once these barriers are overcome, we expect that childhood cancer survivors will live healthier, longer lives.

The Children's Hospital of Philadelphia,                              Anna T. Meadows, MD
Perelman School of Medicine
of the University of Pennsylvania
Philadelphia, PA, USA

# Contents

# Algorithms of Late Effects by Disease

Cindy L. Schwartz, Wendy L. Hobbie, and Louis S. Constine

This chapter provides algorithms designed to facilitate understanding of subsequent chapters. By locating the tumor type, information can be accessed from the algorithms regarding standard tumor therapies, common late effects, and methods of detection. Since the algorithms are relatively inclusive, not all patients will have received all therapies. Availability of the treatment record can assist in determining potential risk and streamlining screening procedures.

Of course, the clinical acumen of the healthcare professional cannot be replaced by algorithms. The recommendations should be used only as guides to potential risks. Information provided in subsequent chapters regarding specific organs is intended to deepen the healthcare provider's understanding of the pathophysiology, manifestations, and methods of detecting late effects.

Abbreviations commonly used in the algorithms are listed below.

| | |
|---|---|
| ACS | American Cancer Society |
| ALL | Acute lymphoblastic leukemia |
| ANLL | Acute nonlymphocytic leukemia |
| ARA-C | Cytosine arabinoside |
| BCNU | 1,3-Bis(2-chloroethyl)-1-nitrosourea |
| BMT | Bone marrow transplant |
| BP | Blood pressure |
| BUN | Blood urea nitrogen |
| CA | Carcinoma |
| CBC | Complete blood count |
| CCNU | Chloroethyl-cyclohexyl-nitrosourea |
| Cr | Creatinine |
| CrCl | Creatinine clearance |
| CXR | Chest radiograph |
| DTIC | Dacarbazine |
| ECHO | Echocardiogram |
| EKG | Electrocardiogram |
| FSH | Follicle-stimulating hormone |
| GFR | Glomerular filtration rate |
| GU | Genitourinary |
| H/P | Hypothalamic/pituitary |
| HD | High dose |
| HiB | *Hemophilus influenzae* type B (vaccine) |
| IT | Intrathecal |
| LFT's | Liver function tests |
| LH | Luteinizing hormone |

C.L. Schwartz, MD (✉)
Division Pediatric Hematology/Oncology,
Rhode Island Hospital, 593 Eddy Street,
Houston, TX 02903, USA
e-mail: Cindy_schwartz@brown.edu

W.L. Hobbie
Division of Oncology, Children's Hospital
of Philadelphia, 34th & Civic Center Boulevard,
Philadelphia, PA 19104, USA
e-mail: hobbie@email.chop.edu

L.S. Constine, MD
Departments of Radiation Oncology and Pediatrics,
University of Rochester Medical Center James
P. Wilmot Cancer Ctr.
601 Elmwood Avenue Box 647,
Rochester, NY 14642, USA
e-mail: Louis_constine@urmc.rochester.edu

© Springer International Publishing 2015
C.L. Schwartz et al. (eds.), *Survivors of Childhood and Adolescent Cancer:
A Multidisciplinary Approach*, Pediatric Oncology, DOI 10.1007/978-3-319-16435-9_1

| | | | |
|---|---|---|---|
| Mg | Magnesium | TSH | Thyroid-stimulating hormone |
| PFT's | Pulmonary function tests | UA | Urinalysis |
| PO$_4$ | Phosphate | VP-16 | Etoposide |
| 6-TG | Thioguanine | | |

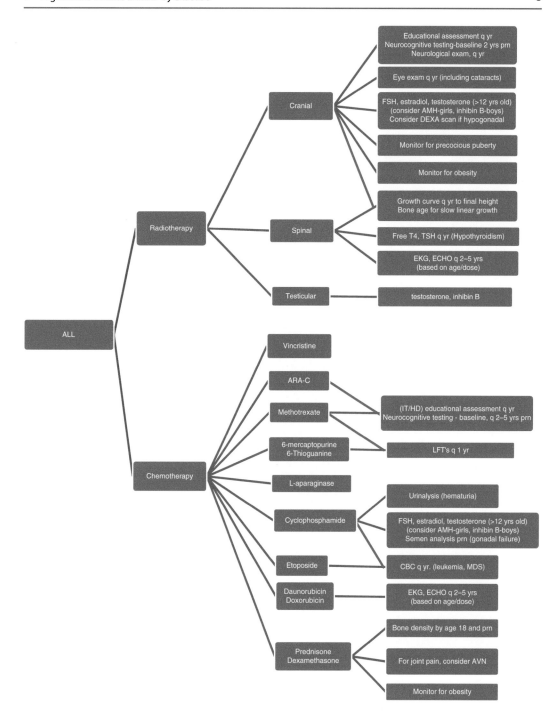

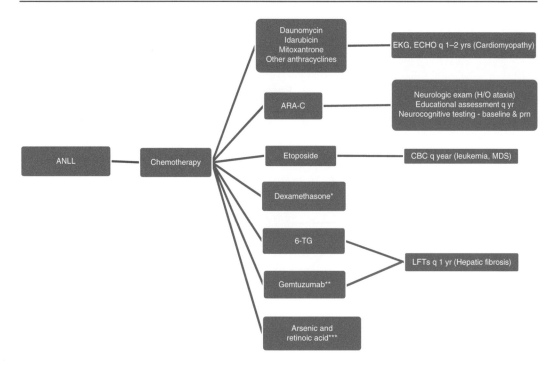

*No longer used in current protocols
**Patients may have received this agent, but it is no longer approved for use in the USA
***APML

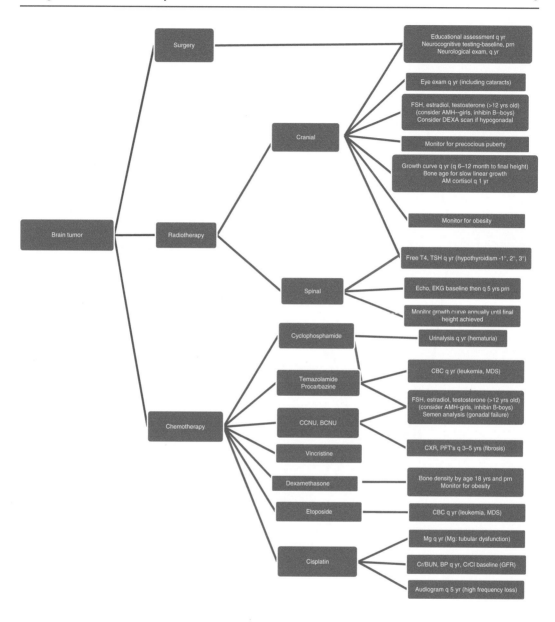

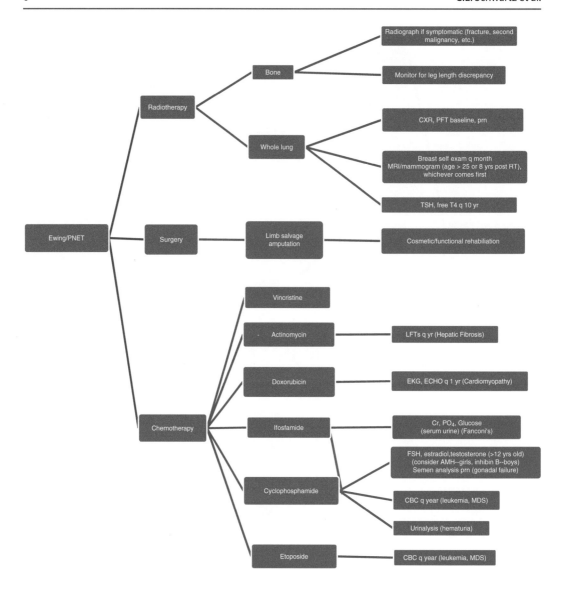

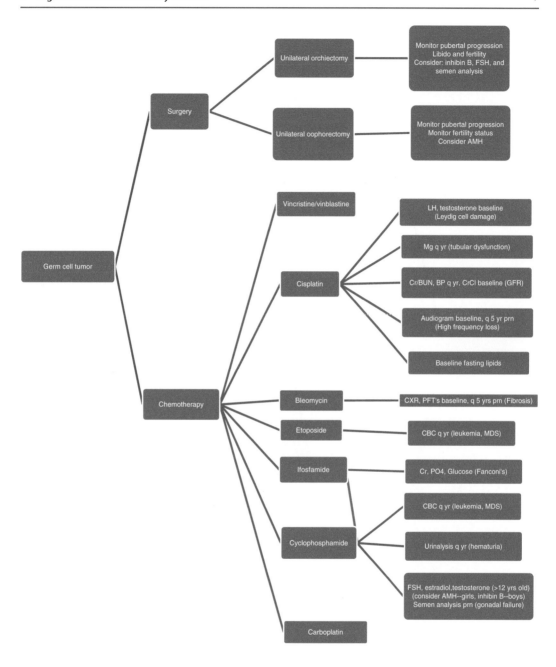

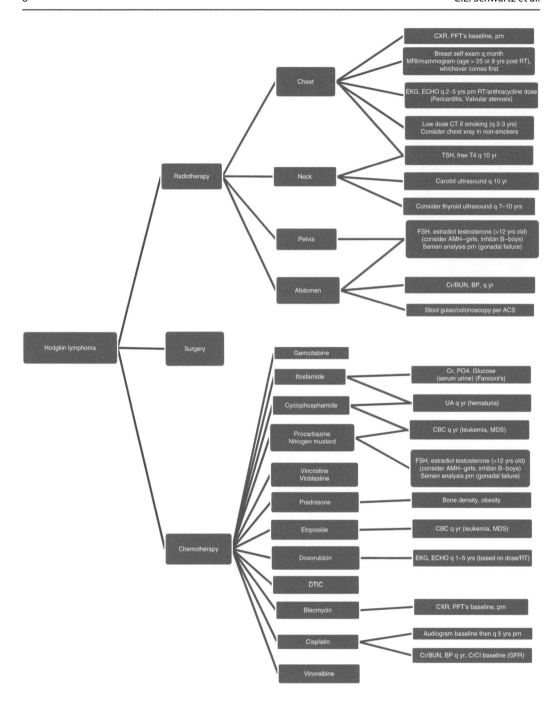

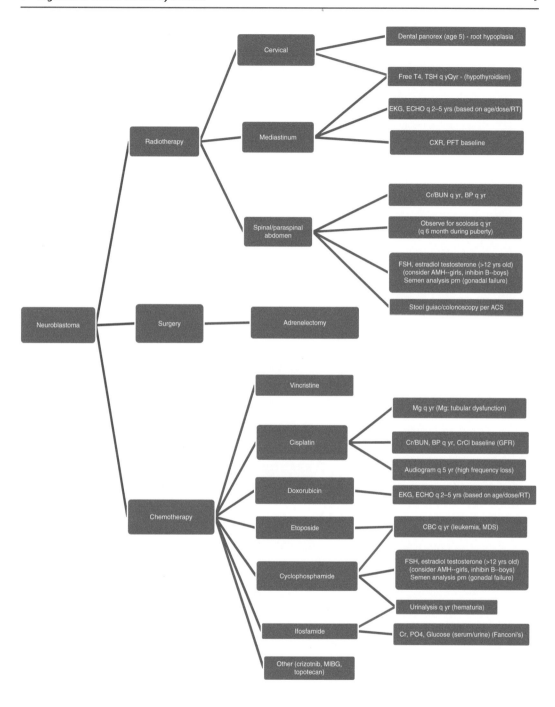

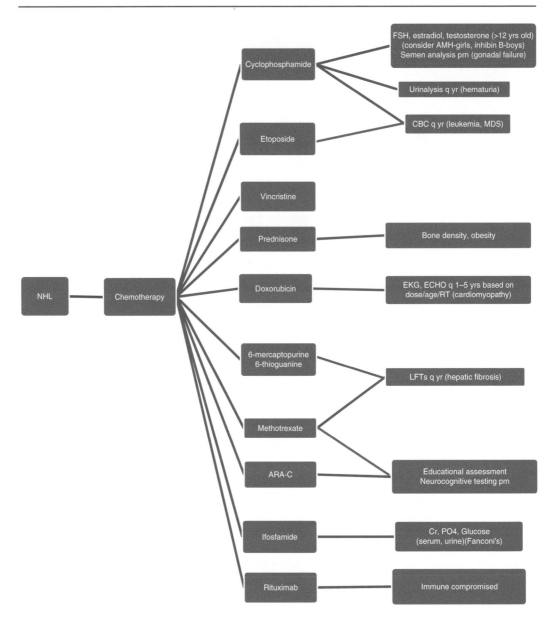

Historical: Cranial, mediastinal or abdominal radiation may have been used (see ALL and HL for recommendation).

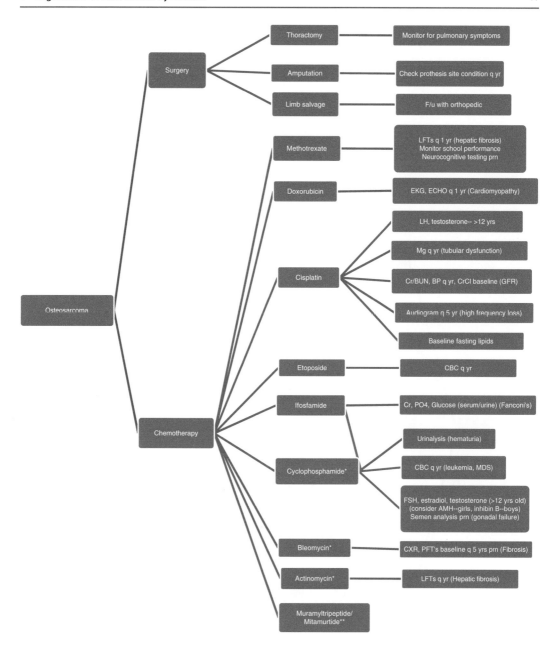

*Not part of most current treatment protocols
**Not approved by US FDA for use yet

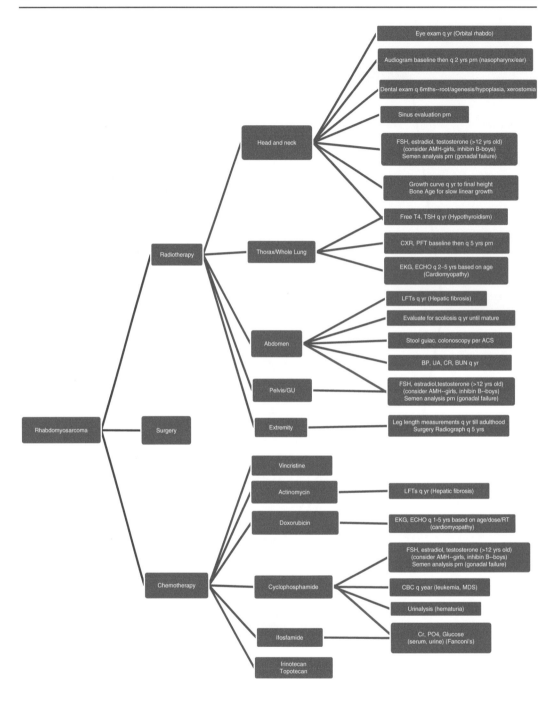

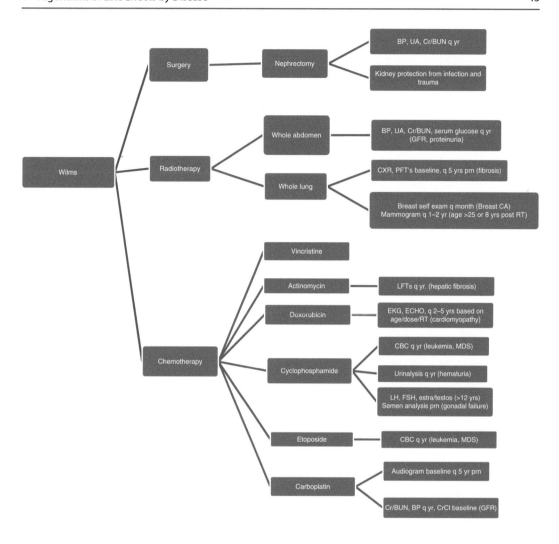

# Facilitating Assessment of Late Effects by Organ System

**2**

Cindy L. Schwartz, Wendy L. Hobbie, and Louis S. Constine

This chapter provides charts by organ system that cover the late effects of various cancer treatments. The healthcare provider for a patient with cardiac symptomatology, for example, can review the cardiac chart to find the common late side effects, causative treatments (chemotherapy, radiation, or surgery), signs and symptoms, screening and diagnostic tests, and appropriate intervention and management procedures. If further information is needed, the reader can refer to the chapter that covers the affected organ for a detailed discussion of the pathophysiology and clinical manifestations, as well as additional information regarding detection, screening, management, and intervention.

The charts (Tables 2.1, 2.2, 2.3, 2.4, 2.5, 2.6, 2.7, 2.8, 2.9, 2.10, 2.11, 2.12, 2.13, and 2.14), in conjunction with the algorithms in Chapter 1, should facilitate planning patient evaluations in preparation for accessing more detailed information in the chapters that follow.

C.L. Schwartz (✉)
Department of Pediatrics,
MD Anderson Cancer Center, Houston, TX, USA
e-mail: clschwartz@mdanderson.org

W.L. Hobbie
Division of Oncology,
Children's Hospital of Philadelphia,
Philadelphia, PA, USA
e-mail: hobbie@email.chop.edu

L.S. Constine
Departments of Radiation Oncology and Pediatrics,
University of Rochester Medical Center James
P. Wilmot Cancer Ctr., Rochester, NY, USA
e-mail: louis_constine@urmc.rochester.edu

© Springer International Publishing 2015
C.L. Schwartz et al. (eds.), *Survivors of Childhood and Adolescent Cancer:
A Multidisciplinary Approach*, Pediatric Oncology, DOI 10.1007/978-3-319-16435-9_2

**Table 2.1** Evaluation of patients at risk for late effects: thyroid

| Late effects | Causative treatment | | | Signs and symptoms | Screening and diagnostic tests | Management and intervention |
|---|---|---|---|---|---|---|
| | Chemotherapy | Radiation | Surgery | | | |
| Overt hypothyroidism (elevated TSH, decreased $T_4$) | | >20 Gy to the neck, cervical spine; >7.5 Gy TBI (total body irradiation) | Partial or complete thyroidectomy | Hoarseness Fatigue Weight gain Dry skin Cold intolerance Dry brittle hair Alopecia Constipation Lethargy Poor linear growth Menstrual irregularities Pubertal delay Bradycardia Hypotension Asymptomatic | Free $T_4$, TSH annually Plot on growth chart | Thyroxine replacement Anticipatory guidance regarding symptoms of hyperthyroidism/ hypothyroidism |
| Compensated hypothyroidism (elevated TSH, normal $T_4$) | | Same as *overt hypothyroidism* | Same as *overt hypothyroidism* | Asymptomatic | Free $T_4$, TSH annually Plot on growth chart | Thyroxine to suppress gland activity |
| Thyroid nodules | | Same as *overt hypothyroidism* | | Same as *overt hypothyroidism* | Free $T_4$, TSH annually Physical exam | Thyroid ultrasound Biopsy/resection |
| Hyperthyroidism (decreased TSH, elevated $T_4$) | | Same as *overt hypothyroidism* | | Nervousness Tremors Heat intolerance Weight loss Insomnia Increased appetite Diarrhea Moist skin Tachycardia Exophthalmos Goiter | Free $T_4$, TSH annually Physical exam $T_3$, antithyroglobulin Antimicrosomal Antibody baseline, then prn symptoms | Refer to endocrinologist (PTU, propranolol, $^{131}$I thyroidectomy) |

**Table 2.2**  Evaluation of patients at risk for late effects: CNS effects

| Late effects | Causative treatment | | | Signs and symptoms | Screening and diagnostic tests | Management and intervention |
|---|---|---|---|---|---|---|
| | Chemotherapy | Radiation | Surgery | | | |
| Neurocognitive deficit | High-dose IV MTX, IT MTX | >18 Gy | Resection of CNS tumor | Difficulty with reading, language, verbal/nonverbal memory, arithmetic, receptive, and expressive language Decreased speed of mental processing Attention deficit Decreased IQ Behavior problems Poor school attendance Poor hand-eye coordination | Neurocognitive testing: psychoeducational, neuropsychologic | Psychoeducation assistance |
| Leukoencephalopathy | MTX Ara-C (IV or IT) | >18 Gy | | Seizures Neurologic impairment Compare with premorbid status | MRI/CT scan baseline and symptoms | Symptom management: Muscle relaxant Anticonvulsants Physical therapy Occupational therapy |
| Focal necrosis | MTX (IT or high-dose IV), BCNU, CDDP | >50 Gy (especially with >21 Gy daily fraction) | Resection of tumor | Headaches Nausea Seizures Papilledema Hemiparesis/other focal findings Speech, learning, and memory deficits | MRI/CT scan baseline, PRN symptoms, PET or SPECT scan | Steroid therapy Debulking of necrotic tissue |
| Large-vessel stroke | | >60 Gy | | Headache Seizures Hemiparesis Aphasia Focal neurologic findings | CT scan/MRI Arteriogram | Determined by specific neurologic impairment |
| Blindness | Intra-arterial BCNU, CDDP | RT (optic nerve chiasm, occipital lobe) | Resection of tumor | Progressive visual loss | Ophthalmic evaluation Visual evoked response | Visual aids |
| Ototoxicity | CDDP, carboplatin | >50 Gy (middle/inner ear) | | Abnormal speech Hearing loss | Conventional pure tone audiogram baseline and prn symptoms | Speech therapy Hearing aid Referral to ENT Feucher amplification |
| Myelitis | Ara-C (IT) | >45–50 Gy | Spinal cord surgery | Paresis Spasticity Altered sensation Loss of sphincter control | MRI | Steroids Physical therapy Occupational therapy |

**Table 2.3** Evaluation of patients at risk for late effects: gastrointestinal

| Late effects | Causative treatment | | | Signs and symptoms | Screening and diagnostic tests | Management and intervention |
|---|---|---|---|---|---|---|
| | Chemotherapy | Radiation | Surgery | | | |
| Enteritis | Doxo and Act-D (RT enhancers) | >40 Gy | Abdominal surgery enhances RT effect | Abdominal pain Diarrhea Decreased stool bulk Emesis Weight loss Poor linear growth | Height and weight q yr Stool guaiac q yr, CBC with MCV q yr Total protein and albumin q 3–5 years (absorption tests, vitamin B12 level, and contrast studies) | Dietary management Refer to gastroenterologist |
| Adhesions | | RT enhances effect | Laparotomy | Abdominal pain Bilious vomiting Hyperactive bowel sounds | Abdominal radiograph | NPO Gastric suction Adhesion lysis |
| Fibrosis: esophagus (stricture) | Doxo and Act-D (RT enhancers) | >40–50 Gy | Abdomen | Dysphagia Weight loss Poor linear growth | Height and weight q yr, CBC q yr | Refer to GI |
| Fibrosis: small intestines | | >40 Gy | Abdomen | Abdominal pain Constipation Diarrhea Weight loss Obstruction | Height and weight q yr, CBC q yr (BA swallow/endoscopy prn) | Esophageal dilation Anti-reflux surgery |
| Fibrosis: large intestine, colon | | >40 Gy | Abdomen | Abdominal colic Rectal pain Constipation Melena Weight loss Obstruction | Height and weight q yr Rectal exam Stool guaiac q yr Lower GI Colonoscopy Sigmoidoscopy | Stool softeners High-fiber diet |

**Table 2.4** Evaluation of patients at risk for late effects: hepatic

| Late effects | Causative treatment | | | Signs and symptoms | Screening and diagnostic tests | Management and intervention |
| | Chemotherapy | Radiation | Surgery | | | |
| --- | --- | --- | --- | --- | --- | --- |
| Hepatic fibrosis/ cirrhosis | MTX, Act-D 6MP, 6TG | >30 Gy | Major resection | Itching<br>Jaundice<br>Spider nevi<br>Bruising<br>Portal hypertension<br>Esophageal varices<br>Hemorrhoids<br>Hematemesis<br>Encephalopathy | LFTs q yr (hepatitis C screen, liver biopsy, endoscopy) | Hepatitis screen (hepatitis A, B, C, CMV)<br>Diuretics<br>Refer to hepatologist |

**Table 2.5** Evaluation of patients at risk for late effects: genitourinary

| Late effects | Causative treatment | | | Signs and symptoms | Screening and diagnostic tests | Management and intervention |
|---|---|---|---|---|---|---|
| | Chemotherapy | Radiation | Surgery | | | |
| Glomerular dysfunction | CDDP, carboplatin, Ifos | >20 Gy or >15 Gy with chemotherapy | | Asymptomatic or fatigue, poor linear growth, anemia, oliguria | Creatinine and BUN q yr; Creatinine clearance baseline and q 3 years; Annual: blood pressure; Height, weight; Hemoglobin; Urinalysis | Low-protein diet; Dialysis; Renal transplant |
| Hypoplastic kidney/renal arteriosclerosis | | 20–30 Gy or 10–15 Gy with chemotherapy | | Fatigue; Poor linear growth; Hypertension; Headache; Edema; Albuminuria; Urinary casts | Same as *glomerular dysfunction* | Same as *glomerular dysfunction* |
| Tubular dysfunction | CDDP, carboplatin, Ifos | | | Seizures ($\downarrow$ Mg); Weakness ($\downarrow$ Po$_4$); Glycosuria; Poor linear growth | Mg, Ca, PO$_4$, Cr, BUN, Hg annually, BP/urinalysis q year, 24-h urine for Ca, Po$_4$ prn for abnormalities | Mg supplement, Po$_4$ supplement |
| Nephrotic syndrome | | 20–30 Gy | | Proteinuria; Edema | Serum protein, albumin, Cr, BUN, q year; Urinalysis q yr; Blood pressure q 1 (24-h urine for protein and Cr) | Low-salt diet; Diuretics |
| Bladder: fibrosis or hypoplasia, reduced bladder capacity | CPM, Ifos, surgical referral | >30 Gy prepubertal >50 Gy postpubertal | | Urgency; Frequency; Dysuria; Incontinence (nocturia); Pelvic hypoplasia | Urinalysis q yr; Cystoscopy, IVP/US, volumetrics | Exercises to increase bladder capacity |

| | Late effect | Chemotherapy | Radiation dose | Signs/symptoms | Screening | Management |
|---|---|---|---|---|---|---|
| | Hemorrhagic and nonhemorrhagic cystitis | CPM, Ifos | 35 Gy (lower doses enhance chemotherapy effect) | Hematuria, or frequency, urgency, dysuria, bladder tenderness | Urinalysis q yr; Cystoscopy if hematuria on 2 exams; Hg q year | Refer to urologist; Maintain Hg; Antispasmodics; Counsel regarding risk of bladder cancer |
| | Prostate | | 40–60 Gy (lower doses inhibit development; higher doses cause atrophy) | Decreased volume of seminal fluid; Hypoplastic or atrophied prostate | Prostate examination q yr; Semen analysis × 1 at maturity. Ultrasound | Counsel regarding possible infertility due to inadequate seminal fluid; Monitor prostate (exam and prostate-specific antigen) |
| | Vagina: fibrosis/diminished growth | Act-D and doxo enhance RT effect | 4–60 Gy (lower doses inhibit development; higher doses cause atrophy) | Painful intercourse; Vaginal bleeding; Small vaginal vault | Pelvic exam (possibly under anesthesia), baseline during puberty and then prn for symptoms | Dilations; Reconstructive surgery; Potential need for cesarean section |
| | Uterus: fibrosis/decreased growth | | >20 Gy (prepubertal); >40–50 Gy (postpubertal) | Spontaneous abortion; Low birth weight infants | Pelvic examination, prn for symptoms or if planning pregnancy | Counsel regarding pregnancy; Refer to gynecologist if considering pregnancy |
| | Ureter: fibrosis | | >50–60 Gy | Frequent UTIs; Pelvic hypoplasia; Hydronephrosis | Urinalysis q yr; Urethrogram | UTI prophylaxis |
| GU | Urethra: strictures | | >50 Gy | Frequent UTIs; Dysuria; Stream abnormalities | Urinalysis q yr; Voiding cystogram | UTI prophylaxis; Surgical intervention |

**Table 2.6** Evaluation of patients at risk for late effects: head and neck

| Late effects | Causative treatment | | | Signs and symptoms | Screening and diagnostic tests | Management and intervention |
|---|---|---|---|---|---|---|
| | Chemotherapy | Radiation | Surgery | | | |
| Xerostomia (decreased salivary gland function) | Doxo and Act D (RT enhances) | >30 Gy (and >50 % of the gland must be radiated) | | Decreased salivary flow Dry mouth Altered taste perception Dental decay Candida (thrush) | Dental examination Salivary flow studies Attention to early caries, periodontal disease | Encourage meticulous oral hygiene Saliva substitute Prophylactic fluoride Dietary counseling regarding avoiding fermentable carbohydrates Nystatin for oral candidiasis Pilocarpine |
| Intranasal scarring | | >40 Gy | | Chronic rhinosinusitis Nasal discharge Postnasal drip Facial pain Headache | Inspection of mucosa Nasopharyngoscopy | Decongestants Drainage procedures Antibiotics prn |
| Epilation (scalp) | | >15–20 Gy | | Thinning of hair Alopecia | Examination | Wigs Compensatory hair styling |
| Eyelash eyebrow | | >50 Gy | | | | |
| Fibrosis | | >40 Gy | | Pain Constriction Facial asymmetry Limitation of jaw motion (TMJ fibrosis) | Examination | Prevention of infection (especially after trauma), "stretching" exercises of TMJ |
| Osteonecrosis | | >50–60 Gy (or interstitial radiation) | Tooth extraction | Ulcers/necrosis | Examination | Prosthetic devices Surgical repair |
| Abnormal facial growth | | >30 Gy | | Facial asymmetry Hypoplastic development of orbit, maxilla, mandible | Examination | Prosthetic devices Surgical repair |
| Craniofacial deformity | | | Surgery | | Examination | Surgical repair |
| Abnormal tooth and root development | VCR, Act-D, CPM, 6MP, PCZ, $HN_2$ | ≥10 Gy | | Enamel appears pale Teeth appear small, uneven Malocclusion | Dental exam q6 months with attention to early caries, periodontal disease, and gingivitis. Panorex/bitewing radiographs baseline (age 5–6) | Careful evaluation prior to tooth extraction, endodontics, and orthodontics Fluoride Antibiotics prn for risk of infection (e.g., trauma) |

| | | | | | |
|---|---|---|---|---|---|
| Sensory neural hearing loss | Cisplatin | ≥35–40 Gy cranial RT enhances the platinum effect | High-frequency hearing loss (bilateral) Tinnitus Vertigo | Conventional pure tone audiogram baseline and then q 2–3 years Bilateral, symmetrical, irreversible | Preferential seating in school Hearing aid and referral ENT teacher amplification |
| Chronic otitis | | ≥40–50 Gy | Dryness and thickness of canal and tympanic membrane Conductive hearing loss Perforation of TM | Otoscopic exam Audiometry | Antibiotic therapy Decongestants Myringotomy PE tubee Perferential seating in school Amplification |
| Decreased production of cerumen | | ≥30–40 Gy | Hard and encrusted cerumen in canal Hearing impairment Otitis externa | Examination of canal | Periodic cleaning of ear canal Cerumen-loosening agents Otic drops for otitis externa Keep ear dry: ear plugs Drying solution |
| Chondritis | | ≥50 Gy | Cauliflower ear | Inspection of auricle | Antibiotics Surgical repair (reconstruction may be hampered by poor blood supply) |
| Chondronecrosis | | ≥60 Gy | | | |

**Table 2.7** Evaluation of patients at risk for late effects: integumentary/breast

| Late effects | Causative treatment | | | Signs and symptoms | Screening and diagnostic tests | Management and intervention |
|---|---|---|---|---|---|---|
| | Chemotherapy | Radiation | Surgery | | | |
| Alopecia | | >40 Gy | | Hair loss involving the scalp, eyelashes, or eyebrows | Examination | Wig Compensatory hair styling |
| Skin hyperpigmentation | Bleo, Bus, DTIC | >30 Gy | | Hyperpigmentation | Examine skin | Cosmetic intervention only |
| Increased benign or malignant melanocytic nevi | | RT | | Increased numbers of pigmented nevi in the field of radiation | Skin examination annually. Photograph involved areas to follow accurately | Refer to dermatologist for close follow-up of multiple or suspicious lesions. Biopsy of suspicious lesions |
| Basal cell carcinoma | | RT | | Lesion | Skin examination annually | Excisional biopsy Refer to dermatology |
| Hypoplasia of soft tissue | Doxo and Act-D (IT enhancers) | >20 Gy (developing child) | | Decreased elasticity Decreased tissue volume Local inability to sweat Dryness | Annual examination of skin elasticity and volume | Avoid sun exposure Use sunscreen a speciality in treated area Moisturizers |
| Telangiectasia | As above | >40 Gy | Enhances risk, compromises blood supply | Skin appears tight with woody texture Spidery pattern of small blood vessels | Annual examination of the skin | Avoid sun exposure. Avoid skin trauma |
| Skin fibrosis/necrosis | As above | >40 Gy | Enhances risk, compromises blood supply | Contractures Discoloration of tissue | Annual skin exam Examination for tissue breakdown | Must be in the care of a dermatologist – may require surgery |
| Hypoplasia of breast tissue | | 10 Gy (pubertal breast very sensitive) | | Reduced breast tissue Failure to lactate in treated breast | Annual breast examination Mammography at later of age 25 years or 8 years post-XRT baseline, then q 1–2 years (annually after age 40) | Teach BSE Anticipatory guidance re: breast nodules Impaired lactation |

**Table 2.8** Evaluation of patients at risk for late effects: musculoskeletal

| Late effects | Causative treatment | | | Signs and symptoms | Screening and diagnostic tests | Management and intervention |
|---|---|---|---|---|---|---|
| | Chemotherapy | Radiation | Surgery | | | |
| Muscular hypoplasia | | >20 Gy (growing child) younger children more sensitive | Muscle loss or resection | Asymmetry of muscle mass when compared with untreated area Decreased range of motion Stiffness and pain in affected area (uncommon) | Careful comparison and measurement of irradiated and unirradiated areas Range of motion | Prevention: exercise program, range of motion Muscle strengthening |
| Spinal abnormalities Scoliosis Kyphosis Lordosis Decreased sitting height | | For young children, RT to hemi-abdomen or spine (especially vertebral), 10 Gy (minimal effect), >20 Gy (clinically notable defect) | Laminectomy | Spinal Curvature Back pain Hip pain Uneven shoulder height Rib humps or flares Gait abnormalities | Standing height by stadiometer. During puberty, examine spine q 5 months if growth is completed Spinal films baseline during puberty then prn curvature (COBB technique to measure curvature) | Refer to orthopedist if any curvature is noted, especially during a period of rapid growth |
| Length discrepancy | | >20 Gy | Involving growth plates | Lower back pain Limp Hip pain Discrepancy in muscle mass and length when compared with untreated extremity Scoliosis | Annual measurement of treated and untreated limb (completely undress patient to assure accurate measurements) Radiograph baseline to assess remaining epiphyseal growth Radiographs annually during periods of rapid growth | Contralateral epiphysiodesis Limb-shortening procedures |
| Pathological fracture | | >40 Gy | Biopsy | Pain Edema Ecchymosis | Baseline radiograph of treated area to assess bone integrity, then prn for symptoms | Consider limitation of activities (e.g., contact sports) Surgical repair of fracture; may require internal fixation |
| Osteonecrosis | Steroids | >40–50 Gy (more common in adults) | | Pain in affected joint Limp | Radiograph, CT scan prn for symptoms | Symptomatic care Joint replacement |
| Osteocartilaginous exostoses | | RT | | Painless lump/mass noted in the field of radiation | Radiograph baseline and prn for growth of lesion | Resection for cosmetic or functional reasons Counsel regarding 10 % incidence of malignant degeneration |
| Slipped capitofemoral epiphysis | High-dose steroids | >25 Gy (at young age) | | Pain in affected hip Limp Abnormal gait | Radiograph baseline to assess integrity of the treated joint(s), then prn for symptoms | Refer to orthopedist for surgical intervention |

**Table 2.9** Evaluation of patients at risk for late effects: ophthalmology

| Late effects | Causative treatment | | | Signs and symptoms | Screening and diagnostic tests | Management and intervention |
|---|---|---|---|---|---|---|
| | Chemotherapy | Radiation | Surgery | | | |
| Lacrimal glands: decreased tear production | 5FU | >40 Gy | | Dry, irritated red eye; Foreign-body sensation | Eye exam/slit-lamp exam; Fluorescein staining | Tear replacement; Occlude lacrimal puncta |
| Lacrimal duct: fibrosis | 5FU | >50 Gy | | Tearing | Ophthalmic exam | Dilation of duct |
| Eyelids: ulceration | | 50 Gy | | Blepharitis; Bleeding/crusted lesion; Previous infections | Eye exam | Topical/oral steroids; Skin balm; Teach: lid hygiene; Radiosensitizing drugs |
| Telangiectasia | | 50 Gy | | Enlarged, tortuous blood vessels; Pigmentary changes | Slit lamp | UV protection; Avoid trauma, harsh soaps, and lotions |
| Conjunctiva: necrosis | | >45 Gy; Radioactive plaque therapy | | Pain, dry irritated eye; Foreign-body sensation | Eye exam; Slit lamp; Fluorescein stain | Steroids/antibiotic drops; Ophthalmology |
| Sclera: thinning | | >50 Gy | | May be asymptomatic; Gray, charred, blue sclera | Eye exam; Slit-lamp exam | Antibiotic drops; Avoid trauma; Protective glasses |
| Cornea: ulceration Keratinization | | >45 Gy | | Pain; Foreign-body sensation; Decreased VA; Photosensitivity | Eye exam; Slit lamp; Fluorescein staining | Antibiotics; Soft bandages; Soft contact lens; Surgery; Ophthalmology |
| Lens: cataract | Steroids (incidence varies with dose) | >6 Gy (single dose) or >10 Gy (fractionated) | | Decreased visual acuity; Opaque lens | Direct ophthalmoscopic exam; Decreased red reflex; Slit lamp; Opaque lens | Prevention by shielding during treatment; Surgical removal; Educate regarding UV protection |

| Condition | Dose | Signs and symptoms | Treatment | Screening | Management |
|---|---|---|---|---|---|
| Iris: neovascularization | >50 Gy | May be asymptomatic / New blood vessels in iris (rubeosis) / Blood in anterior chamber | | Eye exam / Slit lamp | Steroid drops |
| Secondary glaucoma | | Eye pain, headache, nausea/vomiting, decreased peripheral vision, increased IOP | | Measure ocular pressure | Beta-blocker drops, atropine, Acetazolamide |
| Atrophy | >50 Gy | Decreased iris stroma at pupillary margin | | Slit-lamp/penlight exam | Photocoagulation |
| Retina: infarction | >50 Gy | Blanched white cotton spots / Decreased visual acuity / Decreased visual field / Blurred vision (central or peripheral) | | Visual acuity / Visual field | Steroids / Photocoagulation / Education regarding avoiding ASA and bleeding precautions |
| Hemorrhage | >50 Gy | | | | |
| Telangiectasia | >50 Gy | | | | |
| Neovascularization | >50 Gy | | | | |
| Macular edema | >50 Gy | Blister of fluid in the macula | | | |
| Optic neuropathy | >50 Gy | Pale optic disk / Abnormal pupillary responses | Tumor resection | Visual evaluation | Visual aids |

**Table 2.10** Evaluation of patients at risk for late effects: ovarian

| Late effects | Causative treatment | | | Signs and symptoms | Screening and diagnostic tests | Management and intervention |
|---|---|---|---|---|---|---|
| | Chemotherapy | Radiation | Surgery | | | |
| Ovarian failure | CPM, PCB, bus, BCNU, CCNU, Ifos | 4–12 Gy Tolerance decreases with increasing age | Oophorectomy or oophoropexy | Delayed/arrested/absent pubertal development Changes in duration, frequency, and character of menses (cramping) Estrogen deficiency: Hot flashes Vaginal dryness Dyspareunia Low libido Infertility Leg cramping | Tanner stage, LH, FSH, estradiol at: 1. Age 12 years 2. Failure of pubertal development 3. Baseline when fully mature 4. prn for symptoms | Hormone replacement therapy Anticipatory guidance regarding symptoms of estrogen deficiency and early menopause Alternate strategies for parenting |

**Table 2.11** Evaluation of patients at risk for late effects: peripheral system effects

| Late effects | Causative treatment | | | Signs and symptoms | Screening and diagnostic tests | Management and intervention |
|---|---|---|---|---|---|---|
| | Chemotherapy | Radiation | Surgery | | | |
| Peripheral neuropathy | VP-16, VCR, CDDP | 60 Gy | | Weakness Lack of coordination Tingling Numbness | Annual neurologic examination | Protecting affected area from excess heat or cold exposure Physical therapy Occupational therapy Medications |

**Table 2.12** Evaluation of patients at risk for late effects: pulmonary

| Late effects | Causative treatment | | | Signs and symptoms | Screening and diagnostic tests | Management and intervention |
|---|---|---|---|---|---|---|
| | Chemotherapy | Radiation | Surgery | | | |
| Pulmonary fibrosis | Bleo, CCNU, BCNU, CPM, MTX | Pulmonary RT >10 Gy Risk increases with doses, larger volume irradiated, and younger age | | Fatigue Cough Dyspnea on exertion Reduced exercise tolerance Orthopnea Cyanosis Finger clubbing Rales Cor pulmonale | CXR, O$_2$ saturation, PFT with DLCO, baseline then q 3–5 years prn | If symptomatic, refer to pulmonologist Prevention: avoidance of smoking Avoidance of infections: influenza vaccine Pneumovax After bleomycin: avoid FiO2 >30 % (e.g., during surgery) |

**Table 2.13** Evaluation of patients at risk for late effects: testicular

| Late effects | Causative treatment | | | Signs and symptoms | Screening and diagnostic tests | Management and intervention |
|---|---|---|---|---|---|---|
| | Chemotherapy | Radiation | Surgery | | | |
| Germ cell damage: oligospermia/azoospermia | CPM, HN$_2$, CCNU/BCNU, PCB, Ifos | >1–6 Gy to the testes (direct or scatter) | Orchiectomy or surgical manipulation | Testicular atrophy (softer, smaller) Failure to impregnate | Tanner stage Inquire regarding previous sperm banking Assess testicular size and consistency. LH, FSH, consider inhibin B testosterone: 1. For failure of pubertal development 2. Baseline when sexually mature 3. For failure to impregnate, repeat q 3 years for possible recovery Spermoto-analysis at maturity or for failure to impregnate (repeat q 3–5 years prn to assess recovery) | Instruct: testicular self-examination Anticipatory guidance re: infertility counseling, alternate strategies for fathering |
| Leydig cell damage | CPM | >24 Gy to the testes (direct or scattered from pelvis) | Orchiectomy or surgical manipulation | Testicular atrophy (softer, smaller) | At age 13 evaluate: pubertal development Testosterone, CM, consider-inhibin B | Testosterone replacement |
| Testosterone deficiency | Ifos, CCNU, BCNU, HN$_2$ CPM | | | Delayed/arrested/absent pubertal development: pubic and axillary hair (female hair pattern) Lack of penile and testicular enlargement, voice change or body odor, and acne | If sexually mature: Baseline testosterone, LH Consider inhibin B Changes in libido or sexual performance | Anticipatory guidance regarding testosterone deficiency |

**Table 2.14** Evaluation of patients at risk for late effects: cardiac

| Late effects | Causative treatment | | | Signs and symptoms | Screening and diagnostic tests | Management and intervention |
|---|---|---|---|---|---|---|
| | Chemotherapy | Radiation | Surgery | | | |
| Cardiomyopathy (ventricular dysfunction) | Anthracycline >300 mg/m², >200 mg/m² with RT to mediastinum, High-dose CTX (BMT) | >30 Gy, >20 Gy and anthracyclines | | Fatigue, Cough, Dyspnea on exertion, Peripheral edema, Hypertension, Tachypnea/rales, Tachycardia, Cardiomegaly (S3/S4), Hepatomegaly | EKG, ECHO/RNA, and CXR baselines q 1–5 years (depending on risk factors) | Diuretics, Digoxin, Afterload reducers, Antiarrhythmics, Cardiac transplant, Education: risks of smoking, pregnancy, anesthesia, alcohol, drug use, isometric exercise |
| Valvular damage (mitral/tricuspid aortic) | | >30 Gy | | Weakness, Cough, Dyspnea on exertion, New murmur, Pulsating liver | ECHO and CXR baseline, q 3–5 years, and prn for symptoms | Penicillin prophylaxis for surgery/dental procedures |
| Pericardial damage | | >30 Gy | | Fatigue, Dyspnea on exertion, Chest pain, Cyanosis, Ascites, Peripheral edema, Hypotension, Friction rub, Muffled heart sounds, Venous distention, Pulsus paradoxus | EKG (ST–T changes, decreased voltage), ECHO, CXR baseline, q 3–5 years | Pericardial stripping |
| Coronary artery disease | | >30 Gy | | Chest pain on exertion (radiates to arm/neck), Dyspnea, Diaphoresis, Pallor, Hypotension, Arrhythmias | EKG q 3 years, stress test (consider dobutamine stress echocardiography) baseline, q 3–5 years, or prn for symptoms | Diuretics, Cardiac medications, Low-sodium, low-fat diet, Conditioning regimens, Statins |
| Conduction abnormality | Anthracycline >300 mg/m², >200 mg/m² and RT to mediastinum | >30 Gy | | Syncope, Palpitations, Arrhythmias | EKG, Holter monitor after high cumulative anthracycline dose (>300 mg/m²) or symptoms | Cardiology, Anti-arrhythmic |

Abbreviations used in this section are included in the glossary at the end.

Chemotherapy

| | |
|---|---|
| 5FU | 5-Fluorouracil |
| 6MP | 6-Mercaptopurine |
| 6TG | 6-Thioguanine |
| ABVD | Adriamycin, bleomycin, vincristine, actinomycin D |
| Act-D | Actinomycin D |
| Ara-C | Cytosine arabinoside |
| BCNU | 1,3-Bis(2-chloroethyl)-1-nitrosourea) |
| BLEO | Bleomycin |
| Bus | Busulfan |
| Carbo | Carboplatin |
| CCNU | 1,-(2-chloroethyl-3-cyclohexyl-1 nitrosourea) |
| CDDP | Cisplatin |
| Dnm | Daunomycin |
| Doxo | Doxorubicin |
| DTIC | Dimethyl triazine imidazole carboxamide |
| $HN_2$ | Nitrogen mustard |
| HU | Hydroxyurea |
| Ifos | Ifosfamide |
| IT | Intrathecal |
| MTX | Methotrexate |
| PCB, PCZ | Procarbazine |
| VCR | Vincristine |
| VP-16 | Etoposide |

Other Terms

| | |
|---|---|
| Abd | Abdominal |
| ACTH | Adrenocorticotropic hormone |
| ASA | Aspirin |
| B/P | Blood pressure |
| BA | Barium swallow |
| BM | Bone marrow |
| BMT | Bone marrow transplant |
| BSE | Breast self-examination |
| BUN | Blood urea nitrogen |
| Ca | Calcium |
| CBC | Complete blood count |
| CMV | Cytomegalovirus |
| CNS | Central nervous system |
| $CO_2$ | Carbon dioxide |
| Cr | Creatinine |
| CT | Computed tomography |

| | |
|---|---|
| CPM | Cyclophosphamide |
| CXR | Chest radiograph |
| DHEA | Dehydroepiandrosterone |
| DLCO | Diffusing capacity for carbon monoxide (pulmonary) |
| ECHO | Echocardiogram |
| EEG | Electroencephalogram |
| EKG | Electrocardiogram |
| $FiO_2$ | Fractional inspired oxygen |
| Free $T_4$ | Unbound thyroxine |
| FS | Fractional shortening |
| FSH | Follicle-stimulating hormone |
| GFR | Glomerular filtration rate |
| GH | Growth hormone |
| GI | Gastrointestinal |
| GnRH | Gonadotropin releasing hormone |
| GU | Genitourinary |
| GVHD | Graft-versus-host disease |
| Gy | Gray (measure of radiation) |
| H/O | History of |
| H/P axis | Hypothalamic-pituitary axis |
| HD | High dose |
| IOP | Intraocular pressure |
| IQ | Intelligence quotient |
| IT | Intrathecal |
| IV | Intravenous |
| IVP | Intravenous pyelogram |
| LFT | Liver function tests |
| LH | Luteinizing hormone |
| MCV | Mean corpuscle volume |
| Mg | Magnesium |
| MRI | Magnetic resonance imaging |
| NPO | Nothing by mouth |
| PET scan | Positron emission tomography |
| PFT | Pulmonary function test |
| $PO_4$ | Phosphate |
| PRN | As needed |
| PTU | Propylthiouracil |
| QTc | Corrected QT interval |
| R/O | Rule out |
| RNA | Radionuclide angiography |
| RT | Radiation therapy |
| SMN | Second malignant neoplasm |
| SPECT | Single-photon emission computed tomography |
| $T_3$ | Triiodothyronine |
| $T_4$ | Thyroxine |
| TBI | Total body irradiation |

| | | | |
|---|---|---|---|
| TMJ | Temporomandibular joint | UTI | Urinary tract infection |
| TRH | Thyrotropin-releasing hormone | UV | Ultraviolet light |
| TSE | Testicular self-examination | VA | Visual acuity |
| TSH | Thyroid-stimulating hormone | VF | Visual field |
| U/A | Urinalysis | WBC | White blood count |
| US | Ultrasound | | |

# Pediatric Growth and Development: Impact on Vulnerability to Normal Tissue Damage from Cancer Therapy

**3**

Sughosh Dhakal, Arnold C. Paulino, and Louis Constine

## Contents

S. Dhakal, MD (✉)
University of Rochester Medical Center,
Department of Radiation Oncology,
601 Elmwood Ave Box 647, Rochester,
NY 14642, USA
e-mail: sughosh_dhakal@urmc.rochester.edu

A.C. Paulino, MD
MD Anderson Cancer Center, Department of
Radiation Oncology, 1515 Holcombe Blvd Box 97,
Houston, TX 77030, USA
e-mail: apaulino@mdanderson.org

L.S. Constine, MD
Departments of Radiation Oncology and Pediatrics,
University of Rochester Medical Center,
601 Elmwood Ave Box 647, Rochester,
NY 14642, USA
e-mail: louis_constine@urmc.rochester.edu

## 3.1 Introduction

Although increased survival and ultimately cure of cancer remains the primary goal of treatment, our success has shifted our focus to the consequential quality of life. These outcomes are largely dependent on the chronic toxicities of therapies that manifest months to years or even decades after therapy. Recognition of these late effects has been a driving force in the evolution of the treatment of many curable cancers. Surgical techniques, chemotherapeutic regimens, and radiation therapeutic strategies have all evolved with the intention of minimizing toxicities. Advances in diagnostic radiology and radiotherapeutic technologies have led to more conformal radiation treatments that spare adjacent normal structures. In many pediatric malignancies, favorable subsets of patients are now treated with decreased doses of chemotherapy and radiation while still maintaining outstanding overall efficacy.

The development and manifestation of late effects in children differ greatly as compared to adults. While chemotherapy, radiotherapy, and surgery all contribute to development of late effects, most of the existing literature that explores age-related toxicities relates to irradiation. The adverse effects of radiotherapy in adults are primarily a result of inflammatory and fibrogenic processes that are impacted by tissue senescence. While these processes can also occur in children, tissue vulnerability to therapy is heightened by organ growth and normal maturation,

© Springer International Publishing 2015
C.L. Schwartz et al. (eds.), *Survivors of Childhood and Adolescent Cancer:
A Multidisciplinary Approach*, Pediatric Oncology, DOI 10.1007/978-3-319-16435-9_3

and this is more relevant to radiation effects than chemotherapeutic effects. In particular, the biology and kinetics of tissue and organ development explain many of the susceptibilities to and manifestations of radiation-induced injury in the early years of life. In adults, the ability to repair damage is the primary determinant of chronic tissue injury. Furthermore, comorbid illness and prolonged environmental and lifestyle factors are much more likely to affect the development of treatment-related injury in adults.

Many of these principles are illustrated by the example of thoracic irradiation. Both the adult and child will be prone to pulmonary consequences, such as inflammation and fibrosis; however, the child also will be susceptible to a direct restriction of lung compliance from bone hypoplasia and malformation in the developing ribs and spine, as well as indirect effects of compliance due to greater levels of atelectasis and air trapping. Such is not the case in the adult, where the bones are fully grown and hypoplasia and malformation are not an issue. However, co-medical factors generally absent in children but often present in adults, such as smoking or other environment exposures, will affect the risk of treatment-related pneumonitis. In addition, the capacity for tissue repair may be relatively limited in the elderly.

It is important to recognize that growth in children does not occur at a uniform rate or homogenously with regard to individual organ systems. Rather, the tissues and organs that comprise the mosaic of the human body develop and mature at different rates and in different temporal sequences. Since intrinsic radiation sensitivity and vulnerability to radiation-induced normal tissue damage are related to cellular activity and level of maturity, it is important to understand tissue development and consider differing sensitivities to the same insult at any given time in a child's development as this could drastically change the potential for adverse late outcomes. Much less data exist to explore the impact of tissue development on sensitivity to chemotherapeutic agents and thus the differential vulnerabilities of children compared with adults.

This chapter will review organogenesis in the developing human, from the embryo to adulthood, and the complexities involved in manifestation of late effects from radiation therapy, according to stage of development. Similar principles likely exist for sensitivity to the late effects of chemotherapy, although informative data is sparse. In order to more easily conceptualize organ development, we will review the four classic growth curves for normal tissues in children and introduce additional physical and physiologic measures by which to measure growth and human development. We will also briefly discuss a select number of confounding factors that may influence the degree of late effects in the pediatric population. Secondary malignant neoplasms will not be covered in this chapter as they are discussed extensively elsewhere.

## 3.2 Organogenesis: Sensitivity to Late Effects According to Stage of Development

### 3.2.1 Embryo and Fetus

There are three recognized phases of the developmental period in utero: (1) preimplantation, (2) prenatal organogenesis, and (3) fetal period [23].

Preimplantation is the most sensitive phase to the lethal effects of radiation and occurs within the first 2 weeks postconception. The irradiated preimplanted embryo that survives until term grows normally in the prepartum and postpartum periods. When substantial numbers of cells die, the embryo is resorbed.

Prenatal organogenesis occurs immediately after implantation and extends through the first 60 days after conception. Irradiation during this period has resulted in malformations secondary to disruption of morphogenesis. Data acquired predominantly from survivors of Hiroshima suggest that the variable rates of malformations in different organ systems might be related to the length and time of organ development, with the central nervous system, skeletal system, dentition, and genitalia affected more frequently than the gastrointestinal, cardiovascular, or renal systems [16].

The fetal period occurs from 60 days after conception through parturition. Irradiation of an early fetus results in the largest degree of permanent growth retardation, in contrast to an irradiated early embryo which will exhibit greater growth retardation at birth that will largely recover later in life. As can be expected, tissues undergoing the most rapid cell division at the time of exposure are the most susceptible to growth disturbances. For example, the highest incidence of mental retardation in atomic bomb survivors is seen in those exposed at 8–15 weeks of intrauterine life, with a relative risk four times higher than those exposed at 16 weeks or later. Mental retardation was not seen in subjects irradiated before 8 weeks in utero [19]. Similarly, irradiation between 16 and 20 weeks of gestation may also lead to microcephaly and stunting of growth but after 30 weeks of gestation is not likely to produce gross structural abnormalities.

### 3.2.2  Postnatal Period and Childhood

Compared to the prenatal stage, postnatal development after radiation exposure has been less studied, in both in animal models and humans. This period is divided into three growth phases: neogenesis, genesis, and pubogenesis.

Neogenesis refers to the time between birth and approximately 5 years of age, when most normal tissues are newly formed and their development consists of rapid growth of their functional subunits. Brain tissue is rapidly developing during this phase and is hence more susceptible to radiation injury. Musculoskeletal growth, likewise, is more vulnerable when bone growth is most rapid, during neogenesis and pubogenesis; however, mitotic potential is greater for neogenesis rather than pubogenesis. Therefore, it is not surprising that the same dose of radiation would retard bone growth more when administered to a neonate versus an adolescent.

Genesis refers to the time between 5 years of age and just prior to the onset of puberty. Overall, growth is more stable during this period, and the organs have full complement of functional subunits. Irradiation at this time would in general be less detrimental to different organ systems compared to neogenesis as the mitotic potential decreases.

Pubogenesis refers to the time from the onset of puberty to the beginning of adulthood. It is the phase when sexual organs rapidly proliferate and many other organs experience their second growth spurt; however, the brain has essentially attained its full adult size, and so irradiation at this time has less potential detrimental effects on neurocognitive function.

## 3.3  Growth Patterns of Normal Tissues: Influence on Manifestations of Normal Tissue Effects

The growth period for the human body is unusually long among mammalian species, extending for more than a quarter of the normal life span. This long growth period is associated with a delay in most aspects of bodily development, especially skeletal and endocrine maturation. Total body mass continues to increase after maturity, but the rate of increase is slowed considerably after about age 18 years in males and about age 16 years in females.

The growth of specific tissues from birth to adulthood was characterized by Tanner over a half century ago by four classic patterns (Fig. 3.1): (1) lymphoid, with accelerated growth followed by involution at the time of puberty; (2) brain, with rapid postnatal growth that slows and essentially completes by early adolescence; (3) gonadal, with little change during early life but rapid development just before and coincident with puberty; and (4) a more general pattern, epitomized by the musculoskeletal system, characterized by two major periods of rapid growth during the postnatal period and puberty. Figure 3.1 shows the growth relationships according to time and type of organ in the neonatal period and childhood [26], while Table 3.1 provides specific data for a broader number of organs and systems.

In regard to potential late effects from cancer therapy, it is critical to understand that human development is not a linear or homogenous process, but instead that the organs of the body develop and mature at different rates and temporal sequences. Because of this, at any given time during child development, one can expect relative differences in the type and severity of possible late effects, with more pronounced and severe complications occurring if radiation is administered during the periods of increased mitotic activity and relative immaturity. These growth curves provide a context in which to explore and discuss the incidence and differential responses of children with respect to the normal tissue

effects. However, it is important to note that these classic measures of growth and development focused primarily on increases in weight. Additional measures of physical size and physiologic function may in many cases provide more meaning metrics in regard to growth and maturity of organ systems and thus relative vulnerability to therapy in regard to subsequent late effects.

### 3.3.1 Classic Growth Patterns

#### 3.3.1.1 Lymphoid Growth Pattern

This type of growth pattern is characterized by gradual evolution and involution to the time of puberty. An example of an organ that follows this pattern is the thymus. It reaches its greatest relative weight at birth, but its absolute weight continues to increase until the onset of puberty. In fact, in the renewal phase of adulthood, it is estimated that the thymus gland is only about 5–10 % of its original size. No significant late effects from RT occur in the lymphoid system. In particular, there are no age-specific effects, perhaps because the inherent radiation sensitivity of lymphoid tissues outweighs any differential that could be observed due to age.

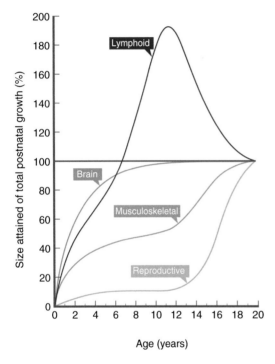

**Fig. 3.1** Four classic growth curves according to age and organ size (Modified with permission from Tanner [26])

#### 3.3.1.2 Brain Growth Pattern

This type of growth pattern is characterized by rapid postnatal growth which slows down and is almost complete in adolescence. Naturally, the head and neck also follow this pattern of growth.

**Table 3.1** Anatomy and physiology: relative rate of development

|                    | Age 0–5 years | Age 5–10 years | Age 10–15 years | Age 15 to adult |
|--------------------|---------------|----------------|-----------------|-----------------|
| Brain              | 4             | 2              | 1               | 1               |
| Thyroid            | 2             | 3              | 3               | 4               |
| GI                 | 4             | 3              | 3               | 2               |
| Gonadal            | 1             | 1              | 4               | 4               |
| Lung               | 3             | 2              | 3               | 4               |
| Urinary system     | 4             | 3              | 3               | 2               |
| Skin               | 3             | 2              | 4               | 4               |
| Lymphoid tissues   | 4             | 4              | Hypoplasia      | Hypoplasia      |
| Liver              | 4             | 2              | 3               | 2               |
| Musculoskeletal    | 3             | 2              | 4               | 2               |
| Head and neck      | 4             | 2              | 2               | 1               |
| Circulatory        | 3             | 2              | 4               | 2               |

*1* static, *2* mild, *3* moderate, *4* significant

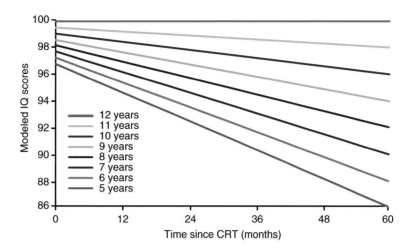

**Fig. 3.2** Intelligence quotient (IQ) scores after conformal radiotherapy in children with low-grade glioma (Reprinted with permission from Merchant et al. [15])

The brain is most sensitive to ionizing radiation in the early fetal period but also postnatally during the first few years of life. Brain growth during the first 3 years of life is not secondary to increase in number of neurons but due to axonal growth, dendritic arborization, and synaptogenesis. Myelinization, though well developed at about the second year of life, is not complete until the second to third decade of life [6]. By 6 years of age, the child's brain has reached adult size. Several studies have shown greater cognitive impairment in younger children compared to older children receiving cranial irradiation [4, 22]. It is for this reason that for many years prior to the era of conformal radiotherapy, in an effort to avoid the deleterious effects of radiotherapy, chemotherapy after surgery was the treatment for children <3 years of age with medulloblastoma, ependymoma, and high-grade gliomas [7]. A report from St. Jude Children's Research Hospital showed cognitive decline after conformal radiotherapy for children under 12 years of age with low-grade glioma (Fig. 3.2). In fact, age at time of irradiation was more important than radiation dose in predicting cognitive decline. Children <5 years old show the most cognitive decline [15]. Consistent with this, most children who are affected with radiation-induced moyamoya syndrome were irradiated when they were <5 years of age, a time when brain growth is rapid [5].

One study attributed a greater degree of deficient development with loss of white matter, and this was presumptively correlated with the impaired cognitive outcome of younger children

[17]. This description of white matter changes is consistent with the classic finding after radiation insult of the normal brain of a focal or diffuse area of white matter necrosis [14]. It is also consistent with the premise that radiotherapy would have more effect during the time when there is greater growth of the brain. Table 3.2 shows the growth and development of the brain according to time of irradiation.

### 3.3.1.3 General Growth Pattern (Musculoskeletal, Heart, Lungs, GI, GU)

This type of growth pattern is characterized by peak growth rates in the early postnatal period and during puberty. It is perhaps best exemplified by the musculoskeletal system; however, the liver and gastrointestinal tract, kidneys and urinary system, and skin also follow this pattern.

Radiation damage to bone is expressed in the epiphysis by arrested chondrogenesis, in the metaphysis by deficient absorptive processes in the calcified bone and cartilage, and in the diaphysis by an alteration in periosteal activity causing abnormal bone modeling [21]. Doses >20 Gy are usually necessary to arrest endochondral bone formation. In a classic study of spinal growth after radiotherapy, the greatest retardation of growth was seen during the periods of most active growth in children <6 years of age and those undergoing puberty [21]. In another study of slipped epiphysis secondary to radiation therapy, doses of >2,500 cGy and young age at time of irradiation were the main risk factors for this complication [24], which occurred

**Table 3.2** Growth and development of the brain with respect to time of irradiation

| Phase | Time | Manifestation after radiation therapy |
|---|---|---|
| Preimplantation | First 2 weeks postconception | Death of preimplanted embryo |
| Prenatal organogenesis and fetal period | 2 weeks to parturition | Microcephaly, mental retardation (greatest risk at 8–15 weeks postconception) |
| Neogenesis | Birth to 6 years | Mental retardation, severe cognitive deficits especially in children <3 years of age when myelin formation is still not nearly complete. Hypoplasia of the portion of the skull and soft tissues which receive radiation therapy |
| Genesis | 6 years to puberty | Mild to moderate cognitive deficits. Mild or no hypoplasia of the skull as the brain reaches its adult size at 6 years of age |
| Pubogenesis | Puberty to 18 years | Mild cognitive deficits. No hypoplasia of the skull |

in 50 % of children <4 years and 5 % of children 5–15 years of age. In contrast to children and adolescents, adult bone is much more tolerant to radiation damage; doses of 6,000 cGy or more are needed to cause osteoradionecrosis.

Muscular growth parallels bone growth, and is bimodal, again occurring during the early postnatal and pubertal periods. Muscular hypoplasia and atrophy have been reported in young children receiving radiotherapy to the spine and extremities.

Another example of the general growth pattern is the urinary system, although its radiosensitivity varies widely, with the ureter being the most resistant, the bladder having intermediate sensitivity, and the kidney the most sensitive. The tolerance of dose for the adult kidney appears to be approximately 23 Gy in 5 weeks to the parenchyma of both kidneys, with 28 Gy to both kidneys in 5 weeks carrying a high risk of severe radiation nephritis [12]. It is not clear whether renal injury is more severe in children than adults or during varying points of the growth curve, with the possible exception of irradiation during neogenesis [2, 20]. This comparison is greatly confounded by the fact that much of the data in regard to the effect of radiation therapy on the pediatric kidney has been collected from survivors of pediatric Wilms tumor, who undergo resection and/or radiation therapy for their primary renal malignancy (and also sometimes present with bilateral disease), as opposed to adults whose kidneys are often only tangentially or incidentally irradiated during the treatment of a range of abdominal/pelvic malignancies. Some data on tolerance doses can be derived from stem cell transplant studies. For example, in one study,

children <5 years of age at the time of total body irradiation had more acute renal dysfunction compared to older children [8]. Overall, in the setting of hematopoietic cell transplantation, fewer than 15 % of children will develop chronic renal insufficiency or hypertension; the risk rises when the patient is an infant (e.g., TBI for neuroblastoma), the total dose exceeds 12 Gy, the individual fraction size is greater than 2 Gy, or the interval fraction is less than 4–6 h [11]. Adults have similar frequencies of chronic renal insufficiency, although the etiology for this may derive from dissimilar comorbid factors.

### 3.3.1.4 Gonadal Growth Pattern

This type of growth pattern is characterized by little change during early life but rapid development just before and coincident with puberty. Examples of organs with this growth pattern are the breast, testicle, and ovary.

As would be expected, children and adults have different manifestations of late radiation injury in the breast, with breast hypoplasia being the most common type of late toxicity in children. In 129 children, <4 years of age receiving a mean dose of 2.3 Gy for hemangioma, breast hypoplasia was observed in 53 % [9]. Others have also observed breast hypoplasia after relatively low doses of radiation, such as for pulmonary metastases from Wilms tumor where children receive bilateral lung irradiation to doses of 10–12 Gy [13]. Although the dose was quite low, the breast in the young has not fully developed, with hyperplasia of the breast not occurring till puberty. The risk of development of secondary breast malignancies is strongly correlated with age (children vs. adults), but it is controversial as to whether irradiation during pubertal development increases the risk for secondary breast cancer. This is discussed in great detail elsewhere in this text.

With regard to the testes, it is important to note that unlike in the ovary, where fertility and hormone production are closely related because of their dependence on the ova and primary follicle, in the testes these functions are carried out separately by the spermatogonia and Leydig cells, which display greatly variable sensitivity to cytotoxic therapy. The germinal epithelium is damaged by much lower dosages (less than 1 Gy) of RT than are Leydig cells (20–30 Gy) [25]. Complete sterilization may occur with fractionated irradiation to a dosage of 1–2 Gy, which would not be expected to have any measurable effect on testosterone levels [1, 10].

### 3.3.2  Complexities in the Association of Growth and Development to the Sensitivity for Late Effects

Although the classic growth curves provide valuable information, these data are limited in that they only describe growth in terms of physical size and more specifically weight. However, it is important to note that changes in the mass of an organ do not necessarily correlate with other physical parameters (such as volume) and moreover that organs grow through a variable combination of parenchymal cell hyperplasia and hypertrophy, as well as stromal development. In regard to the variable sensitivity to late radiation toxicity, growth and physiologic functional development as measured by these parameters may be more important than simple increases in size.

For example, in regard to mass, the ovaries follow the gonadal growth pattern, with little change during early life and rapid development just before and coincident with puberty. However, the organ's sensitivity to late effects from radiation therapy does not follow this pattern, at least in regard to sterility, since the mass

of the ovary as a whole rapidly increases before and during puberty, presumably because of stromal proliferation. The pool of oocytes that are responsible for fertility are continuously decreasing until menopause without replenishment after a maximum number at 5 months gestational age [27].

A classic study showed that the effective sterilizing dose to the ovary after fractionated radiotherapy decreased at increasing age of irradiation: 20.3 Gy at birth, 18.4 Gy at 10 years, 16.5 Gy at 20 years, and 14.3 Gy at 30 years of age [28]. This finding is also supported by the Childhood Cancer Survivor Study, which showed that cyclophosphamide exposure was a risk factor for sterility in older (13–20 years), but not younger (<13 years) children [3]. Finally, data exist showing that ovarian dysfunction may be less in children receiving total body irradiation at an age before menarche, compared with those who were older and received radiotherapy after menarche [18].

This example further highlights the complexity of human growth and development, even at the level of individual tissues and organs, and the need to expand our knowledge of growth patterns beyond simple increases in mass. In addition to expanding our understanding to include additional measures of physical growth, such as volume (Fig. 3.3), and various physiologic parameters, determining differential mechanisms of growth, such as parenchymal cell proliferation and hypertrophy versus stromal development, will enhance our ability to predict and minimize differential late effects from therapy.

## 3.4  Summary

The developing human organism is complex with multiple organ systems developing at different times and rates. Late effects of radiotherapy are influenced not only by total dose, volume, and fractionation but also the stage of normal tissue development, comorbid disease, and various host factors, both intrinsic and extrinsic. While late effects in adults are primarily inflammatory and fibrogenic, in children a major and unique

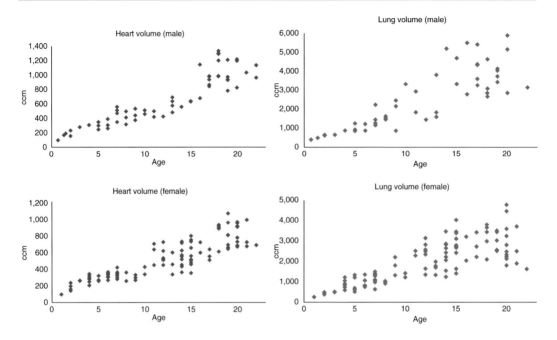

**Fig. 3.3** Heart and lung volumes as function of age, as defined on CT scans from a single institution

contributor to late toxicity is impairment of maturation of the organ. Confounding factors such as comorbid disease, physiologic changes, and environmental factors play a big part in the determination of late toxicity in the adult patient. Knowledge of the growth and development of various organ systems will help the radiation oncologist understand potential degree of late effects both in children and adults.

## References

1. Ash P (1980) The influence of radiation on fertility in man. Br J Radiol 53:271–278
2. Cassady JR (1995) Clinical radiation nephropathy. Int J Radiat Oncol Biol Phys 31:1249–1256
3. Chemaitilly W, Mertens AC, Mitby P (2006) Acute ovarian failure in the childhood cancer survivor study. J Clin Endocrinol Metab 91:1723–1728
4. Conklin HM, Li C, Xiong X, Ogg RJ, Merchant TE (2008) Predicting change in academic abilities after conformal radiation therapy for localized ependymoma. J Clin Oncol 26:3965–3970
5. Desai SS, Paulino AC, Mai WY, Teh BS (2006) Radiation-induced Moyamoya syndrome. Int J Radiat Oncol Biol Phys 65:1222–1227
6. Dobbing J, Sands J (1963) The quantitative growth and development of the human brain. Arch Dis Child 48:757–767
7. Duffner PK, Horowitz ME, Krischer JP, Friedman HS, Burger PC, Cohen ME, Sanford RA, Mulhern RK, James HE, Freeman CR, Seidel FG, Kun LE (1993) Postoperative chemotherapy and delayed radiation in children less than three years of age with malignant brain tumors. N Engl J Med 328:1725–1731
8. Esiashvili N, Chiang KY, Hasselle MD, Bryant C, Riffenburgh RH, Paulino AC (2009) Renal toxicity in children undergoing total body irradiation for bone marrow transplant. Radiother Oncol 90:242–246
9. Furst CJ, Lundell M, Ahlback SO, Holm LE (1989) Breast hypoplasia following irradiation of the female breast in infancy and early childhood. Acta Oncol 28:519–523
10. Izard M (1995) Leydig cell function and radiation: a review of the literature. Radiother Oncol 34:1–8
11. Leiper AD (2002) Non-endocrine late complications of bone marrow transplantation in childhood: part II. Br J Haematol 118:23–43
12. Luxton RW, Kunkler PB (1964) Radiation nephritis. Acta Radiol Ther Phys Biol 66:169–178

13. Macklis RM, Oltikar A, Sallan SE (1991) Wilms' tumor patients with pulmonary metastases. Int J Rad Oncol Biol Phys 21:1187–1193

14. Martins AN, Johnston JS, Henry MJ, Stoffel TJ, Dichiro G (1977) Delayed radiation necrosis of the brain. J Neurosurg 47:336–345

15. Merchant TE, Conklin HM, Wu S, Lustig RH, Xiong X (2009) Late effects of conformal radiotherapy for pediatric patients with low-grade glioma: prospective evaluation of cognitive, endocrine and hearing deficits. J Clin Oncol 27:3691–3697

16. Metler FA, Upton AC (1995) Medical effects of ionizing radiation, 2nd edn. WB Saunders Co, Philadelphia

17. Mulhern RK, Palmer SL, Reddick WE, Glass JO, Kun LE, Taylor J, Langston J, Gajjar A (2001) Risks of young age for selected neurocognitive deficits in medulloblastoma are associated with white matter loss. J Clin Oncol 19:472–479

18. Ogilvy-Stuart AL, Clark DJ, Wallace WH, Gibson BE, Stevens RF, Shalet SM, Donaldson MD (1992) Endocrine deficit after fractionated total body irradiation. Arch Dis Child 67:1107–1110

19. Otake M, Schull WJ, Yoshimura H (1991) Brain damage among the prenatally exposed. J Radiat Res (Suppl) 32:249–264

20. Peschel RE, Chen M, Seashore J (1981) The treatment of massive hepatomegaly in stage IV-S neuroblastoma. Int J Radiat Oncol Biol Phys 7:549–553

21. Probert JC, Parker BP (1975) The effects of radiation therapy on bone growth. Radiology 114:155–162

22. Ris MD, Packer R, Goldwein J, Jones-Wallace D, Boyett JM (2001) Intellectual outcome after reduced-dose radiation therapy plus adjuvant chemotherapy for medulloblastoma: a Children's Cancer Group study. J Clin Oncol 19:3470–3476

23. Russell LB, Russell WL (1954) An analysis of the changing radiation response of the developing mouse embryo. J Cell Physiol 43(Suppl 1):103–149

24. Silverman CL, Thomas PRM, McAlister WH, Walker S, Whiteside LA (1981) Slipped capital femoral epiphysis in irradiated children: dose volume and age relationships. Int J Radiat Oncol Biol Phys 7:1357–1363

25. Sklar CA, Robison LL, Nesbit ME, Sather HN, Meadows AT, Ortega JA, Kim TH, Hammond GD (1990) Effects of radiation on testicular function in long-term survivors of childhood acute lymphoblastic leukemia: a report from the Children's Cancer Study Group. J Clin Oncol 8:1981–1987

26. Tanner JM (1962) Growth at adolescence. Blackwell Scientific Publications, Oxford

27. Wallace WH, Kelsey TM (2010) Human ovarian reserve from conception to menopause. PLoS ONE 5, e8772

28. Wallace WH, Thomson AB, Saran F, Kelsey TW (2005) Predicting age of ovarian failure after radiation to a field that includes the ovaries. Int J Radiat Oncol Biol Phys 62:738–744

# Central Nervous System Effects

# 4

## Nina Kadan-Lottick and Alicia Kunin-Batson

## Contents

N. Kadan-Lottick, MD, MSPH (✉)
Section of Pediatric Hematology-Oncology,
Yale University School of Medicine,
New Haven, CT, USA
e-mail: nina.kadan-lottick@yale.edu

A. Kunin-Batson, PhD
Maternal and Child Health, HealthPartners Institute
for Education and Research, Minneapolis, MN, USA

## 4.1   Introduction

Treatment for childhood cancer can result in damaging effects to the central nervous system (CNS). The spectrum of potential neurological toxicities includes paralysis, neuropathies, blindness, and seizures. Furthermore, survivors may experience decline in intellectual function, learning problems, and emotional-behavior difficulties, contributing to lower levels of educational attainment, unemployment, and impaired quality of life. Though this phenomenon was originally described for children who underwent cranial radiation, subsequent studies have demonstrated that children treated only with chemotherapy are also at risk for neurocognitive deficits. This chapter will review the pathophysiology, clinical presentation, risk factors, diagnosis, and management of late CNS morbidity resulting from the treatment of childhood cancer.

## 4.2   Pathophysiology

### 4.2.1   Postnatal Brain Development

Normal development of the central nervous system begins at conception and is a phenomenon of numerous overlapping processes, thought to be orchestrated by genetic and epigenetic events that are amenable to external influence [1, 2]. The two main periods of development can be divided into

© Springer International Publishing 2015
C.L. Schwartz et al. (eds.), *Survivors of Childhood and Adolescent Cancer:
A Multidisciplinary Approach*, Pediatric Oncology, DOI 10.1007/978-3-319-16435-9_4

(1) the major histogenetic events of neurulation (i.e., the embryonic formation of the neural tube by closure of the neural plate) and (2) reorganization of the human cortex through dendritic and axonal growth, synapse production, neuronal and synaptic pruning, and changes in neurotransmitter sensitivity [2].

The processes of the latter reorganization period continue in the postnatal period into adulthood and thus may be vulnerable to toxic and metabolic insults from pediatric cancer and its therapy. For example, Bergmann glial cells of the Purkinje cell layer of the cerebellar cortex assist in the migration of granule cells even in adulthood [3]. During dendritic proliferation and synaptogenesis in the normal developing brain, an excessive number of synapses are formed which are later eliminated when redundant collateral axons are retracted. Dendritic arborization and synaptic remodeling starts during fetal development but continues through infancy and early childhood [1, 4]. Myelination is another process that is not completed until later in life. The myelination cycle varies for each tract: the medial longitudinal fasciculus is from 24 weeks' gestation to 2 weeks postnatally, the corticospinal tract is from 38 weeks' gestation to 2 years of life, the corpus callosum is from 4 months postnatally to late adolescence, and the ipsilateral association bundle (between the anterior frontal and temporal lobes) is complete at 32 years of age [5].

The central nervous system develops in other important ways during the postnatal period. The whole brain grows enormously in overall size with a fourfold increase in brain volume in the first decade of life [2]. This increase in volume is a function of the number, size, and density of neurons, glia, and dendritic cells. Pruning or normal elimination of neurons contributes to the usual loss of gray matter with age [6]. In contrast, white matter increases during childhood and adolescence. Sensory circuits established in utero may be modified in response to the postnatal environment. Because of the rapid rate of growth early in the postnatal period, infancy may be a period of development which is more vulnerable to damage from external factors such as disease, trauma, or metabolic disturbances. The same exposures occurring in an older child or adult usually results in less impairment in structure and function of the central nervous system [2, 7].

However, not all brain functions experience the same pattern of vulnerability according to age at exposure. Different neurochemical systems or even the same neurochemical system in different locations matures at different rates, extending from the prenatal period to adolescence [8]. For example, it is possible for a neurochemical system within the same cortical area to exhibit different patterns of maturation, according to the cortical level or type of synapse. As Levitt summarized in his review article on primate brain development, "it is not likely that short periods of environmental disruption will uniformly disturb all neurochemical systems or even one system in all brain areas, but rather individual functional domains may be selectively affected" [8]. For example, alterations in dopamine signaling during preadolescence would affect frontal lobe systems, which in turn could affect behavioral inhibition. This is supported by Anderson et al. who found that early brain insult in children younger than 2 years resulted in significant cognitive deficits, while children exposed at ages from 7 to 9 years performed worse in behavioral functioning than younger children [9].

The ability of the brain to recover from postnatal insult is not well understood. Recent studies suggest that there is a potential for neural plasticity manifested by ongoing neurogenesis and synaptogenesis in several areas of the cortex in later childhood and adulthood [2]. The infant brain may recover more easily from some forms of brain injury than occur later in development. This assertion is supported by congenitally deaf children who have a superior response if they receive sensory stimulation from cochlear implants before the age of 5 years [10]. Also, children with early visual deprivation will have less constriction of the visual fields if regular patching was started early [11].

## 4.2.2   Disease Considerations

The late toxicities manifested by the CNS are best considered as a combination of several factors acting in a unique host. Certainly the therapy applied to treat the primary disease can have late manifestations; however, the primary disease process will also impact late effects. Children with leukemia and brain tumors comprise about 51 % of all children with newly diagnosed cancer and comprise the majority of long-term survivors [12]. These children are at risk not only because of the primary site of disease but also because of the need to apply focused CNS-directed therapy.

Although most children with leukemia do not present with CNS manifestations of their disease, a subset of children will. Hyperleukocytosis (characteristically white cell counts of over 100,000 per cubic millimeter) is associated with an increased risk of stroke even prior to the initiation of therapy. Aggressive management of hyperleukocytosis with hydration, exchange transfusion, or cytopheresis is emergently indicated to reduce this risk. Infants and children with T-cell leukemia are more likely to present with high white counts than children with B-precursor ALL. Meningeal infiltration of leukemia, most often diagnosed by examination of the CSF, will occur in less than 5 % of children with newly diagnosed ALL [13]. Although usually not symptomatic, CNS leukemia may lead to infiltration of normal structures and lead to dysfunction of cranial nerves that may in some cases be permanent. Acute promyelocytic leukemia [14] is a distinct type of leukemia with a high risk of coagulopathy, usually hemorrhage, due to the expression of activators of coagulation and fibrinolysis, proteases, and cytokine generation, compounding the usual failure of platelet production due to leukemia marrow invasion. The risk of CNS hemorrhagic complications has been dramatically improved since the use of all-trans retinoic acid (ATRA) but still remains the most frequent cause of mortality.

Children with central nervous system tumors are uniquely at risk. While adults with CNS tumors will frequently present with seizures (as a result of hemispheric tumors), children are more likely to present with features of increased intracranial pressure resulting from obstruction of the normal CSF flow. Tumors involving the fourth ventricle (most commonly PNET/medulloblastoma) are most likely to obstruct CSF flow and lead to hydrocephalus that can present with headache, morning vomiting, ataxia, and ultimately somnolence. The late effects of hydrocephalus are not entirely clear. Studies have shown that children with hydrocephalus severe enough to require a ventriculoperitoneal shunt (VP shunt) have more severe declines in IQ than those that do not [15–17]; however, the need for a VP shunt is likely reflective of the size of the presenting tumor. Another complication unique to children with posterior fossa tumors is the entity of "cerebellar mutism." Mutism will typically be evident in the immediate postoperative period, and although speech may be restored within a few weeks, in some instances it may take up to a year or more to recover and may be incomplete [18]. Children are more frequently affected than adults [19].

Tumors may also directly damage CNS function resulting in both short- and long-term sequelae. Even among children with benign tumors of the CNS treated by surgery alone, only one-third can be expected to have essentially no long-term complications. A Nordic study of children with benign tumors of the CNS (predominately low-grade astrocytomas) found only 31 % of children to be completely without deficits on follow-up and approximately 35 % to have moderate or severe sequelae including ataxia, spastic paresis, vision loss, or epilepsy [20].

## 4.2.3   Radiation

The neurotoxic effects of cranial radiation therapy (CRT) have been well documented and, for many individuals, can be extremely debilitating. CRT is

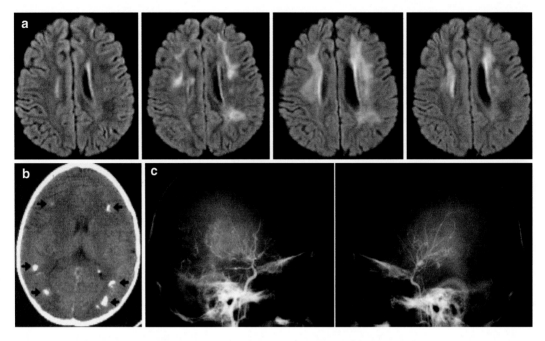

**Fig. 4.1** (**a**) Progressive leukoencephalopathy by MRI fluid-attenuated inversion recovery (FLAIR) in patient with ALL who received high-dose intravenous methotrexate at weeks 7, 18, 44, and 132 of therapy (Reprinted with permission from Mulhern and Palmer [116]). (**b**) Subcortical calcifications on unenhanced computed tomographic (CT) scan in patient with ALL who received cranial irradiation and intrathecal methotrexate central nervous system prophylaxis (Reprinted with permission from Iuvone et al. [133]). (**c**) Moyamoya disease on carotid angiogram in the basal ganglia of an 8-year-old boy with brain stem glioma (Reprinted with permission from Kitano et al. [134])

associated with histological and radiographic abnormalities that have been correlated with clinical findings of impairment. Histological changes associated with CRT consist of subacute leukoencephalopathy, mineralizing microangiopathy, and cortical atrophy, most often becoming apparent several months to years after CRT [21–23]. Corresponding neuroimaging abnormalities after CRT include myelin degeneration, intracerebral calcifications, and ventricular dilatation, respectively [21, 23–25]. Figure 4.1 demonstrates some of these findings on magnetic resonance imaging. White matter seems to be especially vulnerable to CRT exposure (see below) [26].

Ionizing radiation therapy is most commonly administered with photon or electron external beams, but also as charged particles such as protons or carbon ions; they directly or indirectly cause DNA damage through ionization. While radiation therapy may lead to immediate cell death in some instances as a result of the direct ionization of DNA, more commonly cell death is delayed until the cells attempt to move through mitosis. This loss of proliferative capacity eventually leads to tissue death within the irradiated field, ideally leading to death of the tumor target but sparing the normal tissue nearby. To achieve this effect, it is helpful to think of the delivery of radiation therapy within a "therapeutic window," that is, a range in which the therapy will cause death of the tumor cell, but not produce unacceptable damage to the normal tissue of adjacent structures. This therapeutic window varies from site to site within the body, and while the CNS is able to withstand significant doses of ionizing radiation, the "window" within which acceptable normal tissue damage occurs may be quite small. Fractionation, the process of delivering radiation therapy through multiple small doses, is felt to enlarge the therapeutic window by allowing repair of sublethal cell damage by normal tissue. While radiation therapy may result in cellular death through the direct interactions of ionized particle with cellular DNA, late tissue injury from radiation therapy may not be immediately evident, but may become significant as a result of radiation vasculopathy that results from damage to the endothelial cells within the radiation field. This may not become evident for many years following the radiation treatment.

The pathophysiology of radiation injury to the CNS has focused on two major processes: vasculopathy and demyelination. Direct damage to the endothelial cells may initially be evident as increases in vascular permeability but later may be manifested as scarring and wall thickening, ultimately leading to ischemia in the affected area. Demyelination is felt to be the result of radiation damage to the O2A progenitor cell which serves as precursor cell for new oligodendrocytes. The lack of replacement progenitor cells for the existing oligodendrocytes may ultimately lead to the demyelination characteristically associated with radiation injury. A recent study [27] suggests that CRT may affect the cells that create myelin more than it damages existing myelin, which may leave survivors with lower peak levels of white matter density in young adulthood. While these two processes likely account for much of the changes seen following radiation, the exact process of radiation damage is likely much more complex involving many of the other cells of the CNS [28].

Domains of neurocognitive impairment after CRT include short-term memory, distractibility, fine motor coordination, visual-spatial ability, and somatosensory functioning [29–34]. These cognitive impairments have been associated with a significantly reduced intelligence quotient and academic failure [30, 35]. The deficits, which often do not emerge until 4–5 years after diagnosis [36–38], are most severe in those

diagnosed at an age younger than 6 years [30, 39] and among females [40, 41]. Children who received cranial radiation as part of their therapy for acute lymphoblastic leukemia are more likely to be referred to special education services and achieve a lower final level of secondary education, compared to their siblings [42]. There appears to be a dose-response relationship with cranial radiation doses of greater than 2,400 centigray (cGy) resulting in greater impairment [43]. It is not clear that a further decrease to 1,800 cGy is associated with less neurocognitive toxicity, as mixed findings have been reported [37]. However, in one small study of 42 leukemia patients, 1,200 cGy is associated with less impairment than 1,800 cGy [44].

In addition to dose, the age of the child at the time of CRT is strongly associated with neurocognitive performance, with younger age of exposure associated with greater neurocognitive deficit. This relationship is perhaps best illustrated in a report from a longitudinal cohort study, which described cognitive decline after conformal radiation therapy in 78 children with low-grade glioma treated with 54 Gy (see Fig. 4.2) [45]. Age at time of irradiation was more important than radiation dose in predicting cognitive decline, with children younger than 5 years of age showing the most cognitive decline. It should be noted that this decline over time is typically believed to be reflective of the child's failure to acquire new abilities or information at a rate similar to their peers as opposed to representing a progressive loss of skills. Similarly, in childhood ALL survivors, age at treatment also influences the impact of CRT on neurocognitive functioning. Younger age at treatment with 24-Gy CRT was associated with increasing risk for impairment in IQ, academics, and memory [46]. For every age, CRT increased risk, but that risk decreased with increasing age.

Advances in radiotherapy are attempting to deliver the best possible survival rates with the fewest and least severe late effects. Proton-beam radiotherapy is a recent alternative to conventional photon-beam radiotherapy and designed to

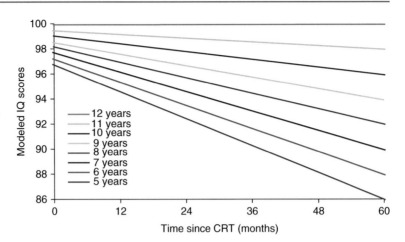

**Fig. 4.2** Modeled intelligence quotient (IQ) scores after conformal radiation therapy (CRT) by age for pediatric low-grade glioma. Age is measured in years, and time is measured in months after the start of CRT (From Merchant et al. [45])

deliver the optimal dose of radiation to the tumor while reducing exposure to surrounding healthy tissue. Compared to conventional photon-beam radiotherapy used in standard CRT, protons have a larger mass and more limited range of penetration, resulting in radiation delivery that is focused on the tumor shape with less impact on structures beyond the tumor target [47]. Currently, there are limited centers in the United States able to deliver proton therapy. Given their scarcity, access to these centers may be influenced by socioeconomic factors (e.g., insurance, ability to travel) that could also play a role in long-term outcomes. Some studies have reported improved clinical disease outcomes with proton-beam radiation therapy [48, 49], but neurocognitive outcome studies are not yet available. While a recent study of health-related quality of life [50] of 142 children with CNS tumors treated with proton-beam radiotherapy found improvements over a 3-year period to levels close to those reported for healthy children, trends in quality of life for children receiving conventional photon-beam radiation therapy were not assessed, and thus direct comparison was not possible.

### 4.2.4 Intrathecal Chemotherapy

Although the effects may be less devastating than those produced by CRT, chemotherapy exposures

are also associated with neurocognitive consequences. Chemotherapeutic agents administered by the intrathecal route for treatment of childhood ALL include methotrexate, cytarabine, and hydrocortisone, often in combination with each other. Acute toxicity of intrathecal methotrexate and intrathecal cytarabine can include chemical arachnoiditis, hallucinations, somnolence, seizures, and neurological signs [51, 52]. Several months to years after termination of intrathecal methotrexate therapy, patients may exhibit radiographic evidence of cortical atrophy, necrotizing leukoencephalopathy, subacute myeloencephalopathy, mineralizing angiopathy, and cerebellar sclerosis [34, 53].

Several studies have investigated proposed mechanisms through which CNS-directed chemotherapy may influence neurocognitive functioning, with intrathecal methotrexate being most widely studied in this regard. These studies have generally implicated white matter abnormalities, which are presumed to result from disruption of the myelinization process during childhood [54]. Specifically, studies have found that MTX can cause leukoencephalopathy, white matter hypodensity, and multiple necrotic lesions in the periventricular white matter [55]. Myelinization in the frontal lobe area of the brain typically occurs later in development, and given that the mature frontal lobe has a high volume of white matter, it is believed to be more vulnerable to damage early in life [54]. Volumetric reductions of the dorsolateral prefrontal cortices and the mammillary bodies have been found in survivors 3 years posttreatment who had received IT chemotherapy [56], and this pattern of abnormality corresponds to noted deficits of memory, processing speed, and attention/distractibility. In addition to white matter damage, other mechanisms underlying neurocognitive late effects after chemotherapy have been proposed, including oxidative stress, neuroinflammation, deregulation of the immune response, and deficits in DNA-repair mechanisms.

Long-term neurocognitive abnormalities have also been observed in children who received systemic and/or intrathecal methotrexate. In a study of patients treated at St. Jude Children's Research Hospital, Ochs et al. concluded that children who received intravenous methotrexate and intrathecal methotrexate had similar neurotoxicity to those who received 1,800 (centigray) cGy CRT and intrathecal methotrexate. Neurocognitive deficits included decreases in full-scale and verbal IQ as well as in arithmetic achievement [32]. These conclusions were confirmed by Mulhern et al. in a longitudinal study which compared children who received 1,800 cGy, 2,400 cGy, and no CRT [36]. There was no statistically significant difference between these groups, but overall, 22–30 % of children experienced a clinically apparent deterioration in neurocognitive function during the period of follow-up (median 7.4 years). The deficits were most marked among females. Cumulative (12–30) IT doses of MTX has also been shown to correlate positively with deficits observed in neuropsychological tests of IQ, attention, and concentration [57].

Raymond-Speden et al. compared ALL patients with chronic asthmatics. This study demonstrated that the detrimental effects of intrathecal chemotherapy are independent of the limitations of having a chronic disease (i.e., missed school, reduced energy levels, etc.) [58]. When compared to children diagnosed with solid tumors who received only systemic chemotherapy, children with leukemia who received systemic and intrathecal CNS-directed therapy

exhibited more severe problems on academic tests of reading, spelling, and arithmetic that only became apparent 3 years post diagnosis [59]. The effects of intrathecal cytarabine and hydrocortisone have not been studied extensively as single agents. However, there is biochemical and autoradiographic evidence for glucocorticoid binding sites in the spinal cord [60]. Given the toxic effects of systemically administered steroids (see below), Kadan-Lottick et al. studied whether patients previously randomized to intrathecal methotrexate vs. "triple" intrathecal therapy (methotrexate with hydrocortisone and cytarabine) had differences in long-term neurocognitive functioning 5.9 years after diagnosis [61]. This study did not show any clinically meaningful differences by intrathecal randomization.

## 4.2.5 Systemic Chemotherapy

Systemic administration of methotrexate may enhance both the acute and late toxicities of other CNS-directed therapies. Among children with ALL treated on a non-radiation containing protocol, acute neurotoxic events occurred significantly more often among those who received IV methotrexate (1,000 mg/m$^2$) in addition to IT methotrexate during consolidation therapy [62]. The presenting acute event was most commonly seizures, which occurred in approximately 80 % of cases. Other observed neurotoxicities included paresthesias, weakness, headaches, aphasia, ataxia, dysarthria, arachnoiditis, and choreoathetosis. CT and MRI findings among those children with acute neurotoxicity were most commonly white matter changes characterized as hypodense areas with or without microangiopathic calcifications. Overall, approximately 10 % of children in this trial who were treated with combined intermediate-dose systemic methotrexate and intrathecal methotrexate developed neurotoxicity. Systemic methotrexate is administered in many other settings in cancer therapy, often at substantial doses. When not combined with intrathecal therapy or cranial radiation, the systemic administration of high doses of methotrexate, as in the treatment of osteosarcoma, has not been consistently associated with CNS sequelae.

Systemic high-dose cytarabine therapy has been associated with acute cerebellar syndrome, seizures, and encephalopathy [25]. Systemic and intrathecal cytarabine have also been associated with spinal cord necrosis [63].

Therapy for acute lymphoblastic leukemia usually includes asparaginase, a chemotherapy agent that results in a hypercoagulable state after prolonged asparagine depletion [64]. A recent review of 548 patients treated on Dana-Farber Consortium protocols from 1991 to 2008 concluded that 1.6 % of patients developed a sinus venous thrombosis [65]. There are limited data regarding long-term outcomes after sinus vein thrombosis in children with cancer and other pediatric populations. However, the available data suggest that most children have mild or no impairment in physical and cognitive functioning [66, 67].

Glucocorticoids have been speculated to contribute to long-term CNS toxicity based on animal experiments and clinical observation in noncancer populations. Rat studies demonstrate that glucocorticoids disrupt the energy metabolism of neurons of the hippocampus, an important organ for memory processing, rendering them more vulnerable to toxic insults [68]. Further experiments in rats demonstrate the impairment of spatial learning in response to chronic corticosteroid treatment [69]. Children with asthma on long-term steroid therapy at higher doses experience greater depression, anxiety, and verbal memory deficits [70]. Associated mood and behavior changes range from irritability to depression and psychosis [71]. The administration of postnatal dexamethasone to preterm infants results in impaired cerebral cortical gray matter growth [72]. Dexamethasone-treated neonates also had a significantly higher incidence of cerebral palsy and developmental delay than those who received placebo [73].

Dexamethasone, instead of prednisone, has been increasingly used in acute lymphoblastic trials because it confers greater event-free survival [74]. In a multisite study, Kadan-Lottick et al. compared neurocognitive functioning in 92 children with standard-risk ALL 9.8 years after previous randomization to prednisone or dexamethasone. No significant overall differences in mean neurocognitive and academic performance scores [61] were found between the prednisone and dexamethasone groups after adjusting for age, sex, and time since diagnosis. However, for the dexamethasone group, older age of diagnosis was associated with worse neurocognitive functioning; for the prednisone group, younger age at diagnosis was associated with worse functioning.

## 4.3 Clinical Presentations

Acute effects of CNS-directed therapy are relatively uncommon. Acute radiation changes to the CNS can result in significant edema at the irradiated site (often following single-dose therapies such as "gamma knife" or "stereotactic radiosurgery") and may present with worsening of the preexisting symptoms (i.e., seizure, weakness, headaches). These symptoms are usually manageable with corticosteroid therapy [75]. Acute effects of chemotherapy on the CNS are also relatively uncommon. Ifosfamide has been associated with changes in mental status, cerebellar function, cranial nerve, and cerebellar and motor system function and seizures [76]. The risk of this acute toxicity may be modified by prior chemotherapy exposure, specifically exposure to cisplatinum [77]. Ara-G, a antimetabolite with selective efficacy against T-cell leukemia, is also associated with acute neurotoxicity. Somnolence and other acute CNS changes may be dose limiting for this new agent [78].

Subacute effects of radiation therapy (those occurring within the first 6 months of exposure) are more common than acute effects. One of the most common of these, the somnolence syndrome, has been described as occurring in up to 50 % of children who receive radiation as CNS prophylaxis for acute lymphoblastic leukemia, but risk decreases with lower radiation doses [79]. The syndrome presents with fatigue, somnolence, anorexia, and nausea, typically occurring 4–8 weeks after the completion of radiation therapy [80]. In some instances the syndrome may include fever and changes on EEG. While usually self-limited, treatment with steroids may ameliorate the symptoms [81]. The somnolence syndrome has also rarely been reported following the use of TBI in the setting of bone marrow transplantation [79]. An analogous condition caused by irradiation of the spinal cord is termed Lhermitte's syndrome and is manifested by shock-like paresthesias of the extremities, following flexion of the neck. While the etiology of these syndromes is unclear, transient demyelinization due to the effects of radiation on the replicating oligodendrocytes has been implicated [82]. Subacute effects of chemotherapy may also occur. Intrathecal cytosine arabinoside and methotrexate have been associated with subacute spinal cord damage that is usually irreversible [63]. As mentioned previously, asparaginase is associated with the occurrence of thrombosis of the CNS, typically occurring days to weeks after therapy [83].

The clinical presentation of the late effects of CNS-delivered therapies is most evident in the learning difficulties experienced by children treated with combinations of radiation and chemotherapy for ALL or brain tumors. While any child receiving CNS-directed therapy is at risk for late effects, the frequency of these two primary diagnoses and the needed application of CNS-directed therapies for them set this group of children apart. Often called "neurocognitive" late effects, these toxicities are characterized by subtle onsets and may not become evident for many years after cancer treatment has ended. While there is no single area of deficit that is diagnostic of neurocognitive late effects, a recent meta-analysis suggests that the most common and severe areas of dysfunction tend to occur in the domains of attention, speed of information processing, and executive functioning [84]. Some other studies have also implicated vulnerabilities in the areas of memory, verbal comprehension, visuospatial skills, and visual-motor function. Neurocognitive late effects are sometimes, but

not consistently, associated with pathological changes such as leukoencephalopathy [85]. Studies have also found survivors of childhood leukemia to experience academic difficulties, which represent downstream manifestations of primary neurocognitive deficits in core domains (e.g., attention, processing speed). Specifically, survivors of ALL have been found to demonstrate slower progress in language skills and mathematics and are more likely to repeat a grade in school [86].

The broader issue of educational attainment among survivors of childhood cancer has been examined within the context of the Childhood Cancer Survivor Study, a large retrospective study of children treated for cancer in the 1970s and early 1980s. In an analysis that included 12,430 survivors and 3,410 full siblings, the use of special education services was reported in 23 % of survivors and 8 % of siblings. The greatest differences were observed among survivors who were diagnosed before age 6 years, most notably survivors of CNS tumors and leukemia. Survivors of leukemia and CNS tumors were also significantly less likely to finish high school compared with siblings [87]. Central nervous system treatments and neurocognitive dysfunction after cancer treatment have also been shown to negatively impact a variety of key functional outcomes in adulthood, including employment [88], marriage rates [89], and the ability to live independently [90].

Beyond the neurocognitive sequelae, survivors of childhood cancer are at risk for other CNS late effects of their therapy. Packer et al. assessed the frequency of self-reported neurosensory and neurologic dysfunctions among 1,607 patients diagnosed between 1970 and 1986 with a primary CNS tumor [91]. Seventeen percent of these patients reported a neurosensory impairment. Relative to a sibling comparison group, patients were at elevated risk for hearing impairments, blindness in one or both eyes, cataracts, and double vision. Radiation exposure greater than 50 Gy to the posterior fossa was associated with a higher likelihood of developing hearing impairment (refer also to the *Hearing* chapter by

Landier et al.), probably due to irradiation of the cochlea and shunting procedures. One would anticipate that hearing complications will be less common in patients treated more recently, with the wider availability of conformal radiation therapy techniques (including intensity-modulated radiation therapy). Packer et al. reported seizure disorders in 25 % of patients, including 6.5 % who had a late first occurrence. Exposure of the CNS to 30 Gy or more to any cortical segment of the brain was associated with a twofold elevated risk for a late seizure disorder among this cohort of patients [91].

Neurocognitive late effects have also been observed status post hematopoietic stem cell transplantation (HCT). In a large follow-up study of 268 patients treated with stem cell transplant, higher risk for neurocognitive difficulty was associated with history of unrelated donor transplantation, total-body irradiation, and graft-versus-host disease (GVHD) [92]. However, these differences were small relative to patient differences in premorbid functioning, particularly those associated with socioeconomic status. Children who are younger at the time of transplant and total-body irradiation (i.e., less than 3 years of age) also appear to be at increased risk for neurocognitive difficulties [93]. In a prospective longitudinal study of children with hematologic malignancies who had undergone HCT, declines in visual-motor and memory skills were noted within the first year posttransplant [94]. By 3 years posttransplant, these scores had improved, but there were new deficits seen in long-term memory scores. By 5 years posttransplant, there were progressive declines in verbal skills, performance skills, and new deficits seen in long-term verbal memory scores. The greatest decline in neurocognitive function occurred in patients who received cranial irradiation either as part of their initial therapy or as part of their HCT conditioning.

Other, less common but more severe sequelae can follow CNS-directed therapies. Radiation necrosis of the CNS is rare, occurring in fewer than 5 % of children treated. Risk of radiation necrosis is increased by larger fractions and larger total doses [95]. The onset of symptoms due to radiation necrosis may be delayed for years following the initial treatment of the child, and in many instances, the symptoms may mimic that of recurrent tumor. Newer imaging modalities, including PET scanning and MR spectroscopy, may be helpful in discriminating radiation necrosis from tumor recurrence, but biopsy may ultimately be needed to establish the diagnosis. Treatment options are limited in their efficacy but include surgery, steroids, pentoxifylline, heparin, and in some instances hyperbaric oxygen [96]. Vascular events are also rare but potentially devastating late effects of radiation therapy. Typically these involve small blood vessel disease, often leading to small strokes. Rarely, large vessel stokes may also occur.

## 4.4 Moderators and Mediators of Central Nervous System Outcomes

While treatment factors (i.e., cranial radiation, radiation dose, intrathecal chemotherapy, methotrexate, neurosurgery) play a role in children's neurocognitive functioning after cancer treatment, it has been increasingly recognized that treatment factors alone are not the sole determinants of outcome. Rather, children who undergo similar treatment regimens for childhood cancer may experience very different neurocognitive outcomes after treatment has ended, leading many to study the influence of other risk factors that may potentially mediate or moderate outcomes. Brouwers has proposed a model to describe the relationships between broad categories of mediators and moderators of neurocognitive late effects in survivors of childhood cancer (Fig. 4.3). Mediators are factors that specify how or by which mechanisms an effect occurs, largely comprised of the therapy exposures described above. Moderators are factors that affect the direction and/or strength of the relation between a mediator and an outcome variable but are not by themselves pathogenic [97]. The following variables have been shown to affect neurocognitive outcome following brain insult for various diseases, including childhood cancer survivors, and have been replicated in a number of studies:

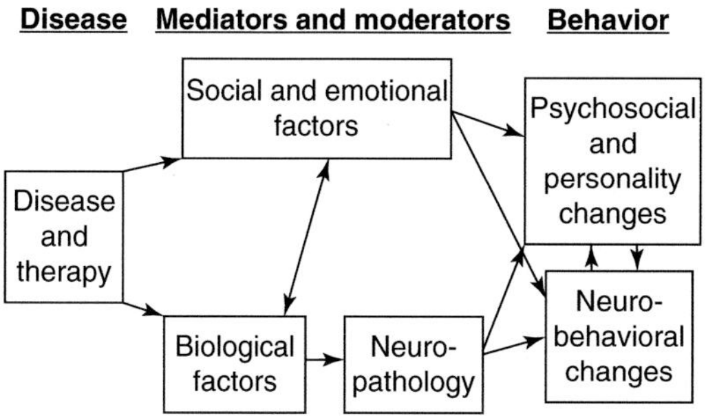

**Disease**   **Mediators and moderators**   **Behavior**

**Fig. 4.3** Mediators and Moderators of Psychosocial and Neurocognitive Outcomes

age at insult, time since insult, gender, socioeconomic/family factors, and genetic polymorphisms. Evidence linking each of these areas to neurocognitive late effects is described below.

The effect of cancer treatment on the brain and on neurocognitive functioning is believed to be progressive. Deficits become more pronounced, both in terms of brain imaging abnormalities [98] and neurocognitive functioning [38, 99], as the time after treatment increases. Additionally, different domains of neurocognitive functioning may show different rates of decline over time. While previous studies have documented an initial decline in nonverbal reasoning skills after CRT, a recent study [100] also found a later decline in verbal IQ. This decline in verbal cognitive skills was associated with current attention and reading problems, but not with the traditional variables associated with early decline in nonverbal cognitive skill (i.e., CRT dose, younger age at diagnosis, and female gender), and was interpreted to represent the progressive neurocognitive sequelae from CRT on the brain. Recent studies of aging adult leukemia survivors have also found progressive impairments in memory correlated with reduced MRI fractional anisotropy (FA) and poorer neurocognitive functioning (i.e., lower intelligence quotient, poorer, visuomotor accuracy, poorer working memory, and sustained attention) for those treated with CRT [27] that may represent accelerated aging. These findings were particularly pronounced after treatment with CRT but also observed among those previously treated with intrathecal chemotherapy only [27]. A dose-response effect of CRT on neurocognitive functioning in older adult survivors of child-

hood cancer [101] has also been reported, with those who had been treated with 24 Gy CRT showing reduced cognitive status and memory and reduced integrity in neuroanatomic regions essential in memory formation.

Gender may moderate the neurocognitive outcome following brain injury, but the direction and magnitude of the effect seems to be dependent on age and on the type and location of the injury. The findings in different patient populations are conflicting. Among children who receive preventive cranial irradiation for ALL, females experience greater neurocognitive deficits [102]. Buizer et al. found that female gender remained a risk factor for attentional dysfunction in survivors of childhood cancer treated without cranial radiation [103]. Other studies of children with ALL treated with chemotherapy only found no association with gender [61, 104, 105].

Studies have suggested that environmental, sociodemographic, and family factors may moderate the neurocognitive outcome following pediatric head injury and thus may affect the neurodevelopmental course of these children. Environmental factors such as family distress, family functioning, family resources, parent adjustment, and family interactions have been investigated. Some studies have concluded that these variables identify children at increased risk for long-term neurocognitive abnormalities following brain injury [106, 107]. While such models have been well studied in the child traumatic brain injury literature, they have been only recently applied to childhood cancer survivors. Beginning with cancer diagnosis, parents of pediatric cancer patients report significant emotional distress and lifestyle adjustments, including the need to take time off work, financial costs, and less time with other family members [108]. Some studies have shown that parent distress and reduced social support can contribute to poor behavioral outcomes in the child survivor [109]. Others have found that family factors (e.g., conflict, support, coping) moderate neurocognitive and academic outcomes after pediatric brain tumor [110, 111]. The role of family factors in neurocognitive functioning of childhood cancer survivors is an important area of study, given that parental distress and family functioning are modifiable factors with the potential to be bolstered by therapy and other psychosocial supports.

Genetic polymorphisms have also been identified as a possible factor contributing to risk for neurocognitive difficulties after cancer treatment. Recent studies have examined the role of genetic polymorphisms affecting key enzyme pathways associated with the pharmacokinetics or pharmacodynamics of cancer treatments (e.g., folate availability, homocysteine levels, oxidative stress), which may impact neurocognitive functioning after therapy. One study [112] found a link between folate pathway polymorphisms (i.e., 10-methyenetetrahydrofolate reductase, MTHFR, and methionine synthase, MS) and parent-reported attention problems and direct performance measures of processing speed and sustained attention in long-term survivors of childhood ALL who were treated with chemotherapy only. A recent study [113] also found that polymorphisms in MS were associated with decreased attentiveness and slow response speed. Specific attention problems after cancer therapy were also associated with polymorphisms in glutathione S-transferases (GSTs). This study further extended the examination of polymorphisms to those outside of the treatment pathways (e.g., apolipoprotein E (APOE) which has been implicated in early-onset dementia and monoamine oxidase A (MAOA) which have been associated with developmental attention deficits) and found associations with specific aspects of attention in survivors, suggesting that a subset of survivors may have genetic predispositions that influence response to physiologic stress and CNS integrity [113].

## 4.5 Prevention and Intervention

### 4.5.1 Prevention: Primary and Secondary

Primary prevention of adverse CNS outcomes largely consists of seeking alternative therapies which are less toxic, but which do not compromise cure. Childhood cancer researchers have been successful in implementing this strategy in several instances. In response to the severity of long-term side effects observed after radiation therapy, intrathecal chemotherapy has replaced CRT for CNS leukemia prophylaxis for most types of ALL [59]. Children with ALL who have poor prognostic features or who have sustained a relapse still require CRT but receive lower doses than was administered previously [114]. In young brain tumor patients, chemotherapy has been administered as neoadjuvant therapy to delay the administration of CRT as long as possible [115]. Refinements in radiation oncology techniques, such as conformal radiation therapy and stereotactic radiotherapy, have further reduced long-term toxicity [13], and emerging technologies (proton-beam radiation) have the potential to result in further reductions in the years to come.

It is commonly recognized that whenever cure is not compromised, less neurotoxic therapy should be used, as neurocognitive functioning is important to optimize quality of life and functional outcomes in adulthood. While primary prevention of CNS late effects is not always possible, secondary prevention is an attainable goal. Caregivers should seek early detection of potential adverse outcomes with the goal of improving prognosis. First, health providers should monitor the patient at clinic visits with a history that includes questions, tailored to the age of the patient, about developmental milestones, school performance, peer relations, need for special education services, and neurological abnormalities (e.g., weakness, seizures). More detailed questions should assess domains of neurocognitive functioning that tend to be impaired specifically in childhood cancer patients. Table 4.1 reviews domains of function as well as possible screening questions that could be included in a history.

Deficits in neurocognitive functioning often do not present until several years after treatment and can be subtle and/or subclinical. For these reasons, presymptomatic neuropsychological assessment should be strongly considered. The timing of neurocognitive assessment depends on the individual patient but may be particularly helpful at school reentry to facilitate transition.

**Table 4.1** Domains of neurobehavioral function potentially affected in survivors of childhood cancer

| Domain[a] | Definition | Screening questions: does the individual… |
|---|---|---|
| Intelligence | Basic reasoning ability | "Get" new concepts that are introduced? |
| | | Have good problem-solving skills? |
| | | Understand things in an age-appropriate way? |
| Processing speed | Rate of mental processing | Take longer than most children to process information? |
| | | Seem slow to respond? |
| | | Seem slow to complete homework or tests? |
| Academic achievement | School performance | Acquire academic skills at a rate similar to that of peers? |
| | | Have grades that are appropriate for the child's ability and grade placement? |
| Attention/ concentration/ distractibility | Ability to focus on task for appropriate amount of time. Distractibility is the degree to which one is sidetracked by internal thoughts or external stimuli | Follow multistep directions? |
| | | Finish schoolwork and other potentially less interesting tasks without getting offtrack? |
| Executive function | Ability to plan, organize, and keep information in mind while processing and manipulating that information | Do well on tests that contain previously studied material that is now presented in a novel format? |
| | | Organize the materials needed for learning? |
| | | Successfully complete projects which require planning of multiple, sequential steps (e.g., book reports)? |
| Language | Ability to understand others and to express oneself | Readily understand what is said to him/her without excessive repetition and rephrasing? |
| | | Explain what he/she is thinking in an understandable way? |
| Visuo-perceptual function | Ability to make sense of what you see and to display spatial skills | Easily get from one place to another in the neighborhood or within the school (e.g., find the cafeteria or a friend's house)? |
| | | Understand when something is *shown* to him/her, even when an explanation is not also verbally provided? |
| Fine motor/ speed/ dexterity | Ability to make small, fine movements | Manipulate small objects without dropping them? |
| | | Button his/her clothes independently? |
| | | Know how to hold a pencil? |
| | | Use scissors well? |
| Visuomotor integration | Ability to copy what you see using your fine motor skills | Have legible handwriting? |
| | | Copy shapes and letters well? |
| | | Tie his/her shoes alone? |
| Memory | Ability to learn and store new information | Retain what he/she has learned? |
| Adaptive function | Ability to display independent functioning in activities of daily living, social skills, and communication with others | Care for himself/herself in an age-appropriate fashion, e.g., teeth brushing, dressing, bathing, etc.? |
| | | Play with other children in an age-appropriate fashion? |
| Emotional and behavioral function | State of your mood and regulation of your emotions and behavior | Seem to lose control of himself or herself? |
| | | Have problems with depression or anxiety? |
| | | Display extreme emotions for the situation (e.g., rage, despair, etc.) or excessive mood swings? |

This table was constructed with the expert input of Fiona Anderson, PhD, Assistant Professor, Division of Pediatric Clinical Neuroscience, University of Minnesota

[a]It should be emphasized there is overlap among these domains, and all should be considered within the developmental context of the child (i.e., are the child's abilities age appropriate?)

For younger patients who are not yet in school or those who attended school during therapy, an evaluation at the end of therapy is recommended but can certainly be done earlier in the treatment course if parents or medical providers express concern about the child's development or behavior. Mulhern and Palmer have suggested that a surveillance plan of formal neuropsychological testing be devised for each individual based on their treatment exposures and premorbid risk factors, even in asymptomatic patients [116]. For example, a child with ALL who did not receive CRT might receive a single neurocognitive evaluation at the completion of therapy and then several years after therapy. In contrast, an infant with a brain tumor would be more frequently evaluated, typically every 6–12 months after diagnosis until school entry. The frequency of follow-up after that point varies by institution and is determined by the child's clinical presentation, with evaluations often occurring (at a minimum) at key developmental transition points (i.e., prior to entry into third grade, middle school, high school, and postsecondary education).

The Children's Oncology Group Long-Term Follow-Up Guidelines suggest that all high-risk survivors undergo neurocognitive assessment at the time of transition into a survivorship or long-term follow-up program, regardless of patient/parent report of concern [117]. This evaluation serves as a baseline for future assessments and can aid in the detection of subtle neurocognitive difficulties that may impact functioning or quality of life. As new studies suggest accelerated aging and mild cognitive impairment in older adult survivors, continued surveillance of neurocognitive problems in adulthood is also recommended, particularly for survivors treated with CRT [46].

Recent efforts are underway within the Children's Oncology Group to streamline and routinize neurocognitive assessments for childhood cancer survivors by embedding brief assessment protocols within cancer treatment protocols to monitor neurocognitive outcomes in response to different treatments [118]. These short, structured assessments measure neuropsychological, social, emotional, and/or behavioral functioning at specific timepoints after completion of therapy. The tools used in the Children's Oncology Group ALTE07C1 battery briefly sample general intellectual ability, auditory attention span, visual-motor processing speed, and learning and memory for verbal and nonverbal information. Also included are measures of parent report of the child's emotional-behavioral functioning, executive functioning, and quality of life (https://clinicaltrials.gov/show/NCT00772200). In a clinical setting, a broader neurocognitive battery may also include child performance measures of executive functioning (e.g., inhibition, response selection, shifting), sustained attention, and fine motor skills (common areas in which cancer survivors may have difficulty) and assessment of academic achievement, depending on the particular needs of the child. With the advent of brief computer-driven neurocognitive assessments (e.g., NIH Toolbox, CogState, etc.), screening of these neurocognitive domains will likely become increasingly available and incorporated into a broader array of clinical trials to measure treatment outcomes. During any neurocognitive assessment, the psychologist should be aware of physical disabilities that could negatively impact performance on standardized tests or warrant modified assessment approaches. Examples include hearing loss after cisplatinum, vision impairment after retinoblastoma, peripheral neuropathy after vincristine treatment, and hemiplegia after a stroke.

## 4.5.2 Interventions

While numerous studies have documented CNS difficulties after cancer treatment in childhood, the empirical literature on the efficacy of interventions to address neurocognitive late effects is still emerging. Comprehensive neurocognitive assessments provide valuable data that can be used to develop tailored intervention strategies for childhood cancer survivors. Approaches to intervention for neurocognitive late effects can include educational accommodations or special education services, medication treatment, and/or cognitive remediation.

For childhood cancer survivors with neurocognitive impairments, educational accommodation and direct learning support in the classroom are an important part of the standard of care, as use of special education services has been shown to improve rates of educational attainment among childhood cancer survivors [87]. Successful translation of the results of neurocognitive assessment requires the clear communication of test findings to the school. In the United States, the rights of children with mental/cognitive and physical limitations to receive special education, accommodations, and related services are protected by three federal laws. The Individuals with Disabilities in Education Act of 1990 (IDEA) requires states that receive federal funding for education to provide a "free appropriate education," including special education and related services, to all disabled *children* 3–21 years (http://idea.ed.gov/explore/view/p/,root,dynamic,TopicalBrief,10). Educational services designed to meet each child's unique needs at no cost to parents are set forth in an individualized education plan (IEP) that details annual measurable goals and the services that will be given. This mechanism for assistance is critical for most childhood cancer survivors with neurocognitive impairment [119].

The second law is Section 504 of the Rehabilitation Act of 1973 which protects individuals with disabilities from being discriminated against, excluded from, or denied benefits of any program or activity (including schools and universities) receiving federal funding (http://www2.ed.gov/about/offices/list/ocr/504faq.html#interrelationship). Childhood cancer survivors may be eligible for classroom accommodations under Section 504 if they have an impairment which substantially limits one or more major life activities. A 504 Plan can be an avenue through which to provide accommodations for physical disabilities (e.g., railing, ramps, one-on-one nursing, FM hearing devices, etc.) or cognitive/learning disabilities (e.g., preferential seating or other accommodations for attention deficits). Eligible students develop a 504 Plan, updated annually, with school officials to ensure that they receive accommodations that will support their academic success and access to the learning environment.

The 504 mechanism does *not* provide for specialized instruction as the IDEA act does. For survivors with learning disabilities, the IDEA process is preferred because it is more involved and requires documentation of specific learning goals and measurable growth in learning and education.

The third law relevant to cognitively impaired childhood cancer survivors is the Americans with Disabilities Act (ADA) which prohibits discrimination based on a disability and requires that persons with disabilities receive "reasonable accommodation" (http://www.ada.gov). This law applies to both the public and private sectors for survivors of all ages which is particularly important for survivors who have completed school and entered the workforce and may need accommodation in such settings where the IDEA and Section 504 do not apply.

Examples of classroom accommodations that are often useful for childhood cancer survivors with neurocognitive difficulties include accommodations to maximize attention and minimize distractions for the child (e.g., positioning the child in the front of the classroom, providing repetition of directions and instructions), support the development of the child's executive skills (e.g., breaking assignments into several smaller steps, assistance organizing information for learning, study skills strategies), and accommodate for slow processing speed (e.g., extended time for completion of tests, reduced homework load) [120]. Survivors with verbal deficits can access speech/language therapy services through their school district, and those with fine motor deficits may benefit from occupational therapy services or accommodations in school. Adapted physical education programs in school are also useful for survivors with poor physical functioning, reduced mobility, or other gross motor difficulties. When feasible, communication with staff at the child's school is benefited by conferences with medical caregivers who can share how areas of neurocognitive impairment are related to the child's cancer treatments. This is particularly helpful to dispel misconceptions about children whose school failure may be incorrectly perceived to be the product of disinterest or laziness in the absence of knowledge about neurocognitive late effects after cancer treatment. Childhood cancer survivors should also be aware that classroom supports do not need to stop for young adults who choose to pursue postsecondary education. Accommodations such as copies of teacher notes or slides from lectures, preferential seating, or testing accommodations (e.g., alternative setting, extended time) are often available in college through the office of disability/student services on campus by providing current assessment results which document this need.

Pharmacotherapy approaches, specifically stimulant medications such as methylphenidate hydrochloride (MPH), have also been proposed as a possible treatment for neurocognitive late effects. Stimulant medications are mixed dopaminergic-noradrenergic agonists which are thought to improve the function of the fronto-striatal attentional network in the brain [120] and commonly used in the treatment of attention deficit hyperactivity disorder (ADHD). Debate exists in the literature as to whether children treated for cancer exhibit symptoms similar to those who have ADHD inattentive type. While some studies [121, 122] have suggested that there is a higher prevalence of inattentive ADHD symptoms, recent studies [121, 123] have found rates of ADHD to be similar to the general population (approximately 9–10 %). Although cognitive problems and inattention are common among childhood cancer survivors, these studies raise speculation that the clinical ADHD profile does not adequately capture the range of neurocognitive late effects experienced by survivors of childhood cancer. Medications commonly used for the treatment of ADHD (i.e., methylphenidate) have been shown to improve attention functioning in survivors of childhood cancer, though not to the extent reported in the broader ADHD literature. In a large randomized double-blind, crossover trial of methylphenidate [124], only 45 % of the sample showed a positive medication response, which is substantially lower than response rates (approximately 75 % in most studies) seen in treatment of developmental ADHD. However, doses were not escalated to efficacious doses as is typically done in the general population. Additionally, there have been some reports of adverse effects in small

subgroups of participants and potential reluctance on the part of parents to consider pharmacologic treatments for their children who have already received numerous medications as part of their cancer therapy [125, 126].

There is also growing interest in the use of cognitive rehabilitation for childhood cancer survivors. Cognitive rehabilitation is an intervention "intended to restore lost cognitive functions or to teach the patient skills to compensate for cognitive losses that cannot be restored" [116]. Butler and colleagues pioneered a program focused on the specific skills areas most relevant for childhood cancer survivors, including attention and executive control. Techniques used included massed practice (i.e., intensive, concentrated, repetitive exercises) for attentional control, metacognitive ("task-approach") strategies for successful completion of tasks (including pre- and post-task strategies), and cognitive-behavioral methods to enhance the ability to withstand distraction. In their large, multisite, clinical trial [127], childhood cancer survivors were randomized to receive center-based cognitive remediation sessions with a therapist every week for 4–6 months or to a no-intervention control group. Results from 161 survivors yielded parent reports of improved attention and academic achievement over the course of the intervention. Despite these improvements, effect sizes were small. A similar intervention using problem-solving skills training was also piloted in a small group ($n = 12$) of survivors [128]. This intervention focused on cognitive, learning, and problem-solving skills for 15 weekly training sessions and also showed preliminary efficacy, with participants who completed the intervention making modest gains [128]. While these studies are promising, clear barriers exist to implementing center-based cognitive remediation, including the time and potential costs involved (for both staff and families) and the inconvenience experienced by families in frequent (often weekly) visits to the study center.

To overcome these limitations, efforts are actively underway to develop and test computer-delivered cognitive rehabilitation programs, which are not constrained to the same degree by time, distance, or cost, and could be more broadly disseminated. Computerized cognitive training programs have an advantage in that they can be completed at home. The programs automatically adjust the difficulty level of the tasks according to the progressing skills of the child, in order to provide an appropriate challenge and maintain the child's interest. Preliminary findings from studies by Hardy et al. [129] and Kessler et al. [130] suggest that such programs are feasible and potentially beneficial for childhood cancer survivors, resulting in improvements on indexes of neurocognitive functioning and in brain activation when neuroimaging (fMRI) is utilized [130, 131].

## 4.6 Future Directions

Currently, it is estimated that about 83 % of all children diagnosed with cancer in the United States will survive five or more years from the time of original diagnosis. Coincident with this success is the realization that "cure" is more than eradication of disease. The ultimate goal of therapy is the return of patients to health and well-being. This includes the most complete realization possible of his or her premorbid potential. The toxicities that modern cancer therapy can impose on the CNS may limit that potential for many of our patients, and multiple strategies designed to understand the pathogenesis of these risk factors are necessary as we move forward. Further studies are needed to help us more readily identify survivors who are at risk and to develop and deliver tailored interventions to those with the greatest need. Further investigation of genetic polymorphisms which may impact on drug or radiation sensitivity is needed, along with studies that provide insight into potential psychosocial risk factors of the child, before, during, and after cancer therapy. New treatment approaches, including new radiation-delivery techniques (e.g., proton beam) and new biologic therapies, must not be assumed to be nontoxic but investigated with the rigor which will allow clear understanding of the outcomes of those children treated. Finally, ongoing research for the recovery and rehabilitation of children who have experience toxicity from

CNS-directed therapies is crucial and could impact positively on thousands of lives. Children with cancer are growing up, entering our workforce, and contributing to our society daily. Our commitment to them must extend beyond the conventional notion of cure to include realization of their maximum potential.

## References

1. Menkes JH (1990) Textbook of child neurology, 4th edn. Lea & Febiger, Philadelphia, xiv, 832 p
2. Webb SJ, Monk CS, Nelson CA (2001) Mechanisms of postnatal neurobiological development: implications for human development. Dev Neuropsychol 19(2):147–171
3. Sarnat HB (1992) Cerebral dysgenesis: embryology and clinical expression. Oxford University Press, New York, x, 473 p
4. Corriveau RA, Huh GS, Shatz CJ (1998) Regulation of class I MHC gene expression in the developing and mature CNS by neural activity. Neuron 21(3): 505–520
5. Minkowski A, Council for International Organizations of Medical Sciences, France (1967) Dâelâegation gâenâerale áa la recherche scientifique et technique. In: Regional development of the brain in early life. F.A. Davis Co., Philadelphia, xii, 539 p
6. Reiss AL et al (1996) Brain development, gender and IQ in children. A volumetric imaging study. Brain 119(Pt 5):1763–1774
7. Taylor HG, Alden J (1997) Age-related differences in outcomes following childhood brain insults: an introduction and overview. J Int Neuropsychol Soc 3(6): 555–567
8. Levitt P (2003) Structural and functional maturation of the developing primate brain. J Pediatr 143(4, Supplement):35–45
9. Anderson V et al (2009) Childhood brain insult: can age at insult help us predict outcome? Brain 132(1): 45–56
10. Robinson K (1998) Implications of developmental plasticity for the language acquisition of deaf children with cochlear implants. Int J Pediatr Otorhinolaryngol 46(1-2):71–80
11. Bowering ER et al (1997) Constriction of the visual field of children after early visual deprivation. J Pediatr Ophthalmol Strabismus 34(6):347–356
12. Grovas A et al (1997) The National Cancer Data Base report on patterns of childhood cancers in the United States. Cancer 80(12):2321–2332
13. Pizzo PA, Poplack DG (2002) Principles and practice of pediatric oncology. Lippincott Williams & Wilkins, Philadelphia, xv, 1692 p
14. Breen KA, Grimwade D, Hunt BJ (2012) The pathogenesis and management of the coagulopathy of acute

promyelocytic leukaemia. Br J Haematol 156(1): 24–36

15. Packer RJ et al (1987) Quality of life in children with primitive neuroectodermal tumors (medulloblastoma) of the posterior fossa. Pediatr Neurosci 13(4): 169–175

16. Reimers TS et al (2003) Cognitive deficits in long-term survivors of childhood brain tumors: identification of predictive factors. Med Pediatr Oncol 40(1): 26–34

17. Hardy KK et al (2008) Hydrocephalus as a possible additional contributor to cognitive outcome in survivors of pediatric medulloblastoma. Psychooncology 17(11):1157–1161

18. Gelabert-Gonzalez M, Fernandez-Villa J (2001) Mutism after posterior fossa surgery. Review of the literature. Clin Neurol Neurosurg 103(2):111–114

19. Steinbok P et al (2003) Mutism after posterior fossa tumour resection in children: incomplete recovery on long-term follow-up. Pediatr Neurosurg 39(4):179–183

20. Sonderkaer S et al (2003) Long-term neurological outcome of childhood brain tumors treated by surgery only. J Clin Oncol 21(7):1347–1351

21. Brouwers P et al (1985) Long-term neuropsychologic sequelae of childhood leukemia: correlation with CT brain scan abnormalities. J Pediatr 106(5):723–728

22. Crosley CJ et al (1978) Central nervous system lesions in childhood leukemia. Neurology 28(7): 678–685

23. Price R (1983) Therapy related central nervous system diseases in children with acute lymphocytic leukemia. In: Mastrangelo R, Poplack D, Riccardi R (eds) Central nervous system leukemia. Martimus Nijhoff Publishers, Netherlands

24. Price RA, Birdwell DA (1978) The central nervous system in childhood leukemia. III. Mineralizing microangiopathy and dystrophic calcification. Cancer 42(2):717–728

25. Peylan-Ramu N et al (1978) Abnormal CT scans of the brain in asymptomatic children with acute lymphocytic leukemia after prophylactic treatment of the central nervous system with radiation and intrathecal chemotherapy. N Engl J Med 298(15):815–818

26. Schultheiss TE et al (1995) Radiation response of the central nervous system. Int J Radiat Oncol Biol Phys 31(5):1093–1112

27. Schuitema I et al (2013) Accelerated aging, decreased white matter integrity, and associated neuropsychological dysfunction 25 years after pediatric lymphoid malignancies. J Clin Oncol 31(27):3378–3388

28. Tofilon PJ, Fike JR (2000) The radioresponse of the central nervous system: a dynamic process. Radiat Res 153(4):357–370

29. Meadows AT et al (1981) Declines in IQ scores and cognitive dysfunctions in children with acute lymphocytic leukaemia treated with cranial irradiation. Lancet 2(8254):1015–1018

30. Cousens P et al (1988) Cognitive effects of cranial irradiation in leukaemia: a survey and meta-analysis. J Child Psychol Psychiatry 29(6):839–852

31. Rogers J et al (1992) Memory after treatment for acute lymphoblastic leukemia. Arch Dis Child 67: 266–268

32. Ochs J et al (1991) Comparison of neuropsychologic functioning and clinical indicators of neurotoxicity in long-term survivors of childhood leukemia given cranial radiation or parenteral methotrexate: a prospective study. J Clin Oncol 9(1):145–151

33. Brown RT, Madan-Swain A (1993) Cognitive, neuropsychological, and academic sequelae in children with leukemia. J Learn Disabil 26(2):74–90

34. Stehbens JA et al (1991) CNS prophylaxis of childhood leukemia: what are the long-term neurological, neuropsychological, and behavioral effects? Neuropsychol Rev 2(2):147–177

35. Radcliffe J et al (1994) Cognitive deficits in long-term survivors of childhood medulloblastoma and other noncortical tumors: age-dependent effects of whole brain radiation. Int J Dev Neurosci 12(4):327–334

36. Mulhern RK, Fairclough D, Ochs J (1991) A prospective comparison of neuropsychologic performance of children surviving leukemia who received 18-Gy, 24-Gy, or no cranial irradiation. J Clin Oncol 9(8): 1348–1356

37. Rubenstein CL, Varni JW, Katz ER (1990) Cognitive functioning in long-term survivors of childhood leukemia: a prospective analysis. J Dev Behav Pediatr 11(6):301–305

38. Jankovic M et al (1994) Association of 1800 cGy cranial irradiation with intellectual function in children with acute lymphoblastic leukaemia. ISPACC. International Study Group on Psychosocial Aspects of Childhood Cancer. Lancet 344(8917): 224–227

39. Robison LL et al (1984) Factors associated with IQ scores in long-term survivors of childhood acute lymphoblastic leukemia. Am J Pediatr Hematol Oncol 6(2):115–121

40. Waber DP et al (1990) Late effects of central nervous system treatment of acute lymphoblastic leukemia in childhood are sex-dependent. Dev Med Child Neurol 32(3):238–248

41. Bleyer WA et al (1990) Influence of age, sex, and concurrent intrathecal methotrexate therapy on intellectual function after cranial irradiation during childhood: a report from the Children's Cancer Study Group. Pediatr Hematol Oncol 7(4):329–338

42. Kingma A et al (2000) Academic career after treatment for acute lymphoblastic leukaemia. Arch Dis Child 82(5):353–357

43. Fuss M, Poljanc K, Hug EB (2000) Full Scale IQ (FSIQ) changes in children treated with whole brain and partial brain irradiation. A review and analysis. Strahlenther Onkol 176(12):573–581

44. Meshref M, ElShazly N, Nasr M, AbdElhai R. (2013). Effect of different doses of prophylactic cranial irradiation in childhood lymphoblastic leukemia on CNS relapse, late cognitive decline and learning disabilities. journal of cancer therapeutics and research, 2(1):10

45. Merchant TE et al (2009) Late effects of conformal radiation therapy for pediatric patients with low-grade glioma: prospective evaluation of cognitive, endocrine, and hearing deficits. J Clin Oncol 27(22): 3691–3697

46. Krull KR et al (2013) Neurocognitive outcomes decades after treatment for childhood acute lymphoblastic leukemia: a report from the St Jude lifetime cohort study. J Clin Oncol 31(35):4407–4415

47. Weber DC et al (2006) Radiation therapy planning with photons and protons for early and advanced breast cancer: an overview. Radiat Oncol 1:22

48. Yock T et al (2010) A phase II trial of proton radiotherapy for medulloblastoma: preliminary results. J Clin Oncol 28(18S):960s

49. Jimenez RB et al (2013) Proton radiation therapy for pediatric medulloblastoma and supratentorial primitive neuroectodermal tumors: outcomes for very young children treated with upfront chemotherapy. Int J Radiat Oncol Biol Phys 87(1):120–126

50. Kuhltau KA et al (2012) Prospective study of health-related quality of life for children with brain tumors treated with proton radiotherapy. J Clin Oncol 30(17): 2079–2086

51. Moleski M (2000) Neuropsychological, neuroanatomical, and neurophysiological consequences of CNS chemotherapy for acute lymphoblastic leukemia. Arch Clin Neuropsychol 15:603–630

52. Ruggiero A et al (2001) Intrathecal chemotherapy with antineoplastic agents in children. Paediatr Drugs 3(4):237–246

53. Prassopoulos P et al (1996) Quantitative assessment of cerebral atrophy during and after treatment in children with acute lymphoblastic leukemia. Invest Radiol 31(12):749–754

54. Moleski M (2000) Neuropsychological, neuroanatomical, and neurophysiological consequences of CNS chemotherapy for acute lymphoblastic leukemia. Arch Clin Neuropsychol 15(7):603–630

55. Mulhern RK, Butler RW (2004) Neurocognitive sequelae of childhood cancers and their treatment. Pediatr Rehabil 7(1):1–14, discussion 15-6

56. Ciesielski KT et al (1999) MRI morphometry of mamillary bodies, caudate nuclei, and prefrontal cortices after chemotherapy for childhood leukemia: multivariate models of early and late developing memory subsystems. Behav Neurosci 113(3):439–450

57. Steinberg S et al (1998) Late sequelae of CNS recurrence of acute lymphoblastic leukemia in childhood. Klin Padiatr 210(4):200–206

58. Raymond-Speden E et al (2000) Intellectual, neuropsychological, and academic functioning in long-term survivors of leukemia. J Pediatr Psychol 25(2):59–68

59. Brown RT et al (1996) A 3-year follow-up of the intellectual and academic functioning of children receiving central nervous system prophylactic chemotherapy for leukemia. J Dev Behav Pediatr 17(6):392–398

60. Orti E, Tornello S, De Nicola AF (1985) Dynamic aspects of glucocorticoid receptors in the spinal cord of the rat. J Neurochem 45(6):1699–1707

61. Kadan-Lottick NS et al (2009) Comparison of neurocognitive functioning in children previously randomly assigned to intrathecal methotrexate compared with triple intrathecal therapy for the treatment of childhood acute lymphoblastic leukemia. J Clin Oncol 27(35):5986–5992

62. Mahoney DH Jr et al (1998) Acute neurotoxicity in children with B-precursor acute lymphoid leukemia: an association with intermediate-dose intravenous methotrexate and intrathecal triple therapy–a Pediatric Oncology Group study. J Clin Oncol 16(5): 1712–1722

63. Watterson J et al (1994) Excessive spinal cord toxicity from intensive central nervous system-directed therapies. Cancer 74(11):3034–3041

64. Raetz EA, Salzer WL (2010) Tolerability and efficacy of L-asparaginase therapy in pediatric patients with acute lymphoblastic leukemia. J Pediatr Hematol Oncol 32(7):554–563

65. Grace RF et al (2011) The frequency and management of asparaginase-related thrombosis in paediatric and adult patients with acute lymphoblastic leukaemia treated on Dana-Farber Cancer Institute consortium protocols. Br J Haematol 152(4):452–459

66. De Schryver EL et al (2004) Long-term prognosis of cerebral venous sinus thrombosis in childhood. Dev Med Child Neurol 46(8):514–519

67. Ross CS et al (2013) Cerebral venous sinus thrombosis in pediatric cancer patients: long-term neurological outcomes. J Pediatr Hematol Oncol 35(4):299–302

68. Sapolsky RM (1993) Potential behavioral modification of glucocorticoid damage to the hippocampus. Behav Brain Res 57(2):175–182

69. Bodnoff SR et al (1995) Enduring effects of chronic corticosterone treatment on spatial learning, synaptic plasticity, and hippocampal neuropathology in young and mid-aged rats. J Neurosci 15(1 Pt 1):61–69

70. Bender BG, Lerner JA, Poland JE (1991) Association between corticosteroids and psychologic change in hospitalized asthmatic children. Ann Allergy 66(5): 414–419

71. Drigan R, Spirito A, Gelber RD (1992) Behavioral effects of corticosteroids in children with acute lymphoblastic leukemia. Med Pediatr Oncol 20(1):13–21

72. Murphy BP et al (2001) Impaired cerebral cortical gray matter growth after treatment with dexamethasone for neonatal chronic lung disease. Pediatrics 107(2):217–221

73. Shinwell ES et al (2000) Early postnatal dexamethasone treatment and increased incidence of cerebral palsy. Arch Dis Child Fetal Neonatal Ed 83(3): F177–F181

74. Bostrom BC et al (2003) Dexamethasone versus prednisone and daily oral versus weekly intravenous mercaptopurine for patients with standard-risk acute lymphoblastic leukemia: a report from the Children's Cancer Group. Blood 101(10):3809–3817

75. Alexander E 3rd, Loeffler JS (1998) Radiosurgery for primary malignant brain tumors. Semin Surg Oncol 14(1):43–52

76. Pratt CB et al (1986) Central nervous system toxicity following the treatment of pediatric patients with ifosfamide/mesna. J Clin Oncol 4(8):1253–1261

77. Pratt CB et al (1990) Ifosfamide neurotoxicity is related to previous cisplatin treatment for pediatric solid tumors. J Clin Oncol 8(8):1399–1401

78. Kurtzberg J et al (1996) 2-Amino-9-B-D-arabinosyl-6-methoxy-9H-guanine (GW506U; compound 506U) is highly active in patients with T-cell malignancies; results of a phase I trial in pediatric and adult patients with refractory hematological malignancies. [abstract]. Blood 88(Suppl 1):699a

79. Miyahara M et al (2000) Somnolence syndrome in a child following 1200-cGy total body irradiation in an unrelated bone marrow transplantation. Pediatr Hematol Oncol 17(6):489–495

80. Freeman JE, Johnston PG, Voke JM (1973) Somnolence after prophylactic cranial irradiation in children with acute lymphoblastic leukaemia. Br Med J 4(5891):523–525

81. Mandell LR et al (1989) Reduced incidence of the somnolence syndrome in leukemic children with steroid coverage during prophylactic cranial radiation therapy. Results of a pilot study. Cancer 63(10):1975–1978

82. van der Kogel A (1991) Central nervous system radiation injury in small animal models. In: Gutin P, Leibel S, Sheline G (eds) Radiation injury to the nervous system. Raven Press, New York, pp 91–112

83. Priest JR et al (1980) Thrombotic and hemorrhagic strokes complicating early therapy for childhood acute lymphoblastic leukemia. Cancer 46(7):1548–1554

84. Campbell LK et al (2007) A meta-analysis of the neurocognitive sequelae of treatment for childhood acute lymphocytic leukemia. Pediatr Blood Cancer 49(1):65–73

85. Montour-Proulx I et al (2005) Cognitive changes in children treated for acute lymphoblastic leukemia with chemotherapy only according to the Pediatric Oncology Group 9605 protocol. J Child Neurol 20(2):129–133

86. Buizer AI et al (2006) Behavioral and educational limitations after chemotherapy for childhood acute lymphoblastic leukemia or Wilms tumor. Cancer 106(9):2067–2075

87. Mitby PA et al (2003) Utilization of special education services and educational attainment among long-term survivors of childhood cancer: a report from the Childhood Cancer Survivor Study. Cancer 97(4):1115–1126

88. Kirchhoff AC et al (2011) Physical, mental, and neurocognitive status and employment outcomes in the childhood cancer survivor study cohort. Cancer Epidemiol Biomarkers Prev 20(9):1838–1849

89. Janson C et al (2009) Predictors of marriage and divorce in adult survivors of childhood cancers: a report from the Childhood Cancer Survivor Study. Cancer Epidemiol Biomarkers Prev 18(10):2626–2635

90. Kunin-Batson A et al (2011) Predictors of independent living status in adult survivors of childhood cancer: a report from the Childhood Cancer Survivor Study. Pediatr Blood Cancer 57(7):1197–1203

91. Packer RJ et al (2003) Long-term neurologic and neurosensory sequelae in adult survivors of a childhood brain tumor: childhood cancer survivor study. J Clin Oncol 21(17):3255–3261

92. Phipps S et al (2008) Cognitive and academic consequences of stem-cell transplantation in children. J Clin Oncol 26(12):2027–2033

93. Mulcahy Levy JM et al (2013) Late effects of total body irradiation and hematopoietic stem cell transplant in children under 3 years of age. Pediatr Blood Cancer 60(4):700–704

94. Shah AJ et al (2008) Progressive declines in neurocognitive function among survivors of hematopoietic stem cell transplantation for pediatric hematologic malignancies. J Pediatr Hematol Oncol 30(6):411–418

95. Rottenberg DA et al (1977) Cerebral necrosis following radiotherapy of extracranial neoplasms. Ann Neurol 1(4):339–357

96. New P (2001) Radiation injury to the nervous system. Curr Opin Neurol 14(6):725–734

97. Baron RM, Kenny DA (1986) The moderator-mediator variable distinction in social psychological research: conceptual, strategic, and statistical considerations. J Pers Soc Psychol 51(6):1173–1182

98. Riccardi R et al (1985) Abnormal computed tomography brain scans in children with acute lymphoblastic leukemia: serial long-term follow-up. J Clin Oncol 3(1):12–18

99. Jannoun L (1983) Are cognitive and educational development affected by age at which prophylactic therapy is given in acute lymphoblastic leukaemia? Arch Dis Child 58(12):953–958

100. Krull K et al (2013) Long-term decline in intelligence among adult survivors of childhood acute lymphoblastic leukemia treated with cranial radiation. Blood 122(4):550–553

101. Armstrong GT et al (2013) Evaluation of memory impairment in aging adult survivors of childhood acute lymphoblastic leukemia treated with cranial radiotherapy. J Natl Cancer Inst 105(12):899–907

102. Waber DP et al (1995) Cognitive sequelae of treatment in childhood acute lymphoblastic leukemia: cranial radiation requires an accomplice. J Clin Oncol 13(10):2490–2496

103. Buizer AI et al (2005) Chemotherapy and attentional dysfunction in survivors of childhood acute lymphoblastic leukemia: effect of treatment intensity. Pediatr Blood Cancer 45(3):281–290

104. Copeland DR et al (1996) Neuropsychologic effects of chemotherapy on children with cancer: a longitudinal study. J Clin Oncol 14(10):2826–2835

105. Kadan-Lottick NS et al (2010) Neurocognitive functioning in adult survivors of childhood non-central nervous system cancers. J Natl Cancer Inst 102(12):881–893

106. Yeates KO et al (1997) Preinjury family environment as a determinant of recovery from traumatic brain

injuries in school-age children. J Int Neuropsychol Soc 3(6):617–630

107. Wade S et al (1995) Assessing the effects of traumatic brain injury on family functioning: conceptual and methodological issues. J Pediatr Psychol 20(6): 737–752

108. Hutchinson KC et al (2009) Adjustment of caregivers of pediatric patients with brain tumors: a cross-sectional analysis. Psychooncology 18(5):515–523

109. Long KA, Marsland AL (2011) Family adjustment to childhood cancer: a systematic review. Clin Child Fam Psychol Rev 14(1):57–88

110. Ach E et al (2013) Family factors associated with academic achievement deficits in pediatric brain tumor survivors. Psychooncology 22(8):1731–1737

111. Carlson-Green B, Morris RD, Krawiecki N (1995) Family and illness predictors of outcome in pediatric brain tumors. J Pediatr Psychol 20(6):769–784

112. Kamdar KY et al (2011) Folate pathway polymorphisms predict deficits in attention and processing speed after childhood leukemia therapy. Pediatr Blood Cancer 57(3):454–460

113. Krull KR et al (2013) Genetic mediators of neurocognitive outcomes in survivors of childhood acute lymphoblastic leukemia. J Clin Oncol 31(17):2182–2188

114. Nesbit ME Jr et al (1981) Presymptomatic central nervous system therapy in previously untreated childhood acute lymphoblastic leukaemia: comparison of 1800 rad and 2400 rad. A report for Children's Cancer Study Group. Lancet 1(8218):461–466

115. Duffner PK et al (1993) Postoperative chemotherapy and delayed radiation in children less than three years of age with malignant brain tumors. N Engl J Med 328(24):1725–1731

116. Mulhern RK, Palmer SL (2003) Neurocognitive late effects in pediatric cancer. Curr Probl Cancer 27(4): 177–197

117. Group CsO (ed) (2008) Long-term follow-up guidelines for survivors of childhood, adolescent and young adult cancers, Version 3.0. Children's Oncology Group, Arcadia

118. Embry, Leanne, et al (2012) Implementation of multi-site neurocognitive assessments within a pediatric cooperative group: Can it be done? Pediatric blood & cancer 59(3):536–539

119. Nathan PC et al (2007) Guidelines for identification of, advocacy for, and intervention in neurocognitive problems in survivors of childhood cancer: a report from the Children's Oncology Group. Arch Pediatr Adolesc Med 161(8):798–806

120. Butler RW, Mulhern RK (2005) Neurocognitive interventions for children and adolescents surviving cancer. J Pediatr Psychol 30(1):65–78

121. Krull KR et al (2008) Folate pathway genetic polymorphisms are related to attention disorders in childhood leukemia survivors. J Pediatr 152(1):101–105

122. Patel SK et al (2007) Attention dysfunction and parent reporting in children with brain tumors. Pediatr Blood Cancer 49(7):970–974

123. Kahalley LS et al (2011) ADHD and secondary ADHD criteria fail to identify many at-risk survivors of pediatric ALL and brain tumor. Pediatr Blood Cancer 57(1):110–118

124. Conklin HM et al (2010) Predicting methylphenidate response in long-term survivors of childhood cancer: a randomized, double-blind, placebo-controlled, crossover trial. J Pediatr Psychol 35(2):144–155

125. Conklin HM et al (2009) Side effects of methylphenidate in childhood cancer survivors: a randomized placebo-controlled trial. Pediatrics 124(1):226–233

126. Charach A et al (2006) Using stimulant medication for children with ADHD: what do parents say? A brief report. J Can Acad Child Adolesc Psychiatry 15(2):75–83

127. Butler RW et al (2008) A multicenter, randomized clinical trial of a cognitive remediation program for childhood survivors of a pediatric malignancy. J Consult Clin Psychol 76(3):367

128. Patel SK et al (2009) Cognitive and problem solving training in children with cancer: a pilot project. J Pediatr Hematol Oncol 31(9):670–677

129. Hardy KK, Willard VW, Bonner MJ (2011) Computerized cognitive training in survivors of childhood cancer a pilot study. J Pediatr Oncol Nurs 28(1):27–33

130. Kesler SR, Lacayo NJ, Jo B (2011) A pilot study of an online cognitive rehabilitation program for executive function skills in children with cancer-related brain injury. Brain Inj 25(1):101–112

131. Zou P et al (2012) Evidence of change in brain activity among childhood cancer survivors participating in a cognitive remediation program. Arch Clin Neuropsychol 27(8):915–929

132. Siegel Rebecca et al (2014) Cancer statistics, CA: a cancer journal for clinicians 64(1):9–29

133. Iuvone L et al (2002). Long-term cognitive outcome, brain computed tomography scan, and magnetic resonance imaging in children cured for acute lymphoblastic leukemia. Cancer 95(12):2562–2570

134. Kitano S et al (2000). Moyamoya disease associated with a brain stem glioma. Child's Nervous System, 16(4):251–255

# Endocrine Complications of Cancer Therapy

**5**

Susan R. Rose, Sarah Lawson,
Karen Burns, and Thomas E. Merchant

## Contents

S.R. Rose, MD (✉) • S. Lawson
Division of Endocrinology and
Metabolism, Cincinnati Children's
Hospital Medical Center
and University of Cincinnati,
3333 Burnet Avenue, MLC 7012,
Cincinnati, OH 45229, USA
e-mail: susan.rose@cchmc.org;
sarah.lawson@cchmc.org

K. Burns
Division of Hematology and Oncology,
Cincinnati Children's Hospital Medical Center
and University of Cincinnati, 3333 Burnet Avenue,
MLC 7012, Cincinnati, OH 45229, USA
e-mail: Karen.burns@cchmc.org

T.E. Merchant
Division of Radiation Oncology, St Jude Children's
Research Hospital, Memphis, TN, USA
e-mail: Thomas.merchant@STJUDE.ORG

© Springer International Publishing 2015
C.L. Schwartz et al. (eds.), *Survivors of Childhood and Adolescent Cancer:
A Multidisciplinary Approach*, Pediatric Oncology, DOI 10.1007/978-3-319-16435-9_5

## Abbreviations

| | |
|---|---|
| ACTH | Adrenocorticotropic hormone |
| ADH | Antidiuretic hormone |
| AM | Morning |
| AMH | Anti-Mullerian hormone |
| BMD | Bone mineral density |
| BMI | Body mass index |
| CNS | Central nervous system |
| CT | Computed tomography |
| DXA | Dual-energy x-ray absorptiometry |
| FSH | Follicular-stimulating hormone |
| GH | Growth hormone |
| GHD | GH deficiency |
| GHRH | GH-releasing hormone |
| GnRH | Gonadotropin-releasing hormone |
| Gy | Gray |
| HPA | Hypothalamic-pituitary axis |
| IGFBP3 | Insulin-like growth factor binding protein |
| IGF-I | Insulin-like growth factor |
| LH | Luteinizing hormone |
| MR | Magnetic resonance |
| OGTT | Oral glucose tolerance test |
| PM | Afternoon |
| PRL | Prolactin |
| RT | Radiation therapy |
| SD | Standard deviation |
| T3 | Triiodothyronine |
| T4 | Thyroxine |
| TRH | Thyrotropin-releasing hormone |
| TSH | Thyroid-stimulating hormone |

## 5.1 Introduction

Endocrinopathy after therapeutic irradiation represents a treatable late effect of successful cancer therapy and highlights the importance of careful follow-up for adults and children. The endocrine effects of irradiation have been extensively studied and demonstrate the systemic manifestations of late effects after localized or large volume irradiation, the differential sensitivity of functional subunits of the hypothalamus and other critical endocrine organs to radiation dose, the low-dose radiation effects in normal tissues, and the benefit of newer radiation methods and modalities.

There is significant morbidity and mortality linked to the late effects of cancer therapy [67]. Despite our understanding of the endocrine effects of cancer therapy, this information is often not considered when models of treatment outcomes and therapy effects are developed. It is possible that the contribution of endocrine deficits to morbidity and mortality is not fully appreciated. Endocrine deficiencies affect patients who do not have pituitary tumors [1] as well as those whose treatment volume encompasses the hypothalamic-pituitary axis. Rare late effects of treatment most often attributed to the volume of irradiation might be linked to the indirect effects of damage to the hypothalamic-pituitary axis or other organs of the endocrine system. A striking example is the link between anticancer therapy for patients with pituitary tumors and craniopharyngioma. These patients are at increased risk for mortality mainly due to radiation-associated vascular disease rather than endocrinologic abnormalities [68]. There needs to be increased recognition of endocrine sequelae of cancer therapy, the contribution of radiation therapy, and an emphasis on early detection and follow-up because of the potential impact on quality of life [72]. Long-term survivors are at increased risk for broad-ranging side effects including metabolic syndrome, growth hormone deficiency, and cardiovascular disease [27]. The field of endocrinology is uniquely capable of intervention to treat the late effects of cancer therapy. Endocrinologists should be consulted early in the management of patients at high risk for preexisting endocrine deficiencies and those likely to develop these common complications.

## 5.2 Pathophysiology

### 5.2.1 Normal Hypothalamic-Pituitary Axis

The hypothalamic-pituitary axis (HPA) is the primary interface between the nervous system and the endocrine system. The actions and interactions of the endocrine and nervous systems constitute the major regulatory mechanisms for virtually all physiologic activities. The hypothalamus has extensive neural communications with other brain regions and regulates brain functions including temperature, appetite, thirst, sexual behavior, and fear. The hypothalamus also contains two types of neurosecretory cells (Fig. 5.1): (1) neurohypophysial neurons, which transverse the hypothalamic-pituitary stalk and release vasopressin and oxytocin from their nerve endings in the posterior pituitary, and (2) hypophysiotropic neurons, which secrete releasing hormones into portal hypophyseal vessels. The releasing hormones regulate secretion of hormones from the anterior pituitary (Table 5.1).

### 5.2.1.1 Growth Hormone

Growth hormone (GH) is a 191-amino-acid polypeptide hormone synthesized and secreted by the somatotrophs in the anterior pituitary gland in response to hypothalamic releasing hormones, primarily GH-releasing hormone (GHRH). In addition, ghrelin secretion from the stomach during fasting also contributes to GH secretion [51]. GHRH levels are usually steady, while somatostatin secretion is interrupted intermittently.

Somatostatin inhibits GH release but paradoxically contributes to synthesis of GH in the pituitary [12]. When somatostatin concentrations decrease, the tonic concentration of GHRH causes release of GH into the systemic circulation. Factors such as neuropeptide Y, leptin, galanin, and ghrelin also affect GH secretion. In healthy children and adults, GH secretion is pulsatile, particularly during sleep, with two to six pulses per night [61]. In adolescents, additional pulses occur during the day, and the pulses have higher peaks than those seen in children and adults (Fig. 5.2a).

Circulating serum GH stimulates production of insulin-like growth factor I (IGF-I) in all tissues. IGF-I mediates GH effects on growth, bone mineralization, and body composition (decreased truncal fat deposition, increased lean muscle mass) [78]. IGF-I is bound to IGF-binding proteins such as IGFBP3 and is transported in the blood. IGF-I and IGFBP3 concentrations are stable during the day, and each reflects the integrated concentration of secreted GH.

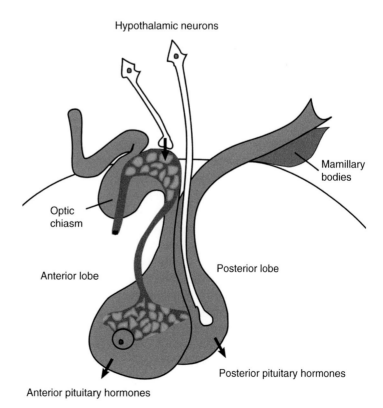

**Fig. 5.1** Diagrammatic representation of the hypothalamic-pituitary axis

**Table 5.1** Anterior pituitary hormones and major hypothalamic regulatory factors

| Pituitary hormone | Hypothalamic factor | Effect |
|---|---|---|
| Growth hormone | Growth hormone-releasing hormone | + |
| | Somatostatin | − |
| Prolactin | Dopamine | − |
| Luteinizing hormone | Gonadotropin-releasing hormone | + |
| Follicle-stimulating hormone | Gonadotropin-releasing hormone | + |
| Thyroid-stimulating hormone | Thyroid-releasing hormone | + |
| | Somatostatin | − |
| Adrenocorticotropin | Corticotropin-releasing hormone | + |
| | Vasopressin | + |

Effects on the hypothalamus were either stimulatory (+) or inhibitory (−)

### 5.2.1.2 Gonadotropins

Luteinizing hormone (LH) and follicle-stimulating hormone (FSH) are glycoprotein hormones both stored in the same cells in the anterior pituitary. Their overall patterns of secretion vary according to the age and gender of the person. The pituitary gland produces and secretes LH and FSH in a pulsatile manner in response to episodic release of GnRH from the hypothalamus (Fig. 5.2a). The hypothalamic stimulus is actively inhibited between 6 months of age and the usual age of onset of puberty (Fig. 5.2b). This inhibition can be disturbed by tumor mass, cranial surgery, or irradiation, thereby resulting in precocious puberty in children. In men, LH stimulates testosterone production in Leydig cells of the testes; normal spermatogenesis requires both LH and FSH. In women, FSH stimulates production of estrogen and LH stimulates production of progesterone in the ovary. The LH surge near the end of the follicular phase of the menstrual cycle is necessary to stimulate ovulation. Development of the ovarian follicles is largely under FSH control, and secretion of estrogen from follicles is dependent on both FSH and LH.

### 5.2.1.3 Thyroid-Stimulating Hormone

Thyrotropin, or thyroid-stimulating hormone (TSH), is a glycoprotein hormone synthesized in the anterior pituitary. Secretion of TSH is stimulated by TSH-releasing hormone (TRH) and inhibited by somatostatin and dopamine secreted from the hypothalamus. In persons older than 12 months of age, there is a circadian pattern to TSH release. TSH concentration is low after 1000 h and in the afternoon, rises dramatically (*surges*) after 1900 h, and reaches highest concentrations between 2200 and 0400 h (Fig. 5.2a) [58]. Thus, at least one third of the trophic influence of TSH on the thyroid gland occurs at night. TRH is necessary for TSH synthesis, posttranslational glycosylation, and secretion of a fully bioactive TSH molecule from the pituitary. Altered TSH glycosylation, resulting in altered bioactivity, is seen in mixed hypothyroidism (central hypothyroidism with mild TSH elevation [5–15 mU/L]) [34, 56].

TSH stimulates the thyroid gland to produce thyroxine (T4) and triiodothyronine (T3). T4 and T3 circulate in the blood stream bound to thyroxine-binding globulin and albumin; only small amounts are free or unbound. Free T4 undergoes intracellular deiodination to form free T3, which interacts with DNA in the cell nucleus to influence cellular mRNA and protein synthesis. Free T4 provides negative feedback at the hypothalamus and pituitary to modulate the secretion of TRH and TSH.

### 5.2.1.4 Adrenocorticotropin

Adrenocorticotropin (ACTH) is a 39-amino-acid peptide hormone processed in the corticotrophs from a large precursor molecule, proopiomelanocortin. In healthy individuals, hypothalamic corticotrophin-releasing hormone and vasopressin released in two or three synchronous pulses per hour synergistically stimulate secretion of ACTH from the pituitary [14]. ACTH secretion is pulsatile and varies throughout the day; it peaks before the person awakens in the morning (Fig. 5.2a), increases with stress, and is inhibited by glucocorticoid medications. Since cortisol secretion is regulated by ACTH, the pattern of cortisol secretion is similar to that of secretion of ACTH. In addition to the negative feedback of glucocorticoids, ACTH inhibits its own secretion (short-loop feedback).

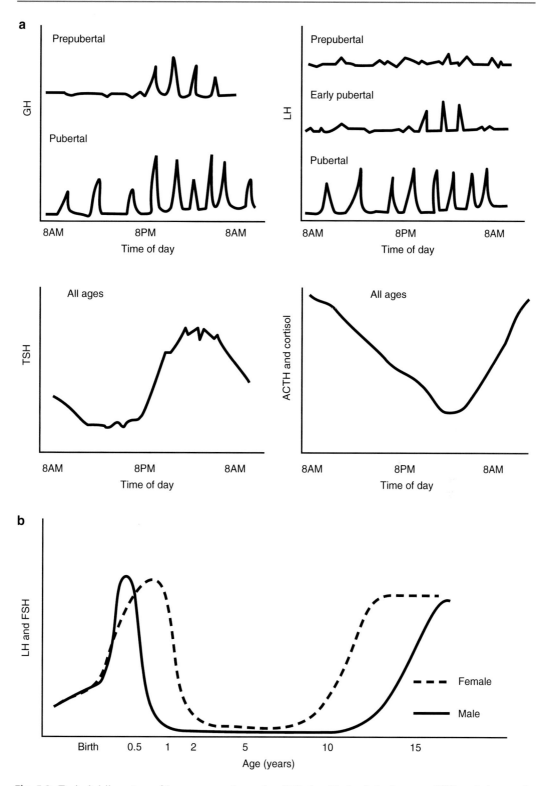

**Fig. 5.2** Typical daily pattern of hormone secretion and changes with pubertal status and time of day in normal individuals (**a**) growth hormone (*GH*), luteinizing hormone (*LH*), thyroid-stimulating hormone (*TSH*), and adrenocorticotropin (*ACTH*) and cortisol secretion. (**b**) Normal changes in LH and FSH levels from infancy to adolescence

### 5.2.1.5 Prolactin

Prolactin (PRL) is a 198-amino-acid polypeptide hormone synthesized and secreted from lactotrophs of the anterior pituitary. A precursor molecule is also secreted and can constitute as much as 10–20 % of the PRL immunoreactivity in the plasma of healthy persons. Hypothalamic control of PRL secretion (primarily through dopamine release) is different than that of the other pituitary hormones in that the hypothalamus inhibits secretion of PRL rather than stimulating it. Thus, elevated PRL levels can be a useful marker of hypothalamic disorders that leave the pituitary intact.

### 5.2.1.6 Antidiuretic Hormone

Antidiuretic hormone (ADH) or vasopressin is a peptide hormone synthesized in the hypothalamic neurohypophyseal neurons, transported through the pituitary stalk in long axons, and released from the nerve terminals in the posterior pituitary. ADH is secreted in response to reduced plasma volume and increased plasma osmolality. In normal individuals, ADH secretion is increased when there is no fluid intake, such as during sleep or in dehydration.

## 5.2.2 Injury of the Hypothalamic-Pituitary Axis in Patients with Cancer

The hypothalamic-pituitary axis (HPA) is vulnerable to damage by certain tumors, surgical trauma, irradiation, chemotherapy, and other common risk factors (Table 5.2) [18, 57]. Patients with tumors in the area of the HPA (e.g., craniopharyngioma or hypothalamic/chiasmatic tumor) are at particular risk for neuroendocrinopathy [23, 42]. Many HPA injuries are attributable to damage caused by radiation therapy (RT) [57]. However, the occurrence of pre-RT neuroendocrinopathies in pediatric patients with brain tumors is high. Of 68 pediatric patients in one study [44], 45 (66 %) showed evidence of neuroendocrinopathy before RT, including 15 of 32 patients with tumors in the posterior fossa not adjacent to the HPA. Seventeen of the 45 patients (38 %) had abnormality in GH, 19 (43 %) in TSH, 10 (22 %) in ACTH, and 6 (13 %) in gonadotropin. In addition, patients who receive chemotherapy alone [with no history of RT or central nervous system (CNS) tumor] may also be at risk for neuroendocrinopathy. Of 31 such patients referred after chemotherapy for evaluation of altered growth and development, 48 % had GH deficiency, 52 % had central hypothyroidism, and 32 % had pubertal abnormalities [62].

GH deficiency is often the first hypothalamic-pituitary deficiency to emerge after injury to the HPA, followed by deficiencies of gonadotropin, TSH, and ACTH [18, 70]; however, these deficiencies can develop in any order [44, 59, 71]. Although the most common neuroendocrinologic abnormality in survivors of childhood cancer is GH deficiency (see Sect. 5.3.1), hypothyroidism is at least as prevalent when sensitive testing methods are used (see Sect. 5.3.4) [59]. The next most common alterations are in pubertal timing (early, rapid, precocious, delayed, or absent) (see Sects. 5.3.2 and 5.3.3). ACTH deficiency, though less common than the other disorders, has more serious consequences if it is not detected (see Sect. 5.3.5). Diabetes insipidus rarely develops after chemotherapy or irradiation, but commonly occurs after surgery in the hypothalamic-pituitary area or in association with histiocytosis or germinoma (see Sect. 5.3.7). Hypothalamic injury resulting from tumor, surgery, or irradiation can result in unrelenting weight gain, termed hypothalamic obesity (see Sect. 5.3.9). Finally, osteopenia may result from hypothalamic-pituitary deficiency, particularly GH deficiency, hypothyroidism, and hypogonadism (see Sect. 5.3.8).

## 5.2.3 Contribution of Radiation to Hypothalamic-Pituitary Axis Injury

Radiation therapy (RT) is a significant contributor to neuroendocrine complications observed after treatment for CNS tumors, CNS preventative therapy for leukemia, and following total

**Table 5.2** Risk factors for endocrine disorders, diagnostic studies, and treatment options

| Disorder | Highest risk | Diagnostic studies[a] | Treatment options[a] |
|---|---|---|---|
| GH deficiency | ≥18 Gy CRT<br>Pretransplant CRT<br>TBI<br>Young age<br>Tumor near HPA<br>Hydrocephalus | IGF-I, IGFBP-3<br>Bone age radiograph<br>GH stimulation tests | Recombinant GH (SC)<br>GnRH agonist (IM)<br>(If pubertal maturity too<br>advanced for height) |
| Gonadotropin deficiency | ≥30 Gy CRT<br>Tumor near HPA | LH, FSH, AMH, inhibin, estradiol,<br>or testosterone (4–8 AM)<br>Bone age<br>GnRH stimulation test | Estrogen/progestin (O or T)<br>(female)<br>Testosterone (IM or T)<br>(male) |
| Precocious puberty | 18–24 Gy CRT<br>Female<br>Young age<br>Tumor near HPA | LH, FSH, estradiol, or testosterone<br>(4–8 AM)<br>Bone age<br>Pelvic ultrasound (female)<br>± GnRH stimulation test<br>± GH stimulation test | GnRH agonist (IM) |
| TSH deficiency | ≥30 Gy CRT<br>TBI<br>Tumor near HPA<br>Hydrocephalus | Free T4, TSH (8 AM)<br>AM-PM TSH ratio<br>Nocturnal TSH surge | L-thyroxine (O) |
| ACTH deficiency | ≥30 Gy CRT<br>Tumor near HPA<br>Hydrocephalus | Cortisol (8 AM)<br>Low-dose ACTH stimulation test | Hydrocortisone (O)<br>Stress dosing (O, IM, or IV) |
| Hyperprolactinemia | ≥50 Gy CRT<br>Tumor near HPA | Prolactin | Dopamine agonists (O) |
| Diabetes insipidus | Histiocytosis<br>Germinomas<br>Tumor or tumor-related<br>cysts near HPA | Simultaneous serum and urine<br>osmolarity after 8–12 h without<br>fluid intake<br>Water deprivation test | Desmopressin (O)<br>DDAVP (SC or IN) |
| Osteopenia | Low GH, TSH, or LH/<br>FSH<br>High prolactin<br>Low vitamin D intake | DXA or quantitative CT<br>25OH-vitamin D level | Calcium + vitamin D (O)<br>± Bisphosphonates (O or IV) |
| Hypothalamic obesity | Young age (<6 years)<br>≥50 Gy (hypothalamus)<br>Tumor near HPA | Fasting insulin and glucose<br>Oral glucose tolerance test with<br>insulin levels | Diet and exercise<br>Ritalin or dexedrine (O)<br>Metformin (O) (monitor for<br>hypoglycemia)<br>Octreotide (SC)<br>Bariatric surgery |

*Abbreviations*: *GH* growth hormone, *CRT* cranial radiation therapy, *TBI* total body irradiation, *HPA* hypothalamic-pituitary axis, *IGF-I* insulin-like growth factor I, *IGFBP3* IGF-binding protein 3, *GHRH* growth hormone-releasing hormone, *GnRH* gonadotropin-releasing hormone, *LH* luteinizing hormone, *FSH* follicle-stimulating hormone, *AMH* anti-Mullerian hormone, *T4* thyroxine, *TSH* thyroid-stimulating hormone, *TRH* thyrotropin-releasing hormone, *ACTH* adrenocorticotropin, O oral, *SC* subcutaneous, *IM* intramuscular, *IN* intranasal, *IV* intravenous, *T* topical
[a]See text for more details

body irradiation. Similar complications are observed when the HPA is incidentally irradiated in the treatment of nasopharyngeal cancer, retinoblastoma, Hodgkin disease with involvement of Waldeyer's ring, and pediatric sarcomas of the head and neck (e.g., parameningeal and orbital rhabdomyosarcoma) (Fig. 5.3). The incidence and time to onset of neuroendocrine sequelae after RT are difficult to predict because of other contributors to HPA dysfunction that may coincide temporally with the administration of RT. A notable example is hydrocephalus which can cause mass effect in the region of the anterior third ventricle and generalized diminished blood

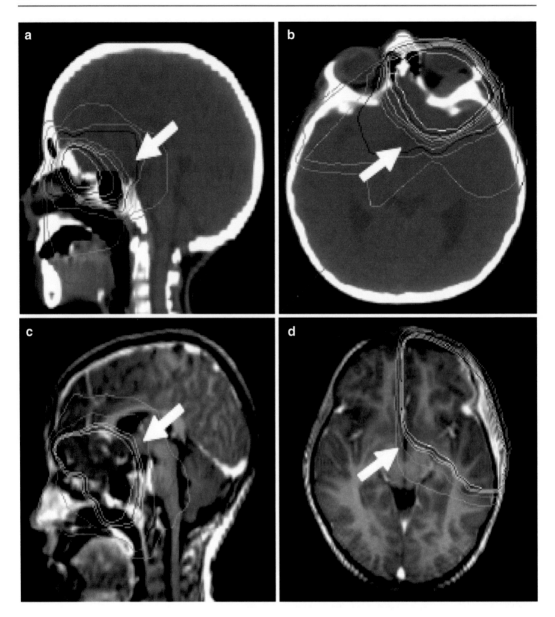

**Fig. 5.3** Radiation dosimetry taken from the treatment of children with orbital (**a**, **b**) and infratemporal fossa rhabdomyosarcoma (**c**, **d**). The images illustrate cases in which the HPA is incidentally irradiated and may receive all or a portion of the prescription dose (*arrow* indicates location of the hypothalamus)

flow to sensitive regions of the brain. In one study, 59 children with infratentorial ependymoma underwent provocative testing for GH, thyroid hormone, and ACTH secretion abnormality prior to RT [43]. Abnormal testing was observed in 27 patients (46 %) with 30 % of the 59 having abnormality in GH secretion. Serial measurements of ventricular size from the time of diagnosis to 1 year after RT were recorded and modeled to show that ventricular size at the time of diagnosis could be used to predict preirradiation endocrinopathy. Change in ventricular size over time could predict GH deficiency prior to irradiation (Fig. 5.4). This study demonstrated a relatively high rate of pre-irradiation endocrinopathy in a well-defined group, confirming

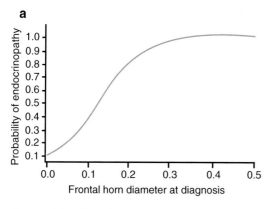

**Fig. 5.4** The effect of hydrocephalus on pre-irradiation endocrinopathy in children with infratentorial ependymoma. (**a**) Probability of pre-irradiation endocrine deficiency based on frontal horn diameter measured at diagnosis. (**b**) Probability of pre-irradiation growth hormone (*GH*) deficiency based on change (slope) in the Evan's index after diagnosis. The Evan's index is the ratio of the distance between the most lateral extent of the frontal horns of the lateral ventricles and the width of the parietal brain at the same level

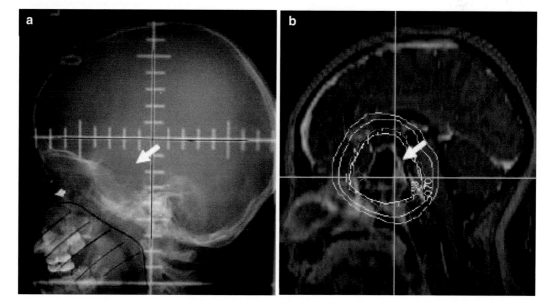

**Fig. 5.5** Homogeneous irradiation of the HPA including (**a**) a traditional treatment portal used for cranial irradiation in ALL and (**b**) dosimetry from focal treatment of craniopharyngioma (*arrow* indicates location of the hypothalamus)

another important tumor-related cause of endocrinopathy. Thus, management of hydrocephalus is important, particularly in children with posterior fossa tumors.

Many reports of neuroendocrine effects of RT have used generalized estimates of radiation dose under conditions where the dose to the HPA was relatively homogeneous and discrete [46]. Examples include patients treated with single-dose or fractionated TBI (8–14 Gy), cranial irradiation for leukemia (18 and 24 Gy) and tumors of the sellar or parasellar region in which the HPA was uniformly included in the volume of prescribed dose (>50 Gy) (Fig. 5.5). For other diseases, the HPA may have been located within the irradiated volume for part or all of the treatment or in the gradient of dose (dose fall off) experiencing only a fraction of the daily dose administered (Fig. 5.6).

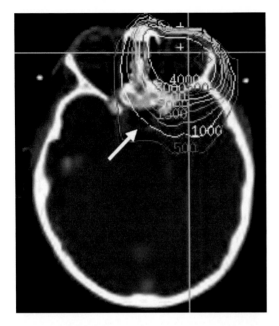

**Fig. 5.6** Dosimetry for a typical patient treated with conventional radiation therapy (40 Gy). This example illustrates that the HPA receives only a portion of the total dose given to the primary tumor (*arrow* indicates location of the pituitary)

These circumstances make it difficult to assign a dose to the HPA and to determine the risk for late effects. When the patient is seen by the endocrinologist years after treatment, retrospective dose calculations may be difficult to perform. Newer radiation techniques employ three-dimensional imaging (computed tomography and magnetic resonance, CT and MR) in the planning process. The HPA and other normal tissues can be contoured on CT or MR data and the dose to the HPA calculated and reported more accurately [33]. This information can be correlated with objective measures of endocrine effects and can be used to predict incidence of specific endocrine effects. Already this type of data has been modeled to predict peak GH secretion after radiation therapy [46] and may in the future be used to optimize RT for children (Fig. 5.7, Table 5.3).

In pediatric radiation oncology, reducing side effects of treatment is an important goal. Reducing side effects can be achieved by limiting CNS irradiation to those for whom indications are clear and

**a**

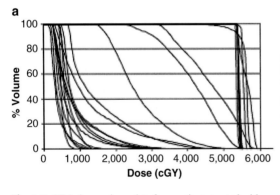

**b**

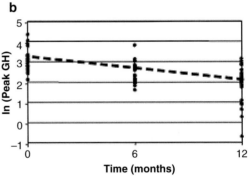

**Fig. 5.7** HPA dose-volume data from patients treated with conformal radiation therapy. (**a**) Dose-volume curves represent the percent-volume of the hypothalamus receiving a specific dose. (**b**) Correlation with change in peak GH (ATT/L-dopa) measured before, 6 and 12 months after radiation therapy results in an estimating equation that can be used to predict GH deficiency up to 12 months after irradiation based on the volume ($V$) received dose over specified intervals. $\ln$ [peak GH] $= 3.072 - (0.00058 \times V_{0-2,000\,cGy} + 0.00106 \times V_{2,000-4,000\,cGy} + 0.00156 \times V_{4,000-6,000\,cGy}) \times$ time

**Table 5.3** Probability of growth hormone deficiency according to hypothalamic radiation dose and according to time since irradiation

| Hypothalamic radiation dose | | | | | | | | | | |
|---|---|---|---|---|---|---|---|---|---|---|
| Time (Gy) | 15 | 20 | 25 | 30 | 35 | 40 | 45 | 50 | 55 | 60 |
| 12 months (%) | 17 | 19 | 22 | 25 | 28 | 31 | 34 | 38 | 42 | 45 |
| 36 months (%) | 26 | 37 | 48 | 59 | 70 | 79 | 86 | 91 | 95 | 97 |
| 60 months (%) | 39 | 57 | 75 | 87 | 95 | 98 | 99 | 100 | 100 | 100 |

Adapted from [46]

benefits outweigh the risks. CNS irradiation has been eliminated from treatment of the majority of children with leukemia and a significant proportion of children with low-grade glioma who may be cured with surgery. However, CNS irradiation will remain a mainstay in treatment of most children with brain tumors. Incidental irradiation of the CNS will continue to be observed in children with ocular tumors or tumors of the head and neck. Increased awareness of the importance of the hypothalamus in radiation-related neuroendocrine sequelae, and use of three-dimensional imaging in planning treatment of these tumors, may lead to a reduction in late endocrine effects. Reducing risk for complications can also be achieved by delaying radiation therapy until the child is older or until chemotherapy has had a chance to shrink the tumor and reduce the field of radiation [5, 70], reducing total dose and by reducing volume of irradiation. Dose reductions have been achieved for many tumors including retinoblastoma, pediatric soft tissue sarcomas of the head and neck, and certain CNS tumors including CNS germinoma. Volume reduction has been an important area of research in the treatment of medulloblastoma, ependymoma, low-grade astrocytoma, craniopharyngioma, and CNS germinoma [41, 45]. The risk of treating smaller volumes must be carefully balanced with objective gains documenting reductions in side effects in prospective clinical trials. To this end, the inclusion of endocrinology and its quantitative and relatively objective measures is essential. The risk of endocrine-related complications should be carefully considered in planning radiation therapy, but should not be used as a reason to avoid curative therapy. Careful follow-up and evaluation will lead to early intervention to mitigate consequences of irradiation.

## 5.3 Clinical Manifestations

### 5.3.1 GH Deficiency

Altered GH secretion leads to poor growth in childhood cancer survivors, particularly in young children after surgery in the suprasellar region, cranial irradiation [≥18 gray (Gy)], or total body irradiation (≥12 Gy). Hypothalamic function is affected more than is pituitary function. In most patients with GH deficiency, altered hypothalamic GHRH and somatostatin secretion lead to loss of the circadian pulsatile pattern of GH secretion. The radiation effect on GH secretion is dependent on fraction size and total hypothalamic dose-volume [46]. A large fraction size of radiation administered over a short period of time is more likely to cause GH deficiency than is the same total dose administered in smaller fractions over a longer period of time. The peak time for clinical identification of slowed growth consistent with GH deficiency is 3–5 years after such an insult, depending on RT dose. In one prospective study, all of the 21 children treated with a total dose of more than 45 Gy for optic pathway tumor experienced GH deficiency and significant slowing of growth rate within 2 years after irradiation [23]. At doses of cranial irradiation higher than 30 Gy (e.g., for suprasellar or posterior fossa tumor), the risk for GH deficiency may be more than 80 % by 10 years after RT [46]. Cranial irradiation doses greater than 24 Gy result in GH deficiency in as many as two thirds of patients who receive this treatment [13]. In many younger children, GH deficiency results from lower doses (>18 Gy). Doses of only 12–14 Gy of total body irradiation combined with chemotherapy and bone marrow transplantation also pose a significant risk for GH deficiency [13, 36, 37] (Table 5.3).

Growth rate is typically slow in children who are undergoing treatment for cancer and usually improves or shows catch-up after completion of cancer therapy (Fig. 5.8). Children whose growth rate does not improve or whose growth rate is less than the mean for age and gender should be evaluated for growth failure (Fig. 5.9). Causes of slow growth other than GH deficiency include hypothyroidism, radiation damage to growth centers of long bones or spine, chronic unresolved illness, poor nutrition, and depression. In individuals who have attained adult height, GH deficiency may be asymptomatic [24, 78], but alternatively may be associated with easy fatigability, decreased muscle with increased fat mass and truncal adiposity, and increased risk for cardiovascular disease [16, 25].

a

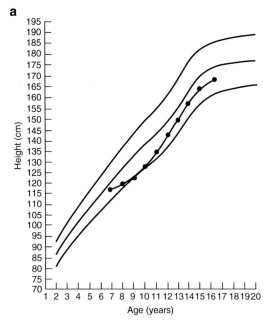

b

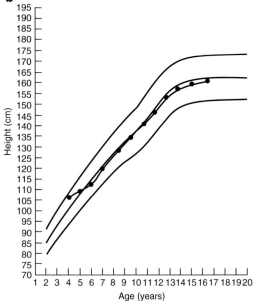

**Fig. 5.8** (**a**) Complete catch-up growth in a boy after cancer therapy. (**b**) Growth in a girl after cancer therapy, without catch-up growth. Normal percentiles (5th, 50th, and 95th) as shown are obtained from the National Center for Chronic Disease Prevention and Health Promotion (2000)

### 5.3.2    LH or FSH Deficiency

High doses of cranial radiation (≥30 Gy) are likely to cause hypothalamic GnRH deficiency and, therefore, gonadotropin deficiency (or in some patients, precocious onset of puberty through loss of inhibition that later progresses to gonadotropin deficiency through loss of GnRH secretory cells). Lower doses of cranial radiation (18–24 Gy) are more likely to cause damage to gamma-aminobutyric-acid-secreting neurons alone (leading to disinhibition and premature activation of GnRH neurons) and, therefore, rapid tempo of puberty or precocious puberty [3, 64]. In girls, the first signs of puberty are growth spurt and breast development (palpable breast buds or thelarche), followed by pubic hair growth and, after about 2 years, by menarche. In boys, the first sign of puberty is testicular enlargement (testes length >2.5 cm), followed by penile and pubic hair growth, followed by a growth spurt. In most studies of normal children, pubertal milestones are attained at ages that are normally distributed, with a standard deviation (SD) of approximately 1 year [76]. Children entering puberty more than 2 SDs earlier or later than average should be considered for endocrine evaluation. The average age that girls experience thelarche is 10 years and that of menarche is about 12 years; the average age when boys experience testicular growth is 11 years.

Patients with gonadotropin deficiency may have delayed, interrupted, or absent puberty. Staging of puberty is usually performed by the criteria of Tanner [76]. In survivors of childhood cancer, we initiate evaluation for delayed puberty in girls with no onset of breast development by 12 years of age or no menarche by 14 years of age and in boys with no sign of testicular growth by 13 years of age. Boys treated with agents that can cause infertility may have normal testosterone and LH concentrations, but reduced testicular volume and elevated FSH because of damage to the seminiferous tubules and reduced sperm production.

### 5.3.3    Precocious or Rapid Tempo of Puberty

Precocious puberty is defined as the onset of secondary sexual development before age

8 years in girls and before age 9 years in boys [9]. Despite controversy that puberty prior to these ages may occur in normal children [7, 69], younger occurrence of puberty than age 8 or 9 years may be the only clue to the presence of pathology and should not be ignored [48]. Pubic hair, acne, and body odor are not usually part of the presentation of precocious puberty in children younger than 4 years. Precocious puberty occurs in childhood cancer survivors who have lost inhibition of hypothalamic GnRH release as a result of tumor presence, raised intracranial pressure, cranial surgery, or low-dose cranial irradiation (18–24 Gy). Female gender and

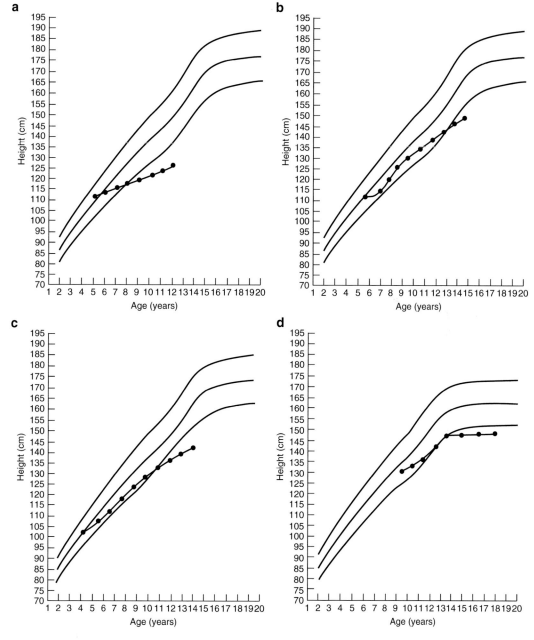

**Fig. 5.9** (**a**) Persistent growth failure in a boy after cancer therapy. (**b**) Later growth failure in a girl after recovery of normal growth. (**c**) Subtle persistent growth failure in a boy. (**d**) Growth in a girl with missed GH deficiency. (**e**) Growth in a boy with missed late onset GH deficiency. (**f**) Growth in a girl with central hypothyroidism

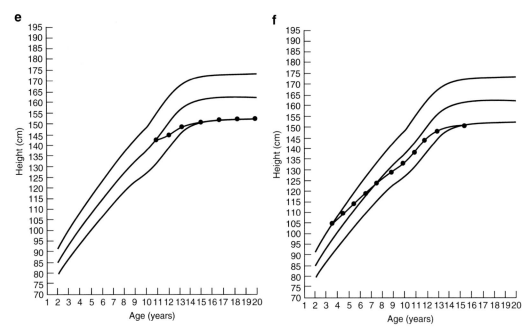

**Fig. 5.9** (continued)

younger age at the time of cancer treatment are risk factors for precocious puberty. In some children who have received cranial irradiation, puberty may start at a normal age and advance rapidly. Thus, tempo of progression as well as timing of onset must be monitored. Rapid tempo of puberty is also caused by loss of inhibition of hypothalamic GnRH secretion. The outcome of early onset and/or rapid tempo of puberty can be short adult height and potential emotional lability; early bony maturation causes the child to lose the opportunity for 1–3 years of height growth (Fig. 5.10).

### 5.3.4 Hypothyroidism

Central hypothyroidism refers to thyroid hormone deficiency caused by a disorder of the pituitary, hypothalamus, or hypothalamic-pituitary portal circulation. In contrast, primary hypothyroidism refers to under-function of the thyroid gland itself.

Primary hypothyroidism is the most common form of hypothyroidism in the general population and may occur in cancer survivors related both to family history and additional contribu-tion from the cancer therapy. In primary hypothyroidism, the thyroid gland may have been injured through irradiation or autoimmune activity, but the central hypothalamic-pituitary-thyroid axis is intact.

In contrast, central hypothyroidism is characterized by blunted or absent nocturnal TSH surge, suggesting the loss of normal circadian variation in TRH release [58]. Central hypothyroidism is difficult to diagnose because of its subtle clinical and laboratory presentation. It is particularly difficult to recognize in patients whose growth is complete, because slowed growth rate can no longer be used as a sign. Symptoms of central hypothyroidism (e.g., asthenia, edema, drowsiness, adynamia, skin dryness) may have a gradual onset and go unrecognized until thyroid replacement therapy is initiated and the patient feels better [22]. In addition to causing delayed puberty and slow growth (Fig. 5.9f), hypothyroidism may cause fatigue, dry skin, constipation, increased sleep requirement, and cold intolerance. Central hypothyroidism was found in as many as 65 % of the survivors of brain or nasopharyngeal tumors, 35 % of bone marrow transplant recipients, and 10–15 % of leukemia survivors [56, 59].

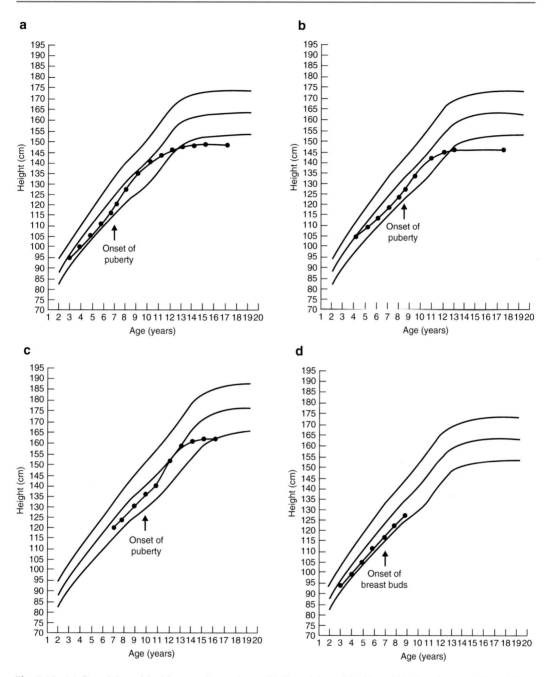

**Fig. 5.10** (**a**) Growth in a girl with precocious puberty. (**b**) Growth in a girl with rapid/early puberty. (**c**) Growth in a boy with rapid/early puberty. (**d**) Growth in a girl with GH deficiency hidden by precocious puberty (no growth spurt)

Secretory dysregulation of TSH after irradiation may precede other endocrine disorders. In one cohort of patients with central hypothyroidism, 34 % had dysregulation of TSH secretion before the development of GH deficiency [58, 59].

In cancer survivors, mixed hypothyroidism reflects separate injuries to the thyroid gland and the hypothalamus (e.g., radiation injury to both structures). TSH values are elevated, but in addition, the secretory dynamics of TSH are abnormal with a blunted or absent TSH surge [58, 59].

This is in contrast to primary hypothyroidism in which TSH is elevated and the TSH surge is normal. In a study of 208 childhood cancer survivors referred for evaluation of possible hypothyroidism or hypopituitarism, mixed hypothyroidism was present in 15 (7 %) [59]. All of the patients with mixed hypothyroidism had free T4 concentrations in the low normal range.

### 5.3.5   ACTH Deficiency

ACTH deficiency is less common than other neuroendocrine deficits but should be suspected in patients who have a history of brain tumor (regardless of therapy modality), cranial irradiation, GH deficiency, or central hypothyroidism [63]. Though uncommon, ACTH deficiency can occur in patients who have received intracranial radiation that did not exceed 24 Gy, but occurs in less than 3 % of patients after chemotherapy alone [62, 63].

Symptoms of central adrenal insufficiency can be subtle and include poor weight gain, anorexia, easy fatigability, and poor stamina. In patients who have ACTH deficiency, as opposed to primary adrenal insufficiency, symptoms of salt craving, electrolyte imbalance, vitiligo, and hyperpigmentation usually are not observed. More overt manifestations of complete ACTH deficiency include weight loss and shakiness that is relieved by eating (hypoglycemia). Signs of adrenal crisis at times of medical stress include weakness, abdominal pain, hypotension, and shock.

Patients with partial ACTH deficiency may have only subtle symptoms unless they become ill. Illness can disrupt these patients' usual homeostasis and cause a more severe, prolonged, or complicated course than expected. As in complete ACTH deficiency, incomplete or unrecognized ACTH deficiency can be life-threatening during concurrent illness. Death during sleep in hypopituitary patients has been proposed to be related to untreated ACTH deficiency [75].

### 5.3.6   Hyperprolactinemia

Hyperprolactinemia has been described in patients who have received doses of radiation larger than 50 Gy to the hypothalamus or surgery disrupting the integrity of the pituitary stalk. Hyperprolactinemia may result in delayed puberty. In adult women, hyperprolactinemia may cause galactorrhea, menstrual irregularities, loss of libido, hot flashes, infertility, and osteopenia; in adult men, impotence and loss of libido. Primary hypothyroidism may lead to hyperprolactinemia as a result of hyperplasia of thyrotrophs and lactotrophs, presumably due to TRH hypersecretion.

### 5.3.7   Diabetes Insipidus

Diabetes insipidus may be caused by histiocytosis, germinomas, surgical trauma, or CNS-involved leukemia. Patients with diabetes insipidus usually present with obvious symptoms of excessive thirst and urination with nocturia or enuresis. However, the diabetes insipidus may not be recognized until the patient has dehydration during an intercurrent illness. The urine remains clear in color throughout the day. In patients with CNS-involved leukemia, severe hypernatremic dehydration can occur if the CNS lesion also affects the centers for thirst regulation.

### 5.3.8   Osteopenia

Osteopenia may result from HPA abnormality (GH deficiency, hypothyroidism, hypogonadism, or hyperprolactinemia) in association with direct effects of glucocorticoid therapy, methotrexate, inactivity, and dietary changes. Osteopenia may present with fractures or may be asymptomatic. Among 141 survivors of childhood leukemia in one study, 30 (21 %) had abnormally low bone mineral density (BMD >1.645 SD below the mean of normal population). Risk factors for bone mineral decrements include male gender, Caucasian race, and cranial irradiation. BMD was inversely correlated with the cumulative dose of cranial irradiation or antimetabolites [31].

### 5.3.9   Hypothalamic Obesity

Hypothalamic damage from a tumor or cancer treatment can also result in hypothalamic obesity – unrelenting appetite or weight gain that does not respond to caloric restriction or exercise – attributable to ventromedial hypothalamus damage and abnormality in leptin, ghrelin, and insulin feedback [5, 30]. In rodents, hypothalamic obesity can be suppressed by pancreatic vagotomy to prevent insulin hypersecretion. Insulin hypersecretion is one of the major mechanisms for the development of hypothalamic obesity [5]. In a study of 148 survivors of childhood brain tumors, the risk factors for hypothalamic obesity included age at diagnosis of cancer (<6 years), tumor location (hypothalamic or thalamic), tumor histology (craniopharyngioma, germinoma, optic glioma, prolactinoma, or hypothalamic astrocytoma), hypothalamic irradiation (>51 Gy), and presence of endocrinopathy (deficiency of GH, sex hormones, ACTH, or vasopressin) [5, 38]. No effects were noted on body mass index from ventriculoperitoneal shunting, steroid use (<6 months), or chemotherapy. Thus, hypothalamic damage, due to tumor, surgery, or RT, is the primary risk factor for development of obesity in this patient population (IRHOD.com registry).

## 5.4 Detection and Screening

### 5.4.1 Signs and Symptoms Prompting Immediate Evaluation

Survivors of childhood cancer with any of the following ten symptoms should be referred for the evaluation of neuroendocrinopathy: (1) slow growth rate or failure to show catch-up growth, (2) failure to thrive, (3) excessive obesity not thought to be related to steroid therapy, (4) persistent fatigue or anorexia, (5) polydipsia and polyuria, (6) severely dry skin or thin and brittle hair, (7) altered timing of onset of puberty (e.g., signs of puberty before age 9 years or in patients with short height, failure to enter puberty by age 12 years in girls and by 13 years in boys), (8) abnormal tempo of puberty (e.g., rapid or interrupted progression of puberty), (9) galactorrhea, and (10) abnormal menstruation or sexual function.

### 5.4.2 Surveillance of Asymptomatic Patients

*Asymptomatic* patients who are at risk for neuroendocrinopathy (Table 5.2) should undergo the following routine yearly surveillance:

- Accurate measurements of height and arm span (an alternative estimate of height, useful if the patient received total body or spinal irradiation or has scoliosis or kyphosis, factors that lead to reduced spinal bone growth or measurement)
- Accurate measurement of weight and assessment of body mass index
- Assessment of nutritional status, adequacy of dietary calcium and vitamin D intake
- Ascertainment of Tanner stage, testicular volume (as measured by Prader orchidometry) or breast development, and interpretation of whether the pubertal status and tempo of progression are appropriate for age and height
- Review of organ systems
- Measurement of serum concentrations of free T4 and TSH
- Low-dose ACTH test if there was tumor in the region of the HPA or cranial irradiation >25 Gy

### 5.4.3 GH Deficiency

GH deficiency (GHD) should be considered in children who have a slow growth rate and a medical history putting them at risk for GHD [26, 81]. Evaluations should include bone maturation, as determined by radiographic analysis of the left hand and wrist and IGF-I and IGFBP3. The combination of previous cranial or total body irradiation, slow growth rate, normal weight gain, no intercurrent illness, delayed bone maturation, and low plasma levels of IGF-I and IGFBP3 (lower than 1 SD below the mean for the child's age group) are highly suggestive of GHD. The diagnosis should be confirmed by GH stimulation testing [39, 61]. Evaluation of the nocturnal profile of GH secretion is rarely necessary to make the diagnosis, but may be abnormal in symptomatic children after cranial irradiation who have normal stimulated GH results [17].

Recognition of GHD in adults is more difficult, because slow growth rate is not available in them as a marker. Recognition depends on clinical suspicion related to medical history. Diagnosis of GHD in adults requires evidence of other hypothalamic-pituitary hormone deficiencies and a low peak response to GH stimulation tests [24].

### 5.4.4 LH or FSH Deficiency

During the range of ages when puberty is normally expected to occur, breast development, pubic hair growth and distribution, and vaginal estrogenization should be monitored every 6 months in girls at risk of having LH or FSH deficiencies. Similarly, testes size, pubic hair growth and distribution, and phallus length should be monitored every 6 months in boys. Testicular size in some boys may be small for their genital maturation because of RT- or chemotherapy-induced damage to the seminiferous tubules.

Measurement of bone age, serum LH, FSH, and sex steroid (testosterone or estradiol) should be performed in children with delayed or interrupted progression of puberty. Markers such as inhibin B and anti-Mullerian hormone (AMH) that examine gonadal preservation and fertility are currently under investigation. Data are promising in adults for using inhibin B and AMH in evaluating gonadal health, but their utility in pediatric clinical medicine is still largely unknown.

Evaluation by an endocrinologist should be prompted by the absence of progression of puberty by 1 year after completion of cancer therapy in girls >13 years of age or in boys >14 years of age. Stimulation testing with synthetic GnRH provides more information than does a single, randomly drawn level of LH and FSH. An alternative to a GnRH stimulation test may be a serum sample for LH, FSH, and testosterone or estradiol drawn between 4 and 8 AM, at the time shortly after nighttime pulses of LH have been occurring (Fig. 5.2a).

### 5.4.5 Precocious Puberty

Precocious puberty is diagnosed if the onset of sexual development is before age 8 years in girls or before age 9 years in boys. A radiograph of the left hand and wrist shows bone age that is advanced compared to chronologic age. However, bone age may be consistent with chronologic age or even delayed in a child who has concurrent GHD or hypothyroidism and who has not undergone a growth spurt (Fig. 5.10d). Since concurrent GHD may not be discovered until after successful treatment of precocious puberty (Fig. 5.10d), we routinely perform provocative GH testing in patients with precocious puberty who have a history of cancer.

### 5.4.6 Hypothyroidism

Yearly measurements of TSH and free T4 should be done in all patients who have received irradiation (cranial, craniospinal, mantle, or total body irradiation), because the symptoms of central hypothyroidism are often subtle and TSH secretory dysregulation after irradiation may precede other endocrine disorders [59]. The diagnosis of hypothyroidism may be delayed in as many as one third of patients, if TSH secretion is not tested until GHD becomes apparent. Such a delay may be acceptable in a minimally symptomatic adult. In children, however, the potential functional implications of hypothyroidism and lost growth opportunity require early intervention [55]. Early diagnosis of mild hypothyroidism permits early intervention to improve growth velocity and quality of life.

Free T4 and serum TSH are the best screening tests for thyroid status. Sex steroids raise thyroid binding in females and lower thyroid binding in males; however, free T4 tends to remain stable throughout life. In primary hypothyroidism, TSH may rise above 3 mU/L before changes in free T4 are observed. Free T4 below the normal range without TSH elevation is strongly suggestive of central hypothyroidism. However, some patients with central hypothyroidism may have free T4 concentrations in the lowest third of the normal range [55, 59]. The first laboratory evidence of central hypothyroidism may be a small decline in free T4. Central hypothyroidism was often present when the free T4 was in the lowest third of the normal range and TSH was not elevated and could be confirmed by measurement of the nocturnal TSH surge (hourly TSH at 1500–1800 h and at 2200–0200 h). However, the TSH surge test requires serial sampling and an inpatient hospital admission [58, 59].

Outpatient screening can be accomplished using measurement of TSH at 0800 h (AM) and in the afternoon (PM; between 12 noon and 1800 h) and calculating the ratio. An AM to PM ratio less than 1.3 is consistent with central hypothyroidism [58]. Suppressed TSH on a modest dose of levothyroxine also confirms central hypothyroidism.

If further testing confirms hypothyroidism, treatment should be initiated even though free T4 is still within the normal range because the FT4 is likely to be below the individual's optimal set point.

### 5.4.7 ACTH Deficiency

For patients at risk for ACTH deficiency (e.g., those who received ≥25 Gy irradiation to HPA), surveillance should include yearly measurement of plasma cortisol concentration at 0800 h and/or a low-dose ACTH test [32]. If cortisol level is below 18 µg/dL (497 nmol/L) at 0800 h, then further evaluation should be directed by an endocrinologist. Measurement of the basal plasma ACTH concentration usually can distinguish primary adrenal disease from central adrenal insufficiency if the ACTH assay is reliable and if there is no urgency in establishing the cause of adrenal insufficiency. Patients with primary adrenal insufficiency have a high concentration of plasma ACTH at 0800 h (as high or higher than 4,000 pg/mL or 880 pmol/L). In contrast, plasma ACTH concentrations are low or low normal in patients with secondary or tertiary adrenal insufficiency. The normal value at 0800 h is usually 20–80 pg/mL (4.5–18 pmol/L).

Patients who present in hypotensive crisis may have adrenal insufficiency or one of several other possible diagnoses. Primary adrenal insufficiency, if present, may have been caused by infection, hemorrhagic diathesis, or metastatic disease to the adrenal gland that requires prompt diagnosis and treatment. In these patients, measurement of basal serum cortisol followed by the low-dose ACTH stimulation test (see below) provides the most rapid and reliable diagnosis. A basal plasma ACTH measurement can be ordered at the same time, but diagnosis and treatment must proceed immediately without waiting for the ACTH and cortisol results.

Patients with partial ACTH deficiency or recent onset of complete ACTH deficiency may have a normal serum cortisol response to high dose of ACTH (250 µg/m² by intravenous infusion over 1 min [60] with cortisol measured 1 h later, normally greater than 20 µg/dL (552 nmol/L)). Thus, ACTH deficiency may not be detected by this test.

As a result, the low-dose ACTH test is the most sensitive test for partial ACTH deficiency [32]. In this test, a more physiologic dose of ACTH (1 µg/m²) is administered by intravenous infusion over 1 min, and blood for a serum cortisol assay is drawn 20 min after the infusion. Peak serum cortisol higher than 20 µg/dL (552 nmol/L) is considered normal, and peak serum cortisol lower than 18 µg/dL (497 nmol/L) is considered low. Patients with cortisol peaks between these values have indeterminate results; these patients should be treated with glucocorticoids when they are ill and will require further evaluation [63]. Further evaluation can include a second low-dose ACTH test or metyrapone administration 2 months to 1 year later.

The low-dose test has supplanted insulin-induced hypoglycemia in many clinical practices. The results are similar to those obtained with insulin-induced hypoglycemia; in addition, ACTH tests can be performed without a physician being present and are less expensive.

### 5.4.8 Hyperprolactinemia

Hyperprolactinemia is diagnosed when the serum level of PRL is elevated. The PRL level should be periodically measured in patients with symptoms outlined above (Sect. 1.2.6) and in those who received more than 50 Gy of irradiation to the hypothalamus. The definitive PRL level should not be drawn in the hour or two after breast examination or nipple stimulation.

### 5.4.9 Diabetes Insipidus

Urine specific gravity of patients with diabetes insipidus is usually lower than 1.010 (<300 mOsm/L), unless the patient is severely dehydrated. In most of these patients, serum osmolarity is slightly increased (>300 mOsm/L), the serum sodium may be increased or high normal, and the plasma concentration of antidiuretic hormone is inappropriately low for the osmolarity. However, patients with an intact thirst mechanism may be able to drink sufficiently to avoid laboratory abnormality. Symptoms of polydipsia, polyuria, and nocturia or enuresis may be the only evidence of diabetes insipidus. In partial diabetes insipidus, a water deprivation test may be needed to establish the diagnosis and to rule out other causes of polyuria.

### 5.4.10 Osteopenia

Osteopenia in cancer survivors may be unrecognized in the absence of fractures unless evaluation is performed. Yearly screening of 25-hydroxyvitamin D may identify dietary vitamin D deficiency, one of the contributors to osteopenia. Identification of low bone mineral requires performance of a dual-energy x-ray absorptiometry (DXA) which offers precise estimates of bone mineral area density (mg/cm$^2$) at multiple sites for the least amount of radiation exposure. DXA results may require adjustment for height age in a short patient [83]. Quantitative computerized tomography measures true volumetric density (mg/cm$^3$) of trabecular or cortical bone at any skeletal site of choice. T- and Z-scores may be calculated in reference to normal young adults (age of peak bone mass, 20–35 years) and age-matched normal individuals of the same gender, respectively. T-score should not be used in children or adolescents. Results of DXA must be adjusted for patient height and age.

### 5.4.11 Hypothalamic Obesity

Clinical symptoms are the basis for diagnosis of hypothalamic obesity. These include rapid weight gain (Fig. 5.11a), voracious appetite, and aggressive food seeking. Patients may have rapid weight gain for other reasons (Fig. 5.11b): exogenous steroid use, inactivity, overfeeding, sympathy of relatives, high thirst, and drinking of sugared drinks. Obesity in adults is defined as having a body mass index (BMI) of ≥30 [BMI = weight (kg)/height (m$^2$)] (http://www.cdc.gov/obesity/adult/defining.html). Overweight in children is defined as having BMI ≥85th percentile, and obesity defined as BMI ≥95th percentile (http://www.cdc.gov/obesity/childhood/basics.html). Evaluation of overweight patients includes blood pressure measurement, fasting lipid profile, fasting glucose and insulin level, and oral glucose tolerance testing with insulin levels (OGTT). In general, fasting glucose is normal and fasting insulin is elevated in patients with hypothalamic obesity. They have high postprandial insulin level as well as early and rapid and excessive insulin excursions to OGTT. However, these results may be seen in any person who becomes obese.

## 5.5 Management of Established Problems

### 5.5.1 GH Deficiency

Growth hormone evaluation usually begins after the first year of treatment completion. Screening labs can help in the diagnosis of growth hormone deficiency, but following a patient's height velocity gives the best insight. There are specific standards for making the diagnosis of growth hormone deficiency. Each varies with age and pubertal status [15, 49].

Standard therapy for GHD is synthetic recombinant human GH (Fig. 5.12a, b). Any patient identified with GHD should be evaluated for possible ACTH deficiency and for central hypothyroidism. If ACTH is deficient, adequate cortisol therapy should be started before GH or thyroid therapy. Patients with GHD who have partial or total ACTH deficiency and are receiving suboptimal hydrocortisone replacement may be at risk of developing symptoms of cortisol deficiency when GH therapy is initiated. This is because of

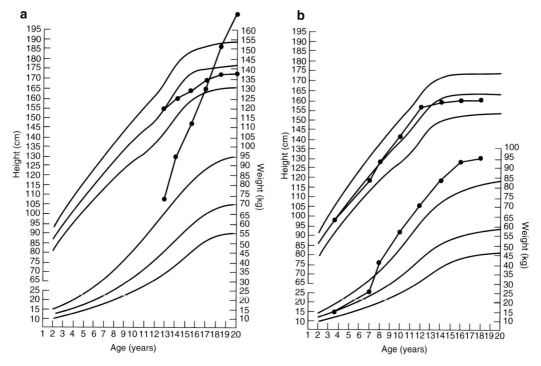

**Fig. 5.11** (**a**) Hypothalamic obesity and GH deficiency in a boy. (**b**) Exogenous obesity in a girl

the inhibitory effect of GH on 11β-hydroxysteroid dehydrogenase type 1, the enzyme that converts cortisone to cortisol [77].

GH treatment is not recommended during the first year after cancer treatment as this is a time of increased recurrence rates for many tumors. If the history is positive for an aggressive tumor, observation for a longer duration is indicated prior to considering GH therapy, up to 2–3 years after tumor treatment [20, 28, 40].

The endocrinologist and oncologist should discuss and agree upon the decision regarding timing of initiation of GH therapy. The usual dose of GH in children is 0.15–0.3 mg/kg per week divided into daily doses and administered subcutaneously in the evening [15]. IGF-I titration is a method of adjusting GH dosing that allows for strict control of statural growth while reducing the risk for possible side effects associated with overtreatment. In patients with a tumor history, maintaining an IGF-I level between the 20th and 80th percentile for age is recommended. This range of GH dosing should support normal growth velocity (not catch-up growth) in patients who could potentially have adverse effects from

even mild overtreatment. Lower doses are used in adults [78].

Each injection of GH produces a pharmacologic level of GH for approximately 12 h. The growth rate in children receiving ongoing GH therapy typically increases to above normal for 1–3 years and then slows to normal velocity. After 4–5 years of GH therapy, the adult height SD scores of leukemia survivors with GHD usually approached the height SD scores at the time of tumor diagnosis [37]. The growth response may be poorer in patients who have received total body or spinal irradiation or in patients with particular diseases such as neuroblastoma [29, 53].

During GH therapy, evaluation of the growth response and adjustment of GH dose should occur every 4–6 months and include measurement of height, weight, and arm span. Arm span is a surrogate measure of height, particularly in patients in whom height measurement may not fully reflect body growth (e.g., those with scoliosis or a history of spinal irradiation). GH dose can be increased as weight gain occurs to maintain a stable dose per kilogram of body weight. Serum IGF-I measurements are recommended every

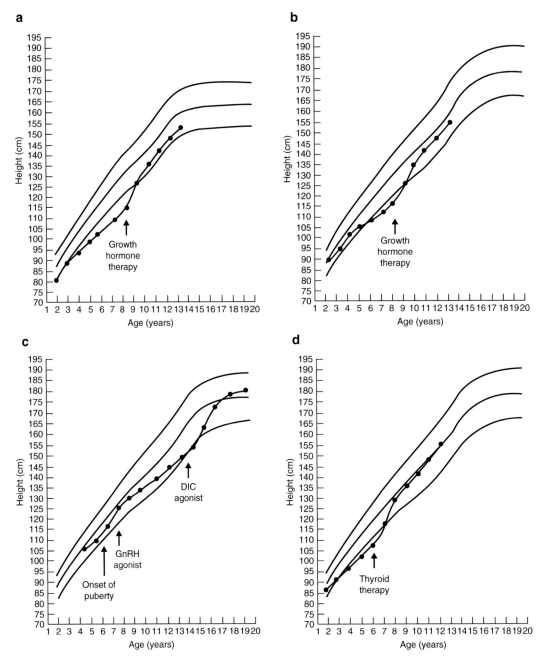

**Fig. 5.12** (**a**) Response to GH therapy in a girl with GH deficiency. (**b**) Response to GH therapy in a boy with GH deficiency. (**c**) Response to GnRH agonist in a boy with precocious puberty. (**d**) Response to thyroid hormone in a boy with central hypothyroidism

4–6 months in the growing years and a minimum of yearly once an adult height has been reached [26]. After the first 1–2 years of GH therapy, if the level of IGF-I surpasses the upper limits of nor- mal for the patient's age and gender, the GH dose should be decreased to achieve an IGF-I near the mean for age and gender. Evaluation of pubertal stage and screening for development of additional endocrinopathies (thyroid, gonadotropins, ACTH) should continue to be performed at least annually. Even with GH therapy, some childhood cancer survivors do not grow as well as expected, a finding that suggests that other factors, such as thyroid hormone deficiency, are present.

GH treatment in children is usually safe [11, 15, 66, 81]. Adverse effects are rare, occur soon after therapy is initiated, and include pancreatitis, benign intracranial hypertension (pseudotumor cerebri), slipped capital femoral epiphysis [50], and carpal tunnel syndrome [8]. Pseudotumor cerebri and carpal tunnel syndrome are probably caused by sodium and water retention. An increase in the growth and pigmentation of nevi also has been described [10]. GH therapy does not increase the risk of brain tumor or leukemia recurrence [4, 20, 37, 74]. GH therapy also did not appear to increase the risk of secondary leukemia or solid malignancy in patients who did not received RT in the Childhood Cancer Survivor Study [20]. Because all of the evaluable patients who developed a second neoplasm in this study had received RT, synergistic effects of GH and irradiation on the development of second malignancy could not be discerned [20]. The absolute number of excess solid tumors attributable to GH (including benign meningiomas), if any, will probably be very small (<4/1,000 person years at 15 years after diagnosis).

### 5.5.2 LH or FSH Deficiency

The use of estrogen or testosterone therapy should not be initiated without careful attention to the pediatric survivor's growth pattern. Replacement of pubertal hormones in a short or slowly growing adolescent can cause fusion of bony growth centers and shorter-than-expected adult height. Such therapy should be provided only in coordination with the pediatric endocrinologist after assessment of growth potential and treatment of GH or thyroid deficiencies. Initiation of sex steroid therapy in a short adolescent may be delayed until age 15 years to permit response to GH or thyroid hormone therapy and taller adult height. In short adolescents with delayed

puberty, a few years of therapy with low-dose sex steroid therapy is preferable to full replacement. Such doses simulate the sex steroid levels observed in the first year or so of puberty and are less likely than full sex steroid replacement to cause inappropriate maturation of bone age. Girls can be treated with the conjugated estrogen tablets Premarin® (0.3 mg every other day), ethinyl estradiol (5 mcg daily, one quarter of a 20-mcg tablet daily), or half of a low-dose estrogen patch changed half as often as in adults [79]. Menstrual spotting can be treated monthly or 3-monthly with medroxyprogesterone 10 mg per day for 10 days without a break in estrogen therapy. Boys can be treated with 45- or 50-mg/m$^2$ testosterone cypionate injected intramuscularly once each month or with topical testosterone gel 0.5–1.25 g daily. After achievement of height acceptable to the patient, both boys and girls may benefit from a gradual increase in hormone replacement therapy to the full replacement dose, if there has been no sex steroid production in recent months. The increase to full replacement should take place in 1- to 3-month steps to permit gradual adjustment to the hormonal effects.

Full hormone replacement in adolescent girls who have reached their adult height is easily achieved with regular use of a standard oral contraceptive (28-day or 3-month pill packet) or estrogen patch (used especially if the girl is on GH therapy). Boys who have attained their adult height can be treated with testosterone (200 mg injected intramuscularly every 2 weeks) or with androgen by patch or by topical gel (about 5 g daily).

One medical risk of delayed puberty is delayed bone mineralization. Adolescents with delayed or interrupted puberty should receive 1,500 mg of elemental calcium and 1,000 IU of vitamin D per day to improve bone mineralization.

### 5.5.3 Precocious Puberty

GnRH analogues are the most effective treatments for precocious puberty, rapid tempo puberty, or normally timed puberty that is inappropriate for height. GnRH analogues suppress

LH and FSH release from the pituitary gland through the provision of a steady rather than a pulsatile level of GnRH; the pituitary gland stops responding to GnRH when GnRH concentrations are steady or unchanging. The use of GnRH analogues to delay pubertal progression optimizes adult height potential by permitting the child to grow taller without experiencing a rapid change in bone maturation [47] (Fig. 5.12c).

Treatment with GnRH analogues should be prescribed and monitored by a pediatric endocrinologist [82]. GnRH analogues can be administered as a daily subcutaneous injection. More commonly, a sustained or depot preparation is used – monthly, every 3 months, every 6 months, or as a yearly subcutaneous implant [35, 52, 54]. GnRH analogue therapy is usually continued at least until patients attain the third percentile for adult height: 152 cm (60 in.) in girls and 162 cm (64 in.) in boys.

### 5.5.4   Hypothyroidism

Standard treatment for central hypothyroidism or for primary hypothyroidism is levothyroxine replacement therapy (Fig. 5.12d). Thyroid hormone replacement can precipitate clinical decompensation in patients with unrecognized adrenal insufficiency, because levothyroxine treatment increases metabolic clearance of cortisol. Thus, it is necessary to evaluate patients for adrenal insufficiency and, if present, treat with hydrocortisone before initiating thyroid hormone therapy. In patients who also have ACTH deficiency, we usually initiate cortisol replacement 3 days before beginning thyroid hormone therapy.

The typical thyroid hormone replacement dose for infants under 3 years of age is levothyroxine 5–10 mcg/kg/day, and for healthy children and adolescents with TSH less than 30 mU/L is 3 mcg/kg by mouth every morning. Children over 3 years of age who have TSH greater than 30 mU/L, or about whom there are concerns about medical stability, can begin levothyroxine at a low dose (0.75 mcg/kg by mouth every morning for a month) and have it further increased by 0.75 mcg/kg per day each month to permit more

gradual physiologic and psychologic adjustment to the new metabolic state. Thyroid hormone concentrations should be measured after 4 weeks of therapy or 4 weeks after any dose change, because levothyroxine has a long half-life (5–6 days).

Unlike primary hypothyroidism, it is not useful to monitor TSH in patients with central hypothyroidism. In one prospective study of 37 patients with central hypothyroidism, free T4 and free T3 were monitored during therapy, and dose was adjusted to achieve free T4 in the midnormal range without free T3 elevation and without symptoms of hypothyroidism or hyperthyroidism [22]. We usually adjust thyroid hormone replacement therapy in patients with central hypothyroidism to maintain the level of free T4 just above the middle of the normal range (e.g., free T4 of 1.4–1.6 ng/dL if the normal range is 0.78–1.85 ng/dL or free T4 of 2.2–2.4 if the normal range is 1.0–2.8 ng/dL).

### 5.5.5   ACTH Deficiency

Patients with ACTH insufficiency require daily hydrocortisone replacement. Hydrocortisone is the preferred glucocorticoid for replacement in children, because it is least likely to impair growth. Patients with ACTH deficiency do not need mineralocorticoid replacement, because these hormones are produced by the adrenal gland under the influence of the renin-aldosterone system rather than under the influence of ACTH. Dexamethasone is not standard for glucocorticoid replacement therapy in children and adolescents because it has greater potential to suppress growth than does hydrocortisone.

The dose of hydrocortisone for replacement therapy is 7–10 mg/m$^2$ per day, divided into two or three doses administered by mouth. For example, a child whose body surface is 0.9 m$^2$ could receive 2.5 mg three times per day, or an adult whose body surface is 1.5 m$^2$ could receive 5 mg at breakfast and at 1500 h plus 2.5 mg at bedtime. The glucocorticoid dose may need to be increased in patients taking drugs that accelerate hepatic steroid metabolism such as phenytoin, barbiturates, newer anticonvulsants, rifampin, mitotane, and aminoglutethimide [19]. Patients with GHD who have partial or total ACTH deficiency and are receiving suboptimal cortisol or cortisone replacement may be at risk of developing symptoms of cortisol deficiency when GH therapy is initiated. This is because of the inhibitory effect of GH on 11β-hydroxysteroid dehydrogenase type 1. Similarly, the initiation of thyroid hormone therapy in a child with unrecognized or undertreated ACTH deficiency also can precipitate adrenal crisis.

Patients with ACTH deficiency must receive "stress dosing": additional glucocorticoid during times of illness or stress (e.g., fever, gastrointestinal illness, injury). The dose of additional hydrocortisone necessary during times of illness is 30 mg/m² per day divided into doses every 8 h administered by mouth. Patients whose illness or injury is severe enough to require emergency care or hospitalization, who are unable to retain oral medication, or who require anesthesia or surgery should urgently receive hydrocortisone (50–100 mg/m² intramuscularly or intravenously), followed by hydrocortisone (10–25 mg/m² intravenously every 6 h) during management of the critical illness [63]. At stress doses, hydrocortisone provides some mineralocorticoid effect. The hydrocortisone dose should be reduced to the usual replacement therapy dose as soon as the event is over or the patient's medical status improves. Tapering of the dose is not necessary if the pharmacologic stress doses are used for less than 10 days.

Patient and family education is an important component of treating patients with ACTH deficiency. The patient and responsible family members should be instructed about the following issues:

- The nature of the hormonal deficit and the rationale for replacement therapy
- Maintenance medications and the need for changes in medications during minor illnesses
- When to consult a physician
- The need to keep an emergency supply of glucocorticoids

- The proper *stress* dose for the patient's body weight
- When and how to inject glucocorticoids for emergencies

Every patient should have at least two pre-prepared syringes of hydrocortisone (Solu-Cortef®): one at home and one at work or school. In addition, it is wise for the patient to carry such a syringe at all times. The syringes can be obtained as 100-mg/2-mL vials ("Activial") or can be prepared by a pharmacist in regular 1-mL syringes from a multidose vial. The patient and parents must be instructed regarding the correct dose. The injectable stress dose is five to ten times the daily hydrocortisone dose. Thus, typical doses for children would be 50 mg (0.5 mL of a 100-mg/2-mL solution). Unused syringes should be replaced each year or if the solution inside becomes cloudy or colored.

The patient and one or more responsible family or household members should be instructed to inject the contents of a syringe subcutaneously or intramuscularly anywhere on the patient's body during any one of the following circumstances:

- The patient has a major injury with substantial blood loss (more than one cup), fracture, or neurogenic shock.
- The patient has nausea and vomiting and cannot retain oral medications.
- The patient has symptoms of acute adrenal insufficiency, such as hypotension or hypoglycemia.
- The patient is found unresponsive.

Instructions should include the need to obtain medical help immediately after the injection of the stress dose. The patient should be instructed to have a low threshold for injecting the hydrocortisone: if the patient feels the injection *might* be necessary, then it *should* be injected, and medical attention should be sought. It is unlikely, however, that a patient will need the stress dose of hydrocortisone more than two or three times per year, and most patients go for years without needing it. Used hydrocortisone syringes should be replaced immediately.

Every patient should wear a medical alert (MedicAlert®) bracelet or necklace and carry the emergency medical information card that is supplied with it. Both should indicate the diagnosis, the daily medications and doses, and the physician to call in the event of an emergency. Patients can enroll in MedicAlert by calling 800-432-5372 or through the internet at www.medicalert.org (USA) or www.medicalert.ca (Canada).

### 5.5.6 Hyperprolactinemia

Prolactin elevation in excess of 100 ng/mL may lead to symptoms. Dopamine agonists such as bromocriptine and cabergoline are the treatment of choice to suppress PRL secretion and to restore normal gonadal function. Cabergoline is, in general, more potent, much longer acting, and better tolerated than bromocriptine. The usual starting dose is 0.25 mg twice a week. High doses such as those used in Parkinson disease have been associated with cardiac valvular problems [2]. However, typical doses used for hyperprolactinemia have not demonstrated such risks [73].

### 5.5.7 Diabetes Insipidus

Hormone replacement in diabetes insipidus is desmopressin acetate or DDAVP®, which can be given by subcutaneous injection, by nasal insufflation, or orally in one or two daily doses. Oral desmopressin is available in tablets containing 0.1 or 0.2 mg. To avoid water intoxication, successive doses should not be given until a brief diuresis has occurred at least once daily. By giving a dose at bedtime, sleep disturbance by nocturia can be avoided. The usual dose of 1.0–5.0 μg intranasally, or 0.1–0.8 mg orally, will usually achieve rapid urinary concentration that lasts approximately 8–24 h (Fig. 5.13). The process of starting desmopressin therapy may require close monitoring of volume of fluid taken in and urine output. Several weeks of dose adjustment may be required before achieving a stable dose (Fig. 5.13). In patients with partial diabetes insipidus, chlorpropamide may be used to enhance the effect of the limited antidiuretic hormone that remains.

### 5.5.8 Osteopenia

Osteopenia after cancer therapy may be prevented by maintaining optimal calcium (1,500 mg daily) and vitamin D (1,000 units daily) in the diet. Nutritional supplements may be needed in cases of osteopenia unresponsive to behavioral and dietary management. In addition, early diagnosis and replacement of hormone deficiencies will benefit bone mineralization. In the event of fractures, bisphosphonate therapy (oral or intravenous) may be beneficial.

### 5.5.9 Hypothalamic Obesity

Part of the therapy for hypothalamic obesity involves early identification and initiation of preventive measures including caloric and dietary control and maintenance of regular exercise. In addition to maintaining these lifestyle choices, several therapies have been used pragmatically or in research efforts. These include dexedrine, ritalin, metformin, and octreotide [6, 21]. Dexedrine and ritalin are taken orally and act as stimulants with the side effect of appetite suppression (in this situation, beneficial). Metformin is taken orally once or twice daily, acts as a sensitizer to insulin effects, and may serve to probe the etiology of obesity in individual patient. If the obesity is exogenous and hyperinsulinemia is a consequence of the obesity and insulin resistance, lifestyle changes with or without metformin may resolve obesity. If the obesity is hypothalamic and the hyperinsulinism is the cause of the increased appetite, metformin use may lead to hypoglycemia and no reduction of striving for food. Octreotide is a somatostatin analogue that binds to the somatostatin receptor. It serves to decrease not only insulin secretion from pancreatic β-cells, but also growth hormone and TSH secretion from the pituitary gland. If the obesity is exogenous and high insulin levels reflect insulin resistance,

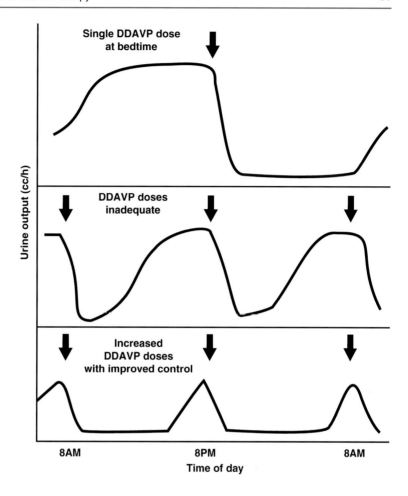

**Fig. 5.13** Urine output with inadequate DDAVP treatment (*top* and *middle panels*) and improved control of urine output with adjusted DDAVP dosing (*bottom panel*)

the patient may become diabetic with octreotide therapy. If the obesity is hypothalamic, octreotide will decrease insulin secretion leading to reduced appetite, weight control, and improved sense of well-being [5, 38]. Octreotide is taken as two or three injections daily. Side effects of octreotide may include gallstones. Patients treated with octreotide may also require therapy with growth hormone and thyroid hormone.

Bariatric surgery has been reported to be beneficial in selected patients [30, 65, 80]. Additional research is needed in order to identify optimal treatment modalities in order to control weight in hypothalamic obesity. An international internet registry (IRHOD.com) has been developed for patients to self-register, in order to be considered for participation in research projects. Investigators can also register on this site to apply for research access to the database.

## References

1. Agha A, Sherlock M, Brennan S et al (2005) Hypothalamic-pituitary dysfunction after irradiation of nonpituitary brain tumors in adults. J Clin Endocrinol Metab 90:6355–6360
2. Antonini A, Poewe W (2007) Fibrotic heart-valve reactions to dopamine-agonist treatment in Parkinson's disease. Lancet Neurol 6:826–829
3. Armstrong GT, Chow EJ, Sklar CA (2009) Alterations in pubertal timing following therapy for childhood malignancies. Endocr Dev 15:25–39
4. Bell J, Parker KL, Swinford RD et al (2010) Long-term safety of recombinant human growth hormone in children. J Clin Endocrinol Metab 95:167–177
5. Bereket A, Kiess W, Lustig RH et al (2012) Hypothalamic obesity in children. Obes Rev. doi:10.1111/j.1467-789X.2012.01004.x
6. Bingham NC, Rose SR, Inge TH (2012) Bariatric surgery in hypothalamic obesity. Front Endocrinol (Lausanne) 3:23
7. Biro FM, Galvez MP, Greenspan LC et al (2010) Pubertal assessment method and baseline characteristics

in a mixed longitudinal study of girls. Pediatrics 126:e583–e950

8. Blethen SL, Allen DB, Graves D et al (1996) Safety of recombinant deoxyribonucleic acid-derived growth hormone: the National Cooperative Growth Study experience. J Clin Endocrinol Metab 81:1704–1710

9. Boepple PA, Crowley WF Jr (1996) Precocious puberty. In: Adashi EY, Rock JA, Rosenwaks Z (eds) Reproductive endocrinology, surgery, and technology, vol 1. Lippincott-Raven, Philadelphia, p 989

10. Bourguignon JP, Pierard GE, Ernould C et al (1993) Effects of human growth hormone therapy on melanocytic naevi. Lancet 341:1505–1506

11. Carel JC, Ecosse E, Landier F et al (2012) Long-term mortality after recombinant growth hormone treatment for isolated growth hormone deficiency or childhood short stature: preliminary report of the French SAGhE study. J Clin Endocrinol Metab 97:416–425

12. Castaño JP, Delgado-Niebla E, Durán-Prado M et al (2005) New insights in the mechanism by which SRIF influences GH secretion. J Endocrinol Invest 28(5 Suppl):10–13

13. Chemaitilly W, Sklar CA (2010) Endocrine complications in long-term survivors of childhood cancers. Endocrinol Relat Cancer 17(3):R141–R159

14. Chrousos GP (1995) The hypothalamic-pituitary-adrenal axis and immune-mediated inflammation. N Engl J Med 332:1351–1362

15. Cook DM, Rose SR (2012) A review of guidelines for use of growth hormone in pediatric and transition patients. Pituitary 15(3):301–310

16. Cummings DE, Merriam GR (2003) Growth hormone therapy in adults. Annu Rev Med 54:513–533

17. Darzy KH, Pezzoli SS, Thorner MO, Shalet SM (2005) The dynamics of growth hormone (GH) secretion in adult cancer survivors with severe GH deficiency acquired after brain irradiation in childhood for nonpituitary brain tumors: evidence for preserved pulsatility and diurnal variation with increased secretory disorderliness. J Clin Endocrinol Metab 90:2794–2803

18. Darzy KH, Shalet SM (2009) Hypopituitarism following radiotherapy. Pituitary 12:40–50

19. Elias AN, Gwinup G (1980) Effects of some clinically encountered drugs on steroid synthesis and degradation. Metabolism 29:582–592

20. Ergun-Longmire B, Mertens AC, Mitby P et al (2006) Growth hormone treatment and risk of second neoplasms in the childhood cancer survivor. J Clin Endocrinol Metab 91:3494–3498

21. Eyal O, Sundararajan S, Inge TH, Rose SR (2006) Obesity in patients with craniopharyngioma. Endocrinologist 16:286–293

22. Ferretti E, Persani L, Jaffrain-Rea ML et al (1999) Evaluation of the adequacy of levothyroxine replacement in patients with central hypothyroidism. J Clin Endocrinol Metab 84:924–929

23. Fouladi M, Wallace D, Langston JW et al (2003) Survival and functional outcome of children with hypothalamic/chiasmatic tumors. Cancer 97:1084–1092

24. Ghigo E, Aimaretti G, Corneli G (2008) Diagnosis of adult GH deficiency. Growth Horm IGF Res 18:1–16

25. Gilchrist FJ, Murray RD, Shalet SM (2002) The effect of long-term untreated growth hormone deficiency (GHD) and 9 years of GH replacement on the quality of life (QoL) of GH-deficient adults. Clin Endocrinol (Oxf) 57:363–370

26. Growth Hormone Research Society (2000) Consensus guidelines for the diagnosis and treatment of growth hormone (GH) deficiency in childhood and adolescence: summary statement of the GH Research Society. J Clin Endocrinol Metab 85:3990–3993

27. Gurney JG, Ness KK, Sibley SD et al (2006) Metabolic syndrome and growth hormone deficiency in adult survivors of childhood acute lymphoblastic leukemia. Cancer 107:1303–1312

28. Hartman ML, Xu R, Crowe BJ et al (2013) Prospective safety surveillance of GH-deficient adults: comparison of GH-treated vs untreated patients. J Clin Endocrinol Metab 98:980–988

29. Hovi L, Saarinen-Pihkala UM, Vettenranta K et al (1999) Growth in children with poor-risk neuroblastoma after regimens with or without total body irradiation in preparation for autologous bone marrow transplantation. Bone Marrow Transplant 24:1131–1136

30. Inge TH, Pfluger P, Zeller M et al (2007) Gastric bypass for treatment of hypothalamic obesity after craniopharyngioma therapy. Nat Clin Pract Endocrinol Metab 3:606–609

31. Kaste SC, Rai SN, Fleming K et al (2006) Changes in bone mineral density in survivors of childhood acute lymphoblastic leukemia. Pediatr Blood Cancer 46:77–87

32. Kazlauskaite R, Evans AT, Villabona CV et al (2008) Corticotropin tests for hypothalamic-pituitary adrenal insufficiency: a metaanalysis. J Clin Endocrinol Metab 93:4245–4253

33. Laughton SJ, Merchant TE, Sklar CA et al (2008) Endocrine outcomes for children with embryonal brain tumors after risk-adapted craniospinal and conformal primary-site irradiation and high-dose chemotherapy with stem-cell rescue on the SJMB-96 trial. J Clin Oncol 26:1112–1118

34. Lee KO, Persani L, Tan M et al (1995) Thyrotropin with decreased biological activity, a delayed consequence of cranial irradiation for nasopharyngeal carcinoma. J Endocrinol Invest 18:800–805

35. Lee PA, Klein K, Mauras N et al (2012) Efficacy and safety of leuprolide acetate 3-month depot 11.25 milligrams or 30 milligrams for the treatment of central precocious puberty. J Clin Endocrinol Metab 97:1572–1580

36. Leung W, Hudson MM, Strickland DK et al (2000) Late effects of treatment in survivors of childhood acute myeloid leukemia. J Clin Oncol 18:3273–3279

37. Leung W, Rose SR, Zhou Y et al (2002) Outcomes of growth hormone replacement therapy in survivors of childhood acute lymphoblastic leukemia. J Clin Oncol 20:2959–2964

38. Lustig RH, Post SR, Srivannaboon K et al (2003) Risk factors for the development of obesity in children surviving brain tumors. J Clin Endocrinol Metab 88:611–616

39. May M, Rose SR (2007) Oral hydration during growth hormone stimulation with clonidine. J Pediatr Nurs 22:383–387

40. Mackenzie S, Craven T, Gattamaneni HR et al (2011) Long-term safety of growth hormone replacement after CNS irradiation. J Clin Endocrinol Metab 96:2756–2761

41. Merchant TE, Pritchard DL, Vargo JA, Sontag MR (2001) Radiation therapy for the treatment of childhood medulloblastoma: the rationale for current techniques, strategies, and dose-volume considerations. Electro Medica 69:69–71

42. Merchant TE, Kiehna EN, Sanford RA et al (2002) Craniopharyngioma: the St. Jude Children's Research Hospital experience 1984–2001. Int J Radiat Oncol Biol Phys 53:533–542

43. Merchant TE, Zhu Y, Thompson SJ et al (2002) Preliminary results from a phase II trial of conformal radiation therapy for pediatric patients with localized low-grade astrocytoma and ependymoma. Int J Radiat Oncol Biol Phys 52:325–332

44. Merchant TE, Williams T, Smith JM et al (2002) Preirradiation endocrinopathies in pediatric brain tumor patients determined by dynamic tests of endocrine function. Int J Radiat Oncol Biol Phys 54:45–50

45. Merchant TE, Kun LE, Krasin MJ et al (2008) Multi-institution prospective trial of reduced-dose craniospinal irradiation (23.4 Gy) followed by conformal posterior fossa (36 Gy) and primary site irradiation (55.8 Gy) and dose-intensive chemotherapy for average-risk medulloblastoma. Int J Radiat Oncol Biol Phys 70(3):782–787

46. Merchant TE, Rose SR, Bosley C et al (2011) Growth hormone secretion after conformal radiation therapy in pediatric patients with localized brain tumors. J Clin Oncol 29:4776–4780

47. Mericq MV, Eggers M, Avila A et al (2000) Near final height in pubertal growth hormone (GH)-deficient patients treated with GH alone or in combination with luteinizing hormone-releasing hormone analog: results of a prospective, randomized trial. J Clin Endocrinol Metab 85:569–573

48. Midyett LK, Moore WV, Jacobson JD (2003) Are pubertal changes in girls before age 8 benign? Pediatrics 111:47–51

49. Molitch ME, Clemmons DR, Malozowski S et al (2011) Evaluation and treatment of adult growth hormone deficiency: an Endocrine Society clinical practice guideline. J Clin Endocrinol Metab 96:1587–1609

50. Mostoufi-Moab S, Isaacoff EJ, Spiegel D et al (2013) Childhood cancer survivors exposed to total body irradiation are at significant risk for slipped capital femoral epiphysis during recombinant growth hormone therapy. Pediatr Blood Cancer 60:1766–1771

51. Nass R, Gaylinn BD, Thorner MO (2011) The role of ghrelin in GH secretion and GH disorders. Mol Cell Endocrinol 340:10–14

52. Neely EK, Lee PA, Bloch CA et al (2010) Leuprolide acetate 1-month depot for central precocious puberty: hormonal suppression and recovery. Int J Pediatr Endocrinol 2010:398639

53. Olshan JS, Willi SM, Gruccio D, Moshang T Jr (1993) Growth hormone function and treatment following bone marrow transplant for neuroblastoma. Bone Marrow Transplant 12:381–385

54. Rahhal S, Clarke WL, Kletter GB et al (2009) Results of a second year of therapy with the 12-month histrelin implant for the treatment of central precocious puberty. Int J Pediatr Endocrinol 2009:812517

55. Rose SR (1995) Isolated central hypothyroidism in short stature. Pediatr Res 38:967–973

56. Rose SR (2001) Cranial irradiation and central hypothyroidism. Trends Endocrinol Metab 12:97–104

57. Rose SR (2008) Mechanisms of hypothalamic-pituitary injury in oncology survivors. Endocrinologist 18:85–89

58. Rose SR (2010) Clinical utility of time-of-day normal ranges for TSH. J Pediatr 157:662–667

59. Rose SR, Lustig RH, Pitukcheewanont P et al (1999) Diagnosis of hidden central hypothyroidism in survivors of childhood cancer. J Clin Endocrinol Metab 84:4472–4479

60. Rose SR, Lustig RH, Burstein S et al (1999) Diagnosis of ACTH deficiency. Comparison of overnight metyrapone test to either low-dose or high-dose ACTH test. Horm Res 52:73–79

61. Rose SR, Municchi G (1999) Six-hour and four-hour nocturnal sampling for growth hormone. J Pediatr Endocrinol Metab 12:167–173

62. Rose SR, Schreiber RE, Kearney NS et al (2004) Hypothalamic dysfunction after chemotherapy. J Pediatr Endocrinol Metab 17:55–66

63. Rose SR, Danish RK, Kearney NS et al (2005) ACTH deficiency in childhood cancer survivors. Pediatr Blood Cancer 45:808–813

64. Roth C, Lakomek M, Schmidberger H, Jarry H (2001) Cranial irradiation induces premature activation of the gonadotropin-releasing-hormone. Klin Paediatr 213:239–243

65. Rottembourg D, O'Gorman CS, Urbach S et al (2009) Outcome after bariatric surgery in two adolescents with hypothalamic obesity following treatment of craniopharyngioma. J Pediatr Endocrinol Metab 22: 867–872

66. Sävendahl L, Maes M, Albertsson-Wikland K et al (2012) Long-term mortality and causes of death in isolated GHD, ISS, and SGA patients treated with recombinant growth hormone during childhood in Belgium, The Netherlands, and Sweden: preliminary report of 3 countries participating in the EU SAGhE study. J Clin Endocrinol Metab 97:E213–E217

67. Shalitin S, Gal M, Goshen Y et al (2011) Endocrine outcome in long-term survivors of childhood brain tumors. Horm Res Paediatr 76:113–122

68. Sherlock M, Ayuk J, Tomlinson JW et al (2010) Mortality in patients with pituitary disease. Endocr Rev 31:301–342

69. Sørensen K, Mouritsen A, Aksglaede L et al (2012) Recent secular trends in pubertal timing: implications for evaluation and diagnosis of precocious puberty. Horm Res Paediatr 77:137–145

70. Spoudeas HA (2002) Growth and endocrine function after chemotherapy and radiotherapy in childhood. Eur J Cancer 38:1748–1759

71. Spoudeas HA, Charmandari E, Brook CG (2003) Hypothalamo-pituitary-adrenal axis integrity after cranial irradiation for childhood posterior fossa tumors. Med Pediatr Oncol 40:224–229

72. Stava CJ, Jimenez C, Vassilopoulou-Sellin R (2007) Endocrine sequelae of cancer and cancer treatments. J Cancer Surviv 1:261–274

73. Steffensen C, Maegbaek ML, Laurberg P et al (2012) Heart valve disease among patients with hyperprolactinemia: a nationwide population-based cohort study. J Clin Endocrinol Metab 97:1629–1634

74. Swerdlow AJ, Reddingius RE, Higgins CD et al (2000) Growth hormone treatment of children with brain tumors and risk of tumor recurrence. J Clin Endocrinol Metab 85:4444–4449

75. Taback SP, Dean HJ (1996) Mortality in Canadian children with growth hormone (GH) deficiency receiving GH therapy 1967–1992. The Canadian Growth Hormone Advisory Committee. J Clin Endocrinol Metab 81:1693–1696

76. Tanner JM, Davies PS (1985) Clinical longitudinal standards for height and height velocity in North American children. J Pediatr 107:317–329

77. Toogood AA, Taylor NF, Shalet SM, Monson JP (2000) Modulation of cortisol metabolism by low-dose growth hormone replacement in elderly hypopituitary patients. J Clin Endocrinol Metab 85:1727–1730

78. Vance ML, Mauras N (1999) Growth hormone therapy in adults and children. N Engl J Med 341(16):1206–1216

79. Walvoord E (2009) Sex steroid replacement for induction of puberty in multiple pituitary hormone deficiency. Pediatr Endocrinol Rev 6(Suppl 2):298–305

80. Weismann D, Pelka T, Bender G et al (2012) Bariatric surgery for morbid obesity in craniopharyngioma. Clin Endocrinol (Oxf). doi:10.1111/j.1365-2265.2012.04409.x

81. Wilson T, Rose SR, Rogol A et al (2003) Update of guidelines for the use of growth hormone in children: the Lawson Wilkins Pediatric Endocrinology Society Drug and Therapeutics Committee. J Pediatr 143:415–421

82. Yanovski JA, Rose SR, Municchi G et al (2003) Treatment with a luteinizing hormone-releasing hormone agonist in adolescents with short stature. N Engl J Med 348:908–917

83. Zemel BS, Leonard MB, Kelly A et al (2010) Height adjustment in assessing dual energy X-ray absorptiometry measurements of bone mass and density in children. J Clin Endocrinol Metab 95:1265–1273

# Ocular Complications Due to Cancer Treatment

**6**

Brad E. Kligman, Jasmine H. Francis, and David H. Abramson

## Contents

B.E. Kligman, MD
Ophthalmic Oncology Service,
Memorial Sloan Kettering Cancer Center,
70 East 66th Street, New York, NY 10021, USA

Department of Ophthalmology,
Edward S. Harkness Eye Institute, Columbia
University College of Physicians and Surgeons,
635 W 165th Street, New York, NY 10032, USA
e-mail: brad.kligman@gmail.com

J.H. Francis, MD
Ophthalmic Oncology Service,
Memorial Sloan Kettering Cancer Center,
1275 York Avenue, New York, NY 10021, USA
e-mail: jasminehfrancis@gmail.com

D.H. Abramson, MD, FACS (✉)
Ophthalmic Oncology Service,
Memorial Sloan Kettering Cancer Center,
70 East 66th Street, New York, NY 10021, USA
e-mail: abramsod@mskcc.org

© Springer International Publishing 2015
C.L. Schwartz et al. (eds.), *Survivors of Childhood and Adolescent Cancer:
A Multidisciplinary Approach*, Pediatric Oncology, DOI 10.1007/978-3-319-16435-9_6

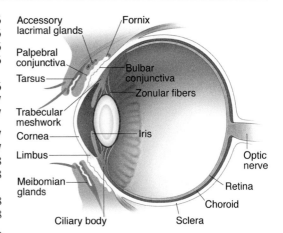

**Fig. 6.1** Cross-sectional anatomy of the eye

## 6.1 Introduction

The eye is a complex organ composed of many tissues that vary greatly in their exposure and sensitivity to cytotoxic therapy. The ocular effects of cancer treatment, ranging from mild discomfort to blindness or loss of an eye, can have a profound effect on the quality of life of long-term cancer survivors. This chapter discusses the known complications of radiation, chemotherapy, and immunosuppressive therapy in the eye. It also considers the effects of graft-versus-host disease (GVHD), which affects the eye in 40–80 % of cases and can be the first or only manifestation of the disease [1, 2]. Each section of the chapter deals with a particular part of the eye and begins with a description of the relevant anatomy (Fig. 6.1). Medical management for the potential complications and indications for referral to an ophthalmologist for specialized care are discussed as well.

## 6.2 Eyelids, Periorbital Skin, and Tear Film

### 6.2.1 Anatomy and Physiology

The thinnest skin in the body is located on the outer surface of the eyelids. It is devoid of subcutaneous fat allowing for the accumulation of fluid to manifest rapidly as swelling. The upper and lower eyelids contain fibrous connective tissue, known as the tarsal plates, which function as structural support. The eyelashes are located on the anterior portion of the eyelids and aid in the protection of the eye.

The tear film covers the anterior surface of the conjunctiva and cornea. It serves the vital role of supplying the cornea with moisture, nutrients, enzymes, immunoglobulins, and protein signals, as well as allowing the maintenance of a clear, nonkeratinized epithelium in the visual axis. Furthermore, the tear film comprises the smooth outer refractive coating essential to vision by filling in corneal irregularities. The tear film consists of three layers. The aqueous layer is produced by the accessory lacrimal glands found in the conjunctiva. Meibomian glands located within the tarsal plates produce an oily layer that sits on top of and acts to stabilize the aqueous layer. The goblet cells of the conjunctiva produce the third, or mucous, layer. The overall function of the tear film is vitally dependent on each of these individual layers, and a deficiency in any layer will adversely affect the entire ocular surface.

The tears drain from the ocular surface via two puncta located on the medial aspect of the upper and lower lid margin. The puncta lead to the canaliculi that empty into the lacrimal sac and, ultimately, into the nose via the nasolacrimal duct.

### 6.2.2 Acute Radiation Effects

Madarosis, or loss of eyelashes, and erythema are the first side effects of radiation therapy

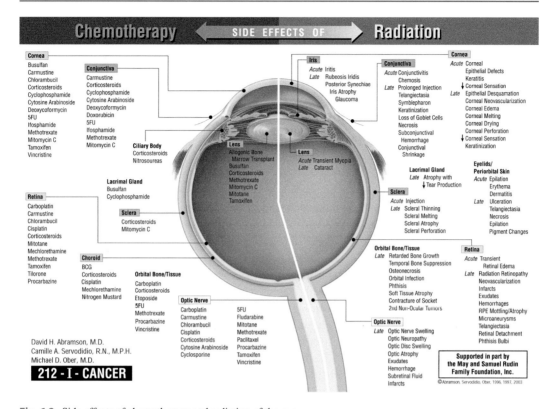

**Fig. 6.2** Side effects of chemotherapy and radiation of the eye

(RT) involving the eye. Usually, eyelashes will grow back; however, permanent loss does occur. Erythema can occur within days of treatment (generally after doses of at least 20–30 Gy) and usually persists for a few days. Dermatitis is the most common acute side effect of RT. Dry dermatitis of irradiated skin can occur with doses greater than 20 Gy and often leads to desquamation. Moist dermatitis, with exposure of the dermis and associated serum leakage, can occur after the fourth week of RT following doses of 40 Gy or more, fractionated over a 4-week period. Blisters and edema may precede moist dermatitis. Symptoms include redness, peeling, burning, itching, and pain [3] (Fig. 6.2).

### 6.2.3   Chronic Radiation Effects

The late effects of RT to the eyelids following doses from 30 to 60 Gy include madarosis, telangiectasia (dilated, tortuous blood vessels; Fig. 6.3), hyperpigmentation, depigmentation,

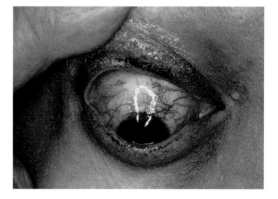

**Fig. 6.3** Telangiectasia of the conjunctival blood vessels

ectropion, hyperkeratosis, atrophy, necrosis, ulceration, and punctal occlusion. Although rarely seen today, lid deformities, such as ectropion (out-turning of eyelid margin), entropion (in-turning of eyelid margin), and atrophy or contracture, are seen when the tarsus has been included in the radiation field. The time of onset ranges from 2 months to greater than 5 years after treatment. Destruction or occlusion of the puncta may occur when the medial portions of the eyelid are irradiated, which leads to impaired tear drainage. Lid necrosis, exacerbated by excess sun exposure in areas previously irradiated, may develop months to years after treatment [4, 5].

### 6.2.4 Chemotherapy and Immunosuppressive Agents

Many chemotherapeutic agents, such as cyclophosphamide, ifosfamide, and methotrexate, alter the normal tear film physiology either by causing inflammation of the lacrimal glands or by being excreted directly into tears. This leads to dry eye symptoms including irritation, foreign body sensation, and photophobia, as well as inflammation around the eyelids and anterior segment of the eye [6]. Patients treated with alkyl sulfonates, including busulfan and nitrosourea, have also reported developing dry eye [7]. Both 5-fluorouracil [8] (5-FU) and docetaxel [9] can cause stenosis of the puncta and tear drainage system leading to excessive tearing called epiphora. 5-FU does so through squamous metaplasia and narrowing of the canalicular lumen [10], while docetaxel induces stromal fibrosis [11]. Some patients receiving 5-FU also develop cicatricial eyelid malpositioning [12]. Intravenous doxorubicin is associated with excessive lacrimation as well.

Paleness of the periorbital skin can occur following mithramycin infusion, while drooping of the upper eyelid, known as ptosis, has been reported following long-term corticosteroid use [13]. Vincristine can also cause unilateral or bilateral ptosis alone or as part of a cranial polyneuropathy [14–16].

### 6.2.5 Graft-Versus-Host Disease

The eye is primarily affected in the chronic phase of graft-versus-host disease (cGVHD), generally defined as greater than 100 days after transplant while the patient is being tapered off immunosuppressive therapy. Keratoconjunctivitis sicca, inflammation of the ocular surface secondary to insufficient tear film, is the most common manifestation of cGVHD. It is caused, in part, by lacrimal gland dysfunction from T-cell infiltration leading to scarring and decreased tear production [2, 17]. These patients are also more prone to developing dry eye because of conditioning regimens with total body irradiation and high-dose chemotherapy used to prepare the patient's body to receive donor stem cells.

Dermatitis of the lid skin in cGVHD can lead to erythema, scaling, and ultimately lichenification or stiffening of the lids causing entropion or ectropion, lagophthalmos (incomplete lid closure), and trichiasis, all of which can worsen the symptoms of dry eye. The inflammatory response within the lids can also manifest as edema, hyperkeratosis, telangiectasias, or periorbital hyperpigmentation [2, 18]. Cicatricial occlusion of the lacrimal puncta may occur leading to epiphora [19].

### 6.2.6 Medical and Nursing Management

The management for eyelid complications due to cancer treatment consists mainly of skin care, including the use of ultraviolet protection, meticulous hygiene with mild soaps, use of skin lubricants, avoiding skin-sensitizing drugs (i.e., tetracycline), and occasionally corticosteroid and/or antibiotic creams. Ptosis, nasolacrimal duct obstruction, or eyelid malposition may require minor surgical manipulation by an ophthalmologist and should be referred in clinically significant cases [20]. At the first sign of epiphora secondary to punctal occlusion, prompt diagnosis and management by an ophthalmologist can prevent complete fibrosis of the canaliculi, which would require more invasive surgical intervention such as dacryocystorhinostomy. If identified early on, less invasive procedures such as punctoplasty or canalicular intubation with silicone tubes can be performed, which may prevent future occlusion [9]. In advanced cases of canalicular obstruction where surgery is contraindicated or not desired by the patient, botulinum toxin injection into the lacrimal gland can serve as a palliative option to alleviate epiphora [21].

Many cases of chemotherapy-induced ptosis eventually resolve after discontinuing the offending agent. Vincristine-induced ptosis, however, has been treated successfully with combined pyridoxine and pyridostigmine therapy [14–16].

The mainstay of dry eye therapy consists of tear replacement with artificial tears drops and ointment. Patients with symptoms or at risk should be encouraged to use liberal amounts of artificial tears. Unpreserved artificial tears are preferred, especially when they are used more than four times per day, due to the fact that the preservatives themselves can be irritating to the cornea, conjunctiva, and eyelids. Further aids include punctal occlusion, warm compresses to the eyelids, and, in advanced cases, cyclosporine drops [22]. Topical cyclosporine A, which inhibits T-cell activation and downregulates inflammatory cytokines in the conjunctiva, may even be effective in preventing or lessening the severity of dry eye when used prophylactically for cGVHD [23]. Patients with continued symptomatic or refractory dry eyes should be referred to an eye care professional without delay, as the consequences of hesitating could be permanent vision loss.

## 6.3   Conjunctiva

### 6.3.1   Anatomy and Physiology

The conjunctiva is a thin, transparent mucous membrane that lines both the posterior aspect of the eyelids (palpebral conjunctiva) and the anterior surface of the eye (bulbar conjunctiva). The folds between the palpebral and bulbar conjunctiva are known as the superior and inferior fornices, respectively. Tissue is redundant in the fornices to allow for adequate movement of the globe. The main lacrimal gland, which functions during reflex tearing, empties into the superior fornix, while the accessory lacrimal glands, supplying basal tear secretion, are found throughout the conjunctiva, concentrating in the fornices.

The conjunctiva contains a stratified nonkeratinized epithelium overlying a stroma, known as the substantia propria. Goblet cells supplying the mucin layer of the tear film are found intermixed with the epithelial cells. Besides acting as a physical barrier, the conjunctiva aids in host defenses by hosting immune cells as well as colonizing bacteria.

### 6.3.2   Acute Radiation Effects

Conjunctival inflammation (conjunctivitis), which manifests as vascular injection with clear or mucoid discharge, tends to occur 1–3 weeks after the start of radiation treatment. Edema of the conjunctiva, known as chemosis, may occur simultaneously or in isolation and usually lasts for a few days. The affected conjunctiva may also ulcerate leading to an increased risk of infection. The duration of these signs may be prolonged when RT doses over 30 Gy are used [3, 4, 24].

### 6.3.3   Chronic Radiation Effects

Late effects of RT to the conjunctiva include prolonged injection, telangiectasis, symblepharon (adhesions between the bulbar and palpebral conjunctiva), subconjunctival hemorrhage, shortening of the fornices, loss of goblet cells, keratinization, and necrosis. Exposure to 30–50 Gy results in prolonged conjunctival injection, which develops in 1–2 years, followed by telangiectatic vessels 3–6 years later. These fragile vessels tend to rupture with minor trauma, resulting in subconjunctival hemorrhage [5].

Chronic ulceration of the conjunctiva can be seen following treatment with 60 Gy. This leads to symblepharon formation. The definition of symblepharon is clarified in the paragraph above, resulting in shortening of the fornices, eyelid malpositioning, and trichiasis (turning of lashes onto the ocular surface). Goblet cell loss occurs at relatively low doses, resulting in tear film instability and dry eye symptoms, while doses over 50 Gy may result in keratinization of the conjunctiva. These keratin plaques constantly irritate the adjacent cornea, occasionally causing scarring and visual loss. Necrosis may occur after radioactive plaque therapy for retinoblastoma patients, where doses to the conjunctiva can reach between 90 and 300 Gy [3, 4, 24].

### 6.3.4 Chemotherapy and Immunosuppressive Agents

Conjunctivitis is a commonly reported symptom following induction therapy with many chemotherapeutic agents, including cyclophosphamide, ifosfamide, nitrosoureas, cytosine arabinoside, doxorubicin, methotrexate, deoxycoformycin, and mitomycin. 5-Fluorouracil is also associated with conjunctivitis and eye irritation. This usually occurs concurrently with the initiation of therapy, and it resolves within 2 weeks of treatment cessation. The immunosuppressive effects of corticosteroids are believed to facilitate opportunistic infections throughout the eye, including bacterial, viral, and fungal conjunctivitis, and can also lead to delayed wound healing [25]. Periocular carboplatin injections, a treatment sometimes used for intraocular tumors, can lead to fibrosis of the conjunctiva and underlying tissues [26].

### 6.3.5 Graft-Versus-Host Disease

In cGVHD, histological studies have demonstrated that there is a severe decline in Meibomian gland function as well as reduction in the total number of goblet cells in the conjunctiva [18, 27]. These two factors contribute to tear film deficiency and dry eye symptoms as described in the previous section. Keratinization of the conjunctival epithelium, conjunctival hyperemia with chemosis and serosanguineous exudate, subtarsal fibrosis, and conjunctival necrosis can also be seen in cGVHD [18]. Pseudomembranous conjunctivitis is a sign of severe systemic involvement in acute graft-versus-host disease, which occurs prior to tapering of immunosuppressive therapy [28]. Although not life-threatening, dry eye as a result of cGVHD has a significant effect on quality of life.

### 6.3.6 Medical and Nursing Management

Antibiotic eyedrops, sometimes in combination with corticosteroids, are used for prolonged conjunctivitis and for conjunctival ulceration. Artificial tears often aid chronic conjunctival irritation by providing the lubrication necessary to replace lost tear volume and dilute toxic chemotherapeutic metabolites excreted into the tear film. Vitamin A ophthalmic ointment (tretinoin 0.01 % or 0.1 %) may reverse squamous metaplasia and loss of vascularization from scar formation [29]. Patients with infectious conjunctivitis should be instructed to wash their hands frequently and take great care in interactions with others to prevent the spread of communicable diseases. In addition, sunglasses for protection from the sun and wind may be helpful in reducing symptoms. Severe conjunctival reactions, such as symblepharon and forniceal shortening, may require ophthalmologic manipulations such as symblepharon lysis on a repeated basis, or mucous membrane grafting with forniceal reconstruction. Ophthalmologic referral is therefore indicated.

## 6.4 Cornea

### 6.4.1 Anatomy and Physiology

The cornea is the transparent, avascular, anterior structure of the eye that refracts and transmits light to the inner structures of the eye. Along with the overlying tear film, it provides approximately two thirds of the refracting power of the eye. The conjunctiva borders the cornea in an area known as the limbus. This region contains corneal stem cells. Therefore, compromising this zone leads directly to the loss of corneal transparency and often its integrity. The cornea is an avascular tissue and thus depends on the limbal vessels along with the tear film and aqueous fluid from the anterior chamber for nutrients and waste removal.

The cornea consists of five specialized layers, including, from anterior to posterior: epithelium, Bowman's membrane, stroma, Descemet's membrane, and endothelium. The epithelium is stratified and nonkeratinized and replaces itself every 5–7 days. The stroma contains approximately 90 % of the overall corneal thickness, including a specialized superficial region known as the

Bowman's membrane. Descemet's membrane is a tough, thickened basement membrane secreted by the endothelium. The endothelial cells form a monolayer, which controls corneal hydration via ionic pumps. Small changes in corneal hydration (thickness) drastically change the optical properties of the cornea; thus, the endothelial pumps are essential to maintaining clear vision. Endothelial cells can migrate to fill an area with damage, but they do not regenerate. Therefore, all loss of endothelial cells is permanent. Inflammation of the cornea, known as keratitis, also increases the corneal thickness and blurs vision.

### 6.4.2   Acute Radiation Effects

The corneal epithelium is adversely affected after RT doses of 10–20 Gy. Early effects include epithelial defects, keratitis, and decreased corneal sensation. When the tear film production or integrity is reduced, the epithelial cells become fragile and loosely adherent to themselves and the underlying stromal bed, resulting in epithelial defects. Patients with this problem will complain of ocular discomfort, foreign body sensation, excess reflex tearing, and blurry vision. Acute keratitis is often self-limited following exposure to 30 Gy, but following treatment with up to 50 Gy, it may persist for months along with conjunctivitis. Decreased corneal sensation may result from nerve damage and be exacerbated by impaired reflex tearing which, in turn, diminishes the blink rate and delays complaints from the patient [3, 24].

### 6.4.3   Chronic Radiation Effects

Late RT effects on the cornea include chronic epithelial defects, neovascularization, keratinization, edema, ulceration, and perforation. Epithelial defects may persist for months when radiation causes damage to corneal epithelial stem cells, accessory tear glands, goblet cells, and/or corneal nerves. The cornea responds to these nonhealing areas with neovascularization and keratinization, both of which temporarily or permanently decrease visual acuity. Abnormal

blood vessels and chronic inflammation may lead to lipid deposition within the corneal stroma, further worsening vision. Damage to lacrimal glands, goblet cells, and corneal sensation impairs host defenses by limiting the cornea's contact with tears and their accompanying nourishment, lubrication, immunoglobulins, and enzymes. Colonization and invasion of the corneal surface by bacteria may accelerate ulceration and perforation [3, 5, 24, 30].

### 6.4.4   Chemotherapy and Immunosuppressive Agents

Patients develop keratitis following treatment with many intravenous chemotherapeutic agents, including chlorambucil, cyclophosphamide, methotrexate, nitrosoureas, 5-fluorouracil, and deoxycoformycin [6]. Punctate corneal opacities and keratitis will occur acutely with cytosine arabinoside therapy, usually resolving approximately 4 weeks after completion. Intravitreal methotrexate, a treatment for intraocular lymphoma, can also cause a corneal epitheliopathy of varying severity, generally developing after three doses [31]. Both vincristine and vinblastine have been associated with corneal hypoesthesia, which may lead to neurotrophic corneal ulceration [32]. Patients undergoing long-term tamoxifen treatment may acquire whorl-like corneal epithelium deposits known as verticillata [33]. The immunosuppressive effects of corticosteroids facilitate opportunistic infections throughout the eye, resulting in bacterial, viral, and fungal keratitis as well as in corneal ulcers.

### 6.4.5   Graft-Versus-Host Disease

Chronic graft-versus-host disease can affect the cornea both directly via infiltration by macrophages and release of proinflammatory molecules and indirectly as a result of keratoconjunctivitis sicca and lagophthalmos [34]. The combination of tear film insufficiency and corneal exposure with a background inflammatory response can lead to a wide spectrum of corneal disorders. Punctate keratopathy, corneal epithelial sloughing, filamentary keratitis, or superior limbic keratoconjunctivitis may be seen as effects on the superficial structures of the cornea. Once the protective epithelial layer is compromised, the deeper structures of the cornea may become involved leading to corneal erosion, thinning, and ulceration. If untreated, perforation of the cornea can occur rapidly. Often in these cases, stromal infiltration by neutrophils is seen, but no microorganism is isolated [18]. Chronic inflammation of the cornea in GVHD can cause permanent stromal scarring, corneal vascularization [35], and calcification [2].

### 6.4.6 Medical and Nursing Management

Artificial tears and ointment are important in maintaining a healthy cornea following insults from cancer treatment. Patients using these solutions more than four times daily should consider unpreserved formulations. Autologous or allogeneic serum eyedrops made from the patient or a relative's blood may be used for refractory cases. These contain epidermal growth factor, vitamin A, transforming growth factor-β, and fibronectin, which are all important for corneal and conjunctival health and are not present in artificial tears [36, 37]. Antibiotic drops are recommended for epithelial defects. Corticosteroid (dexamethasone) eyedrops are often given prophylactically with antimetabolite treatment, especially cytosine arabinoside, to reduce corneal and conjunctival irritation. Steroid drops may also be used with specific types of sterile infiltrates for keratitis, but should initially be avoided if active infectious causes are suspected. Corneal infections and ulcerations are treated with administration of antibiotic eyedrops as frequently as every 15 min. Bandage contact lenses, particularly gas-permeable silicone hydrogel lenses [38] or gas-permeable scleral lenses [39], along with antibiotic drops, may be used for nonhealing epithelial defects. Systemic immunosuppressive therapy with FK506 (tacrolimus) and corticosteroids

have been used successfully to treat highly refractive dry eye cases, but this modality is limited by the potential for opportunistic infection or relapse of leukemia with long-term use [40]. It must also be noted that tacrolimus can cause a reversible toxic posterior leukoencephalopathy with cortical blindness [41]. Emergency surgical intervention with partial to complete tarsorrhaphy (sewing the eyelids shut to protect the cornea) or corneal transplantation may be required when corneal perforation is pending or apparent or with the formation of a central corneal scar [18]. Patients should be instructed to avoid factors that may contribute to eye irritation or dryness, such as fans, wind, smoke, or low-humidity situations. Moisture goggles at night and protective eyewear that reduces airflow over the eyes for outdoor activities can be beneficial [42].

## 6.5 Lens

### 6.5.1 Anatomy and Physiology

The lens is the second clear, avascular refracting surface of the eye. It lies posterior to the iris and is suspended circumferentially by a ring of fibrous bands known as the zonule. This encapsulated structure is devoid of nerves and vasculature and thus depends on the aqueous and vitreous humor for nutrients. Throughout life, the mitotically active cells located within the anterior periphery of the lens migrate inward toward the denser nucleus in the center. The cells of the lens are never shed; rather, they are incorporated into the nucleus. Thus, injured cells leave permanent, visible defects. For this reason, the crystalline lens is particularly susceptible to the formation of a cataract after cancer treatment. A cataract simply refers to the loss of optical clarity within the lens, a condition that can vary widely in severity.

### 6.5.2 Acute Radiation Effects

On rare occasions, transient myopia may occur in the weeks following RT as a result of increased water content within the lens.

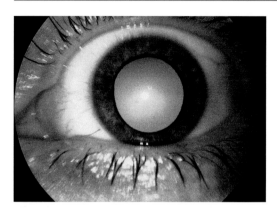

**Fig. 6.4** Radiation-induced cataract

### 6.5.3  Chronic Radiation Effects

The posterior subcapsular cataract is the characteristic late complication of RT (Fig. 6.4). The lens is the most radiosensitive structure within the eye because of its perpetual mitotic activity and inability to remove injured cells or disperse heat efficiently. The report on cataracts following radiation therapy in 1957 by Merriam and Focht yielded results that remain clinically relevant today. They found the threshold for cataract development to be a single exposure to 200 rads, fractionated doses of 400 rads over 3 weeks to 3 months, or a total dose of 550 rads divided over more than 3 months. Furthermore, they reported that patients receiving a single treatment of 200 rads, fractionated doses of >1,000 rads over 3 weeks to 3 months, or 1,100 rads over greater than 3 months developed cataracts 100 % of the time [43]. The lens in children less than 1 year of age is more sensitive to radiation, as compared to the adult lens, presumably due to higher mitotic activity [24].

### 6.5.4  Chemotherapy and Immunosuppressive Agents

Cataract is the most frequently reported side effect associated with corticosteroid use. The incidence of steroid-induced cataracts ranges from 15 to 52 %, depending on dose and duration of treatment [44]. Although variable, the approximate threshold for cataract formation is 10 mg prednisone daily for 1 year [45]. It should be noted that steroid-induced cataracts have been reported following treatment with systemic, inhaled, topical, and skin formulations. Some patients treated with busulfan [46] also acquire cataracts, as do those receiving topical mitomycin C. Patients taking tamoxifen have been found to have a higher proportion of a specific class of cataract (posterior subcapsular) following years of treatment, which also may be indicative of lenticular toxicity [6, 47].

### 6.5.5  Medical and Nursing Management

At the present time, there are no known medical treatments for the reversal of cataracts. Prevention of cataracts is best accomplished by fractionation of the RT dose, lens shielding during treatment, and limiting exposure to toxic medications. Once a clinically significant cataract develops, surgical extractions and observation become the only options. Cataract extraction is elective in the vast majority of situations and depends upon the patient's and family's desires.

Cataract formation in young children is particularly significant, as visual pathways in the brain develop only during a finite period of time. When the central nervous system is presented with altered visual stimuli during this critical period, such as through an opaque lens, the potential visual acuity is reduced. When this phenomenon occurs, it is termed amblyopia. The vital time begins before or at birth and is believed to end between age 7 and 13. Once development is complete, alterations in the visual system no longer change the potential vision. When identified early in its course, amblyopia is potentially reversible. Visually impairing complications in children such as cataracts must therefore be recognized and treated early.

### 6.6  Uvea: Iris, Ciliary Body, and Choroid

### 6.6.1  Anatomy and Physiology

The uvea consists of three structures with a common embryologic origin: the iris, ciliary body, and choroid. The iris acts as the light aperture of the eye. It is a muscular membrane with a central circular opening (the pupil). Despite the wide variation in iris color on the anterior surface, the posterior surface of the normal iris characteristically contains a thick layer of heavily pigmented cells that act to absorb and thus limit the influx of light. The size of the pupil is controlled by the autonomic nervous system with input from both sympathetic and parasympathetic systems.

The ciliary body is a muscular structure located posterior to the iris and peripheral to the lens. The ciliary body produces the aqueous humor, the fluid that fills the anterior segment of the eye. This fluid drains through a structure known as the trabecular meshwork located anterior to the iris. As a result, the fluid must travel through the pupil in order to exit the eye. Any disruption to this flow will result in a backup of fluid and increased pressure within the eye. This may lead to a condition called glaucoma, wherein prolonged elevation of intraocular pressure can lead to damage of the optic nerve and irreversible vision loss. The muscles within the ciliary body are also responsible for adjusting the tension on the zonule that allows for lens accommodation. The choroid, located between the retina and sclera, is the posterior segment of the uveal tract. It is a highly vascular structure that supplies the outer retina with oxygen.

### 6.6.2  Acute Radiation Effects

Uveitis (inflammation of the uvea) is an early effect of RT. It is caused by an increase in vascular permeability, which leads to a leakage of protein and inflammatory cells [4]. Iritis (inflammation of the iris) is dose related and can occur after a fractionated dose of greater than 60 Gy over 5–6 weeks.

### 6.6.3  Chronic Radiation Effects

Iris neovascularization, posterior synechiae (adhesions between the iris and the lens), and iris atrophy are the major long-term complications of RT. Iris neovascularization, also known as rubeo-

sis iritis, occurs several months to years following RT with fractionated doses of 70–80 Gy over 6–8 weeks. The abnormal vessels that result from this condition can grow into the trabecular meshwork, thereby causing intractable glaucoma. Rubeosis iritis is believed to be caused by retinal ischemia, resulting in the liberation of vascular growth factors throughout the eye. Posterior synechiae can also cause glaucoma by preventing fluid produced behind the iris from reaching the trabecular meshwork located anterior to the iris. Iris atrophy has been reported 3 years after high doses of beta irradiation with 170–250 Gy [4, 5].

### 6.6.4  Chemotherapy and Immunosuppressive Agents

Corticosteroid treatment is known to cause an elevation in intraocular pressure with a moderate elevation in 30 % of patients and a severe elevation in 5 % of patients [48]. Several factors may influence a patient's susceptibility to steroid-induced glaucoma, including older age, genetic predisposition to glaucoma, and length and increased dose of treatment [49–51]. Generally, therapy for at least 2 weeks is required for increased intraocular pressure to manifest. Although the increased pressure induced by corticosteroids usually resolves with cessation of the therapy, irreversible glaucoma has also been demonstrated [52]. In addition, corticosteroids have been implicated in facilitating infectious uveitis.

Severe uveal reactions have been reported following intracarotid treatment with chemotherapeutic agents, including one case of choroidal effusion and exudative retinal detachment with intracarotid cisplatin infusion [53]. Intracarotid carboplatin can cause a severe choroidal vasculitis with exudative retinal detachment, glaucoma, and permanent loss of vision if there is inadvertent backflow of the drug into the ophthalmic artery [54]. In addition, one report found that 25 % of patients treated with intracarotid mechlorethamine, a nitrogen mustard compound, developed an ipsilateral necrotizing uveitis [55].

### 6.6.5   Graft-Versus-Host Disease

Occasionally, graft-versus-host disease can manifest as uveitis. Both nongranulomatous iridocyclitis and mild choroiditis have been reported to occur in GVHD, usually in the acute phase [18, 56].

### 6.6.6   Medical and Nursing Management

The medical management of noninfectious uveitis includes steroid ophthalmic drops and dilation drops (often Cyclogyl) to reduce inflammation, paralyze the ciliary body for pain control, and pull the iris away from the lens. Beta-blocker, alpha-agonist, carbonic anhydrase inhibitors, and prostaglandin analog eyedrops all aid in lowering intraocular pressure. Photocoagulation of the iris (peripheral iridotomy) is occasionally needed to restore aqueous flow from production by the ciliary body posterior to the iris to drainage in the trabecular meshwork anterior to the iris. In cases of neovascular glaucoma, intravitreal injection of anti-VEGF agents may facilitate regression of the abnormal blood vessels blocking the trabecular meshwork. Severe, unresponsive glaucoma may require surgical intervention to create an alternative pathway for aqueous drainage. Enucleation, surgical removal of the globe, is the last resort for end-stage glaucoma causing a blind, painful eye.

## 6.7   Sclera

### 6.7.1   Anatomy and Physiology

The sclera is an acellular, avascular, collagenous protective layer of the eye. It is continuous with the cornea at the limbus and is covered anteriorly by the conjunctiva. The superficial coating of the sclera, known as the episclera, consists of a loose, transparent, vascular coating.

### 6.7.2   Acute Radiation Effects

The sclera may become inflamed (scleritis) 2–4 weeks after the initiation of RT. This condition is transient and usually resolves on its own.

### 6.7.3   Chronic Radiation Effects

The sclera is able to tolerate doses of RT up to 900 Gy from an iodine or cobalt plaque when administered over a period of 4 days to 1 week for the treatment of intraocular tumors. Thinning, melting, or atrophy of the sclera can occur several years after fractioned RT doses of 20–30 Gy. These conditions are uncommon after RT for childhood tumors treated with external beam radiation, unless extremely high doses are used. Scleral perforation may also occur, although it is rare [4].

### 6.7.4   Chemotherapy and Immunosuppressive Agents

There are no reported scleral complications when chemotherapy agents are used systemically. However, mitomycin C, which is used topically as adjunct treatment for ocular surface tumors, may lead to scleral ulceration, scleritis, and scleral calcification [6].

### 6.7.5   Graft-Versus-Host Disease

Rarely, episcleritis or scleritis may be seen as a manifestation of cGVHD [2].

### 6.7.6   Medical and Nursing Management

Episcleritis typically resolves on its own and may be treated symptomatically with artificial tears and cool compresses. For more persistent cases that do not quickly resolve, short-term therapy with NSAIDs, including ibuprofen and indomethacin, may be employed. NSAIDs are also the first-line treatment for scleritis. For refractory cases, systemic corticosteroids or immunomodulatory agents such as methotrexate, cyclophosphamide, mycophenolate, or infliximab may be necessary to control the inflammation. More severe reactions, such as scleral melting and ulceration, require close observation, treatment with antibiotic drops, and surgical repair with scleral patch grafting. Eye protection and the importance of avoiding trauma should be emphasized to patients.

## 6.8 Optic Nerve and Retina

### 6.8.1 Anatomy and Physiology

The retina is a thin, transparent structure that functions to convert light energy into electrical stimuli for the brain to interpret. It receives nutrients from the underlying retinal pigment epithelium and choroidal blood vessels. Separation from these supporting tissues, known as a retinal detachment, can lead to permanent vision loss. The macula, located temporal to the optic disk, is responsible for central vision and contains the highest concentration of photoreceptors. The blood–retina barrier, which is analogous to the blood–brain barrier, protects the retina. It is very sensitive to changes in vascular permeability that can lead to swelling of the retinal layers (i.e., macular edema).

The optic nerve contains 1,100,000 axons from the superficial layer of the retina. These axons leave the eye through an area known as the optic disk and comprise the pathway through which visual stimuli reach the brain, terminating in the occipital lobe.

### 6.8.2 Acute Radiation Effects

Radiation therapy, with 20–35 Gy fractionated over 2–4 weeks or in doses in excess of 50 Gy, has been reported to produce a transient retinal edema [3, 4].

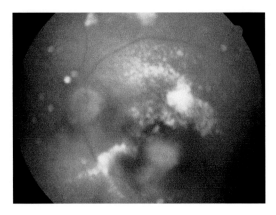

**Fig. 6.5** Radiation retinopathy

### 6.8.3 Chronic Radiation Effects

Radiation retinopathy (Fig. 6.5) is a well-documented consequence of radiation treatment that leads to an irreversible reduction in visual acuity. It is characterized by specific examination findings, including microaneurysms, hard exudates, cotton-wool spots, optic disk swelling, vascular occlusion, hemorrhages, and neovascularization. These changes are clinically indistinguishable from retinal changes due to diabetes. Radiation retinopathy can develop as soon as 3 weeks and as late as 15 years, following RT, although typically it occurs between 1 and 3 years. While as little as 15 Gy of external beam radiation has led to signs of retinopathy, 30–60 Gy is usually required. In the authors' experience, fewer than 5 % of children treated with external beam radiation for retinoblastoma develop radiation retinopathy. Fifty gray is regarded as the threshold for the development of retinopathy following radioactive plaque exposure. Either a history of diabetes mellitus or concurrent treatment with chemotherapy is believed to increase susceptibility to radiation retinopathy [5, 57].

### 6.8.4 Chemotherapy and Immunosuppressive Agents

The optic nerve and retina are common sites for chemotherapeutic complications. Retinal hemorrhages, cotton-wool spots, and optic disk edema have all been reported following systemic nitrosoureas [58], while intracarotid infusion has been implicated in optic neuritis and atrophy [59]. In some patients treated systemically, cisplatin can produce optic neuritis, papilledema, and retinal toxicity that manifests as color blindness [60]. Intravenous carboplatin may lead to visual loss due to retinopathy and optic neuropathy [61]. Intracarotid infusion of platinum-based chemotherapeutics can cause visual loss from severe retinal and/or optic nerve ischemia, pigmentary retinopathy, or exudative retinal detachment [53]. Intrathecal methotrexate has been reported to cause optic nerve atrophy, optic neuropathy, retinal pigment changes, and retinal edema [62]. Patients treated with tamoxifen for a period greater than 9 months are susceptible to a crystalline retinopathy and visual impairment, although the visual impairment is generally reversible with cessation of treatment. In addition, bilateral optic neuritis with retinal hemorrhages has been reported within 3 weeks of initiating tamoxifen therapy [63].

Plant alkaloids vincristine and vinblastine may lead to visual loss and double vision secondary to optic neuropathy, optic atrophy, and cranial nerve palsies [32, 64]. Acute optic neuropathy, along with cranial nerve palsy, may also follow 5-fluorouracil treatment [6]. In addition, visual loss in the form of optic nerve damage has been attributed to fludarabine, cyclosporine, paclitaxel, nitrogen mustards, and intrathecal cytosine arabinoside [65–68]. In the three reported cases, fludarabine led to rapid, irreversible vision loss as a result of direct neurotoxicity to the retinal ganglion and bipolar cells. This was a harbinger of more generalized CNS dysfunction and death in each case [69].

Corticosteroids have been implicated in the development of pseudotumor cerebri and its associated optic nerve swelling. In addition, the immunosuppressive effects of corticosteroids may lead to opportunistic retinal infections.

### 6.8.5 Graft-Versus-Host Disease

Retinal hemorrhage occurs in 3.5–20 % of patients with GVHD as a result of GVHD vasculopathy, CMV retinitis, or recurrence of leukemic disease. Optic disk edema and cotton-wool spots are also occasionally seen [28].

### 6.8.6 Medical and Nursing Management

Retinal hemorrhages and cotton-wool spots as part of radiation retinopathy will resolve without treatment. However, they are clear indications of retinal damage and are causes for ophthalmologic referral. Retinal edema manifests as blurred vision when it affects the macula. It is diagnosed by careful slit lamp biomicroscopy with the aid of optical coherence tomography (OCT) and fluorescein angiography. Current treatment options include laser photocoagulation and corticosteroids. Intravitreal injection of bevacizumab (Avastin), an antibody to vascular endothelial growth factor, has been studied extensively in the treatment of radiation retinopathy with limited success. In the majority of studies, there is a short-term improvement in retinal edema and visual acuity, but these changes are not sustained in the long term [70]. Neovascularization, both of the iris and retina, is a manifestation of chronic retinal ischemia and is also treated with laser photocoagulation. Because diabetes mellitus and hypertension can mimic and/or potentiate radiation retinopathy, strict control of blood sugar and blood pressure should be emphasized.

The treatment of optic disk edema and optic neuropathy is controversial. While the use of systemic corticosteroids and pressure-lowering medications may be effective, discontinuing the offending agent and observation is also a viable option.

The use of OCT for screening of patients on long-term tamoxifen therapy may help to detect early signs of foveal pseudocyst formation, the cause of visual disturbance in tamoxifen retinopathy. At that point the drug should be discontinued to prevent retinal damage and visual disturbance [71].

## 6.9 Orbital Bones and Tissue

### 6.9.1 Anatomy and Physiology

The orbital cavity is composed of seven bones: the maxilla, palatine, frontal, sphenoid, zygomatic, ethmoid, and lacrimal bones. They form the shape of a quadrilateral pyramid with the

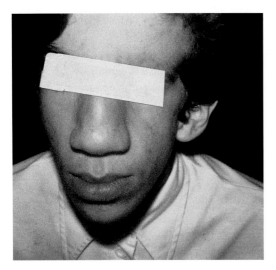

**Fig. 6.6** Orbital bone suppression

apex forming posteriorly and the medial walls parallel. The soft tissues of the orbit consist of the extraocular muscles, orbital fat, fascia, and vascular structures. The function of the orbital bones is to protect the eye, while the soft tissues act to cushion the eye and optic nerve during movement.

### 6.9.2 Acute Radiation Effects

There are no known acute radiation effects to the orbital bones.

### 6.9.3 Chronic Radiation Effects

Suppression of bony growth remains the most common chronic orbital complication of RT. The result is especially noticeable in patients treated at a young age for retinoblastoma or rhabdomyosarcoma. A hollowing of the temporal bone, stunted vertical growth of the orbit, and saddle nose (flattening and shortening of the bridge of the nose) are typical features which occur years after a dose of 40–70 Gy to the orbit, fractionated over a 3- to 7-week time period [4] (Fig. 6.6). The bony effects of radiation are reduced when treatment is delayed until 6 months or, even more so, until 1 year of age [5]. Furthermore, advanced radiation techniques, such as brachytherapy with

radioactive plaques applied directly to the eye, allow greater precision in tissue localization, thus sparing the anterior segments of the eye and uninvolved bone.

Anophthalmic socket syndrome, or soft tissue atrophy, and contracture of the socket following removal of the eye have been documented after radiotherapy in patients treated for retinoblastoma [72]. Osteonecrosis rarely results after very high doses of radiotherapy, but may be associated with concurrent orbital infections. Most devastatingly, second, non-ocular cancers may also develop in the radiation field, especially in retinoblastoma patients who are predisposed to tumor formation [73].

### 6.9.4 Chemotherapy and Immunosuppressive Agents

Intracarotid carboplatin alone or concurrent with intravenous etoposide may produce ocular pain, motility disturbance, or severe visual loss secondary to severe orbital inflammation and optic nerve ischemia [54, 74]. Periocular injection of carboplatin can cause inflammation and fibrosis of orbital tissues [26].

Both 5-fluorouracil and methotrexate therapy have also led to clinically significant periorbital edema. Corticosteroids have been shown to cause a protrusion of the globe known as exophthalmos [75]. Paralysis of the eye muscles (ophthalmoplegia) has been reported with cyclosporine [76] and vincristine, due to cranial nerve palsy [32].

### 6.9.5 Medical and Nursing Management

There is no medical treatment to reverse the retardation of bone growth due to RT. Osteonecrosis may require surgical debridement and antibiotics. Anophthalmic socket syndrome is very difficult to treat and sometimes requires orbital reconstruction surgery. Anophthalmic sockets with ocular prosthesis require regular care and cleaning with gentle soaps. The orbit itself must be examined by a medical professional periodically for the development of second malignancies. Finally, counseling should be available to patients regarding the disfiguring effects of radiation on bone growth.

Inflammation of the orbital soft tissues may be managed with intravenous corticosteroids. This could control the acute inflammatory symptoms; however, the effects on vision are often irreversible.

### Conclusion

With the advent of newer, more durable treatment options for childhood cancer, there is more incentive than ever to identify reversible ocular complications and correct them before they lead to permanent vision loss. Improvements in radiation techniques for tumors in and around the ocular structures provide the ability to conserve vision and spare the noninvolved bone, reducing the long-term effects of this highly effective treatment modality. With close follow-up and prompt referral to an ophthalmologist in necessary cases, quality of life can be vastly improved by preserving any amount of salvageable vision. Unfortunately, prolonging life often trumps sparing vision, and loss of sight is sometimes an unavoidable side effect of treating a systemic cancer. In such situations, referral to services for the blind and visually impaired can greatly improve the quality of life of long-term cancer survivors.

**Acknowledgments** Adapted from Ober MD, Servididio C, Abramson DH. Ocular Complications due to Cancer Treatment. In Schwartz C, Hobbie W, Constine L, Ruccione K., eds. Survivors of Childhood Cancer. Springer-Verlag Heidelberg

# References

1. Inamoto Y, Chai X, Kurland BF et al (2012) Validation of measurement scales in ocular graft-versus-host disease. Ophthalmology 119(3):487–493. doi:10.1016/j.ophtha.2011.08.040
2. Dietrich-Ntoukas T, Cursiefen C, Westekemper H et al (2012) Diagnosis and treatment of ocular chronic graft-versus-host disease: report from the German-Austrian-Swiss Consensus Conference on Clinical Practice in chronic GVHD. Cornea 31(3):299–310. doi:10.1097/ICO.0b013e318226bf97

3. Haik B, Jereb B, Abramson D (1983) Ophthalmic radiotherapy. In: Iliff NT (ed) Complications in ophthalmic surgery. Churchill Livingstone, New York, pp 4449–4485
4. Brady LW, Shields J, Augusburger J, Markoe A, Karlsson UL (1989) Complications from radiation therapy to the eye. Front Radiat Ther Oncol 23:238–250; discussion 251–254
5. Ober M, Beaverson K, Abramson D (2004) Ocular complications. In: Wallace H, Green D (eds) Late effects of childhood cancer. Arnold, London
6. Al-Tweigeri T, Nabholtz JM, Mackey JR (1996) Ocular toxicity and cancer chemotherapy. A review. Cancer 78(7):1359–1373. doi:10.1002/(SICI)1097-0142(19961001)78:7<1359::AID-CNCR1>3.0.CO;2-G
7. Sidi Y, Douer D, Pinkhas J (1977) Sicca syndrome in a patient with toxic reaction to busulfan. JAMA 238(18):1951
8. Prasad S, Kamath GG, Phillips RP (2000) Lacrimal canalicular stenosis associated with systemic 5-fluorouracil therapy. Acta Ophthalmol Scand 78(1):110–113. doi:10.1034/j.1600-0420.2000.078001110.x
9. Esmaeli B, Valero V, Ahmadi MA, Booser D (2001) Canalicular stenosis secondary to docetaxel (taxotere): a newly recognized side effect. Ophthalmology 108(5):994–995
10. Agarwal MR, Esmaeli B, Burnstine MA (2002) Squamous metaplasia of the canaliculi associated with 5-fluorouracil: a clinicopathologic case report. Ophthalmology 109(12):2359–2361
11. Esmaeli B, Burnstine MA, Ahmadi MA, Prieto VG (2003) Docetaxel-induced histologic changes in the lacrimal sac and the nasal mucosa. Ophthal Plast Reconstr Surg 19(4):305–308. doi:10.1097/01.IOP.0000075016.29682.E0
12. Straus DJ, Mausolf FA, Ellerby RA, McCracken JD (1977) Cicatricial ectropion secondary to 5-fluorouracil therapy. Med Pediatr Oncol 3(1):15–19
13. Miller D, Peczon JD, Whitworth CG (1965) Corticosteroids and functions in the anterior segment of the eye. Am J Ophthalmol 59:31–34
14. Dejan S, Dragana B, Ivana P, Borivoje B, Marko P (2009) Vincristine induced unilateral ptosis. J Pediatr Hematol Oncol 31(6):463. doi:10.1097/MPH.0b013e3181a7153e
15. Bay A, Yilmaz C, Yilmaz N, Oner AF (2006) Vincristine induced cranial polyneuropathy. Indian J Pediatr 73(6):531–533
16. Müller L, Kramm CM, Tenenbaum T, Wessalowski R, Göbel U (2004) Treatment of vincristine-induced bilateral ptosis with pyridoxine and pyridostigmine. Pediatr Blood Cancer 42(3):287–288. doi:10.1002/pbc.10301
17. Ogawa Y, Yamazaki K, Kuwana M et al (2001) A significant role of stromal fibroblasts in rapidly progressive dry eye in patients with chronic GVHD. Invest Ophthalmol Vis Sci 42(1):111–119
18. Franklin RM, Kenyon KR, Tutschka PJ, Saral R, Green WR, Santos GW (1983) Ocular manifestations of graft-vs-host disease. Ophthalmology 90(1):4–13

19. Kamoi M, Ogawa Y, Dogru M et al (2007) Spontaneous lacrimal punctal occlusion associated with ocular chronic graft-versus-host disease. Curr Eye Res 32(10):837–842. doi:10.1080/02713680701586409

20. Seiff SR, Shorr N, Adams T (1985) Surgical treatment of punctal-canalicular fibrosis from 5-fluorouracil therapy. Cancer 56(8):2148–2149

21. Tu AH, Chang EL (2005) Botulinum toxin for palliative treatment of epiphora in a patient with canalicular obstruction. Ophthalmology 112(8):1469–1471. doi:10.1016/j.ophtha.2005.02.022

22. Rao SN, Rao RD (2006) Efficacy of topical cyclosporine 0.05 % in the treatment of dry eye associated with graft versus host disease. Cornea 25(6):674–678. doi:10.1097/01.ico.0000208813.17367.0c

23. Malta JB, Soong HK, Shtein RM et al (2010) Treatment of ocular graft-versus-host disease with topical cyclosporine 0.05 %. Cornea 29(12):1392–1396. doi:10.1097/ICO.0b013e3181e456f0

24. Donnenfeld E, Ingraham H, Abramson D (1993) Effects of ionizing radiation on the conjunctiva, cornea, and lens. In: Alberti W, Sagerman R (eds) Radiotherapy of intraocular and orbital tumors, Medical Radiology. Springer, Berlin, pp 261–270

25. Palmer M, Hyndiuk R (2000) Toxicology of corticosteroids and other antiinflammatory agents. In: Albert D, Jakobiec F (eds) Principles and practice of ophthalmology, 2nd edn. Saunders, Philadelphia, pp 399–416

26. Marr BP, Dunkel IJ, Linker A, Abramson DH (2012) Periocular carboplatin for retinoblastoma: long-term report (12 years) on efficacy and toxicity. Br J Ophthalmol 96(6):881–883. doi:10.1136/bjophthalmol-2011-300517

27. Ogawa Y, Okamoto S, Wakui M et al (1999) Dry eye after haematopoietic stem cell transplantation. Br J Ophthalmol 83(10):1125–1130

28. Ogawa Y, Kuwana M (2003) Dry eye as a major complication associated with chronic graft-versus-host disease after hematopoietic stem cell transplantation. Cornea 22(7 Suppl):S19–S27

29. Tseng SC (1986) Topical tretinoin treatment for severe dry-eye disorders. J Am Acad Dermatol 15(4 Pt 2):860–866

30. Blodi FC (1958) The late effects of x-radiation on the cornea. Trans Am Ophthalmol Soc 56:413–450

31. Frenkel S, Hendler K, Siegal T, Shalom E, Pe'er J (2008) Intravitreal methotrexate for treating vitreoretinal lymphoma: 10 years of experience. Br J Ophthalmol 92(3):383–388. doi:10.1136/bjo.2007.127928

32. Albert DM, Wong VG, Henderson ES (1967) Ocular complications of vincristine therapy. Arch Ophthalmol 78(6):709–713

33. Kaiser-Kupfer MI, Lippman ME (1978) Tamoxifen retinopathy. Cancer Treat Rep 62(3):315–320

34. Inagaki E, Ogawa Y, Matsumoto Y, Kawakita T, Shimmura S, Tsubota K (2011) Four cases of corneal perforation in patients with chronic graft-versus-host disease. Mol Vis 17:598–606

35. Mohammadpour M (2007) Progressive corneal vascularization caused by graft-versus-host disease. Cornea 26(2):225–226. doi:10.1097/01.ico.0000243956.22275.8c

36. Ogawa Y, Okamoto S, Mori T et al (2003) Autologous serum eye drops for the treatment of severe dry eye in patients with chronic graft-versus-host disease. Bone Marrow Transplant 31(7):579–583. doi:10.1038/sj.bmt.1703862

37. Chiang C-C, Lin J-M, Chen W-L, Tsai Y-Y (2007) Allogeneic serum eye drops for the treatment of severe dry eye in patients with chronic graft-versus-host disease. Cornea 26(7):861–863. doi:10.1097/ICO.0b013e3180645cd7

38. Russo PA, Bouchard CS, Galasso JM (2007) Extended-wear silicone hydrogel soft contact lenses in the management of moderate to severe dry eye signs and symptoms secondary to graft-versus-host disease. Eye Contact Lens 33(3):144–147. doi:10.1097/01.icl.0000244154.76214.2d

39. Takahide K, Parker PM, Wu M et al (2007) Use of fluid-ventilated, gas-permeable scleral lens for management of severe keratoconjunctivitis sicca secondary to chronic graft-versus-host disease. Biol Blood Marrow Transplant 13(9):1016–1021. doi:10.1016/j.bbmt.2007.05.006

40. Ogawa Y, Okamoto S, Kuwana M et al (2001) Successful treatment of dry eye in two patients with chronic graft-versus-host disease with systemic administration of FK506 and corticosteroids. Cornea 20(4):430–434

41. Mejico LJ, Bergloeff J, Miller NR (2000) New therapies with potential neuro-ophthalmologic toxicity. Curr Opin Ophthalmol 11(6):389–394

42. Townley JR, Dana R, Jacobs DS (2011) Keratoconjunctivitis sicca manifestations in ocular graft versus host disease: pathogenesis, presentation, prevention, and treatment. Semin Ophthalmol 26(4–5):251–260. doi:10.3109/08820538.2011.588663

43. Merriam GR Jr, Focht EF (1957) A clinical study of radiation cataracts and the relationship to dose. Am J Roentgenol Radium Ther Nucl Med 77(5):759–785

44. Braver DA, Richards RD, Good TA (1967) Posterior subcapsular cataracts in steroid treated children. Arch Ophthalmol 77(2):161–162

45. Loredo A, Rodriguez RS, Murillo L (1972) Cataracts after short-term corticosteroid treatment. N Engl J Med 286(3):160. doi:10.1056/NEJM197201202860317

46. Podos SM, Canellos GP (1969) Lens changes in chronic granulocytic leukemia. Possible relationship to chemotherapy. Am J Ophthalmol 68(3):500–504

47. Gorin MB, Day R, Costantino JP et al (1998) Long-term tamoxifen citrate use and potential ocular toxicity. Am J Ophthalmol 125(4):493–501

48. Becker B (1965) Intraocular pressure response to topical corticosteroids. IOVS 4(2):198–205

49. Armaly MF (1966) The heritable nature of dexamethasone-induced ocular hypertension. Arch Ophthalmol 75(1):32–35

50. Armaly MF (1963) Effect of corticosteroids on intraocular pressure and fluid dynamics: I. The effect of dexamethasone* in the normal eye. Arch Ophthalmol 70(4):482–491. doi:10.1001/archopht.1963.00960050484010

51. Armaly MF (1963) Effect of corticosteroids on intraocular pressure and fluid dynamics: II. The effect of dexamethasone in the glaucomatous eye. Arch Ophthalmol 70(4):492–499. doi:10.1001/archopht.1963.00960050494011

52. Spaeth GL, Rodrigues MM, Weinreb S (1977) Steroid-induced glaucoma: A. Persistent elevation of intraocular pressure B. Histopathological aspects. Trans Am Ophthalmol Soc 75:353–381

53. Margo CE, Murtagh FR (1993) Ocular and orbital toxicity after intracarotid cisplatin therapy. Am J Ophthalmol 116(4):508–509

54. Watanabe W, Kuwabara R, Nakahara T et al (2002) Severe ocular and orbital toxicity after intracarotid injection of carboplatin for recurrent glioblastomas. Graefes Arch Clin Exp Ophthalmol 240(12):1033–1035. doi:10.1007/s00417-002-0573-9

55. Anderson B, Anderson B Jr (1960) Necrotizing uveitis incident to perfusion of intracranial malignancies with nitrogen mustard or related compounds. Trans Am Ophthalmol Soc 58:95–104

56. Hettinga YM, Verdonck LF, Fijnheer R, Rijkers GT, Rothova A (2007) Anterior uveitis: a manifestation of graft-versus-host disease. Ophthalmology 114(4):794–797. doi:10.1016/j.ophtha.2006.07.049

57. Brown GC, Shields JA, Sanborn G, Augsburger JJ, Savino PJ, Schatz NJ (1982) Radiation retinopathy. Ophthalmology 89(12):1494–1501

58. Shingleton BJ, Bienfang DC, Albert DM, Ensminger WD, Chandler WF, Greenberg HS (1982) Ocular toxicity associated with high-dose carmustine. Arch Ophthalmol 100(11):1766–1772

59. Miller DF, Bay JW, Lederman RJ, Purvis JD, Rogers LR, Tomsak RL (1985) Ocular and orbital toxicity following intracarotid injection of BCNU (carmustine) and cisplatinum for malignant gliomas. Ophthalmology 92(3):402–406

60. Ostrow S, Hahn D, Wiernik PH, Richards RD (1978) Ophthalmologic toxicity after cis-dichlorodiammine-platinum(II) therapy. Cancer Treat Rep 62(10):1591–1594

61. Rankin EM, Pitts JF (1993) Ophthalmic toxicity during carboplatin therapy. Ann Oncol 4(4):337–338

62. Millay RH, Klein ML, Shults WT, Dahlborg SA, Neuwelt EA (1986) Maculopathy associated with combination chemotherapy and osmotic opening of the blood-brain barrier. Am J Ophthalmol 102(5):626–632

63. Ashford AR, Donev I, Tiwari RP, Garrett TJ (1988) Reversible ocular toxicity related to tamoxifen therapy. Cancer 61(1):33–35

64. Shurin SB, Rekate HL, Annable W (1982) Optic atrophy induced by vincristine. Pediatrics 70(2):288–291

65. Porges Y, Blumen S, Fireman Z, Sternberg A, Zamir D (1998) Cyclosporine-induced optic neuropathy, ophthalmoplegia, and nystagmus in a patient with Crohn disease. Am J Ophthalmol 126(4):607–609

66. Chun HG, Leyland-Jones BR, Caryk SM, Hoth DF (1986) Central nervous system toxicity of fludarabine phosphate. Cancer Treat Rep 70(10):1225–1228

67. Capri G, Munzone E, Tarenzi E et al (1994) Optic nerve disturbances: a new form of paclitaxel neurotoxicity. J Natl Cancer Inst 86(14):1099–1101

68. Margileth DA, Poplack DG, Pizzo PA, Leventhal BG (1977) Blindness during remission in two patients with acute lymphoblastic leukemia: a possible complication of multimodality therapy. Cancer 39(1):58–61

69. Bishop RJ, Ding X, Heller CK 3rd et al (2010) Rapid vision loss associated with fludarabine administration. Retina (Philadelphia, Pa) 30(8):1272–1277. doi:10.1097/IAE.0b013e3181d20589

70. Wen JC, McCannel TA (2009) Treatment of radiation retinopathy following plaque brachytherapy for choroidal melanoma. Curr Opin Ophthalmol 20(3):200–204. doi:10.1097/ICU.0b013e328329b62d

71. Mauget-Faÿsse M, Martine M-F, Gambrelle J, Joël G, Quaranta-El Maftouhi M, Maddalena Q-EM (2006) Optical coherence tomography in tamoxifen retinopathy. Breast Cancer Res Treat 99(1):117–118. doi:10.1007/s10549-006-9187-y

72. Abramson DH (1988) The diagnosis of retinoblastoma. Bull N Y Acad Med 64(4):283–317

73. Abramson DH, Frank CM (1998) Second nonocular tumors in survivors of bilateral retinoblastoma: a possible age effect on radiation-related risk. Ophthalmology 105(4):573–579. doi:10.1016/S0161-6420(98)94006-4; discussion 579–580

74. Lauer AK, Wobig JL, Shults WT, Neuwelt EA, Wilson MW (1999) Severe ocular and orbital toxicity after intracarotid etoposide phosphate and carboplatin therapy. Am J Ophthalmol 127(2):230–233

75. Van Dalen JT, Sherman MD (1989) Corticosteroid-induced exophthalmos. Doc Ophthalmol 72(3–4):273–277

76. Bixenman WW, Nicholls JV, Warwick OH (1977) Oculomotor disturbances associated with 5-fluorouracil chemotherapy. Am J Ophthalmol 83(6):789–793

# Head and Neck

# 7

## Chrystal U. Louis and Arnold C. Paulino

## Contents

C.U. Louis, MD
Division of Pediatric Hematology/Oncology, Department
of Pediatrics, Texas Children's Cancer Center, Baylor
College of Medicine, Houston, TX, USA

A.C. Paulino, MD (✉)
Division of Pediatric Hematology/Oncology, Department
of Pediatrics, Texas Children's Cancer Center, Baylor
College of Medicine, Houston, TX, USA

Department of Radiation Oncology, MD Anderson
Cancer Center, 1515 Holcombe Blvd., Box 97,
Houston, TX 77030, USA
e-mail: apaulino@mdanderson.org

## 7.1 Introduction

Most head and neck neoplasms require a combination of chemotherapy and radiation therapy for cure as their anatomic location makes local control by surgical resection difficult. Approximately 40 % of rhabdomyosarcomas arise in this region. Ewing sarcoma, osteosarcoma, non-rhabdomyosarcoma soft tissue sarcoma, nasopharyngeal carcinoma, lymphoma, neuroblastoma, hemangioma, and histiocytosis also occur in the head and neck. However, the head and neck region is composed of multiple sensitive tissues, including the major organs for sensation (eyes, ears, nose, and mouth), mucous membranes, salivary glands, teeth, larynx, pharynx, skull base, and associated regions of the brain and the hypothalamic-pituitary axis, in which treatment-related toxicity can be associated with significant acute and long-term morbidity. The current chapter reviews the pathophysiology and clinical manifestations of the late effects in the head and neck region, outlines methods for screening and detection, and suggests interventions that can be used in their management.

## 7.2 Pathophysiology

### 7.2.1 Normal Organ Development

By the time of birth, the skin and mucous membranes, salivary glands, taste buds, bones and connective tissues, deciduous incisor crowns, and auditory apparatus are all formed. These tissues of the head and neck region arise in the embryo from branchial arches, beginning in the fourth week of gestation. Ectoderm, mesoderm, and endoderm, along with migrating neural crest cells and myoblasts, give rise to the specialized structural and functional components of this region [61].

Sixty-five percent of the growth of the mandible, maxilla, and alveolar ridge takes place from birth to puberty, with the remaining development completed by age 20. During childhood (age 4 through adulthood), mandibular growth is primarily forward, while the maxilla grows vertically. The permanent dentition and vocal cords are forming as well. The more visible front teeth develop during the preschool years, while the remaining dentition continues to develop until 16 years of age [18]. Likewise, formal differentiation of the vocal cords occurs from 2 months when the first sign of bilaminar structure of distinct cellular population appears to approximately 13 years when both elastin and collagen fibers are present [38]. Thus, therapy anytime during childhood can affect dentition and phonation. Long-term effects are dependent upon developmental status at the time of systemic therapy and radiotherapy.

## 7.2.2 Organ Damage and Developmental Effects of Cytotoxic Therapy

The head and neck comprise a complex region with multiple tissue types, including the mucosa, skin, subcutaneous tissue, salivary gland tissue, teeth, bone, and cartilage. Each has a unique response to cytotoxic therapy. In general, two types of effects are seen: (1) acute effects occur during or shortly after a course of treatment and usually involve tissues that divide rapidly, resulting in erythema and ulceration of mucosa, erythema and desquamation of skin, reduced serous output from salivary glands, and reduction of taste acuity, and (2) late effects may not manifest until months or years after therapy, in tissues that proliferate slowly. Early changes within slowly

proliferating tissues may also occur, but are usually not detected by standard methods of observation. Table 7.1 shows some of the more common late toxicities in relation to radiotherapy dose and type of systemic therapy.

### 7.2.2.1 Skin and Mucous Membranes

The skin and mucosa exhibit early epithelial damage and delayed permanent vascular injury that are dependent on the total radiation dose, the fraction size, and the volume of irradiated tissue. Early radiation injury to the skin is directly attributable to the effect of ionizing radiation on the stratum germinativum cells [27]. Release of vasoactive substances results in increased capillary permeability and dilatation that manifest as skin erythema [78]. An increase in melanin-containing cells at 2–3 weeks enhances pigmentation. Moist desquamation that occurs 3–4 weeks from the initiation of treatment has been found to correlate with the development of severe delayed telangiectasias [3]. In some situations when patients are neutropenic from chemotherapy, the acute effects of radiotherapy on the skin and mucous membranes may be more pronounced.

Late radiation effects are primarily caused by fibrosis and vascular damage, particularly to small vessels. Arterioles become narrow as a result of myointimal proliferation and destruction of capillaries and sinusoids [25]. Delayed histologic manifestations of these changes include fibrin deposition, ulceration, and fibrosis. Telangiectasias are caused by endothelial cell depletion and basement membrane damage that cause capillary loops to contract into distorted sinusoidal channels. While the incidence of mucositis in patients being treated with chemotherapy approaches 40 %, stomatotoxicity resulting from individual chemotherapeutic agents, such as methotrexate, doxorubicin, 5-fluorouracil, bleomycin, and cytosine arabinoside, has not been associated with long-term effects [77]. However, when administered in conjunction with radiotherapy, or when given in high doses as required prior to stem cell transplantation, acute injury may be enhanced, resulting in an increased risk for long-term damage. Mucositis is the end result of a multistep

**Table 7.1** Radiotherapy doses and types of chemotherapy attributed to late effects in the head and neck region

| Late effect | Radiotherapy dose | Type of systemic therapy |
|---|---|---|
| **Bone and muscle** | | |
| Hypoplasia | RT dose ≥18–24 Gy (lower dose for younger children, lower for soft tissue/muscle compared to bone) [30, 37, 44, 68, 80] | Bisphosphonates [93] |
| Trismus | RT dose >40 Gy to pterygoid and masseter muscles [51] | |
| Osteoradionecrosis | RT dose ≥60 Gy (maybe lower, >40 Gy, with dental extraction after RT) [34, 53, 55] | |
| **Skin** | | |
| Severe dermatitis | RT dose ≥40 Gy [50] | |
| Permanent epilation | Mean RT dose >46 Gy to hair follicles [53] | |
| Necrosis/ulceration | RT dose ≥70 Gy [10] | |
| **Teeth** | | |
| Growth disturbances | RT dose ≥20 Gy [44, 49, 80, 83] | Cyclophosphamide Vincristine Vinblastine [24, 40, 44, 54, 63, 66, 75, 82] |
| **Vocal cords** | | |
| Vocal cord dysfunction secondary to head and neck RT | Mean RT dose to the larynx, and lateral pharyngeal wall >65 Gy [20] | |
| Vocal cord dysfunction secondary to recurrent laryngeal nerve injury | RT dose >44 Gy [45, 46] | |
| **Salivary gland** | | |
| Xerostomia | Mean RT dose ≥24 Gy for both parotid glands treated. If one parotid gland receives <20 Gy, salivary gland dysfunction is usually not seen [16, 22, 30] | Stem cell transplantation [15] |
| **Ear** | | |
| Sensorineural hearing loss | Mean RT dose ≥35 Gy to the cochlea [33, 41, 67, 87] | Cisplatin (cumulative dose ≥360 mg/m$^2$) Carboplatin [9, 18, 90] |

process that begins with direct damage to the DNA of basal epithelial cells by chemotherapeutics and/or radiation and the generation of reactive oxygen species [81]. This damage leads to upregulation of transcription factors (i.e., nuclear factor-kappa beta proteins, NF-KB; wnt; and p53) causing the production of proinflammatory cytokines and enzymes (i.e., tumor necrosis factor-alpha, TNF-α). Mucosal injury is then amplified by both feedback loops and activation of macrophages by bacteria colonized within the mouth. Once ulcers have formed, the majority will heal on their own within 2 weeks if caused by standard chemotherapy. Those patients with mucositis secondary to radiotherapy and/or chemoradiotherapy may require 4 or more weeks after therapy is completed for recovery.

### 7.2.2.2 Bone and Connective Tissue

Irradiation of the growing bone causes injury to actively dividing mesenchymal cells, osteoblasts, and endothelial cells [26]; it also causes impairment of the osteoid formation. The long-term injury observed in irradiated growth centers includes atrophy, fibrosis of marrow spaces, and lack of osteocytes. Impaired vascularity and fibrosis of both the periosteum and endosteum can occur.

Rat models have been used to determine the mechanism of action that chemotherapeutics have on bone formation. Doxorubicin administration leads to thinning of the growth plates [27, 86]. Corticosteroids alter bone formation by suppressing osteoblastic activity [27, 91]. Historically, bone alterations secondary to methotrexate have been better investigated and are caused by disruptions of the growth plate because of reduced cartilage formation and decreased bone formation by direct toxicity of the agent to osteoblasts and bone marrow osteoprogenitor cells [27].

Toxicity within the soft tissues may also be affected by radiation. Fibrosis occurs as a consequence of increased fibroblast proliferation, combined with collagen deposition, in children whose craniofacial structures are irradiated [28]. Hypoplasia also occurs. Mucosal atrophy, reduced tissue vascularity, and tumor effects predispose to osteoradionecrosis, chondronecrosis, and soft tissue necrosis, particularly with high radiation dose/time and large irradiated volume. Interstitial implants and intraoral techniques further enhance the likelihood of such outcomes. In children receiving conventional fractionation radiotherapy (1.8–2 Gy per day), the dose of radiation to cause musculoskeletal impairment varies from approximately 20 Gy where hypoplasia of the developing muscle and bone can occur to 60 Gy where osteonecrosis and fracture may develop.

### 7.2.2.3 Salivary Glands and Taste Buds

The parotid, submandibular, and sublingual glands are the major salivary glands. Other (minor) salivary glands are variably distributed throughout the oral cavity and pharynx. In the resting state, saliva production comes primarily from the submandibular gland. With food intake, 60 % of the saliva may originate from the parotid gland. The composition of saliva produced is characteristic of the specific gland. Parotid saliva production is primarily serous, while the minor salivary glands secrete a predominantly mucous fluid that is more viscous. The submandibular and sublingual glands produce mixed mucous and serous secretions. Radiation damages the serous cells to a greater extent than it does the mucous cells and epithelium of ducts. Histopathologic changes 10–12 weeks after initiation of RT to doses of 50–70 Gy consist predominantly of serous acini loss, mild fibrosis, dilatation and distortion of ducts, and aggregation of lymphocytes and plasma cells [10]. Clinically, however, a decrease in the amount of salivary production can be seen at lower RT doses. When the salivary flow rates were measured in 88 patients with head and neck cancer, most glands that received a mean dose >24–26 Gy produced no saliva after 1 month and had no improvement in salivary production by 1 year after RT [22]. There is little evidence that standard doses of chemotherapy have a long-term effect on salivary gland function; however, a recent study noted the presence of xerostomia in the long-term survivors of stem cell transplantation in which busulfan, not radiation, was used in the preparative regimen [15, 58].

Modification in taste occurs as a result of changes in oral mucosa and saliva [57]. Patients retain the perception of sweet and salt more readily than that of sour and bitter. Dietary changes thus enhance dental decay in an environment already conducive to caries production [5]. Although the taste buds are considered relatively radioresistant, some taste alterations may be caused by damage to the microvilli.

### 7.2.2.4 Teeth

Radiotherapy (RT) effects on dentition are influenced by the developmental stage of the tooth, with the most severe disturbances occurring in children younger than 6 years of age [12, 47, 80]. Prior to morphodifferentiation and calcification, irradiation may result in agenesis. Direct irradiation at a later stage may cause microdontia, enamel hypoplasia, incomplete calcification of enamel, and arrested root development. Chemotherapeutic agents, such as cyclophosphamide, vincristine, and vinblastine, have also been shown to affect dentition, resulting in hypodontia, enamel hypoplasia, microdontia, and root malformation with the greatest individual risk factor for dental abnormalities being treated prior to the age of 5 [1, 14, 24, 40, 44, 48, 63, 66, 75, 82]. A report from the Childhood Cancer Survivor Study showed that RT dose ≥20 Gy was associated with dental abnormalities [49].

### 7.2.2.5 Ear

Children who present with primary tumors of the head and neck area or brain frequently encounter radiation to the external, internal, and middle ear during the course of their treatment [64]. Hearing loss may occur secondary to tumor involvement and extension to the auditory apparatus and may

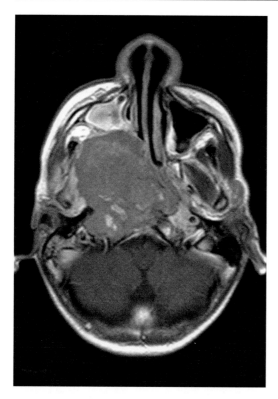

**Fig. 7.1** A 13-year-old male who presented with hearing loss (right > left), headaches, and nasal bleeding. Axial, T1-weighted, post-contrast MRI shows a large right-sided nasopharyngeal mass. Hearing loss was exacerbated after cisplatin chemotherapy radiation to the primary tumor site

effects that are most prominent in the high-frequency ranges (which can be affected significantly by radiation – see Chap. 8). For cisplatin, approximately 40–60 % of children may experience bilateral, irreversible hearing loss [62], and toxicity has been reported within 72 h of drug infusion [6]. Changes in hearing are thought to be secondary to both direct DNA damage and the generation of reactive oxygen species within the cochlea. However, as the presentation and degree of toxicity varies in patients treated with similar doses of platinum-based compounds, many groups have begun to investigate the role of pharmacogenomics and genetic variants in cisplatin-associated ototoxicity [62].

Although rare, retinoids (i.e., isotretinoin) have also been implicated in acute and permanent hearing abnormalities ranging from tinnitus to hearing loss [76].

### 7.2.2.6 Vocal Cords

There are a limited number of studies that have evaluated the progression of pediatric vocal cord development. Hartnick et al. described the pathologic changes seen in necroscopy sections from children 0 to 18 years of age and noted that at birth, only a hypercellular monolayer within the lamina propria exists [38]. It was not until the ages of 11–12 that three distinct layers could be found on the autopsy samples: a hypocellular superficial layer, a middle layer consisting of elastin, and a deeper layer of collagen fibers (Table 7.2). Although only microscopic analysis was studied, the assumption proposed by the authors was that an increasing complexity of mechanical stimulation required of the vocal cords as children grow leads to cellular differentiation [38]. This suggests that patients with head and neck tumors may be more at risk for vocal cord injuries secondary to direct tissue toxicity or neuronal toxicity during early development.

To date, the most common cause of unilateral or bilateral vocal cord paralysis is trauma to the recurrent laryngeal nerves. Due to its longer length and proximity to many thoracic structures, unilateral paralysis is more likely to occur on the left. Patients with unilateral paralysis are typically hoarse, but may present with symptoms of stridor. For patients with bilateral paralysis,

be treatment related (Fig. 7.1). There can be effects on the otic structures, both during the treatment sessions and months to years following therapy. The immediate effect on the ear is desquamation of the columnar epithelium, which lines the ears and covers the ossicles, leading to edema of the mucosa within the ear. Altered production of cerumen, in conjunction with epithelial desquamation, leads to plugging of the ear canals that may persist long after completion of therapy. More chronic effects from fibrosis and scarring can lead to chronic radiation otitis and hearing loss. Hearing loss secondary to radiation therapy is usually permanent and can be sensorineural or conductive, depending on the structures affected by the radiation. Direct effects of radiation on the cartilaginous structures can lead to stenosis or necrosis of the ear canal and external ear.

As noted in Table 7.1, cisplatin and carboplatin have dose-dependent, long-term sensorineural

**Table 7.2** Development and maturation of the vocal cord according to age

| Age | Developmental event |
| --- | --- |
| Birth | Hypercellular monolayer within the human vocal fold lamina propria |
| 2 months | Cellular differentiation and development of bilaminar structure (hypocellular superficial layer and deeper hypercellular layer) |
| 11 months | Three-layer structure (superficial hypocellular layer below by epithelial layer and a deeper hypercellular layer) is first noted and found in approximately 20 % of subjects |
| 7 years | Three-layer lamina propria structure seen in all cases |
| 11–12 years | Classic vocal ligament is identified with maturation of vocal folds and fiber deposition. There now exists the classic pattern of a hypocellular superficial layer followed by a middle layer of predominantly elastin fibers and a deeper layer of predominantly collagen fibers |

From Ref. [38]

clinical symptomatology is directly related to the position of the cords: airway obstruction occurs if the cords are closer together (near midline), as compared to aspiration, hoarseness, or the inability to speak if the cords are further apart (lateral positioning). Patients that suffer from vocal cord paresis, in which some function of the cords is maintained, may present with high-pitched stridor and a normal voice as the adductor muscles typically work better than the abductor muscles with this type of injury.

Although rare, acute vocal cord paralysis has been reported after treatment with vinca alkaloids and includes both unilateral [7] and bilateral [2] paralyses. It is speculated that the neuropathogenesis secondary to vincristine is due to the disruption of microtubule formation after it binds to $\alpha$-tubulin [2].

## 7.3 Clinical Manifestation of Late Effects

### 7.3.1 Skin and Mucous Membranes

Mucosal atrophy after conventionally fractionated doses of 60–70 Gy over a period of 6–7 weeks is common, but necrosis, chronic ulceration, and bone exposure rarely occur unless large daily doses are delivered or the total dose exceeds 70 Gy in 7 weeks [10]. Thrombosis of small blood vessels in the submucosa results in ischemia and the consequent appearance of ulcers and telangiectasias. This condition may become apparent as soon as 6 months after irradiation or as late as 1–5 years and is irreversible. Scarring and fibrosis of the nasal mucosa can alter sinus drainage and predispose patients to persistent rhinosinusitis. Children may complain of symptoms of chronic sinusitis, which include chronic nasal discharge, postnasal drip, headache, and facial pain. Smell acuity is significantly affected by radiation treatment of the olfactory mucosa, and, although this is not usually voiced as a specific complaint, it can contribute to decreased appetite and poor nutrition.

Severe skin reactions, including permanent hyperpigmentation, telangiectasias, and skin ulcerations, are rarely seen with the use of modern-day megavoltage RT, unless the skin is intentionally treated with a high dose. A recent study showed that increasing RT dose and skin volume receiving >40 Gy were associated with the severity of radiation dermatitis in children receiving RT for sarcoma [49]. Another study compared children with nasopharyngeal carcinoma treated with conventional and intensity-modulated RT (IMRT). Both grade 3 skin (47.1 % vs. 5.3 %) and mucous membrane (52.9 % vs. 15.8 %) were found to be higher in the conventional RT compared to IMRT-treated patients [51]. Doxorubicin and actinomycin can interact with radiation to produce severe skin reactions and may contribute to late skin effects. When these drugs are given early in the course of radiation, such reactions may be seen after low doses of 20–30 Gy. These and other chemotherapeutics (i.e., capecitabine, gemcitabine, melphalan, docetaxel), if delivered after radiation, can be associated with either "radiation sensitivity" or "radiation recall," in which skin reactions appear in the treated field [8, 19, 35]. Typically radiation sensitivity is defined by a time interval of <7 days between the end of radiation and the start of chemotherapy, and recall is reserved for intervals greater than 1 week apart [8]. The skin often remains chronically dry due to damage to the sebaceous and eccrine glands. The sebaceous glands are as radiosensitive as the basal epithelial cells of hair follicles; eccrine glands are less sensitive [36].

Epilation within the treatment field usually occurs 2–3 weeks into the course of radiation treatment. The permanency of the hair loss depends on the total dose of radiation delivered to the hair follicles, and this, in turn, depends on the treatment technique and beam energy. Single fraction doses of 7–8 Gy or more and total doses (after fractionated therapy) of greater than 45 Gy can result in permanent hair loss [53]. Hair loss is common with chemotherapy. After chemotherapy treatments have been concluded, hair begins to regrow within 1–2 months. It may be lighter in color and have a finer texture [26]. Microscopic analysis of hair samples of patients receiving chemotherapy has shown fracture and splitting of the hair cortex and decrease in diameter and depigmentation of the hair shaft, all of which may account for the changes in color and texture [65].

## 7.3.2 Bone and Connective Tissue

Clinical manifestations of radiation include hypoplasia, deformities, fracture, and necrosis [39, 73]. The age at which RT is given is the most important factor determining orbital growth retardation in tumors like retinoblastoma. As the orbit has three growth spurts, the first between 0 and 2 months, the second between 6 and 8 months, and the third during adolescence, radiation in children younger than 6 months of age is more damaging to orbital growth than if administered at an older age [43].

The craniofacial development of children is affected, resulting in reduced temporomandibular joint mobility, growth retardation, and osteoradionecrosis [13]. Impaired growth of the mandible and facial bones can contribute to malocclusion. Eventual fibrosis of the temporomandibular joint results in muscle pain and headaches [14]. Tumor invasion of the temporomandibular joint, surgery, and the use of large daily fractions further increase the risk of radiation-induced trismus. Combined modality therapy has a greater impact on facial structures when radiation doses are high as children receiving doses of 24 Gy or less to the temporomandibular joint have not demonstrated

clinical signs of trismus [56]. Maxillary and mandibular hypoplasias are also common dento-maxillofacial defects after chemoradiation. Linear cephalometric values suggest that the growth of the mandible may be more affected than that of the maxilla [60].

Overall, the facial skeleton appears to be the most susceptible to high radiation doses before age 6 and at puberty, which are critical times of skeletal development. In a study of 26 children receiving a mean dose of 54 Gy for either nasopharyngeal cancer or rhabdomyosarcoma, cephalometric measurements utilizing CT showed deviations in the cranial vault, anterior and mid-interorbital distances, and lateral orbital wall length, compared with normal skulls [17]. Figure 7.2 shows an example of bony and muscular hypoplasia after surgery and two radiotherapy courses for rhabdomyosarcoma.

Chemotherapy may also affect the growing skeleton. A recent review of the alterations in height for long-term survivors of acute lymphoblastic leukemia noted that chemotherapy administration was associated with a decrease in height during treatment; that the use of intensive chemotherapy leads to a long-term decrease in height that can be worsened if patients also received radiotherapy; and that young children are more at risk for severe height loss [88].

Rhabdomyosarcoma of the head and neck is a condition in which the long-term side effects of combined modality therapy have been extensively studied. Late side effects in children treated with combined modality therapy for head and neck rhabdomyosarcoma are usually seen within the first 10 years after treatment [68], given that the most will have experienced their pubertal growth by that time. Clinical or radiographic dentofacial abnormalities have been observed in 80 % of long-term survivors [24]. Abnormalities including enamel defects, bony hypoplasia/facial asymmetry, trismus, velopharyngeal incompetence, tooth/root agenesis, and disturbance in root formation were the most common findings. The largest report on the late effects in pediatric head and neck rhabdomyosarcoma comes from IRS II and IRS III, in which 213 patients were followed for a median length of 7 years. Seventy-seven percent had one or more late sequelae, including poor statural growth,

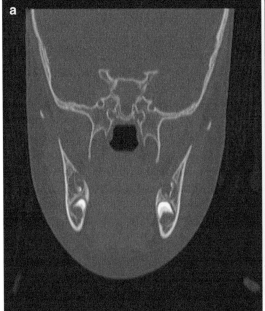 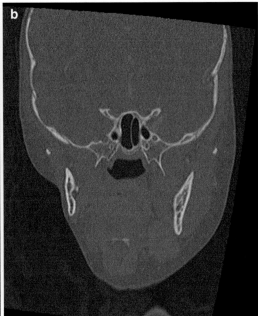

**Fig. 7.2** (**a**) Reformatted CT with contrast of the neck in a 3.5-year-old female prior to therapy. (**b**) The image details both bony and soft tissue changes including hypoplasia of the right hemi-mandible and pterygoid and masseter muscles in a 7.5-year-old female with a history of recurrent right cheek rhabdomyosarcoma. She received 5,040 cGy to the area at 2 years of age, and after a local recurrence, with positive post-resection margins, she received another 4,140 cGy to the right cheek

facial and nuchal asymmetry, dental abnormalities, and vision/hearing dysfunction [74].

Cosmetic effects become more apparent as normal growth proceeds in adjacent unirradiated areas. In 1983, Guyuron et al. reported on 41 patients who had been treated as children with RT to the head and face. They noted that hypoplastic development of the soft tissue and bone was a common finding [37]. Irradiation of the cranial base was often correlated with soft tissue deficits in the upper face and midface. Soft tissue was more vulnerable to RT than growing facial bones, with a threshold dose as low as 4 Gy (in contrast to 30 Gy for facial bones). In 1984, Jaffe reported on the maxillofacial abnormalities seen in 45 patients who had been treated as children with megavoltage RT for lymphoma, leukemia, rhabdomyosarcoma, and miscellaneous tumors [44]. Forty-three of the 45 patients also received chemotherapy (including vincristine, actinomycin D, cyclophosphamide, methotrexate, 6-mercaptopurine, prednisone, procarbazine, or nitrogen mustard in various combinations). In 82 % of the radiated patients, dental and maxillofacial abnormalities were detected, including trismus, abnormal occlusal relationships, and facial deformities. The most severe radiation deformities were seen in younger patients who received higher radiation doses.

Paulino found that 11 of 15 children treated for head and neck rhabdomyosarcoma with RT and chemotherapy developed facial asymmetry in the RT field at doses between 44 and 60 Gy [68]. Sonis studied 97 patients with acute lymphoblastic leukemia (ALL) who received either chemotherapy alone or with 18–24 Gy cranial RT [80]. The treatment fields routinely included the temporomandibular joints, posterior tooth buds, and the ramus of the mandible. A significant dose-effect relationship was seen between 18 and 24 Gy (2 Gy/fraction). Children under the age of 5 who received 24 Gy of cranial RT and chemotherapy had a 90 % incidence of craniofacial abnormalities, but no craniofacial abnormalities were seen in children over the age of 5 or in those receiving only 18 Gy of cranial RT and chemotherapy. No craniofacial abnormalities were noted after chemotherapy alone. It is unlikely that chemotherapy alone contributes to bony or soft tissue abnormalities, although it clearly does affect dental development in relation to age at treatment [59, 63]. Although amifostine, a radio-protective agent, has been demonstrated to reduce craniofacial growth inhibition in immature rabbits, evidence for its applicability in humans is lacking [29].

Radiation therapy also has an effect on wound healing that may be critical for those who require a surgical procedure in the irradiated region [18]. RT may also affect the connective tissues and bone, leading to fibrosis and osteoradionecrosis. In the Fromm series, two patients developed temporomandibular joint fibrosis with limitation of jaw motion [30]. While many studies have documented the appearance of bone hypoplasia in the dose range of 18–24 Gy, limited information is available regarding RT dose to the mandibular muscles (pterygoid and masseter) and its effect on jaw dysfunction including trismus. Krasin and colleagues found that for each 10 % of mandibular muscle volume treated above 40 Gy, a 2 mm reduction in jaw depression was seen [50]. Osteoradionecrosis has been well described in the adult head and neck literature; however, little has been written on its incidence in the pediatric population. Osteoradionecrosis usually develops in the mandible, and its risk is directly correlated with total radiation dose, fractionation dose, tumor size, and bony involvement by the tumor. In the adult literature, osteoradionecrosis is uncommon at mandibular doses <60 Gy. The incidence of osteoradionecrosis for adult head and neck cancer patients ranges from 5 % to 10 % in most series [54]. In one study, the incidence was 1.2 % for all head and neck and 5.5 % for oral cavity sites using IMRT. Maximum mandibular dose >70 Gy and mean mandibular dose >40 Gy correlated with dental extractions after IMRT [34]. In a small single-center review of the long-term effects of IMRT and platinum-based chemotherapy in pediatric patients with nasopharyngeal carcinoma (NPC), Louis et al. noted that while all patients experienced toxicity in at least three body systems, two of the five patients developed osteoradionecrosis of the mandible [55]. Historically, this risk is increased in patients who received postirradiation dental extraction, compared with pre-irradiation extraction. It is believed that radiation is associated with decreased blood flow and oxygen levels, consequently compromising tissue repair. An example of osteoradionecrosis in a nasopharyngeal patient treated with radiotherapy is shown in Fig. 7.3.

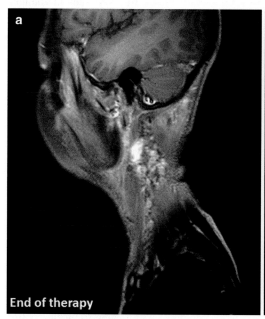
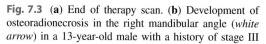
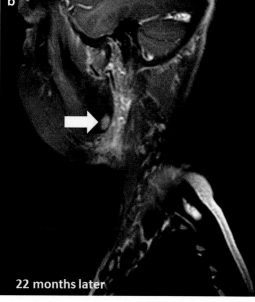

**Fig. 7.3** (**a**) End of therapy scan. (**b**) Development of osteoradionecrosis in the right mandibular angle (*white arrow*) in a 13-year-old male with a history of stage III nasopharyngeal carcinoma 22 months after treatment with induction chemotherapy and cisplatin-based chemoradiotherapy, delivering 61.2 Gy in 34 fractions

Bisphosphonate-related osteonecrosis of the jaw has also been reported. The median onset of bisphosphonate-related osteonecrosis of the jaw was 21 months with zoledronic acid, 30 with pamidronate, and 36 with zoledronic acid and pamidronate [93].

### 7.3.3 Salivary Glands and Taste Buds

Salivary gland dysfunction may occur when one or more of the major salivary glands are irradiated. Permanent damage can lead to xerostomia, predisposing to dental caries, decay, and osteoradionecrosis. Studies of salivary function in children after RT are limited [52]. Fromm found that 8 of 11 parotid glands that received >45 Gy to more than 50 % of the gland volume failed to secrete saliva, whereas all parotid glands receiving 40 Gy retained the ability to secrete [30]. More recent studies in adult patients have shown a lower dose-response effect. In 2010, Deasy summarized the data from published manuscripts evaluating salivary function as related to radiation dose-volume parameters and noted that a minimal reduction of function is seen with doses to the parotid glands of <10–15 Gy, a gradual decrease in function with doses between 20 and 40 Gy, and severe (>75 %) reduction with doses >40 Gy [16]. The use of amifostine, as a radioprotector for xerostomia, is gaining popularity in the pediatric oncology community despite limited experience in children. Currently, patients on Children's Oncology Group Protocol ARAR0331, treatment of nasopharyngeal cancer with neoadjuvant chemotherapy followed by concomitant chemoradiotherapy, are given amifostine prior to their daily RT dose. This practice is an extrapolation of results from randomized trials in adult oncology which shows the efficacy of amifostine in reducing acute and late xerostomia without compromising locoregional disease control [79, 92].

Chemotherapy for children with acute leukemia alters salivary function [58]. Mansson-Rahemtulla and colleagues showed decreased thiocyanate concentration in saliva following cyto-toxic chemotherapy, which can lead to alteration in function of the salivary peroxidase system, as well as increased oral complications. Patients who undergo bone marrow transplantation are also at risk. Xerostomia, as has been noted in patients with chronic graft-versus-host disease, can persist for as long as a year and results in a high risk for developing dental caries [4]. Although only one of five children with NPC reported in the Louis et al. cohort reported xerostomia immediately after chemotherapy, four of five had symptoms noted during their long-term follow-up [55].

### 7.3.4 Teeth

Late effects on dentition in children can be attributed directly to the cytotoxic effects on the growing tooth buds and indirectly to salivary gland damage. Salivary gland damage results in a pronounced shift toward highly acidogenic and cariogenic oral microflora, which promotes dental caries [10]. The severity and frequency of long-term dental complications due to RT are related to the type of RT given, the total dose, the size and location of RT fields, and the age of the patient. Growing tooth buds may be arrested with <10 Gy, while doses >10 Gy can completely destroy buds [57]. Root shortening, abnormal curvature, dwarfism, and hypocalcification are noted with doses of 20–40 Gy [44, 80].

Age at the time when chemotherapy is administered does influence the degree of dental effects, which is most pronounced in children treated at less than 5 years of age. All such children <5 years have V-shaped roots, compared with 36 % of those older than 5 years. Blunted roots occur in 12 % of children treated when less than 5 years old as compared to 9 % of those older than 5 years [80]. Jaffe reported that 5 of 23 children treated with chemotherapy for non-head and neck tumors had acquired amelogenesis imperfecta, microdontia of bicuspid teeth, and thinning of roots with an enlarged pulp chamber [44]. Similarly, Alpaslan found significant differences in plaque index, enamel hypoplasias, discolorations, and agenesis in 30 chemotherapy-treated survivors, compared with matched healthy control subjects [1]. Age at the time of RT is likewise important in the development of dental complications. A recent study showed that the most severe dental toxicity using proton therapy was seen in children receiving >20 Gy CGE at ages <4 years during treatment [83]. Children treated with both RT and chemotherapy likewise may develop dental complications. One study showed that all children with head and neck rhabdomyosarcoma receiving RT to developing teeth, the alveolar portion of the mandible, or the lingual surface of the maxilla developed dental abnormalities, including microdontia, root stunting, and dental caries [68]. Kaste found radiographically identifiable dental abnormalities, including agenesis, microdontia, and root stunting in 77 % of children with head and neck rhabdomyosarcoma treated with chemotherapy and RT [47].

Information regarding dental outcome after bone marrow transplantation (BMT) is limited [11, 21, 40, 85]. Neuroblastoma patients who received 12 Gy fractionated total body irradiation (TBI)-based or non-TBI-based transplants were not different in the incidence of microdontia and missing teeth [40], although TBI was associated with more severe root defects and a higher chance of permanent damage to teeth. The incidence of tooth abnormalities, including agenesis, was 62.9 % in another study in which most of the children were treated with a TBI-based BMT regimen [85].

### 7.3.5  Ear

RT has long been associated with various forms of ototoxicity. The exact mechanism of radiation-induced ototoxicity is unknown. Some physicians hypothesize that direct damage to the ossicles and tympanic membrane may lead to conductive hearing loss and fibrosis. Direct damage to the cochlea may also be seen. Other physicians believe that late radiation effects to small vessels cause hypoxia to inner ear structures, leading to hearing loss. Damage to the brainstem through radiation may also lead indirectly to hearing loss.

In categorizing deleterious effects of radiation on the ear, three clinical syndromes are found [33, 67]. The first of these is acute radiation otitis.

The effects of acute radiation otitis can be seen during or shortly after the completion of radiation. It is associated primarily with erythema of the tympanic membrane and external canal and occasionally with middle ear effusion and tinnitus. Radiation doses equal to or greater than 30 Gy have been implicated. According to some studies, 15–30 % of pediatric patients will be affected. Acute radiation otitis is usually self-limiting but in severe cases requires further therapy. The second, and most common, clinical syndrome is that of chronic radiation otitis. Clinically, patients present with dry cerumen, thickened tympanic membrane, and, occasionally, slight hearing loss (both conductive and sensorineural) several months after RT has been completed. Radiation doses of 45–65 Gy are required, and in some studies this syndrome has been found in up to 70 % of patients receiving radiation therapy [67]. The third and most rarely seen clinical syndrome is late radiation-associated deafness. In this case, patients have been treated with radiation to the brainstem or the ear. They experience an irreversible, unilateral, profound hearing loss, which may progress over weeks or months to the contralateral ear. Symptoms tend to occur 3–10 years following RT [67].

Specific antineoplastic agents have been shown to enhance the ototoxic effects of radiotherapy. In particular, the platinum-based agents, cisplatin and carboplatin, have well-documented effects on hearing with radiation having been shown to be synergistic in terms of ototoxicity. Children with primary brain tumors, NPC, osteosarcoma, germ cell tumors, and neuroblastoma are most at risk for this added ototoxicity, because they are more likely to receive platinum-based chemotherapy, and some may require RT as well. The mechanisms of ototoxicity related to platinum-based chemotherapy are thought to be secondary to direct damage to the cochlea [62]. Cisplatin ototoxicity has been reported in 9–91 % of patients, depending on the dose, duration, and circumstances surrounding its use. The initial effects are on high-frequency hearing (above 8,000 Hz), but lower frequencies can also be affected at higher doses. In one study, 14 of 25 children who received a cumulative cisplatin dose of 474 mg/m$^2$ developed hearing loss in the 250–2,000 Hz range, while only 4 of 29 children had hearing loss in the same range with a cumulative dose of 410 mg/m$^2$ [9]. Hearing loss with cisplatin is generally irreversible and bilateral. Cohen et al. have shown that the threshold for high-frequency hearing loss in patients receiving cisplatin is lower than for patients who have brain tumors treated with RT [9]. Information regarding the effects of timing the treatment with platinum-based chemotherapy and RT on patients has not been well characterized. Walker hypothesized that RT given concurrently with or prior to cisplatin administration was associated with a worsening of hearing [90].

More recent advances in RT and newer generation platinum compounds like oxaliplatin may lead to fewer ear-related, treatment-induced effects. Due to the precise delivery of RT with the conformal techniques, patients can receive full doses to the target volume while receiving lower doses to the auditory structures [31, 70]. Intensity-modulated radiation therapy (IMRT) and 3D conformal radiotherapy (3D CRT) have been associated with reduced ototoxicity in pediatric patients receiving RT and cisplatin for the treatment of medulloblastoma [42, 69], although the projected estimate for hearing loss in NPC patients being treated with cisplatin-based chemoradiotherapy (using either IMRT or CRT) approach is 60 %. Paulino and colleagues found that patients without ototoxicity after cisplatin and IMRT for medulloblastoma all received mean cochlear doses <43 Gy. The mean cochlear dose also correlated with the degree of ototoxicity; the mean cochlear dose was 34.3, 35.6, 36.8, 37.0, and 47.9 for grades 0, 1, 2, 3, and 4, respectively [69]. In the absence of chemotherapy, Hua and colleagues reported that a mean cochlear dose of ≤30 Gy was found to have a low incidence, while mean doses of >40–45 Gy were associated with increased incidence of hearing loss. The authors recommend a cumulative cochlear mean dose of <35 Gy for brain tumor patients receiving 54–59.4 Gy in 30–22 fractions [41]. The high-frequency range is likewise more likely to be affected than the low-frequency range in radiation-induced ototoxicity [41].

## 7.3.6　Vocal Cords

Long-term toxicity to the vocal cords, larynx, and pharynx after treatment for cancer has been linked to curative doses of radiotherapy. Voice quality is related to proper functioning of the vocal cords, pharyngeal lubrication, as well as the presence of adequate saliva. Vocal dysfunction is thought to be secondary to doses delivered to the larynx, pharynx, and oral cavity [32]. Radiotherapy just to the vocal cords at doses 60–66 Gy without chemotherapy usually results in good voice outcome in adult patients with stage I laryngeal cancer [89]. Dornfeld and colleagues found that doses >66 Gy to the false vocal cords and lateral pharyngeal walls were associated with decrease in speech-related quality of life scores [20].

Another mechanism for vocal cord dysfunction is recurrent laryngeal nerve injury. Unilateral vocal cord paralysis was identified in 5 % of patients treated with 44 Gy to parasternal, axillary, and supraclavicular lymph nodes after radical mastectomy in patients with breast cancer [46]. All of the patients presented with hoarseness and had left-sided involvement based on visual exam. Of note, the first patient presented 10 years after therapy was completed and the last 25 years of posttreatment. The authors felt that the etiology was radiation-induced damage to the mediastinal portion of the recurrent laryngeal nerve leading to left-sided vocal cord paralysis [46]. However, Jaruchinda et al. found a quicker time of onset in their cohort of 70 patients with head and neck carcinoma treated with ≥60 Gy. They reported a 10 % incidence of vocal cord palsy (five with paralysis and two with paresis) that developed within 14–35 months of completing radiotherapy. But, similar to the breast cancer patients, all had unilateral involvement, and 100 % presented with a hoarse voice [45]. Although there is almost a 10-year difference in the time to presentation, these papers do stress the importance of direct laryngoscopy in patients presenting with voice changes at any point after radiation therapy.

Two other symptoms reported in 28 % of those with vocal cord palsy in the Jaruchinda study were dysphagia and aspiration [45]. In 2010, Rancati et al. summarized the recent publications specific to radiation dose-volume effects in dysphagia and aspiration [72]. The authors noted that as swallowing is a complex procedure, it has been difficult to determine how to assess which radiation fields and anatomic locations are the most important to study. But based on the limited data available, the risk for dysphagia and aspiration increases with increasing volumes of the larynx and pharyngeal constrictor muscles that receive ≥60 Gy, and decreasing volumetric exposure to ≥50 Gy, when possible, is associated with less symptomatology [72].

## 7.4 Detection and Screening

The successful evaluation, diagnosis, and management of late effects require a multidisciplinary approach. All children with head and neck cancers need prolonged follow-up by a pediatric oncologist and radiation oncologist. They must also have access to specialists in endocrinology, ophthalmology, otolaryngology, and dentistry. In addition, psychological counseling should be available, as some of these children have suffered trauma secondary to cosmetic changes from tumor and/or treatment. Abnormalities in any of the head and neck or dental structures should be noted at diagnosis and prior to treatment. In general, it is preferable to perform tooth extractions prior rather than after RT to decrease the chance of osteoradionecrosis. Children with head and neck cancers should receive at least an annual assessment of growth, pubertal status, endocrine and growth function, as well as frequent ophthalmologic and dental exams.

The initial dental exam for children who have received chemotherapy and RT should consist of a full series of radiographs, including periapical, bitewing, and panoramic views of the teeth. Asymptomatic patients are often found on radiographic exam to have dental disease. Horizontal and vertical alveolar bone loss, retained root tips, deep caries, and periapical pathology can usually be visualized only on intraoral radiographs [71]. It is critical to assess crown and root development, as abnormalities can predispose a tooth to premature loss. Changes in root development are critically important to recognize, as they may affect decisions to recommend the removal of permanent teeth prior to the initiation of radiation therapy. To assess abnormal tooth and root development, it is recommended that patients receive a dental exam every 6 months, with special attention to early caries, periodontal disease, and gingivitis. Careful evaluation of root and crown status is required before tooth extraction and endodontic and orthodontic procedures. With time, the risk of periodontal bone loss increases, and it is, therefore, critical that proper periodontal prophylaxis be offered to patients, including professional cleaning with fluoride applications and meticulous oral hygiene [94]. When areas of the periodontium exposed to radiation are treated, or in cases where the risk of infection is increased with trauma, antibiotics may be given.

Radiation-induced changes in salivary pH and quantity produce an environment conducive to the development of caries. Xerostomia and a high-carbohydrate diet can predispose the pediatric cancer patient to radiation-induced caries. Frequent dental visits to identify early caries, periodontal disease infection, gingival recession, and soft tissue ulcers are important. Salivary flow studies are helpful in assessing xerostomia, and salivary substitutes containing the enzymes (lactoperoxidase, glucose oxidase, and lysozyme) such as mouthwashes, aerosolized sprays, toothpaste, chewing gums, and sialogogues like pilocarpine may be offered to symptomatic patients. Nutritional counseling on the importance of avoiding fermentable carbohydrates and maintaining excellent oral hygiene is critical. Mouth rinsing is essential, and daily topical fluoride applications (i.e., solution for mouth rinsing) are all effective in reducing the risk of radiation caries [23].

In children who have received high doses of radiation to the developing facial bones and soft tissues, the use of screening to identify craniofacial abnormalities and problems with jaw movement is important for early detection and management. Trismus, crepitus, limited mandibular movement, and abnormal growth associated with the temporomandibular joint may be present

[56] and should be evaluated at both clinical follow-up and dental visits.

Routine ear, nose, and throat evaluation, including inspection of the oral mucosa for ulcers, indirect and direct laryngoscopy, and nasopharyngoscopy may be included in the screening process to ensure a thorough assessment of the mucosa. It is important to look for nasal scarring, as this may interfere with the normal movement of mucus and sinus drainage, leading to recurrent sinusitis. The soft tissue of the head and neck should be evaluated for muscle hypoplasia, fibrosis, and ulceration. Irradiated skin often has impaired vascularity, and the resultant "thin skin" is highly susceptible to minor trauma.

Both an otoscopic exam and inspection of the auricle are necessary to rule out the presence of otitis externa and chondronecrosis, respectively. Detailed inspection of the ear canal can detect cerumen impaction and tympanic scarring, both of which can lead to conductive hearing loss. In addition, the patient should be evaluated for the possible presence of otitis media or tympanic membrane perforation. Children who received cisplatin, high-dose carboplatin, or radiation doses ≥30 Gy to the inner ear should have complete audiology examinations, with hearing screening, upon starting long-term follow-up and at least yearly, or as determined per the audiologist, if hearing loss is detected [94]. Finally, the physician following a child cured from cancer should always be aware of the possibility of secondary malignancies, particularly in irradiated fields.

## 7.5 Management of Established Problems and Rehabilitation

### 7.5.1 Oral Cavity

One of the best ways to manage late effects of the teeth is preventative care. Ideally, all patients should undergo a dental evaluation and treatment of any existing dental problems prior to undergoing treatment for cancer. Patients who are younger at diagnosis and who have received higher radiation doses will require more watchful attention for future problems. Patients should

have dental exams and cleanings every 6 months, and these should include fluoride applications [23]. For those who develop malocclusion or other structural abnormalities and/or the need for tooth extraction, consultation with an orthodontist who has experience in the management of childhood cancer survivors who have undergone irradiation is preferred. All patients should have at least a baseline panorex examination prior to dental procedures to evaluate their root development, since root thinning and shortening occur fairly frequently. Symptomatic treatment of temporomandibular joint dysfunction may be required and involve exercises and pain control.

When major periodontal disease is present, care should be taken to minimize trauma to the oral cavity. Oral infections that occur after procedures should be aggressively treated with antibiotics. Care should be taken to avoid tight sutures and trauma during use of orthodontics.

Patients should be evaluated yearly for xerostomia, and symptomatic care with saliva substitutes, moistening agents, and sialogogues may be required. Fungal infections are more likely to occur in patients with xerostomia, so special care should be taken to treat with appropriate antifungal medications, either topically or systemically.

### 7.5.2 Bone and Connective Tissue Disease

Many bone and connective tissue late effects may require extensive surgical correction, often staged procedures, spanning many months to years. A craniofacial team, consisting of a head and neck plastic surgeon and neurosurgeon, may be necessary in restoring function and cosmesis to an affected child.

Patients who have experienced radiation to the region requiring operation will also experience poor wound healing and increased susceptibility to infection. Patients who develop infections of the soft tissue regions will require not only aggressive antibiotic therapy, but also possible surgical debridement and supportive care of pain and swelling. Soft tissue and bone necrosis can be devastating to the patient, both physically and psychologically, so measures should be taken to prevent trauma to the areas affected by radiation.

Chronic sinusitis is more likely to occur in patients who have a history of atopy or hypogammaglobulinemia. Aggressive management of sinus infections with the guidance of ENT specialists is required. Patients should have their sinuses evaluated at least yearly by history and physical exam, and CT of the sinuses should be obtained as clinically indicated.

### 7.5.3 Ears

Younger patients and those who have received higher radiation doses are more likely to experience sclerotic side effects and eustachian tube dysfunction. They are also at greater risk for developing sensorineural hearing loss. Patients should have audiograms or brainstem auditory-evoked response (BAER) tests performed yearly or as clinically indicated. Speech and language evaluations should be performed at the end of treatment and as needed for clinical concerns. Those children with hearing loss will require routine speech and language therapies. Special educational interventions may be required as well, including alternative learning methods, individualized education plans (IEP), and preferential seating in the classroom. Table 7.3 lists various amplification and assisted living devices currently available. The

Table 7.3 Amplification and assisted listening devices for children with hearing loss

| Amplification |
| --- |
| Conventional analog hearing aid |
| Digital hearing aid |
| Bone conduction hearing aid |
| Bone anchored hearing aid |
| Bone and air conduction spectacles/eyeglasses |
| Assisted listening devices and personal systems |
| FM trainers |
| Telephone devices with volume controls and couplers for hearing aids |
| Closed captioning television |
| Signaling devices |
| Bluetooth wireless devices |

use of a hearing aid can help amplify any residual hearing. Personal devices, such as FM trainers, can aid in reducing the signal-to-noise ratio in various listening situations like the classroom, where there may be significant background noise.

For those suffering with chronic otitis, ENT referral is indicated. Treatment usually includes antibiotic therapy, myringotomy, and/or the placement of pressure-equalizing tubes. Chronic cerumen and obstruction of the ear canal will require routine cleaning and the use of agents to soften the cerumen. Some patients may require treatment for otitis externa with the use of topical otic drops. These patients should avoid submersion in water without protective earplugs.

### 7.5.4 Vocal Cord Dysfunction

Little is known about the management of vocal dysfunction in children. In adults, voice rehabilitation has been employed in some patients after RT. A Swedish trial investigated the utility of voice rehabilitation consisting of a 10-week protocol of relaxation, respiration, posture, and phonation exercises. There was a trend toward better improvement of voice quality and self-perceived function in patients who received voice rehabilitation compared to a control group that did not [84]. Some of the other measures that may improve voice quality in patients whose larynx has been irradiated include avoiding smoking or secondhand smoke which can make laryngeal edema worse and decreasing the amount of talking during the treatment course as this seems to affect the amount of time for voice recovery [92].

### References

1. Alpaslan G et al (1999) Disturbances in oral and dental structures in patients with pediatric lymphoma after chemotherapy: a preliminary report. Oral Surg Oral Med Oral Pathol Oral Radiol Endod 87:317–321
2. Anghelescu DL et al (2002) Vincristine-induced vocal cord paralysis in an infant. Paediatr Anaesth 12:168–170
3. Bentzen SM, Overgaard M (1991) Relationship between early and late normal-tissue injury after

postmastectomy radiotherapy. Radiother Oncol 20:159–165

4. Berkowitz RJ, Feretti GA, Berg JH (1988) Dental management of children with cancer. Pediatr Ann 17(11):715–725

5. Bonanni G, Perazzi F (1965) Variations in taste sensitivity in patients subjected to high energy irradiation for tumors of the oral cavity. Nucl Radiol 31:383–397

6. Buhrer C et al (1990) Acute onset deafness in a 4-year-old girl after a single infusion of cisplatinum. Pediatr Hematol Oncol 7(2):145–148

7. Burns BV, Shotton JC (1998) Vocal fold palsy following vinca alkaloid treatment. J Laryngol Otol 112:485–487

8. Burris HA 3rd, Hurtig J (2010) Radiation recall with anticancer agents. Oncologist 15(11):1227–1237

9. Cohen BH et al (1990) Ototoxic effect of cisplatin in children with brain tumors. Pediatr Neurosurg 16(6):292–296

10. Cooper JS et al (1995) Late effects of radiation therapy in the head and neck region. Int J Radiat Oncol Biol Phys 31(5):1141–1164

11. Dahllöf G et al (1988) Disturbances in dental development after total body irradiation in bone marrow transplant recipients. Oral Surg Oral Med Oral Pathol 65:41–44

12. Dahllöf G et al (1989) Effect of chemotherapy on dental maturity in children with hematological malignancies. Pediatr Dent 11:303–306

13. Dahllöf G et al (1994) Disturbances in the oral cavity in pediatric long-term survivors after different forms of anti-neoplastic therapy. Pediatr Dent 16:217–223

14. Dahllöf G et al (1994) Histologic changes in dental morphology induced by high dose chemotherapy and total body irradiation. Oral Surg Oral Med Oral Pathol 77(1):56–60

15. Dahllöf G et al (2011) Xerostomia in children and adolescents after stem cell transplantation conditioned with total body irradiation or busulfan. Oral Oncol 47:915–919

16. Deasy JO et al (2010) Radiotherapy dose-volume effects on salivary gland function. Int J Radiat Oncol Biol Phys 76:S58–S63

17. Denys D et al (1998) The effects of radiation on craniofacial skeletal growth: a quantitative study. Int J Pediatr Otorhinolaryngol 45:7–13

18. Donahue B et al (1994) Head and neck. In: Schwartz CL, Hobbie WL, Constine LS, Ruccione KS (eds) Survivors of childhood cancer. Mosby, St. Louis

19. Donaldson SS, Glick JM, Wilbur JR et al (1974) Adriamycin activating a recall phenomenon after radiation therapy. Ann Intern Med 81:407–408

20. Dornfeld K et al (2007) Radiation doses to structures within and adjacent to the larynx are correlated with long-term diet- and speech-related quality of life. Int J Radiat Oncol Biol Phys 68:750–757

21. Duggal MS et al (2003) Root surface areas in long-term survivors of childhood cancer. Oral Oncol 39:178–183

22. Eisbruch A et al (1999) Dose, volume, and function relationships in parotid salivary glands following conformal and intensity-modulated irradiation of head and neck cancer. Int J Radiat Oncol Biol Phys 45:577–587

23. Epstein JB et al (1996) Effects of compliance with fluoride gel application on caries and caries risk in patients after radiation therapy for head and neck cancer. Oral Surg Oral Med Oral Pathol Oral Radiol Endod 82:268–275

24. Estilo CL et al (2003) Effects of therapy on dentofacial development in long-term survivors of head and neck rhabdomyosarcoma: the Memorial Sloan-Kettering Cancer Center experience. J Pediatr Hematol Oncol 25:215–222

25. Fajardo LF, Berthrong M (1988) Vascular lesions following radiation. Pathol Annu 23:297–330

26. Fajardo LG et al (2001) Radiation pathology. Oxford University Press, New York

27. Fan C et al (2011) Methotrexate toxicity in growing long bones of young rats: a model for studying cancer chemotherapy-induced bone growth defects in children. J Biomed Biotechnol 2011:903097. doi:10.1155/2011/903097, Epub 2011 Mar 17

28. Fiorillo A et al (1999) Radiation late effects in children treated for orbital rhabdomyosarcoma. Radiother Oncol 53:143–148

29. Forrest CR et al (2002) Efficacy of radioprotection in the prevention of radiation-induced craniofacial bone growth inhibition. Plast Reconstr Surg 109:1311–1323

30. Fromm M et al (1986) Late effects after treatment of twenty children with soft tissue sarcomas of the head and neck. Experience at a single institution with a review of the literature. Cancer 57:2070–2076

31. Fukunaga-Johnson N et al (1998) The use of 3D conformal radiotherapy (3D CRT) to spare the cochlea in patients with medulloblastoma. Int J Radiat Oncol Biol Phys 41:77–82

32. Fung K et al (2001) Vocal function following radiation for non-laryngeal versus laryngeal tumors of the head and neck. Laryngoscope 111:1920–1924

33. Goldwein JW et al Late radiation-associated deafness in children treated for medulloblastoma and brainstem tumors, a newly recognized sequelae of radiation treatment. Oncolink website, University of Pennsylvania. http://www.virtualtrials.com/btlinks/lradeaf.htm

34. Gomez DR et al (2011) Correlation of osteoradionecrosis and dental events with dosimetric parameters in intensity-modulated radiation therapy for head-and-neck cancer. Int J Radiat Oncol Biol Phys 81:e207–e213

35. Greco FA et al (1976) Adriamycin and enhanced radiation reaction in normal esophagus and skin. Ann Intern Med 85:294–298

36. Guggenheimer J et al (1977) Clinicopathologic effects of cancer chemotherapeutic agents on human buccal mucosa. Oral Surg Oral Med Oral Pathol 44:58–63

37. Guyuron B et al (1983) Effect of irradiation on facial growth: a 7- to 25-year follow-up. Ann Plast Surg 11:423–427

38. Hartnick CJ, Rehbar R, Prasad V (2005) Development and maturation of the pediatric human vocal fold lamina propria. Laryngoscope 115:4–15

39. Heyn R et al (1986) Late effects of therapy in orbital rhabdomyosarcoma in children. A report from the Intergroup Rhabdomyosarcoma Study. Cancer 57:1738–1743

40. Holtta P et al (2002) Long-term adverse effects on dentition in children with poor-risk neuroblastoma treated with high-dose chemotherapy and autologous stem cell transplantation with or without total body irradiation. Bone Marrow Transplant 29:121–127

41. Hua C et al (2008) Hearing loss after radiotherapy for pediatric brain tumors: effect of cochlear dose. Int J Radiat Oncol Biol Phys 72:892–899

42. Huang E et al (1998) Intensity—modulated radiation therapy for pediatric medulloblastoma: early report on the reduction of ototoxicity. Int J Radiat Oncol Biol Phys 41:77–82

43. Imhof SM et al (1996) Quantification of orbital and mid-facial growth retardation after megavoltage external beam irradiation in children with retinoblastoma. Ophthalmology 103:263–268

44. Jaffe N et al (1984) Dental and maxillofacial abnormalities in long term survivors of childhood cancer: effects of treatment with chemotherapy and radiation to the head and neck. Pediatrics 73:816–823

45. Jaruchinda P, Jindavijak S, Singhavarach N (2012) Radiation-related vocal fold palsy in patients with head and neck carcinoma. J Med Assoc Thai 95:S23–S28

46. Johansson S, Svensson H, Denekamp J (2000) Timescale of evolution of late radiation injury after postoperative radiotherapy of breast cancer patients. Int J Radiat Oncol Biol Phys 48:745–750

47. Kaste SC et al (1995) Dental abnormalities in long-term survivors of head and neck rhabdomyosarcoma. Med Pediatr Oncol 25:96–101

48. Kaste SC et al (1998) Dental abnormalities in children treated for neuroblastoma. Med Pediatr Oncol 30:22–27

49. Kaste SC et al (2009) Impact of radiation and chemotherapy on risk of dental abnormalities. A report from the Childhood Cancer Survivor Study. Cancer 115:5817–5827

50. Krasin MJ et al (2009) Incidence and correlates of radiation dermatitis in children and adolescents receiving radiation therapy for the treatment of pediatric sarcomas. Clin Oncol 21:781–785

51. Krasin MJ et al (2012) Jaw dysfunction related to pterygoid and masseter muscle dosimetry after radiation therapy in children and young adults with head-and-neck sarcomas. Int J Radiat Oncol Biol Phys 82:355–360

52. Laskar S et al (2008) Nasopharyngeal carcinoma in children: comparison of conventional and intensity-modulated radiotherapy. Int J Radiat Oncol Biol Phys 72:728–736

53. Lawenda BD et al (2004) Permanent alopecia after cranial irradiation: dose-response relationship. Int J Radiat Oncol Biol Phys 60:879–887

54. Lee IJ et al (2009) Risk factors and dose-effect relationship for mandibular osteoradionecrosis in oral and oropharyngeal cancer patients. Int J Radiat Oncol Biol Phys 75:1084–1091

55. Louis CU et al (2007) A single institution experience with pediatric nasopharyngeal carcinoma: high incidence of toxicity associated with platinum-based chemotherapy plus IMRT. J Pediatr Hematol Oncol 29(7):500–505

56. Maguire A et al (1987) The long-term effects of treatment on the dental condition of children surviving malignant disease. Cancer 60:2570–2575

57. Marcial V (1989) The oral cavity and oropharynx. In: Moss WT, Cox JD (eds) Radiation oncology. Mosby-Year Book, St. Louis

58. Månsson-Rahemtulla B et al (1992) Analysis of salivary components in leukemia patients receiving chemotherapy. Oral Surg Oral Med Oral Pathol 73:35–46

59. Minicucci EM et al (2003) Dental abnormalities in children after chemotherapy treatment for acute lymphoid leukemia. Leuk Res 27:45–50

60. Möller P, Perrier M (1998) Dento-maxillofacial sequelae in a child treated for a rhabdomyosarcoma in the head and neck. A case report. Oral Surg Oral Med Oral Pathol Oral Radiol Endod 86:297–303

61. Moore K (1977) The developing human, 2nd edn. Saunders, Philadelphia

62. Mukherjea D, Rybak LP (2011) Pharmacogenomics of cisplatin-induced ototoxicity. Pharmacogenomics 12(7):1039–1050

63. Nunn JH et al (1991) Dental caries and dental anomalies in children treated by chemotherapy for malignant disease: a study in the north of England. Int J Paediatr Dent 1:131–135

64. Ondrey FG et al (2000) Radiation dose to otologic structures during head and neck cancer radiation therapy. Laryngoscope 110:217–221

65. Pai GS et al (2000) Occurrence and severity of alopecia in patients on combination chemotherapy. Indian J Cancer 37:95–104

66. Pajari U, Lanning M et al (1988) Prevalence and location of enamel opacities in children after antineoplastic therapy. Community Dent Oral Epidemiol 16:222–226

67. Parsons JA (1984) The effect of radiation on normal tissues of the head and neck. In: Million RR, Cassisi NJ (eds) Management of head and neck cancer. A multi-disciplinary approach. Lippincott, Philadelphia, pp 173–207

68. Paulino AC et al (2000) Long-term effects in children treated with radiotherapy for head and neck rhabdomyosarcoma. Int J Radiat Oncol Biol Phys 48:1489–1495

69. Paulino AC et al (2010) Ototoxicity after intensity-modulated radiation therapy and cisplatin-based chemotherapy in children with medulloblastoma. Int J Radiat Oncol Biol Phys 78(5):1445–1450

70. Paulino AC et al (2000) Posterior fossa boost in medulloblastoma: an analysis of dose to surrounding structures using 3-dimensional (conformal) radiotherapy. Int J Radiat Oncol Biol Phys 46:281–286

71. Peterson D, Sonis S (1983) Oral complications of cancer chemotherapy. Nijhoff, Boston
72. Rancati T et al (2010) Radiation dose-volume effects in the larynx and pharynx. Int J Radiat Oncol Biol Phys 76:S64–S69
73. Raney RB et al (1999) Late complications of therapy in 213 children with localized, nonorbital soft-tissue sarcoma of the head and neck: a descriptive report from the Intergroup Rhabdomyosarcoma Studies (IRS)-II and – III. IRS Group of the Children's Cancer Group and the Pediatric Oncology Group. Med Pediatr Oncol 33:362–371
74. Raney RB et al (2000) Late effects of therapy in 94 patients with localized rhabdomyosarcoma of the orbit: report from the Intergroup Rhabdomyosarcoma Study (IRS)-III, 1984–1991. Med Pediatr Oncol 34:413–420
75. Rosenberg SW (1987) Altered dental root development in long-term survivors of pediatric acute lymphoblastic leukemia. Cancer 59:1640–1648
76. Rosende L et al (2011) Hypoacusia in a patient treated by isotretinoin. Case Rep Med 2011:789143. doi:10.1155/2011/789143, Epub 2011 Nov 24
77. Rosenthal C, Karthaus M et al (2000) New strategies in the treatment and prophylaxis of chemo- and radiotherapy-induced oral mucositis. Antibiot Chemother 50:115–132
78. Rubin P, Casarett G (1968) Clinical radiation pathology. Saunders, Philadelphia
79. Sasse AD et al (2006) Amifostine reduces side effects and improves complete response rate during radiotherapy: results of a meta-analysis. Int J Radiat Oncol Biol Phys 64:784–791
80. Sonis AL et al (1990) Dentofacial development in long-term survivors of acute lymphoblastic leukemia. A comparison of three treatment modalities. Cancer 66:2645–2652
81. Sonis ST (2009) Mucositis: the impact, biology and therapeutic opportunities of oral mucositis. Oral Oncol 45(12):1015–1020
82. Stene T et al (1976) The effect of vincristine on dentinogenesis in the rat incisor. Scand J Dent Res 84:342–344
83. Thompson RF et al (2013) Dose to the developing dentition during therapeutic irradiation: organ at risk determination and clinical implications. Int J Radiat Oncol Biol Phys 86:108–113
84. Tuomi L, Bjorkner E, Finizia C (2014) Voice outcome in patients treated for laryngeal cancer: efficacy of voice rehabilitation. J Voice 28:62–68
85. Uderzo C et al (1997) Long-term effects of bone marrow transplantation on dental status in children with leukaemia. Bone Marrow Transplant 20:865–869
86. van Leeuwen BL et al (2000) Effect of single chemotherapeutic agents on the growing skeleton of the rat. Ann Oncol 11(9):1121–1126
87. van Leeuwen BL et al (2003) The effect of chemotherapy on the morphology of the growth plate and metaphysis of the growing skeleton. Eur J Surg Oncol 29:49–58
88. Viana MB, Vilela MI (2008) Height deficit during and many years after treatment for acute lymphoblastic leukemia in children: a review. Pediatr Blood Cancer 50(2 Suppl):509–516
89. Waghmare CM, Agarwal J, Bachher GK (2010) Quality of voice after radiotherapy in early vocal cord cancer. Expert Rev Anticancer Ther 10:1381–1388
90. Walker DA et al (1989) Enhanced cis-platinum ototoxicity in children with brain tumors who have received simultaneous or prior cranial irradiation. Med Pediatr Oncol 17:48–52
91. Walsh S et al (2001) High concentrations of dexamethasone suppress the proliferation but not the differentiation or further maturation of human osteoblast precursors in vitro: relevance to glucocorticoid-induced osteoporosis. Rheumatology (Oxford) 40(1):74–83
92. Wasserman TH, Brizel DM, Henke M et al (2005) Influence of intravenous amifostine on xerostomia, tumor control and survival after radiotherapy for head-and neck cancer: 2-year follow-up of a prospective, randomized, Phase III trial. Int J Radiat Oncol Biol Phys 63:985–990
93. Watters AL et al (2013) Intravenous biphosphonate-related osteonecrosis of the jaw: long-term follow-up of 109 patients. Oral Surg Oral Med Pathol Oral Radiol 115:192–200
94. www.survivorshipguidelines.org

# Adverse Effects of Cancer Treatment on Hearing

**8**

Wendy Landier and David R. Freyer

## Contents

W. Landier PhD, CRNP (✉)
Division of Pediatric Hematology/Oncology,
Institute for Cancer Outcomes and Survivorship,
School of Medicine, University of Alabama at
Birmingham, Birmingham, AL, USA
e-mail: wlandier@peds.uab.edu

## 8.1 Introduction

Curative therapy for pediatric malignancies often requires the use of therapeutic modalities that have the potential to adversely impact hearing. Monitoring of audiologic function during and after treatment is therefore an essential component of care for patients treated with potentially ototoxic therapy. Since hearing loss can have a significant impact on social, emotional, and cognitive function, timely and appropriate interventions should be employed to mitigate the effects of hearing loss in survivors at risk for this common treatment-related complication. Emerging areas of investigation in ototoxicity include genetic risk and prevention.

## 8.2 Pathophysiology

### 8.2.1 Normal Anatomy and Physiology

The ears are completely formed in utero, and auditory brainstem responses are present at 28 weeks of gestation. Newborns are capable of

D.R. Freyer DO, MS
LIFE Cancer Survivorship and Transition Program,
Children's Center for Cancer and Blood Diseases,
Children's Hospital Los Angeles,
Los Angeles, CA, USA

Department of Clinical Pediatrics, Keck School of
Medicine, University of Southern California,
Los Angeles, CA, USA

© Springer International Publishing 2015
C.L. Schwartz et al. (eds.), *Survivors of Childhood and Adolescent Cancer:*
*A Multidisciplinary Approach*, Pediatric Oncology, DOI 10.1007/978-3-319-16435-9_8

processing sound and analyzing loudness and pitch; however, continued maturation of auditory structures, related neuronal pathways, and the auditory cortex continue throughout infancy and early childhood. Interhemispheric sensory transfer through the corpus callosum takes several years to fully mature [86]. The processing of sounds occurs in the external, middle, and inner ears (Fig. 8.1). The pinna funnels environmental sound into the external auditory canal, where it is amplified and directed toward the middle ear. The tympanic membrane then vibrates in proportion to the frequency and intensity of the acoustic wave and transmits the sound to the ossicles, which serve as impedance matching transformers, converting the sound into mechanical energy and transmitting it to the inner ear through the oval window. In the inner ear, sound is transmitted through the cochlea by hydraulic waves that stimulate specialized sensory hair cells lining the basilar membrane of the organ of Corti. The hydraulic waves cause displacement of the basilar membrane and bending of the sensory hair cells, resulting in depolarization and release of neurotransmitters, which then stimulate the cochlear branch of the VIIIth cranial nerve. These neural

impulses are subsequently transmitted through the medulla, midbrain, and thalamus to the auditory cortex of the temporal lobe. In most people, the right ear is dominant; therefore, speech processing usually occurs in the left temporal lobe.

Sound is described in terms of its *intensity* or loudness (measured in decibels) and *frequency* or pitch (measured in Hertz). Normal hearing thresholds are between −10 and 25 dB, and hearing loss is graded on a scale of "mild" to "profound" (Table 8.1). The speech frequencies are between 250 and 2,000 Hz, but higher frequencies (>2,000–8,000 Hz) are critical for speech discrimination, since many of the consonant sounds are in the high-frequency range; therefore, even a "mild" degree of high-frequency hearing loss can have a profound effect on a young child who is just acquiring language. *Conductive hearing loss* occurs when transmission of sound from the environment is impaired due to a pathological process in the outer or middle ear. *Sensorineural hearing loss* occurs as a result of pathology involving the cochlea or auditory nerve. *Mixed hearing loss* encompasses elements of both conductive and sensorineural hearing loss. In general, hearing loss occurring as a consequence of ototoxic pharmacologic agents is sensorineural in

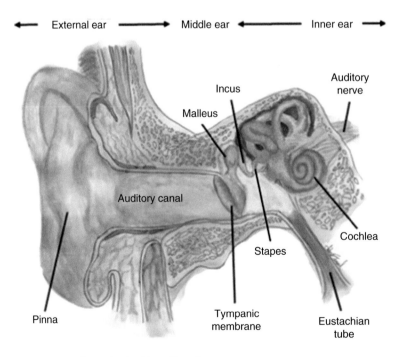

**Fig. 8.1** Anatomy of the ear (Illustration by Aimee Ermel)

**Table 8.1** Degrees of hearing loss

| Hearing threshold | Degree of loss |
| --- | --- |
| −10 to 25 dB | Normal |
| 26–40 dB | Mild |
| 41–55 dB | Moderate |
| 56–70 dB | Moderately severe |
| 71–90 dB | Severe |
| >90 dB | Profound |

Data from: Stach [88], pp. 208–209

nature, whereas hearing loss resulting from radiation, tumor, or surgical procedures is often multifactorial and may include both conductive and sensorineural components.

### 8.2.2 Ototoxic Effects of Tumor and Therapy: Risk Factors and Prevalence

#### 8.2.2.1 Surgery and Tumor

Hearing loss is rarely a presenting symptom in tumors that affect children. Exceptions include nasopharyngeal cancer, parameningeal rhabdomyosarcoma, tumors of the base of skull (chordoma), vestibular schwannoma, and metastases that affect the temporal bone, most notably neuroblastoma. Although CNS tumors may come in contact with vital aspects of the auditory system (including the VIIIth nerve and associated vasculature and the brainstem and vestibular nuclei, as well as cortical tracts essential to hearing), hearing loss is not commonly recorded at diagnosis. Surgical management of CNS tumors or musculoskeletal tumors of the head and neck can have a profound and irreversible effect on hearing, especially when essential components of the auditory system are involved with the tumor and surgical resection is required. Transcranial surgery in the region of the middle cranial fossa and suboccipital region can result in bony complications that may lead to mastoiditis and infections. Fortunately, most pediatric head and neck tumors are sensitive to radiation and chemotherapy. Tumors of the CNS account for nearly 20 % of all neoplasms in children, with the posterior fossa one of the most common locations. Children with medulloblastoma, ependymoma, cerebellar astrocytoma, and other tumors that

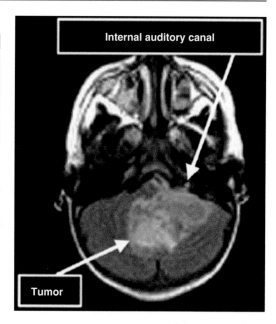

**Fig. 8.2** Left cerebellopontine angle ependymoma encasing CN VIII with extension into the internal auditory meatus

gain access to the lateral recesses and cranial nerves are at risk for transient or permanent hearing loss at the time of resection. Great skill is required to remove tumor from the lateral aspect of the brainstem, through which the VIIIth nerve and vessels may run (Fig. 8.2). Recent efforts in surgery include intraoperative neurophysiologic monitoring of cranial nerves during tumor resection to limit neurologic impairment [84].

Children with CNS tumors often present with hydrocephalus that requires emergent evaluation and treatment with temporary ventriculostomy and resection. When the natural flow of CSF cannot be reestablished, permanent ventriculoperitoneal shunting may be required. Rapid loss of intracranial pressure, which may occur after profound blood loss, lumbar puncture, ventriculostomy, and tumor resection, has been associated with hearing loss. The mechanism is likely related to the anatomic connection between the CSF spaces and the perilymph of the cochlea (cochlear aqueduct) (Fig. 8.3). Hydrocephalus and its management can influence radiation and chemotherapy-related hearing loss. In one study that included children with localized brain tumors treated with conformal radiation therapy, patients with CSF shunts and pre-irradiation ototoxic chemotherapy had the greatest change in hearing thresholds. Patients with shunts and supratentorial tumors who received radiation doses exceeding 32 Gy (without chemotherapy) over a 6-week period had hearing impairment at low and intermediate frequencies. Additionally, patients with shunts and suprasellar, hypothalamic, or thalamic tumors developed intermediate-frequency hearing loss after radiation regardless of dose [54]. In a recent study of children with medulloblastoma with and without ventriculoperitoneal shunting, the odds of hearing loss for patients with a CSF shunt were 23.5-fold higher (95 % confidence interval, 4.21–131.15) than for those without a shunt, suggesting an independent association between shunting and hearing loss [26].

### 8.2.2.2 Radiation Therapy

Hearing loss is a potential complication of radiation therapy in children. Serous otitis media, with associated conductive hearing loss, may be noted as a complication in patients receiving radiation in doses ≥30 Gy to the posterior nasopharynx and mastoid [95]. The problem can be long-standing, as in the case of patients with nasopharyngeal carcinoma or rhabdomyosarcoma, although the risk appears to be increased in those with middle ear effusions prior to irradiation [48] (Fig. 8.4). Mucociliary dysfunction is thought to be the primary cause of middle ear effusions during and after radiation therapy; this can be self-limited in nature or, in severe cases, may require treatment with myringotomy [100]. Direct structural damage to the conductive system, including osteoradionecrosis, is rare with modern radiation therapy, although patients who receive high-dose irradiation to the ear and temporal bone may be at high risk for complications from localized bone and soft tissue infections arising in the region of the external auditory canal. For this reason, soft tissue infections of the ear should be treated aggressively and instrumentation of the external auditory canal should be undertaken cautiously. Clinical experience suggests that patients treated with irradiation encompassing the ear canals may have chronic difficulty with production of excessive and/or dry cerumen, leading to accumulation of inspissated debris that can interfere with hearing and require periodic removal.

Sensorineural hearing loss can occur as a result of radiation effects from the auditory cortex to the cochlea. Because the doses administered to neural tissue directly or indirectly are

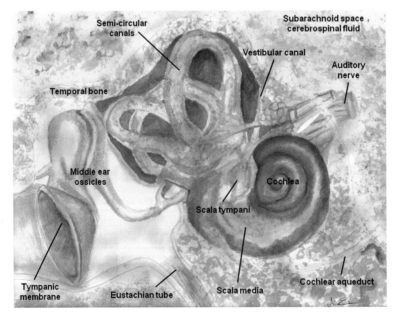

**Fig. 8.3** Drawing of cochlear duct and anatomic relationships with CSF spaces and auditory system (Illustration by Aimee Ermel)

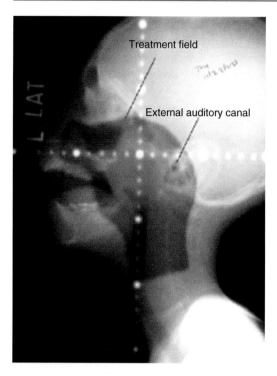

**Fig. 8.4** Lateral radiation portal film of a child with naso-pharyngeal rhabdomyosarcoma

generally accepted as safe and below the threshold for neurologic impairment, sensorineural effects of radiation are most likely to occur in the cochlea and are usually noted months or years after treatment. Despite recognition of the cochlea as the primary component in sensorineural hearing loss [23], the prevalence and time course for injury due to radiation is unknown. Because most children at risk for radiation-related hearing loss also receive ototoxic chemotherapy, the pathophysiology and clinical course of hearing loss is most often described after combined modality therapy. Similar to the effects of ototoxic chemotherapy, the effects of radiation appear to be dose related, with a threshold dose for sensorineural hearing loss in the range of 35–45 Gy [31, 54]. The combined effects of radiation and chemotherapy – specifically cisplatin and carboplatin – for the treatment of medulloblastoma and other CNS tumors is better understood, with the high prevalence of hearing loss reported among children receiving combined modality therapy [82].

### 8.2.2.3 Pharmacologic Therapy

The primary pharmacologic agents implicated in ototoxicity include platinum chemotherapy, aminoglycoside antibiotics, and loop diuretics. These agents are all capable of causing sensorineural hearing loss; however, ototoxicity related to carboplatin alone is uncommon [15, 34, 43, 89], except when administered at myeloablative doses [44, 67], in combination with cisplatin [37, 42], or possibly in very young children when dosed according to body surface area rather than weight [72]. The mechanism of aminoglycoside and platinum-related ototoxicity is oxidative stress resulting in destruction of cochlear sensory hair cells [16, 81]. These specialized hair cells are arranged tonotopically (in order of pitch) in four rows (one inner and three outer rows) along the organ of Corti, and each hair cell is sensitive to a limited frequency range [51].

Cisplatin and aminoglycoside antibiotics damage the outer hair cells, whereas carboplatin selectively damages only inner hair cells [92]. The initial hearing loss associated with ototoxic pharmacologic agents usually affects the high-frequency ranges. This is because destruction of the sensory hair cells typically begins at the base of the cochlea, where high-frequency sounds are processed, and proceeds toward the apex, where the processing of low-frequency sound occurs [77]. Individuals are generally born with a full complement of auditory sensory hair cells. Once destroyed, these cells cannot regenerate; therefore, hearing loss occurring as a result of sensory hair cell loss is almost always irreversible.

The mechanism of ototoxicity associated with loop diuretics is thought to be related to changes in the fluid and electrolyte balance within the inner ear, resulting in tissue edema within the cochlea and decreased endocochlear potential [16, 79]. Hearing loss resulting from diuretics typically occurs following rapid intravenous administration. Fortunately, this type of hearing loss is usually transient. However, if loop diuretics are administered simultaneously with or shortly after the administration of platinum chemotherapy or aminoglycosides, the likelihood of permanent auditory damage increases as a result of synergism between these agents [3, 90].

Factors placing survivors at highest risk for hearing loss related to pharmacologic therapy include very young age (less than 5 years) at the time of cancer therapy, diagnosis of central nervous system tumor, treatment with multiple ototoxic agents, and/or treatment with platinum chemotherapy in combination with radiation to the ear or brain [33, 47, 65, 67, 82, 97]. Many childhood malignancies, including germ cell tumors, central nervous system tumors, osteosarcoma, and neuroblastoma, frequently require treatment with platinum-based chemotherapy protocols, and supportive care regimens often employ aminoglycoside antibiotics and loop diuretics [27, 42, 46, 65]. Therefore, the index of suspicion for treatment-related hearing loss should be high for any survivor who received potentially ototoxic therapy, including patients treated for malignancies such as acute myeloid leukemia, where administration of platinum compounds is rare, but use of aminoglycosides for infectious complications is common.

Factors contributing to the risk for ototoxicity include diminished renal function at the time of treatment [25], rapid intravenous administration of ototoxic agent(s) [73], prolonged elevated serum trough drug levels [90], coadministration of other ototoxic drugs (e.g., chelating agents, quinine, salicylates [16, 77]), and excessive noise exposure [7]. Further, the potential impact of new agents with ototoxic properties (e.g., oxaliplatin [16]) should be kept in mind when assessing patient risk.

The prevalence of ototoxicity is well documented in children receiving cisplatin chemotherapy [83] and is dose related, with an inverse relationship to age at therapy [96]. Brock et al. [5] studied 29 children off therapy for at least 2 years who had received "standard-dose" (60–100 mg/m$^2$/course) cisplatin-containing chemotherapy regimens without brain or ear irradiation. Median age at diagnosis was 2 years, 2 months (range: 1 month–13.5 years) and median cumulative dose was 540 mg/m$^2$ (range: 400–1,860 mg/m$^2$). Moderate to severe sensorineural hearing loss was detected in 48 % of these children, with 33 % requiring hearing aids; no child demonstrated any recovery of hearing at median 4-year

follow-up. Schell et al. [82] studied 177 children and young adults receiving cisplatin (median cumulative dose 360 mg/m$^2$, range 90–1,260 mg/m$^2$) with and without prior cranial radiation (median dose: 5,050 cGy; range 2,880–8,260 cGy). In irradiated patients, doses as low as 270 mg/m$^2$ were associated with a high probability of substantial hearing loss, whereas nonirradiated patients demonstrated negligible loss at doses up to 360 mg/m$^2$; however, as cumulative doses increased to 720 mg/m$^2$, the risk of substantial shifts in hearing threshold increased to 25 %. In a study of 49 patients with osteosarcoma receiving 400 mg/m$^2$ cisplatin with or without ifosfamide, Meyer et al. [55] reported a significant increase in the incidence of hearing loss ($\geq$30 dB at 2,000 or 3,000 Hz) in the cisplatin/ifosfamide group, indicative of a synergistic effect between the two agents. Although a small early study of patients receiving carboplatin reported that 11 of 22 children who received carboplatin at a median dose of 2,409 mg/m$^2$ demonstrated sensorineural hearing loss at 4,000–12,000 Hz [50], most subsequent studies of carboplatin in pediatric oncology populations have demonstrated only rare, isolated cases of moderate to severe hearing loss at conventional doses [43, 58, 68, 89]. However, in one recent study, sustained ototoxicity was documented in 10 of 60 (17 %) infants and toddlers treated with carboplatin for retinoblastoma, a finding potentially explained by the relatively large exposure of 3,850 mg/m$^2$ (range, 2,580–4,580 mg/m$^2$) that resulted from dose calculation by body surface area rather than weight [72]. In children receiving myeloablative doses of carboplatin and in those receiving carboplatin in combination with cisplatin, moderate to severe hearing loss is commonly seen [42, 67, 85].

Ototoxicity is also a potential complication of therapy with aminoglycoside antibiotics [53] and loop diuretics [79]. Prospective studies by Fee [19] and Smith et al. [87] reported ototoxic rates of 10–16 % for gentamicin and tobramycin. Lerner et al. [45] reported an 11 % incidence of ototoxicity associated with gentamicin and a 13 % incidence in amikacin-treated patients. An augmented ototoxic effect has been reported with the concurrent administration of cisplatin and gentamicin [76]. Brookhouser [7] described a 6.4 % incidence of furosemide-associated oto-toxicity and a 0.7 % incidence for ethacrynic acid; however, the risk increased significantly when loop diuretics were administered concur-rently with aminoglycoside antibiotics [3].

### 8.2.3   Genetic Susceptibility

Variations in individual susceptibility suggest that genetic factors may play a role in predispos-ing certain patients to drug-induced ototoxicity [2, 64, 69, 75, 78]. Currently, only a few studies have explored genetic variants that may render certain patients at high risk for ototoxicity. Early work is based on candidate genes linked plausi-bly to the physiologic mechanisms of cisplatin ototoxicity (i.e., generation of reactive oxygen species (ROS) leading to depletion of the nor-mally protective cochlear antioxidant enzymes involved in detoxification of superoxides). Polymorphisms of genes coding for glutathione $S$-transferase (GST) proteins (crucial enzymes involved in detoxification) have been implicated in cisplatin-related ototoxicity. For example, Peters et al. reported a protective effect of the GSTM3*B allele on ototoxicity [69], and Oldenburg et al. reported the presence of both alleles of 105Val-GSTP1 to be protective against ototoxicity, while the GSTM1 variant was asso-ciated with increased susceptibility to cisplatin-related hearing loss in testicular cancer patients [64]. Recently, Rednam et al. reported an increased risk for radiation-associated ototoxic-ity among patients with the GSTP1-105G allele in pediatric medulloblastoma, as well as a strong interaction with radiation dose [74]. In a discov-ery cohort of 54 children, strong associations between cisplatin-induced ototoxicity and genetic variants in thiopurine $S$-methyltransferase (TPMT) and catechol-$O$-methyltransferase (COMT) have also been reported; for the com-bined mutation, the odds ratio was 42.2 ($p = 1.1 \times 10e9$), with positive and negative pre-dictive values of 92.9 % and 48.6 %, respec-tively [78]. Additional plausible candidate genes

identified to date include megalin, a low-density lipoprotein-related protein 2 strongly expressed within the stria vascularis in the cochlea; ERCC1, a nucleotide excision repair gene; and mutations in mitrochonrial DNA associated with aminoglycoside-induced deafness [6, 57]. A genome-wide approach to identification of genetic variants associated with susceptibility to ototoxicity is also underway [57]. In principle, identification of genetic variants that place patients at high risk for ototoxicity could inform future strategies to tailor chemotherapy and/or utilize preventive measures in order to maximize efficacy while minimizing risk. However, there are currently contradictory findings, and further validation of data is needed in larger groups in order to make informed recommendations.

### 8.2.4   Preventive Measures

The administration of platinum chemotherapy prior to, rather than following, cranial irradia-tion in children with CNS tumors has been shown to reduce ototoxicity [40, 82]. Newer radiation delivery techniques (e.g., intensity-modulated and proton beam radiation) hold the promise of reducing radiation-related ototoxic-ity by conforming the prescribed dose to the region at risk and sparing the cochlea [31, 54, 56]. Using these techniques, the dose to the cochlea can be estimated more accurately to optimize treatment and to collect dose informa-tion, which can be correlated with other factors that influence hearing after treatment [31, 32, 54, 56] (Fig. 8.5).

Careful monitoring and appropriate dose modification earlier in the course of therapy, before severe hearing loss has been sustained, are effective in decreasing auditory morbidity; how-ever, decisions regarding dose modification or substitution of alternate therapeutic agents in the face of identified hearing loss must be weighed carefully against concerns regarding disease con-trol and survival [47, 91]. Thus, identification of effective otoprotective strategies holds promise for reducing ototoxicity without compromising potentially curative therapy.

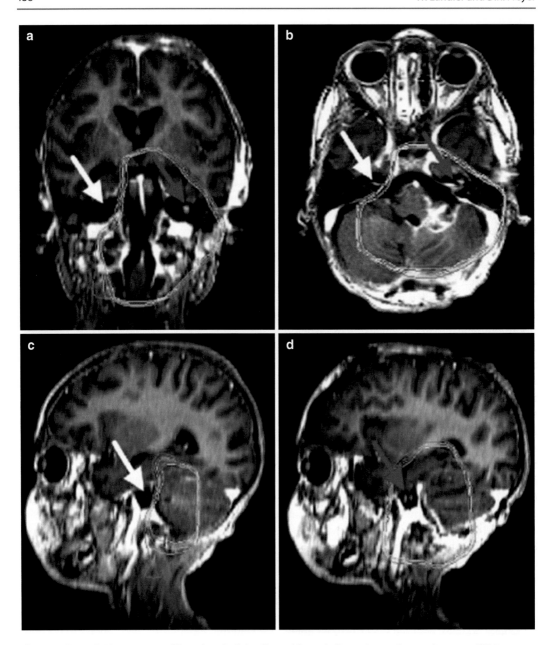

**Fig. 8.5** Coronal (**a**), transverse (**b**), and sagittal (**c, d**) MR images with three-dimensional radiation dosimetry, showing the ability of conformal treatment techniques to spare auditory structures not adjacent to tumor bed in a child with cerebellopontine angle ependymoma. (*White arrows* represent spared cochlea; *red arrows* represent irradiated cochlea)

To date, only two agents have been the subject of study in clinical trials. Amifostine, a reactive oxygen scavenger, was originally developed as a radiation protectant [80] and has been evaluated in several recent trials to assess its potential for otoprotection. Although otoprotec-tion was observed in a study of amifostine in adults with advanced ovarian cancer [36], studies of amifostine in children receiving platinum chemotherapy for hepatoblastoma [35], germ cell tumors [52], and osteosarcoma [22, 70] failed to demonstrate significant otoprotection.

However, a recent comparative cohort study using a more dose-intensive amifostine schedule demonstrated a significant protective effect against severe ototoxicity in children receiving cisplatin for average-risk medulloblastoma [20]. Studies of sodium thiosulfate, a free-radical scavenger thiol compound, have been reported to provide otoprotection in limited institution studies [17, 63], and pediatric cooperative group otoprotection studies of this agent are currently underway [21, 91]. Other potential otoprotectants at various stages of investigation include N-acetyl-cysteine [62, 93, 99], D-methionine [10], and ebselen [49]. Another approach that is conceptually appealing is the intratympanic administration of otoprotectants as compartmental therapy to avoid risks attributed to systemic exposure, but to date experience with this has been limited [30, 98].

Additional otoprotective strategies include counseling patients regarding the importance of avoiding other potentially ototoxic agents, including medications (e.g., chelating agents, salicylates) and loud noises (especially $\geq 85$ dB). Patients should also be advised to use protective measures (e.g., ear plugs) when in noisy environments and avoid excessively loud volumes with headphones in order to prevent comorbid noise-induced hearing loss [24, 71].

## 8.3    Clinical Manifestations

### 8.3.1    Clinical Manifestations of Ototoxicity Related to Surgery or Tumor

Tumor-related hearing loss is not a common presenting symptom. Notable exceptions include patients with nasopharyngeal tumors or rhabdomyosarcoma involving the middle and inner ear, patients with eustachian tube dysfunction secondary to mass effect or lymphadenopathy, and the rare patient with neurofibromatosis type II who develops a neurofibroma involving the otoacoustic nerve (CN VIII). In the scope of possible side effects and complications first noted after surgery for brain tumors, hearing loss is usually not a pri-

ority. Children at risk for hearing loss from surgery often have acquired other deficits that are more apparent or life-threatening, which can delay the diagnosis of surgery-related hearing loss. These patients often have deficits involving the abducens (CN VI) or facial nerve (CN VII) and, in extreme cases, lower cranial nerves affecting speech and swallowing. Children who require temporary or permanent CSF shunting may experience altered hearing, either temporary or permanent loss, or heightened sensitivity (hyperacusis). Recovery from surgery-related hearing deficits can occur in some cases despite adjuvant irradiation, provided that the nerve has not been transected or the vascular supply permanently disrupted.

### 8.3.2    Clinical Manifestations of Radiation-Related Ototoxicity

Radiation-related effects on the auditory system may occur during or after treatment. Acute effects are more likely to involve the external auditory canal (radiation dermatitis of the epithelium lining the canal leading to otitis externa) and middle ear (otorrhea with otalgia or mucociliary dysfunction of the middle ear with resultant eustachian tube dysfunction). Cerumen production appears to be increased in some patients during and after radiation, although the contribution from other causes cannot be excluded. Atrophy of the sebaceous glands may occur and is dose dependent. Soft tissue fibrosis, otosclerosis, and even cholesteatoma have been reported. Because radiation therapy is often given in conjunction with ototoxic chemotherapy, separating the effects of the two treatments can be difficult. Since most instances of treatment-related hearing loss occur in close temporal proximity to chemotherapy or combined modality therapy, more ototoxicity is known or observed in this setting. However, radiation therapy alone may result in hearing loss with an onset many years following treatment; therefore, long-term survivors remain at risk for hearing loss. Radiation-related hearing loss may occur during the first year after treatment in patients who also received chemotherapy and is usually seen 2 or more years after treatment in patients treated with radiation alone. With newer means of delivering radiation therapy, namely, noncoplanar, individually shaped beams to avoid the middle ear and cochlea, some of the acute and late effects of treatment appear to be reduced. With additional considerations regarding the timing of radiation and chemotherapy, further reductions in ototoxicity seem to be feasible.

### 8.3.3 Clinical Manifestations of Ototoxicity Related to Pharmacologic Agents

Hearing loss resulting from ototoxic medications is generally bilateral and symmetrical, progressive with continued therapy, and irreversible. Early symptoms may include tinnitus, vertigo, and difficulty hearing in the presence of background noise, which is indicative of vestibular injury and high-frequency (>2,000 Hz) hearing loss. Because consonant sounds are primarily high frequency and vowel sounds are primarily low frequency, a person with high-frequency hearing loss will be able to hear vowel sounds better than consonants. The English language relies heavily on high-frequency consonant sounds (such as "th," "f," "s," and "k,") to convey the meaning of words (Fig. 8.6); therefore, the inability to hear high-frequency sounds often results in poor speech discrimination, or a perception of "hearing but not understanding." For people with high-frequency hearing loss, understanding high-pitched voices (e.g., females and children) may be particularly problematic. Increasing the volume of the speaker's voice (e.g., by shouting) is generally not helpful, since this raises the intensity level of vowels but not consonants. As hearing loss progresses, patients may experience difficulty in hearing sounds within the speech ranges (250–2,000 Hz). It is important to understand that even mild high-frequency hearing loss is clinically significant, particularly in young children. It may result in difficulties with speech discrimination and language acquisition that adversely affect both cognitive and social development.

## 8.4 Detection and Screening

### 8.4.1 Auditory Screening

It is important to distinguish between auditory "screening" and "testing." Conventional auditory screening typically evaluates the patient's ability to hear pure tones at 1,000, 2,000 and 4,000 Hertz (Hz) in each ear; a score of "pass" or "fail" is given (hearing threshold ≤20 or >20 decibels [dB], respectively). Measurement of otoacoustic emissions (OAEs) is another auditory screening technique often utilized for newborns or very young children. OAEs are sounds generated by the cochlea's outer hair cells in response to stimulation by auditory signals [88]. A score of "pass" on OAE screening verifies that a patient has near-normal hearing (threshold ≤30 dB). However, inasmuch as carboplatin selectively damages inner rather than outer hair cells, OAE screening is not appropriate for monitoring carboplatin-related ototoxicity [28]. In general, auditory screening is used to select individuals who need referral for formalized testing, and OAEs may be more sensitive in detecting initial ototoxic damage; however, the gold standard for ototoxicity monitoring is formal diagnostic audiometric assessment using measurement of pure-tone thresholds [38].

### 8.4.2 Diagnostic Audiometry

#### 8.4.2.1 Pure-Tone Audiometry

The standard method used for diagnostic evaluation of hearing in cooperative patients is pure-tone audiometry. The aim is to establish hearing thresholds across a wide range of sound frequencies (usually 250–8,000 Hz, up to 12,000 or even higher with ultra-high-frequency testing). This testing is generally done in a soundproof booth; air and bone conduction thresholds are measured and results graphed on an audiogram (Fig. 8.7a), which indicates the sound intensity needed to produce a response (the hearing threshold, dB) at a given frequency (Hz). Often, a "stairstep" pattern of hearing loss, progressing from the high frequencies down to the speech ranges, is evident on the

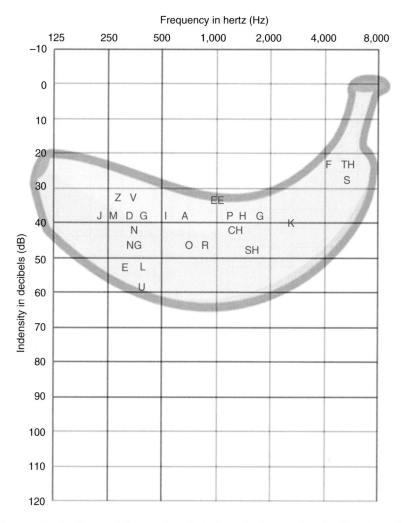

**Fig. 8.6** Audiogram showing the speech frequencies, which cluster in a banana-shaped region, often referred to as the "speech banana"

audiogram of patients with sensorineural hearing loss resulting from ototoxic therapy (Fig. 8.7b). For patients with a developmental age less than 4–5 years, pure-tone audiometric testing can be performed using behavioral modification techniques, such as conditioned play audiometry or visual-reinforcement audiometry [9].

### 8.4.2.2 Brainstem Auditory-Evoked Response

For patients unable to cooperate with behavioral testing due to young age, cognitive impairment, and/or medical illness, hearing can be assessed via brainstem auditory-evoked response (BAER, ABR). Electrodes are placed on the skull, and sound is presented at intensity levels that elicit an electrophysiological response, recorded as a waveform. The intensity of the stimulus is then lowered until the response is no longer measurable; this level corresponds roughly to the threshold measurements used in pure-tone audiometry. In order to determine hearing sensitivity for purposes of ototoxicity monitoring, frequency-specific tone-burst stimuli (rather than broadband clicks) should be used during the assessment [11]. The patient must remain motionless

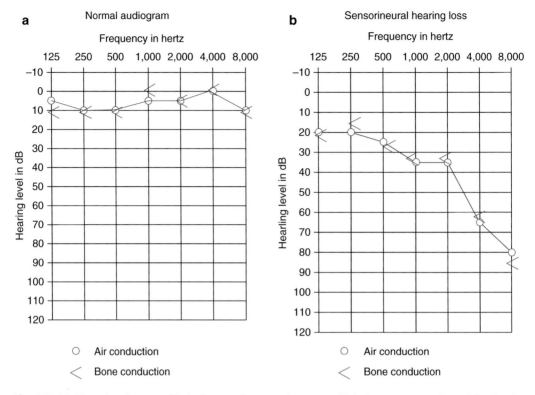

**Fig. 8.7** (**a**) Normal audiogram. (**b**) Audiogram demonstrating severe high-frequency sensorineural hearing loss (85 dB at 8,000 Hz and 60 dB at 4,000 Hz). *Hz* Hertz, *dB* decibels

throughout this test; therefore, sedation is almost always required for infants and young children (as reviewed in [88]).

### 8.4.3  Guidelines for Audiologic Monitoring

The importance of ongoing audiologic monitoring for patients receiving ototoxic therapy cannot be overemphasized, to allow for early detection of hearing loss, dose modification when appropriate, and auditory intervention when indicated. Audiologic evaluation is recommended as a baseline measure for all patients scheduled to receive ototoxic therapy and then at appropriate intervals prior to platinum-based courses based on patient age, dose per course, cumulative platinum exposure, and contributing factors such as concurrent aminoglycoside therapy and history of middle ear dysfunction [1, 18].

Survivors who received ototoxic therapy also require ongoing monitoring [4, 39]. Because of its latency in causing hearing loss, patients who received radiation at a dose of 30 Gy or higher to the ear, infratemporal or nasopharyngeal areas, or to the brain or craniospinal axis should receive audiologic monitoring on an annual basis for 5 years following completion of therapy and, if stable, every 5 years and as clinically indicated. Patients younger than 10 years of age should continue annual monitoring until they are at least 5 years off therapy *and* at least 10 years old. Patients who received treatment with platinum chemotherapy (particularly at cumulative cisplatin doses of $\geq 360$ mg/m$^2$ or myeloablative doses of carboplatin), those treated with radiation involving the ear at doses less than 30 Gy (including the infratemporal or nasopharyngeal areas, whole brain, craniospinal axis and/or total body irradiation), and patients who received significant exposure to nonplatinum ototoxic agents (e.g., aminoglycosides or loop diuretics) should have a baseline audiogram at entry into long-term follow-up. Patients with abnormal audiograms should be referred to an audiologist for evaluation and management and should continue to receive, at minimum, annual monitoring until hearing loss stabilizes. Testing should be done more frequently if there is evidence of progressive hearing loss, in order to allow for continued adjustment of hearing aids or other assistive devices and referral for additional interventions as indicated [14].

### 8.4.4 Ototoxicity Grading

Grading of the severity of treatment-induced ototoxicity is important for guiding therapeutic decisions and facilitating comparison of toxicity among treatment regimens. Several grading systems are currently in use (Table 8.2). The commonly used Brock system [5] and the more recent Chang scale [12] were designed to detect high-frequency hearing loss associated with platinum agents and are applied to single audiometric determinations. In contrast, the National Cancer Institute Common Terminology Criteria for Adverse Events (NCI-CTCAE) [59, 60] and the American Speech-Language-Hearing (ASHA) [1] systems incorporate threshold shifts and require comparison with baseline values. This has implications for conducting research and for management of children where baseline audiometry could not be obtained due to debilitation or inability to cooperate. Concern has been expressed regarding the variability in grading between these systems and the resultant inability to effectively compare the extent of ototoxicity associated with various clinical trial regimens [61]. A new grading system (the SIOP-Boston Ototoxicity Scale) has been proposed for use internationally in pediatric trials that incorporate potentially ototoxic agents; validation of this system is currently ongoing [6]. The quest for improved pediatric ototoxicity grading scales is driven by the need for them to be both predictive and sensitive enough to detect clinically important hearing loss at an early stage.

**Table 8.2** Common ototoxicity grading scales

| Grading scale | Description |
|---|---|
| Brock [5] | 5-point scale designed to grade hearing loss configuration commonly associated with platinum-related ototoxicity (i.e., progression from high to low frequencies). Baseline assessment not required |
| Chang [12] | 7-point modification of Brock scale addresses functional deficits and includes additional interval frequencies (i.e., 3,000 and 6,000 Hz). Baseline assessment not required |
| NCI-CTCAE [59, 60] | 4-point scale incorporates both objective and subjective criteria. Baseline assessment required, except when hearing loss is severe. Not specifically designed for pediatrics or for the hearing loss configuration commonly associated with platinum-related ototoxicity |
| ASHA [1] | Grades hearing compared to baseline in absolute terms. Degree of hearing loss cannot be quantified; only the presence/absence of hearing loss is rated |
| SIOP-Boston [6] | Proposed in 2012 through the consensus of an international working group, designed to be widely applicable to clinical research settings. Uses absolute hearing levels; baseline assessment not required. Currently lacks reliability and validity testing |

## 8.5 Management of Hearing Loss

The impact of deafness goes beyond the loss of hearing; at its core is the problem of impaired communication that can result in loss of social interaction, with devastating cognitive and emotional consequences for the survivor. While hearing loss reduces quality of life for patients of all ages, its potential impact is especially profound in prelingual children (infants and toddlers) where not only communication is impaired but also language acquisition, hearing-based learning, and social adjustment. Children with hearing loss are more likely to develop behavioral difficulties due to ineffectual communication and resultant barriers to the establishment of normal discipline and relationships at home and in the classroom.

## 8.5.1 Hearing Aids

Hearing aids are an integral component of the management of hearing loss; however, it is important for the clinician to understand that hearing aids *do not* restore normal hearing [94]. Although recent advancements in digital hearing aid technology have resulted in significant improvements, hearing aids amplify *all* environmental sounds to some extent, including background noise, and the quality of aided sound for a patient with sensorineural hearing loss remains distorted due to sensory hair cell destruction and inability to process sounds.

All hearing aids have three basic parts. The *microphone* picks up sound waves from the environment and converts them into electrical current. The *amplifier* increases the intensity (volume) of the sound and then sends it to the *receiver*, which converts the amplified electrical impulse back into sound waves and delivers them to the ear. Newer digital hearing aids incorporate digital signal processing, which allows tailoring of amplification to the child's specific pattern of hearing loss, with attendant reduction in sound distortion and improvement in speech recognition.

There are a variety of hearing aids styles available. To accommodate rapid growth, most preadolescent children are fitted with a behind-the-ear model. In addition to the hearing aid components, which are contained in a case located behind the ear, the model also has an ear mold, which is fitted into the ear canal. As the child grows, the only component that requires refitting is the ear mold; this is done approximately every 6 months through the age of about 9 years.

Other types of hearing aids include in-the-ear, in-the-canal, and completely-in-the-canal models; digital technology has resulted in smaller, more discreet devices, some with customized programmability, wireless communication, and advanced speech processing. The future holds promise for sophisticated hearing aids that will be able to restore near-normal hearing, including sound localization and the ability to hear speech in noisy environments, which current devices are unable to provide (as reviewed in [8, 29, 41]).

Patients and parents should be counseled regarding the importance of hearing aid maintenance. Frequent cleaning of the aid is important, and batteries must be changed regularly (usually every 7–14 days). Since young children typically will not report a nonfunctional hearing aid, use of a calendar or other reminder system for battery changes is imperative; parents should also check to be certain that the hearing aid is switched to the "on" position on a daily basis. Close follow-up by an experienced audiologist is essential to provide for ongoing adjustment and fine-tuning of the hearing aid best suited for the patient's needs. Many children, especially teenagers, need significant encouragement to wear their hearing aids at a time when being "different" carries a social stigma. Newer devices are considerably smaller, are less visible, and come in a variety of colors some teens find appealing.

## 8.5.2 Other Assistive Devices

Besides hearing aids, there are a number of other assistive devices available for patients with hearing impairment. Auditory trainers are particularly helpful in the classroom or daycare setting; these devices employ a microphone (worn by the teacher or caregiver) and a receiver (worn by the patient). The speaker's voice is transmitted over FM radio waves to a receiver that can either be plugged into the hearing aid or worn as a stand-alone device. The system significantly reduces background noise and is ideal for classroom use.

Additional assistive devices include telephone amplifiers and telephone devices for the deaf (TDD), text pagers, and modified appliances, such as vibratory alarm clocks and smoke detectors. Closed captioning for television is widely available, and the Internet also provides significant communication options for the hearing impaired, including texting and social media (as reviewed in [8, 29]).

## 8.5.3 Cochlear Implants

Unlike hearing aids that amplify sound, cochlear implants use electronic impulses to stimulate auditory neural pathways in the cochlea, circumventing damaged sensory hair cells and allowing transmission of sound impulses to the brain. Cochlear implants are indicated only for patients with severe to profound hearing loss who are unable to benefit from powerful, well-fitted hearing aids. The implant's receiver is surgically placed in the mastoid bone and an electrode array is threaded into the cochlea. A microphone worn behind the ear is used to collect environmental sounds that are filtered and digitalized by an external speech processor. The digital impulses then travel across the skull and into the receiver by way of a magnetized transmitter. The signal is relayed to the electrodes that in turn stimulate the auditory nerve, allowing for sound perception by the brain. Sounds processed through a cochlear implant tend to be distorted and mechanical; however, patients with severe to profound hearing loss not amenable to correction with hearing aid technology may derive significant benefit from the procedure. Intensive postoperative speech therapy is always required (as reviewed in [41, 66]).

### 8.5.4  Communication Methods

Several communication options are available for patients with significant hearing loss. The *auditory-verbal method* is an in-depth educational approach that teaches children to use residual hearing in order to learn to listen and speak. Intensive involvement on the part of the family and the school are required.

*Cued speech* is a communication method that combines speech-reading (lipreading) with hand signs, clarifying certain words.

*Sign language* is a unique form of communication with its own grammar and syntax and is communicated entirely via signs, gestures, and facial expressions.

*Total communication* is a method that combines auditory training with hand signs correlating exactly with the child's primary language (e.g., English). The decision regarding which communication method is best suited for an individual patient is an intensely personal one that should be made by the family. However, for patients whose hearing loss occurs after they have attained substantial language development, the use of methods based on preexisting language (e.g., the auditory/verbal or total communication methods) are often most practical, as reviewed in [13].

### 8.5.5  Community and Educational Resources

The Individuals with Disabilities Education Act (IDEA), a public law (PL 105–17) in the United States, recognizes hearing loss as a disability. As a result of the IDEA law, children in the United States diagnosed with hearing loss are legally entitled to receive a free and appropriate public education that meets their special needs in the "least restrictive" (e.g., regular or modified classroom) environment. "Part B" of this law provides for other related services, such as speech therapy and assistive devices. All services covered by the IDEA legislation must be provided at public expense under the supervision of the state's educational agency. If the local public school is unable to accommodate the child's needs, services may be provided through a referral agency. A second US law, the Americans with Disabilities Act (ADA; PL 101–336), guarantees people with hearing loss equal access to public events, spaces, and opportunities. It is this law that provides the basis for text telephones and telephone amplifiers in public venues, closed captioning for television programs, and assistive listening devices in theaters.

---

### Conclusion

Hearing loss resulting from cancer therapy during childhood can have a profound impact on the survivor's cognitive, social, and emotional functioning. Appropriate surveillance and intervention for deficits in audiologic function are an integral part of care for survivors at risk for this potentially debilitating complication.

# References

1. American Speech-Language-Hearing Association (1994) Guidelines for the audiologic management of individuals receiving cochleotoxic drug therapy. ASHA 36(Suppl 12):11–19
2. Bates DE (2003) Aminoglycoside ototoxicity. Drugs Today (Barc) 39:277–285
3. Bates DE, Beaumont SJ, Baylis BW (2002) Ototoxicity induced by gentamicin and furosemide. Ann Pharmacother 36:446–451
4. Bertolini P, Lassalle M, Mercier G et al (2004) Platinum compound-related ototoxicity in children: long-term follow-up reveals continuous worsening of hearing loss. J Pediatr Hematol Oncol 26:649–655
5. Brock PR, Bellman SC, Yeomans EC et al (1991) Cisplatin ototoxicity in children: a practical grading system. Med Pediatr Oncol 19:295–300
6. Brock PR, Knight KR, Freyer DR et al (2012) Platinum-induced ototoxicity in children: a consensus review on mechanisms, predisposition, and protection, including a new International Society of Pediatric Oncology Boston ototoxicity scale. J Clin Oncol 30:2408–2417
7. Brookhouser PE (2000) Diseases of the cochlea and labyrinth. In: Wetmore RF, Muntz HR, McGill TJ (eds) Pediatric otolaryngology: principles and practice pathways. Thieme, New York, pp 327–354
8. Brookhouser PE, Beauchaine KL, Osberger MJ (1999) Management of the child with sensorineural hearing loss. Medical, surgical, hearing aids, cochlear implants. Pediatr Clin North Am 46:121–141
9. Campbell KC, Durrant J (1993) Audiologic monitoring for ototoxicity. Otolaryngol Clin North Am 26:903–914
10. Campbell KC, Meech RP, Klemens JJ et al (2007) Prevention of noise- and drug-induced hearing loss with D-methionine. Hear Res 226:92–103
11. Chang KW (2011) Clinically accurate assessment and grading of ototoxicity. Laryngoscope 121:2649–2657
12. Chang KW, Chinosornvatana N (2010) Practical grading system for evaluating cisplatin ototoxicity in children. J Clin Oncol 28:1788–1795
13. Cherow E, Dickman DM, Epstein S (1999) Organization resources for families of children with deafness or hearing loss. Pediatr Clin North Am 46:153–162
14. Children's Oncology Group (2008) Children's Oncology Group long-term follow-up guidelines for survivors of childhood, adolescent, and young adult cancers. Children's Oncology Group, Arcadia
15. Dean JB, Hayashi SS, Albert CM et al (2008) Hearing loss in pediatric oncology patients receiving carboplatin-containing regimens. J Pediatr Hematol Oncol 30:130–134
16. Ding D, Allman BL, Salvi R (2012) Review: ototoxic characteristics of platinum antitumor drugs. Anat Rec (Hoboken) 295:1851–1867
17. Doolittle ND, Muldoon LL, Brummett RE et al (2001) Delayed sodium thiosulfate as an otoprotectant against carboplatin-induced hearing loss in patients with malignant brain tumors. Clin Cancer Res 7:493–500
18. Durrant JD, Campbell K, Fausti S et al (2009) American Academy of Audiology position statement and clinical practice guidelines: ototoxicity monitoring. American Academy of Audiology, Reston
19. Fee WE Jr (1980) Aminoglycoside ototoxicity in the human. Laryngoscope 90:1–19
20. Fouladi M, Chintagumpala M, Ashley D et al (2008) Amifostine protects against cisplatin-induced ototoxicity in children with average-risk medulloblastoma. J Clin Oncol 26:3749–3755
21. Freyer DR, Sung L, Reaman GH (2009) Prevention of hearing loss in children receiving cisplatin chemotherapy. J Clin Oncol 27:317–318, author reply 318–319
22. Gallegos-Castorena S, Martinez-Avalos A, Mohar-Betancourt A et al (2007) Toxicity prevention with amifostine in pediatric osteosarcoma patients treated with cisplatin and doxorubicin. Pediatr Hematol Oncol 24:403–408
23. Gamble JE, Peterson EA, Chandler JR (1968) Radiation effects on the inner ear. Arch Otolaryngol 88:156–161
24. Gratton MA, Salvi RJ, Kamen BA et al (1990) Interaction of cisplatin and noise on the peripheral auditory system. Hear Res 50:211–223
25. Grewal S, Merchant T, Reymond R et al (2010) Auditory late effects of childhood cancer therapy: a report from the Children's Oncology Group. Pediatrics 125:e938–e950
26. Guillaume DJ, Knight K, Marquez C et al (2012) Cerebrospinal fluid shunting and hearing loss in patients treated for medulloblastoma. J Neurosurg Pediatr 9:421–427
27. Hale GA, Marina NM, Jones-Wallace D et al (1999) Late effects of treatment for germ cell tumors during childhood and adolescence. J Pediatr Hematol Oncol 21:115–122
28. Hall JW (2000) Handbook of otoacoustic emissions. Singular, San Diego
29. Helt-Cameron J, Allen PJ (2009) Cisplatin ototoxicity in children: implications for primary care providers. Pediatr Nurs 35:121–127
30. Hill GW, Morest DK, Parham K (2008) Cisplatin-induced ototoxicity: effect of intratympanic dexamethasone injections. Otol Neurotol 29:1005–1011
31. Hua C, Bass JK, Khan R et al (2008) Hearing loss after radiotherapy for pediatric brain tumors: effect of cochlear dose. Int J Radiat Oncol Biol Phys 72:892–899
32. Huang E, Teh BS, Strother DR et al (2002) Intensity-modulated radiation therapy for pediatric medulloblastoma: early report on the reduction of ototoxicity. Int J Radiat Oncol Biol Phys 52:599–605
33. Ilveskoski I, Saarinen UM, Wiklund T et al (1996) Ototoxicity in children with malignant brain tumors

treated with the "8 in 1" chemotherapy protocol. Med Pediatr Oncol 27:26–31

34. Jehanne M, Lumbroso-Le Rouic L, Savignoni A et al (2009) Analysis of ototoxity in young children receiving carboplatin in the context of conservative management of unilateral or bilateral retinoblastoma. Pediatr Blood Cancer 52:637–643

35. Katzenstein HM, Chang KW, Krailo M et al (2009) Amifostine does not prevent platinum-induced hearing loss associated with the treatment of children with hepatoblastoma: a report of the Intergroup Hepatoblastoma Study P9645 as a part of the Children's Oncology Group. Cancer 115: 5828–5835

36. Kemp G, Rose P, Lurain J et al (1996) Amifostine pretreatment for protection against cyclophosphamide-induced and cisplatin-induced toxicities: results of a randomized control trial in patients with advanced ovarian cancer. J Clin Oncol 14:2101–2112

37. Knight KR, Kraemer DF, Neuwelt EA (2005) Ototoxicity in children receiving platinum chemotherapy: underestimating a commonly occurring toxicity that may influence academic and social development. J Clin Oncol 23:8588–8596

38. Knight KR, Kraemer DF, Winter C et al (2007) Early changes in auditory function as a result of platinum chemotherapy: use of extended high-frequency audiometry and evoked distortion product otoacoustic emissions. J Clin Oncol 25:1190–1195

39. Kolinsky DC, Hayashi SS, Karzon R et al (2010) Late onset hearing loss: a significant complication of cancer survivors treated with Cisplatin containing chemotherapy regimens. J Pediatr Hematol Oncol 32:119–123

40. Kretschmar CS, Warren MP, Lavally BL et al (1990) Ototoxicity of preradiation cisplatin for children with central nervous system tumors. J Clin Oncol 8:1191–1198

41. Kulkarni K, Hartley DE (2008) Recent advances in hearing restoration. J R Soc Med 101:116–124

42. Kushner BH, Budnick A, Kramer K et al (2006) Ototoxicity from high-dose use of platinum compounds in patients with neuroblastoma. Cancer 107:417–422

43. Lambert MP, Shields C, Meadows AT (2008) A retrospective review of hearing in children with retinoblastoma treated with carboplatin-based chemotherapy. Pediatr Blood Cancer 50:223–226

44. Laverdiere C, Cheung NK, Kushner BH et al (2005) Long-term complications in survivors of advanced stage neuroblastoma. Pediatr Blood Cancer 45:324–332

45. Lerner SA, Schmitt BA, Seligsohn R et al (1986) Comparative study of ototoxicity and nephrotoxicity in patients randomly assigned to treatment with amikacin or gentamicin. Am J Med 80:98–104

46. Lewis MJ, DuBois SG, Fligor B et al (2009) Ototoxicity in children treated for osteosarcoma. Pediatr Blood Cancer 52:387–391

47. Li Y, Womer RB, Silber JH (2004) Predicting cisplatin ototoxicity in children: the influence of age and the cumulative dose. Eur J Cancer 40: 2445–2451

48. Low WK, Fong KW (1998) Long-term post-irradiation middle ear effusion in nasopharyngeal carcinoma. Auris Nasus Larynx 25:319–321

49. Lynch ED, Gu R, Pierce C et al (2005) Combined oral delivery of ebselen and allopurinol reduces multiple cisplatin toxicities in rat breast and ovarian cancer models while enhancing anti-tumor activity. Anticancer Drugs 16:569–579

50. Macdonald MR, Harrison RV, Wake M et al (1994) Ototoxicity of carboplatin: comparing animal and clinical models at the Hospital for Sick Children. J Otolaryngol 23:151–159

51. Mann ZF, Kelley MW (2011) Development of tonotopy in the auditory periphery. Hear Res 276:2–15

52. Marina N, Chang KW, Malogolowkin M et al (2005) Amifostine does not protect against the ototoxicity of high-dose cisplatin combined with etoposide and bleomycin in pediatric germ-cell tumors: a Children's Oncology Group study. Cancer 104(4): 841–847

53. Matz GJ (1993) Aminoglycoside cochlear ototoxicity. Otolaryngol Clin North Am 26:705–712

54. Merchant TE, Gould CJ, Xiong X et al (2004) Early neuro-otologic effects of three-dimensional irradiation in children with primary brain tumors. Int J Radiat Oncol Biol Phys 58:1194–1207

55. Meyer WH, Ayers D, McHaney VA et al (1993) Ifosfamide and exacerbation of cisplatin-induced hearing loss. Lancet 341:754–755

56. Moeller BJ, Chintagumpala M, Philip JJ et al (2011) Low early ototoxicity rates for pediatric medulloblastoma patients treated with proton radiotherapy. Radiat Oncol 6:58

57. Mukherjea D, Rybak LP (2011) Pharmacogenomics of cisplatin-induced ototoxicity. Pharmacogenomics 12:1039–1050

58. Musial-Bright L, Fengler R, Henze G et al (2011) Carboplatin and ototoxicity: hearing loss rates among survivors of childhood medulloblastoma. Childs Nerv Syst 27:407–413

59. National Cancer Institute (2006) Common terminology criteria for adverse events, version 3.0, http://ctep.cancer.gov/protocolDevelopment/electronic_applications/docs/ctcaev3.pdf

60. National Cancer Institute (2010) Common terminology criteria for adverse events, version 4.0, http://evs.nci.nih.gov/ftp1/CTCAE/About.html

61. Neuwelt EA, Brock P (2010) Critical need for international consensus on ototoxicity assessment criteria. J Clin Oncol 28:1630–1632

62. Neuwelt EA, Pagel MA, Kraemer DF et al (2004) Bone marrow chemoprotection without compromise of chemotherapy efficacy in a rat brain tumor model. J Pharmacol Exp Ther 309:594–599

63. Neuwelt EA, Brummett RE, Doolittle ND et al (1998) First evidence of otoprotection against

carboplatin-induced hearing loss with a two-compartment system in patients with central nervous system malignancy using sodium thiosulfate. J Pharmacol Exp Ther 286:77–84

64. Oldenburg J, Kraggerud SM, Cvancarova M et al (2007) Cisplatin-induced long-term hearing impairment is associated with specific glutathione s-transferase genotypes in testicular cancer survivors. J Clin Oncol 25:708–714

65. Orgel E, Jain S, Ji L et al (2012) Hearing loss among survivors of childhood brain tumors treated with an irradiation-sparing approach. Pediatr Blood Cancer 58:953–958

66. Papsin BC, Gordon KA (2007) Cochlear implants for children with severe-to-profound hearing loss. N Engl J Med 357:2380–2387

67. Parsons SK, Neault MW, Lehmann LE et al (1998) Severe ototoxicity following carboplatin-containing conditioning regimen for autologous marrow transplantation for neuroblastoma. Bone Marrow Transplant 22:669–674

68. Pecora Liberman PH, Schultz C, Schmidt Goffi-Gomez MV et al (2011) Evaluation of ototoxicity in children treated for retinoblastoma: preliminary results of a systematic audiological evaluation. Clin Transl Oncol 13:348–352

69. Peters U, Preisler-Adams S, Hebeisen A et al (2000) Glutathione S-transferase genetic polymorphisms and individual sensitivity to the ototoxic effect of cisplatin. Anticancer Drugs 11:639–643

70. Petrilli AS, Oliveira DT, Ginani VC et al (2002) Use of amifostine in the therapy of osteosarcoma in children and adolescents. J Pediatr Hematol Oncol 24:188–191

71. Portnuff CD, Fligor BJ, Arehart KH (2011) Teenage use of portable listening devices: a hazard to hearing? J Am Acad Audiol 22:663–677

72. Qaddoumi I, Bass JK, Wu J et al (2012) Carboplatin-associated ototoxicity in children with retinoblastoma. J Clin Oncol 30:1034–1041

73. Reddel RR, Kefford RF, Grant JM et al (1982) Ototoxicity in patients receiving cisplatin: importance of dose and method of drug administration. Cancer Treat Rep 66:19–23

74. Rednam S, Scheurer ME, Adesina A et al (2013) Glutathione S-transferase P1 single nucleotide polymorphism predicts permanent ototoxicity in children with medulloblastoma. Pediatr Blood Cancer. 60:593–598

75. Riedemann L, Lanvers C, Deuster D et al (2008) Megalin genetic polymorphisms and individual sensitivity to the ototoxic effect of cisplatin. Pharmacogenomics J 8:23–28

76. Riggs LC, Brummett RE, Guitjens SK et al (1996) Ototoxicity resulting from combined administration of cisplatin and gentamicin. Laryngoscope 106:401–406

77. Roland JT, Cohen NL et al (1998) Vestibular and auditory ototoxicity. In: Cummings CW, Fredrickson JM, Harker LA (eds) Otolaryngology head and neck surgery, 3rd edn. Mosby, St. Louis, pp 3186–3197

78. Ross CJ, Katzov-Eckert H, Dube MP et al (2009) Genetic variants in TPMT and COMT are associated with hearing loss in children receiving cisplatin chemotherapy. Nat Genet 41:1345–1349

79. Rybak LP (1993) Ototoxicity of loop diuretics. Otolaryngol Clin North Am 26:829–844

80. Rybak LP, Whitworth CA, Mukherjea D et al (2007) Mechanisms of cisplatin-induced ototoxicity and prevention. Hear Res 226:157–167

81. Schacht J, Talaska AE, Rybak LP (2012) Cisplatin and aminoglycoside antibiotics: hearing loss and its prevention. Anat Rec (Hoboken) 295:1837–1850

82. Schell MJ, McHaney VA, Green AA et al (1989) Hearing loss in children and young adults receiving cisplatin with or without prior cranial irradiation. J Clin Oncol 7:754–760

83. Schweitzer VG (1993) Ototoxicity of chemotherapeutic agents. Otolaryngol Clin North Am 26:759–789

84. Simon MV (2011) Neurophysiologic intraoperative monitoring of the vestibulocochlear nerve. J Clin Neurophysiol 28:566–581

85. Simon T, Hero B, Dupuis W et al (2002) The incidence of hearing impairment after successful treatment of neuroblastoma. Klin Padiatr 214:149–152

86. Sininger YS, Doyle KJ, Moore JK (1999) The case for early identification of hearing loss in children. Auditory system development, experimental auditory deprivation, and development of speech perception and hearing. Pediatr Clin North Am 46:1–14

87. Smith CR, Lipsky JJ, Laskin OL et al (1980) Double-blind comparison of the nephrotoxicity and auditory toxicity of gentamicin and tobramycin. N Engl J Med 302:1106–1109

88. Stach BA (1998) Clinical audiology: an introduction. Singular, San Diego

89. Stohr W, Langer T, Kremers A et al (2004) Hearing function in soft tissue sarcoma patients after treatment with carboplatin: a report from the late effects surveillance system. Oncol Rep 12:767–771

90. Stringer SP, Meyerhoff WL, Wright CG (1991) Ototoxicity. In: Paparella MM, Shumrick DA (eds) Otolaryngology, 3rd edn. Saunders, Philadelphia, pp 1653–1669

91. Sullivan MJ (2009) Hepatoblastoma, cisplatin, and ototoxicity: good news on deaf ears. Cancer 115:5623–5626

92. Takeno S, Harrison RV, Ibrahim D et al (1994) Cochlear function after selective inner hair cell degeneration induced by carboplatin. Hear Res 75:93–102

93. Thomas Dickey D, Muldoon LL, Kraemer DF et al (2004) Protection against cisplatin-induced ototoxicity by N-acetylcysteine in a rat model. Hear Res 193:25–30

94. Turner CW (2006) Hearing loss and the limits of amplification. Audiol Neurootol 11(Suppl 1):2–5

95. Walker GV, Ahmed S, Allen P et al (2011) Radiation-induced middle ear and mastoid opacification in skull base tumors treated with radiotherapy. Int J Radiat Oncol Biol Phys 81:e819–e823

96. Weatherly RA, Owens JJ, Catlin FI et al (1991) cis-platinum ototoxicity in children. Laryngoscope 101:917–924

97. Whelan K, Stratton K, Kawashima T et al (2011) Auditory complications in childhood cancer survivors: a report from the childhood cancer survivor study. Pediatr Blood Cancer 57:126–134

98. Wimmer C, Mees K, Stumpf P et al (2004) Round window application of D-methionine, sodium thiosulfate, brain-derived neurotrophic factor, and fibroblast growth factor-2 in cisplatin-induced ototoxicity. Otol Neurotol 25:33–40

99. Yildirim M, Inancli HM, Samanci B et al (2010) Preventing cisplatin induced ototoxicity by N-acetylcysteine and salicylate. Kulak Burun Bogaz Ihtis Derg 20:173–183

100. Young YH, Lu YC (2001) Mechanism of hearing loss in irradiated ears: a long-term longitudinal study. Ann Otol Rhinol Laryngol 110:904–906

# The Thyroid Gland

# 9

Michael T. Milano, Sughosh Dhakal,
Cindy L. Schwartz, and Louis S. Constine

## Contents

M.T. Milano (✉) • S. Dhakal
Department of Radiation Oncology, University of
Rochester, 601 Elmwood Ave., Box 647, Rochester,
NY 14642, USA
e-mail: michael_milano@urmc.rochester.edu

L.S. Constine
Departments of Radiation Oncology and Pediatrics,
University of Rochester, 601 Elmwood Ave.,
Box 647, Rochester, NY 14642, USA

C.L. Schwartz
The University of Texas MD Anderson Cancer Center,
1515 Holcombe Blvd, Houston, TX 77030, USA

Thyroid dysfunction or deregulation is a clinically significant sequelae of cancer therapy due to the spectrum of physiologic consequences; subsequent thyroid neoplasia is uncommon but potentially serious and raises issues of surveillance strategies. The thyroid gland may be intentionally or incidentally exposed to therapeutic radiation dose in the treatment of many malignancies, such as with prophylactic or therapeutic irradiation of the cervical lymphatics in the treatment of Hodgkin lymphoma and non-Hodgkin lymphoma. Primary hypo- or hyperthyroidism may result from this thyroid gland radiation exposure. Cranio-spinal axis irradiation, as used for some central nervous system (CNS) tumors, may also cause hypo- or hyperthyroidism due to thyroid gland exposure and/or radiation exposure to the hypothalamic-pituitary axis. Additionally, the increased rates of development of both benign nodules and malignant thyroid tumors are a well-documented late effect after cancer therapy. This chapter will focus on the late effects of radiation exposure to the thyroid gland, resulting in increased risks of hyperthyroidism, hypothyroidism, thyroiditis, benign nodule formation, and malignancy [1–3].

© Springer International Publishing 2015
C.L. Schwartz et al. (eds.), *Survivors of Childhood and Adolescent Cancer:*
*A Multidisciplinary Approach*, Pediatric Oncology, DOI 10.1007/978-3-319-16435-9_9

## 9.1 Anatomy and Pathophysiology

### 9.1.1 Anatomy

The thyroid gland is a bilobed, butterfly-shaped endocrine gland, with right and left lobes connected by a narrow isthmus. In some people, there may be a vestigial pyramidal lobe, which is a remnant of the lower end of the thyroglossal duct. The gland is surrounded by a fibrous capsule which attaches to the pretracheal fascia. It is situated in the low anterior neck, partially encircling the larynx and trachea anteriorly, extending superiorly from the thyroid cartilage and inferiorly to the tracheal rings [2] (Fig. 9.1).

The thyroid gland consists of follicles, lined with a single layer of epithelial cells that actively transport iodine into the follicle as well as generate and secrete thyroid hormones, T3 and T4 (Fig. 9.2a, b). The follicles are filled with colloid, rich with the high-molecular-weight protein thyroglobulin necessary for thyroid hormone synthesis as well as the hormonally inactive monoido- and diiodo-tyrosines [2].

### 9.1.2 Thyroid Endocrine Dysfunction

Generally, radiation changes in the thyroid gland result from damage to small vessels (remote branches off of the superior and inferior thyroid arteries) and presumably less so from direct damage to the fully differentiated follicular epithelial cells. This relates to their slow proliferative rate that makes them relatively less sensitive to radiation injury [2, 3]. The endothelial cells of the thyroid gland vasculature may have proliferation cycles shorter than those of endocrine cells. Thus, Rubin and Cassarett postulated that the initial radiation injury to the thyroid gland was more specifically to the endothelium of small vessels, and with additional radiation exposure, the follicular epithelial cells degenerate as a result of further damage to the vasculature [1], a concept further supported by Fajardo [4].

Histopathologic changes in an irradiated thyroid gland include progressive obliteration of the fine vasculature, degeneration of follicular cells and follicles, and atrophy of the stroma [1]. Because radiation damage is dependent on the

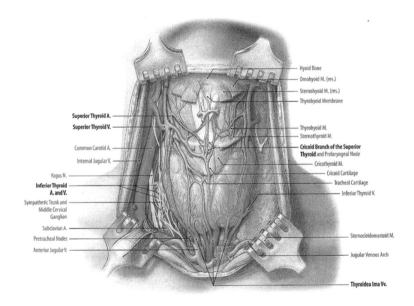

**Fig. 9.1** Gross anatomy of the neck showing the thyroid gland in relation to nerves, vasculature, and muscles [81]

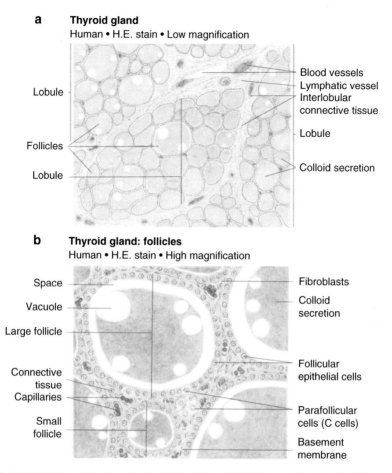

**Fig. 9.2** Histologic appearance of the thyroid gland at low (**a**) and high (**b**) magnification. At high magnification, the follicular epithelial cells and parafollicular cells are readily apparent [82]

degree of the mitotic activity and because the thyroid of a developing child grows in parallel with the body, this gland might be expected to show an age-related degree of injury and repair. Late changes are primarily attributable to vascular damage, while acute and subacute changes may be more affected by repairable damage to the epithelioid cells [3]. Acute radiation changes to the thyroid include diminished follicle size with low cuboidal epithelium lining residual follicles. With high radiation doses, including therapeutic I131 exposure, there is follicular necrosis, vasculitis, thrombosis, and hemorrhage followed by vascular sclerosis and lymphocytic infiltration [2]. Chronic changes after relatively

low-dose exposure include focal and irregular follicular hyperplasia, hyalinization, fibrosis beneath the vascular endothelium, lymphocytic infiltration, thyroiditis, cellular and nuclear atypia, infarction, and necrosis [2, 5].

### 9.1.3 Thyroid Nodules and Malignancy

Ionizing radiation can cause DNA damage that leads to somatic mutations. Double-strand breakage can result in genomic rearrangements, which can cause deactivation of tumor suppressor genes or activation of proto-oncogenes. This ultimately increases the risk of development of both benign and malignant tumors.

Investigators studying radiation-induced papillary thyroid cancer have indentified specific translocations in the RET gene which when altered in this manner is referred to as the RET/PTC oncogene; this translocation results in constitutive expression and activation. Molecular and biologic studies of pathologic specimens of papillary thyroid carcinoma from individuals exposed to radiation following the Chernobyl accident in 1986 have found an increased incidence in several isoforms of the RET/PTC rearrangements compared to those from papillary thyroid cancer specimens as a whole [6, 7]. The frequency of RET translocations also has been found to be increased in thyroid cancer cases associated with external radiation treatment for benign and malignant condition [7, 8].

Further support for this etiology of radiation-induced thyroid malignancy is provided by the observation that point mutations in the BRAF gene, a common genetic activation in papillary thyroid cancer in the general population, are rarely found in radiation-related cases [9]. Additionally, the role of radiation-related translocations is further supported by the occurrence of TRK oncogenes [10].

It is not entirely clear whether radiation-related papillary thyroid cancers containing translocations behave differently from cancers without them; however, one of the above noted studies did find that cancers with the RET/PTC rearrangements had more aggressive behavior than BRAF-positive tumors or PTC without gene alterations [6].

## 9.2    Clinical Manifestations

Hypothyroidism may manifest with classic symptoms, including weight gain, cold intolerance, dry skin, brittle hair, constipation, menstrual irregularities, muscle cramping, and slower mentation; classic signs include periorbital and peripheral edema, hypotension, bradycardia, pericardial effusions, pleural effusions, and prolonged relaxation of deep tendon reflexes. Hypothyroidism may be occult, detected only by low thyroxine levels and/or elevated TSH [11]. This is often referred to as subclinical or covert hypothyroidism, as opposed to clinical or overt hypothyroidism, in which the hypothyroidism is associated with clinical symptomatology. Compensated hypothyroidism occurs when the pituitary gland releases high levels of TSH and thus overworks the thyroid gland to maintain adequate levels of circulating thyroid hormones. With uncompensated hypothyroidism, T4 remains low despite elevated TSH. Radiation-induced occult hypothyroidism is likely to progress to clinical hypothyroidism [2], though TSH levels can spontaneously normalize over long time intervals [2, 12].

Hyperthyroidism can manifest with classic symptoms including palpitations, heat intolerance, anxiety, fatigue and insomnia, diarrhea, menstrual irregularities, weight loss, and weakness. Clinical signs include goiter, tachycardia, tremor, warm moist skin, thinner skin, fine hair and alopecia, and infiltrative ophthalmopathy. Grave's disease is an autoimmune form of hyperthyroidism resulting from the production of antibodies which bind to and chronically stimulate the receptor for thyroid-stimulating hormone (expressed on the follicular cells of the thyroid gland) causing increased production of the T3 and T4 hormones.

Thyroid cancer usually presents as a solitary, asymptomatic nodule [13]. The vast majority of children and adults with thyroid nodules have normal thyroid function. Sparse data exist on the presenting characteristics of children with secondary thyroid cancer. However, it is worth noting that children with de novo thyroid cancer, especially those who are prepubescent, more often present with advanced disease as compared with adolescents and adults [13, 14]. A review of over 500 pediatric patients from nine large referral centers found that the great majority of cases presented with only an isolated neck mass. However, after careful physical examination, over half of patients had palpable lymph nodes. Postoperative pathology revealed microscopic regional lymph node involvement in 71–90 %, extracapsular extension with invasion of the trachea in 20–60 %, and involvement of the recurrent laryngeal nerve in 30 %. The most common site of distant metastases was the lung (10–28 %), followed by the bones and brain [13]. These and other data suggest that thyroid carcinoma in the pediatric age group is a biologically independent and more aggressive entity than in adults.

## 9.2.1 Hypothyroidism

### 9.2.1.1 Radiation for Childhood Malignancies

Because of the incidental radiation to the thyroid gland in the treatment of Hodgkin lymphoma, many studies have specifically addressed late thyroid complications in this group. The incidence of hypothyroidism noted following therapeutic irradiation for Hodgkin lymphoma varies, depending on the report [3]. If an elevated serum TSH concentration is the determinant, then 4–79 % of patients become affected. This large range exists because parameters relevant to the induction of hypothyroidism – such as radiation dose, technique, and the frequency and types of follow-up testing – differ in the various reports. Most studies show the incidence of hypothyroidism progressively rising in the first 3–5 years after radiation, with most patients manifesting clinical signs or symptoms 2–4 years after radiotherapy [15–17]. Some studies demonstrate additional cases of hypothyroidism beyond 5 years [15–18], and rare and unexpected new cases can occur more than 20 years after diagnosis of Hodgkin lymphoma [16, 17].

A classic study by Hancock and colleagues [16] of 1,677 children and adults with Hodgkin lymphoma in whom the thyroid had been irradiated showed that the actuarial risk at 26 years for overt or subclinical hypothyroidism was 47 % (Table 9.1), with the peak incidence occurring 2–3 years after treatment. There are several reports specifically addressing the incidence of hypothyroidism in children as a function of radiation dose (Table 9.2) [12, 16, 17, 19–21]. Constine and colleagues [12] noted thyroid abnormalities in 4 of 24 children (17 %) who received mantle irradiation of 26 Gy or less and in 74 of 95 children (78 %) who received greater than 26 Gy. The abnormality in all but three children (one with hyperthyroidism and two with thyroid nodules) included an elevated serum TSH concentration with or without low serum T4 concentration. The spontaneous return of TSH to normal limits was observed in 20 of the 75 patients (27 %).

A report by Sklar [17] of 1,791 patients from the Childhood Cancer Survivor Study (CCSS) cohort showed that the relative risk of hypothyroidism in Hodgkin lymphoma survivors was 17.1, with 28 % of the cohort affected. The average time to developing hypothyroidism was 5 years. In patients who were treated with chemotherapy alone, the incidence of hypothyroidism was 7.6 %. In a multivariate analysis, the major risk factors associated with the development of hypothyroidism were radiation dose, female sex, and older age at diagnosis. The actuarial risk of developing hypothyroidism 20 years after a diagnosis of Hodgkin lymphoma was 30 % for patients whose thyroid received 35≤45 Gy and 50 % for patients whose thyroid received ≥45 Gy. Elapsed time since diagnosis was a risk factor, where the risk increased in the first 3–5 years after diagnosis [17]. Figure 9.3 shows, from this study, the time dependence of hypothyroidism, grouped by radiation dose to the thyroid [17].

The cumulative incidence of hypothyroidism among survivors 15 years following leukemia diagnosis has also been evaluated in the CCSS and was 1.6 %. In multivariate analysis, survivors who received ≥20 Gy cranial radiotherapy plus any spinal radiotherapy had the highest risk of subsequent hypothyroidism (hazard ratio 8.3) compared with those treated with chemotherapy alone. In radiation dosimetry analysis, pituitary doses ≥20 Gy combined with thyroid doses ≥10 Gy were associated with hypothyroidism [22]. In another study of 95 patients with childhood cancer [19] elevated TSH 5–34 years after radiation was seen in 68 % of patients who received ≥30 Gy to the thyroid versus 15 % of patients who received <30 Gy ($p = 0.007$). In the recent RiSK study of 404 childhood cancer survivors [20], compared to those who received prophylactic cranial RT (median dose 12 Gy), the relative risk of elevated TSH was 3.1 ($p = 0.002$) and 3.8 ($p = 0.009$) after doses of 15–25 Gy and >25 Gy to the thyroid gland, respectively; the relative risk was 5.7 ($p < 0.001$) for those who underwent cranio-spinal radiation.

**Table 9.1** Thyroid disease after treatment of Hodgkin's disease

| Disease | No. of patients/ total no.[a] | Actuarial risk (%) | | Time to occurrence (year) | |
|---|---|---|---|---|---|
| | | 20 year | 26 years | Median | Range |
| At least one thyroid disease | 573/1,787//> | 50 | 63 | 4.6 | 0.2–25.6 |
| | 570/1,677//> | 52 | 67 | 4.6 | 0.2–25.6 |
| Hypothyroidism | 513/1,787//> | 41 | 44 | 4.0 | 0.2–23.7 |
| | 512/1,677//> | 43 | 47 | 4.0 | 0.2–23.7 |
| Graves' disease[b] | 34/1,787//> | 3.1 | 3.1 | 4.8 | 0.1–17.6 |
| | 32/1,677//> | 3.3 | 3.3 | 4.9 | 0.1–17.6 |
| Graves' ophthalmopathy[b] | 21/1,677//> | – | – | – | – |
| Silent thyroiditis | 6/1,677//> | 1.6 | 0.6 | 3.7 | 0.8–15.3 |
| Hashimoto's thyroiditis | 4/1,677//> | 0.7 | 0.7 | 7.9 | 3.5–15.2 |
| Thyroidectomy | 26/1,677//> | 6.6 | 26.6 | 14.0 | 1.5–25.6 |
| Thyroid cancer | 6/1,677//> | 1.7 | 1.7 | 13.3 | 9.0–18.9 |
| Benign adenoma | 10/1,677//> | – | – | 12.0 | 1.5–25.6 |
| Adenomatous nodule | 6/1,677//> | – | – | 17.4 | 12.7–24.4 |
| Multinodular goiter | 4/1,677//> | – | – | 14.8 | 10.8–19.4 |
| Clinically benign nodule | 12/1,677//> | 3.3 | 5.1 | 12.6 | 2.4–22.6 |
| Clinically benign cyst | 4/1,677//> | 0.7 | 0.7 | 8.1 | 1.6–16.7 |
| Multinodular goiter[c] | 2/1,677//> | 0.5 | 0.5 | 13.8 | 10.5–17 |

From [16], with permission
[a]The total refers either to all 1,787 patients at risk or to the 1,677 patients who underwent irradiation of the thyroid region
[b]Thirty of the 34 patients who had been given a diagnosis of Graves' disease had hyperthyroidism; ophthalmopathy developed in three during a period of hypothyroidism and in one during a period of euthyroidism
[c]Identified by clinical examination

Uncompensated hypothyroidism (decreased serum T4 and elevated serum TSH concentration) occurs in 6–27 % of children receiving radiation to the thyroid. In the study by Constine and colleagues, age did not affect the incidence of hypothyroidism but was weakly correlated with the degree of abnormality, as suggested by higher serum TSH concentrations in adolescents compared with younger children [12]. In reports from Hancock [16], Sklar [17], and Constine [12] older age at treatment of Hodgkin lymphoma was a major risk factor for future development of an underactive thyroid. This may reflect the greater sensitivity of the thyroid gland in rapidly growing pubertal children, compared with preadolescents, or it may reflect the fact that the older children generally received a higher radiation dose than the younger children.

### 9.2.1.2 Influence of Chemotherapy

The role of chemotherapy in producing thyroid abnormalities is less understood. The influence of chemotherapy on the development of thyroid dysfunction among Hodgkin patients appears to be negligible in most reports [12, 17–19, 21, 23, 24], although some data of patients with brain tumors (most of whom received cranial-spinal radiation) suggest that chemotherapy may add to the frequency of compensated hypothyroidism [25]. Notably, the thyroid gland in many chemotherapy-treated brain tumor patients (i.e., medulloblastoma) receives higher doses of radiation than in non-chemotherapy-treated patients.

### 9.2.1.3 Stem Cell Transplantation

Patients undergoing a bone-marrow transplant who receive total body irradiation (TBI) are also at risk for thyroid injury due to direct injury to the thyroid gland. Sklar [26] found that a single dose of 7.5 Gy caused a decrease in serum T4 concentration in 9 % patients and an elevated serum TSH concentration in 35 %. The frequency of

Table 9.2 Radiation dose to the thyroid gland and the risk of hypothyroidism

| Institution | Patient population | # | Risk of hypothyroidism |
|---|---|---|---|
| Stanford U [12] | Children with Hodgkin lymphoma | 119 | Thyroid disorders (mostly hypothyroidism): 78 % for >26 Gy versus 17 % for ≤26 Gy |
| Stanford U [16] | Adults and children with Hodgkin lymphoma | 1,787 | Clinical hypothyroidism: 20 % for ≥30 Gy versus 5 % for 7.5–30 Gy at 20 years, $p=0.001$ |
|  |  |  | Subclinical or clinical hypothyroidism: 44 % for ≥30 Gy versus 27 % for 7.5–30 Gy at 20 years, $p=0.008$ |
| Childhood Cancer Survivor Study [17] | Children with Hodgkin's disease | 1,791 | Patient reports "underactive thyroid" 50 % for ≥45 Gy versus 30 % for 35–45 Gy versus ~20 % for <35 Gy at 15 years |
| Joint Center for Radiation Therapy [19] | Childhood cancer | 95 | Elevated TSH: 68 % for ≥30 Gy versus 15 % for <30 Gy $p=0.007$ |
| RiSK Study [20] | Childhood cancer | 404 | Elevated TSH versus prophylactic cranial RT |
|  |  |  | 15–25 Gy to thyroid gland, RR 3.1 ($p=0.002$) |
|  |  |  | >25 Gy to thyroid gland, RR 3.8 ($p=0.009$) |
|  |  |  | Cranio-spinal radiation, RR 5.7 ($p<0.001$) |
| Turkey [21] | Children with Hodgkin's disease | 55 | Abnormal thyroid function: |
|  |  |  | 27 % (6 of 22) after 25.2 Gy |
|  |  |  | 7 % (1 of 14) after 30.6 Gy |
|  |  |  | 83 % (5 of 6) after 36 Gy |

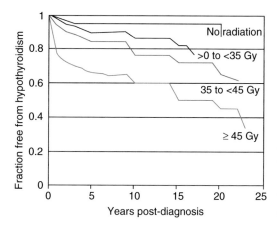

Fig. 9.3 Dose dependence of hypothyroidism risk from a study of 1,791 survivors of childhood cancer (Data and figure was derived from reference [17], in which actuarial rates of hypothyroidism were calculated among 377 patients who received no radiotherapy and 1,210 patients for whom sufficient data were available to estimate the dose of radiation to the thyroid gland (median 35 Gy and range 0.004–55 Gy))

overt hypothyroidism following transplantation is highly variable and depends largely on the conditioning regimen. Hypothyroidism after a 10 Gy, single dose of TBI can occur in up to 90 % of patients [27] versus 14–15 % in patients treated with fractionated TBI [28, 29]. Previously, regimens that did not involve whole-body irradiation were not associated with an increased risk, or at least a smaller risk [30]. However, in a report from the Fred Hutchinson Cancer Research Center, the increased risk of thyroid dysfunction was not different between children receiving cyclophosphamide and whole-body irradiation and those receiving a busulfan-based chemotherapy regimen ($p=0.48$), while those who received cyclophosphamide conditioning alone experienced significantly lower risks (HR 0.32, $p=0.03$) The highest risk of thyroid dysfunction was in the cohort treated with both busulfan and TBI (HR 1.7, $p=0.009$) Although these data suggest that both TBI and busulfan may contribute to risk for thyroid dysfunction, the magnitude of the risk associated with the chemotherapy-only treatment is likely confounded by clinical selection of chemotherapy only for younger children [31].

## 9.2.2  Hyperthyroidism

Hyperthyroidism occurs less commonly after radiation than does hypothyroidism. Thirty of 1,787 (1.7 %) Hodgkin lymphoma patients (1,677 treated with radiation) at Stanford developed hyperthyroidism at a mean of 5.3 years (0–18 years) post treatment [16]. Ten had previously been treated for hypothyroidism. In addition, four clinically hypo- or euthyroid patients developed infiltrative ophthalmopathy consistent with Grave's disease. Overall, this study showed a 7.2–20.4-fold increased risk of Grave's disease [16]. In the CCSS cohort, including 1,791 patients with childhood Hodgkin lymphoma, hyperthyroidism developed in 4.5 % (RR = 8) at 0–22 (mean of 8) years after diagnosis [17]. Significantly increased risk was associated with doses ≥35 Gy.

Because hyperthyroidism and thyroiditis are much less common late effects after radiation than hypothyroidism, the risk factors associated with these complications are not well documented. Univariate analysis did not find gender, radiation dose, or chemotherapy exposure to be significant risk factors for hyperthyroidism [16]. An immunologic basis has been hypothesized based on the higher frequency noted in Hodgkin lymphoma patients versus others treated with incidental neck irradiation and is consistent with finding of a Hungarian study that noted a fourfold increase in the prevalence of serum antithyroglobulin antibodies in irradiated females with Hodgkin lymphoma [18]. Similarly, investigators at Roswell Park noted that the addition of chemotherapy to radiation significantly reduced the risk of thyroid autoantibodies (to 17 % versus 48 %, $p < 0.01$), bringing the baseline prevalence to that seen in the general population [15].

## 9.2.3  Thyroid Nodules and Malignancy

Thyroid radiation results in an increased risk of benign adenoma formation as well as thyroid cancer. When evaluating the incidence of thyroid nodules after radiation therapy, it is important to note the high baseline frequency of asymptomatic thyroid nodules in the general population: upon careful physical exam, clinically palpable nodules are found in 4–7 % of normal adults and in as many as 35–50 % of pathologic specimens following surgery or autopsy [32].

In a series of 87 patients treated with radiation to the neck for childhood cancer at the Joint Center for Radiation Therapy, 32 developed palpable thyroid abnormalities including nodules ($n = 25$) and diffuse enlargement ($n = 7$) [19]. The risk of palpable abnormalities was independent of radiation dose and more commonly seen in patients with longer follow-up, who were more likely to have received orthovoltage radiation. Resections in 10 of the 32 patients revealed hyperplastic follicular adenomas ($n = 8$), papillary thyroid cancer ($n = 3$), and an atypical malignant schwannoma ($n = 1$).

Roughly one-tenth to one-third of thyroid nodules developing in adult patients years to decades after radiation after childhood radiation proved to be malignant [17, 19, 33, 34]. This translates into a greater than 10 to 50-fold increased risk of thyroid cancer [17, 35–42]. In a study of 5,379 patients treated with radiation for benign conditions of the head and neck, incidences for thyroid nodules were 6 % for malignant and 8–12 % for benign lesions after low-dose (<15 Gy) external beam radiation [43]. Generally, radiation-induced thyroid malignancies are localized to the thyroid or regional lymph nodes and readily curable.

Historically, low-dose radiation (as low as 0.1 Gy) for benign disease (such as tinea capitis, thymic enlargement, lymphoid hyperplasia, lice, acne) has been a well-established risk factor for thyroid nodules and malignancy, with higher dose [44–46] and younger age at exposure associated with increased risk [46]. Overall, in this setting (low-dose radiation, generally 2–5 Gy, for benign conditions) new nodules develop at a rate about 2 % per year, with a peak incidence at 15–25 years [47].

In the 1970s–1980s, case reports were published suggesting that the higher therapeutic radiation doses used to treat malignancy could also induce thyroid nodules and thyroid cancer [48]. The vast majority of radiation-induced solid tumors occur within the radiation field [35, 49]. In a study by Schneider and colleagues [43], 318 of 5,379 patients who had received RT for benign conditions of the head and neck developed thyroid cancer 3–42 years later. The most common type of cancer after thyroid radiation is papillary carcinoma, which, fortunately, has a high cure rate if detected early [50]. The course of the cancer in these patients appears to be the same as that of thyroid cancer found in other settings [43].

A report from the Late Effects Study Group [36] found that, in 9,170 childhood cancer survivors (≥2 years after diagnosis), the risk for thyroid cancer was increased (RR = 53) in association with both increasing dose and the time from treatment. The majority (68 %) of the cancers occurred within a field exposed to at least 1 Gy (via scatter for some patients). A US population-based study of 7,670 survivors of childhood showed that radiation treatment increased (compared to the general population) thyroid cancer risk 4.5-fold for brain tumor survivors and 1.8 to 2-fold for leukemia and lymphoma survivors [51].

A CCSS analysis of 12,547 5-year survivors of childhood cancer diagnosed between 1970 and 1986, and followed through 2005 [52], identified 119 pathologically confirmed thyroid cancer cases; the standardized incidence ratio of thyroid cancer versus the general population was 14.0 (95 % CI 11.7–16.8). The British Childhood Cancer Survivor Study demonstrated a standardized incidence ratio of 18.0 in their cohort of 17,980 childhood cancer survivors treated between 1940 and 1991 [42], The mean period of latency from time of primary malignancy diagnosis in this study was 20.7 years with a trend of increased risk when the radiation exposure occurred at <10 years of age.

Among the general population of pediatric cancer survivors, those treated for Hodgkin lymphoma appear to have the greatest risk of thyroid adenoma [53] and carcinoma [54], either due to a greater likelihood of undergoing thyroid radiation, inherent genetic susceptibility, or a combination of factors. In a nested-case control study of 69 survivors of childhood cancer, those with Hodgkin lymphoma were more likely to develop smaller (<1 cm) thyroid cancers and have no nodal involvement versus survivors of other cancers [54], perhaps a result of more rigorous screening. However, the CCSS analysis of 12,547 5-year survivors of childhood cancer did not demonstrate a statistically significant difference in tumor size between survivors of HL and with other cancers [55].

In Stanford's series of pediatric Hodgkin lymphoma survivors, palpable thyroid nodules were appreciated in 44 of 1,677 irradiated patients (2.6 %) from 1.5 to 25 years after radiation [16]. Eighteen patients had clinically benign disease, including nodules that concentrate radioiodine (n = 12), cysts (n = 4, based on ultrasound and aspiration) and multinodular goiter (n = 2). Twenty-six had pathologically benign disease (which was clinically worrisome for malignancy given the lowered radioiodine uptake), including adenoma (n = 10), adenomatous nodule (n = 6), and multinodular goiter (n = 4). Six patients had thyroid cancer 9–19 years after radiation therapy, with a relative risk of 15.6 (p < 0.00001) and absolute risk of 33.9 per 100,000 person years. The risk for developing thyroid cancer >19 years after radiotherapy was 1.7 % (versus an expected 0.7 %). All patients with cancer remained without evidence of disease recurrence at last follow-up.

In the CCSS of 1,791 patients with childhood Hodgkin lymphoma, thyroid nodules developed in 146 patients (8.2 %) 0–22 years (mean 14 years) after diagnosis, with a relative risk of 27 compared with sibling controls [17]. The relative risk of developing thyroid cancer was 18.3, compared with the general population. Eleven of the 146 patients with thyroid nodules had thyroid cancer; in addition 9 patients developed thyroid cancer which was not associated with thyroid nodularity.

Two other reports found a >30-fold relative risk for developing thyroid cancer among childhood Hodgkin lymphoma survivors following radiation [39, 56]. In a multicenter Late Effects Study Group [36], patients treated for neuroblastoma and Wilms' tumor were more likely to develop thyroid cancer than those treated for Hodgkin lymphoma; however, patients with neuroblastoma and Wilms' tumor were generally younger in age at the time of treatment, which may be associated with an increase in risk for second malignant thyroid cancers.

In MD Anderson's series of 145 child and adult patients treated with radiation for Hodgkin lymphoma, seven patients developed palpable thyroid tumors, of which two were malignant [57]. In Roswell Park's series of 126 adult patients treated for Hodgkin lymphoma and non-Hodgkin lymphoma, 12 patients (11 of whom were women) developed thyroid nodules 1–6 years after treatment, 5 of whom did not undergo prior neck radiation [15]. No patient underwent thyroidectomy and two underwent biopsy, which revealed adenoma in one patient and thyroiditis in another.

### 9.2.3.1 Gender

Gender appears to influence the incidence of thyroid cancer. In a multi-institutional retrospective study, 1.5 % of 930 childhood Hodgkin lymphoma survivors developed thyroid cancer at a median of 14.4 (range 8.5–23) years after HL diagnosis, with ~4 times as many females developing thyroid cancer as compared to males [58]; this is not surprising since spontaneous thyroid carcinoma occurs in US females approximately two and a half times more commonly than in males. Several studies indicate an increased incidence of thyroid cancer in females survivors of childhood Hodgkin lymphoma [35, 37, 41, 58–60]. In a study by Metayer et al., 6 of 3,188 male survivors had thyroid cancer while 16 of 2,737 female survivors developed thyroid cancer [37]. In a smaller series by Bhatia et al., males and females had an incidence rate of 0.9 % and 2.3 %, respectively [35]. It is unclear whether or not gender influences the absolute excess risk or relative risk of thyroid cancer after radiation.

### 9.2.3.2 Chemotherapy

In most studies, chemotherapy does not appear to increase thyroid cancer risk or modify the risk-effect of radiation [54, 61], although one study suggested that perhaps chemotherapy reduces the effect of radiation [52]. A CCSS analysis of 12,547 childhood cancer survivors demonstrated that alkylating agents increased thyroid cancer risk 2.4-fold, but only with radiation doses of <20 Gy; at higher radiation doses, there was no effect of chemotherapy [55].

### 9.2.3.3 Radiotherapy and Duration After Radiotherapy

Although the risk of cancer induction appears to increase with dose [36, 40, 54, 61], incremental dose exposure beyond 20–30 Gy apparently reduces the risk of cancer induction [40, 52, 53, 54, 61]. Figure 9.4 shows the dose-response curve from CCSS. Perhaps this effect reflects cell killing at higher radiation doses [40, 52, 54, 61]. Analyses have shown that the dose-response relationship seen in Hodgkin survivors (who account for a greater number of pediatric survivors who develop thyroid cancer) is similar to that among those treated for other pediatric cancers [52, 54].

In the CCSS of 12,547 patients [52], the excess relative risk of thyroid cancer was modified by age at exposure (higher radiation risk with younger age) ($p < 0.001$) while excess absolute risk was modified by sex (higher radiation risk among females) ($p = 0.008$) and time since exposure (higher radiation risk with longer time) ($p < 0.001$).

Interestingly, a recent study of 3,254 survivors of childhood cancer demonstrated a similar relationship of radiation dose to risk of thyroid adenoma [53]. Younger age at time of radiation increased thyroid adenoma risks as did chemotherapy exposure in the absence of radiation; among those who received chemotherapy and radiation, chemotherapy appeared to reduce the effect of radiation dose.

For thyroid cancer induction, the risk appears to persist beyond 40 years postradiation treatment [37]. In the multivariate analysis from the CCSS of 1,791 patients with childhood Hodgkin lymphoma, an interval ≥10 years since diagnosis,

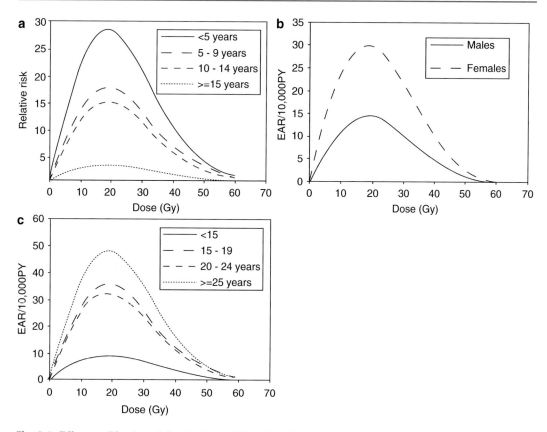

**Fig. 9.4** Effect modification of fitted relative risk and excess absolute risk dose responses. (Panel **a**) relative risk by age at radiation exposure; (panel **b**) excess absolute risk by sex; (panel **c**) excess absolute risk by time since radiation exposure

female sex, and radiation dose ≥25 Gy were independently associated with future development of thyroid nodules. Many studies demonstrate that a younger age at therapeutic radiation exposure is also associated with a greater risk of cancer induction [35, 37, 38, 52, 54, 61]. One study suggests that the relative risk increases with earlier age of treatment, but that the absolute risk is relatively constant across pediatric age groups, and perhaps younger children, who tend to receive lower radiation doses, are actually more susceptible to lower radiation doses [36].

In an Italian study of children receiving total body irradiation with >10 years follow-up, the regimen using larger fraction size (9.9 Gy in 3.3 Gy daily fractions versus 12 Gy in 2 Gy twice daily fractions) was associated with a significantly greater risk of nodule formation (80 % versus 2.7 %, $p = 0.002$) [62]. In that study, 60 %

of patients developed nodules, of which one-quarter proved to be malignant.

Radiation-induced thyroid cancer does not appear to have a different survival rate from that of sporadic thyroid cancer [63]. In general, most thyroid cancers induced by radiation are well-differentiated papillary adenocarcinomas, with a small percentage being follicular. Radiation-induced thyroid cancers do not usually include the anaplastic and medullary types; thus the fatality rate of radiation-induced thyroid tumors may be even lower than for sporadic cancers.

At least several cases of anaplastic thyroid tumors have been reported following radiation exposure [64, 65], though it is uncertain whether these were fortuitous or whether they were indeed radiation induced. It is possible that they may have resulted from the degeneration of better differentiated radiogenic tumors.

## 9.3    Detection and Screening

A comprehensive history and physical examination is necessary for all patients who received direct or scattered radiation to the neck. Laboratory screening evaluations for asymptomatic patients should include serum concentrations of TSH and thyroxine (usually, free T4) tests. The measurement of free T4 is recommended (e.g., versus total T4 by radioimmunoassay) because it is not affected by changes in binding proteins. Although some patients with normal serum-free T4 and TSH concentrations might show an exaggerated TSH response to provocative testing with TRH, the clinical significance of this finding is unclear and this testing is not routinely recommended. Screening for immunologic abnormalities (antimicrosomal and antithyroglobulin antibodies) is of uncertain clinical significance.

Although a careful physical exam should be performed in all patients, one study comparing thyroid palpation versus high-resolution thyroid ultrasonography found that only 21 % of nodules found by ultrasound were noted on physical exam. Detection by examination was dependent on size, with a rate of 6.4 % for nodules <0.5 cm, 40 % for nodules >1.5 cm, but still only 48 % for nodules >2.0 cm [66]. Patients with palpable abnormalities of the thyroid gland should undergo ultrasonography to evaluate the number, location, and density of nodules and 99mTc scanning to evaluate the functional status of the nodules. Whether all patients who have received radiation to the thyroid gland should undergo periodic screening with one or the other of these techniques is controversial.

Ultrasound is a more sensitive test than physical exam in regard to thyroid nodule detection, but specificity for thyroid malignancy is suboptimal, even in high-risk populations. An analysis by Eden et al. concluded that if 10,000 survivors were screened with ultrasound, 150 additional cases of thyroid carcinoma would be detected compared to screening by palpation alone and 1,689 patients would undergo surgery for a nonmalignant nodule compared to 480 patients if screened by palpation alone [67]. Sonographic findings that are more commonly associated with malignancy and can help guide management decisions include microcalcifications, border irregularity, hypoechogenicity, central flow, and size [68].

Stewart and colleagues performed thyroid ultrasound on 30 patients treated with mantle radiation for Hodgkin lymphoma who did not have palpable abnormalities and found unilateral or bilateral atrophy in 8 patients, multiple hypoechoic lesions smaller than 0.75 cm in 18, and dominant cystic solid or complex lesions larger than 0.75 cm in 7 patients [69]. Biopsies were not performed. Soberman [70] performed ultrasonography on 18 long-term survivors of Hodgkin lymphoma who had received a mean dose of 34 Gy to the neck 1–16 years (mean 6.4) previously; 16 patients (89 %) had abnormalities, including diffuse atrophy (nine cases), solitary nodules (five cases), multiple nodules (six cases), and gland heterogeneity (one case). Only two patients had palpable nodules. Biopsies in four patients revealed multifocal papillary carcinoma in one patient and adenomas in three patients.

In a study from the University of Rochester, 99mTc scanning was performed in 34 euthyroid patients without palpable thyroid abnormalities who had been irradiated at least 5 years earlier to the cervical region for Hodgkin lymphoma or other malignancies [50]. Seven patients (21 %) had abnormal scans, and two of these patients were diagnosed with thyroid cancer. Patient numbers are currently too small to make firm recommendations. Although 99mTc scanning is less sensitive than ultrasonography, its specificity for detecting clinically significant nodules is greater.

Neither the American Thyroid Association [71] nor the American Association of Clinical Endocrinologists (AACE) [72] recommends ultrasound for initial screening of patients who do not have an increased risk of thyroid malignancy. They both recognize, however, that radiation exposure is a risk factor, and the AACE therefore endorses ultrasound screening for high-risk populations [72], while the ATA makes no recommendations [71]. The Children's Oncology Group is currently developing long-term follow-up guidelines for screening for thyroid malignancy in childhood cancer survivors.

## 9.4 Management

Efforts to minimize radiation dose exposure to the thyroid may prevent postradiation thyroid sequelae. Historically, clinicians attempted to further decrease the risk of thyroid injury in the setting of radiotherapy for Hodgkin lymphoma by shielding the gland from irradiation [73] or administering thyroxine during irradiation [74]. The former approach was found to place patients at risk for the inadvertent shielding of diseased cervical lymph nodes, and the latter approach did not prevent subsequent hypothyroidism. Therefore, these approaches are not recommended. More conformal delivery of radiation, using novel technologies such as intensity-modulated radiation and/or image-guided radiotherapy, may be beneficial. However, as previously discussed, it is important to note that the risk of secondary thyroid cancers occurs at relatively low doses and peaks at approximately 20–30 Gy, so the increased risk is difficult to eliminate even with careful and sophisticated treatment planning.

After radiation exposure to the neck, routine examination of the neck should be performed to assess for nodularity and/or growth. Free T4 and TSH should be used to monitor thyroid function after therapeutic radiation exposure to the neck. The NCI recommends annual laboratory assessment up to 10 years postradiation, although the risk for first demonstrating abnormality may extend beyond this time point [75]. The functions regulated by the thyroid gland are particularly important in a growing child. Therefore, early diagnosis and treatment of hypothyroidism, even when subclinical, is required to optimize growth, cognition, and progression to puberty [76].

### 9.4.1 Hypothyroidism

Hypothyroidism can be managed with thyroxine replacement therapy. Levothyroxine is a synthetic form of thyroxine (thyroid hormone), used for hormone replacement for patients with radiation-induced hypothyroidism. Patients with uncompensated hypothyroidism (low serum concentration of thyroxin) require thyroid replacement therapy. In most institutions, patients with compensated hypothyroidism (elevated serum concentrations of TSH but normal thyroxine) also are treated with thyroid replacement therapy. The rationale for this approach is based on animal studies, which have demonstrated that elevated levels of TSH in the presence of irradiated thyroid tissue can lead to the development of thyroid carcinoma.

The rationale for replacement therapy includes restoration of clinical well-being for patients with symptoms, prevention of potential symptomatology, but also diminishing the risks for cardiovascular sequelae and carcinogenesis from persistently elevated TSH.

### 9.4.2 Hyperthyroidism

Hyperthyroidism can be managed with propylthiouracil, I131, or thyroidectomy. Propylthiouracil inhibits the enzyme thyroperoxidase, which is involved in thyroxine synthesis, and enzyme 5′-deiodinase which converts T4 to the active form T3.

### 9.4.3 Patients with Palpable Thyroid Abnormalities

Patients with palpable thyroid abnormalities should undergo ultrasonography or 99mTc scanning and be evaluated by an endocrinologist and surgeon. If nodules are discovered, then biopsy is necessary. Fine-needle aspiration of newly diagnosed thyroid nodules particularly those that do not demonstrate I125 uptake is suggested. Interpretation of the fine-needle aspiration may be confounded by radiation-induced atypia.

The approach for patients who are not receiving replacement hormone and have clinically normal thyroid glands, but who also have nodules detected by ultrasonography or 99mTc scanning, is not well defined. Multiple small 2–3 mm carcinomas have been found in irradiated thyroid glands [29], and autopsies have shown a high incidence of occult (less than 1 mm) papillary carcinomas. The significance of cancer found in clinically occult lesions is arguable. It would seem appropriate that suspicious nodules should be aspirated even if small (<1.5 cm) in patients with prior radiation exposure [77–79]. Researchers from University of Illinois and Michael Reese Hospitals have investigated thyroid abnormalities in a cohort of 4,296 patients irradiated between the 1939 and 1962 for benign conditions, of whom 1,059 developed thyroid nodules and were evaluable for study [79]. If only one or two of the largest nodules were aspirated, 42 % and 17 % of cases would have been misdiagnosed, respectively. Suspicious nodules or biopsy-proven thyroid cancer should be resected. In the study from Chicago, more than half of patients with thyroid cancer had multiple cancer nodules, and more than half of these patients had cancer involving both lobes necessitating total thyroidectomy as suggested by these authors as well as the American Thyroid Association [78, 79]. It is crucial to review the pathology of any biopsied nodule carefully, because an adenomatous nodule with cytologic atypia can be difficult to distinguish from thyroid carcinoma [5].

Despite the fact that thyroid carcinomas that develop following radiation show signs of greater aggressiveness and tend to be more multifocal [47], with an increased incidence of both locoregional invasion and distant metastases, overall prognosis is very good [80]. Guidelines by the American Thyroid Association and the American Association of Clinical Endocrinologists recommend that treatment for differentiated thyroid tumors following exposure to radiation should be treated in the same manner as those treated absent the exposure [71, 72].

# References

1. Rubin P, Cassarett G (1968) Clinical radiation pathology. WB Saunders Co. Philadelphia, PA
2. Hancock SL, McDougall IR, Constine LS (1995) Thyroid abnormalities after therapeutic external radiation. Int J Radiat Oncol Biol Phys 31:1165–1170
3. Jereczek-Fossa BA, Alterio D, Jassem J et al (2004) Radiotherapy-induced thyroid disorders. Cancer Treat Rev 30:369–384
4. Fajardo L, Berthrong M, Anderson R (2001) Radiation pathology. Oxford University Press, New York, pp 337–343
5. Carr RF, LiVolsi VA (1989) Morphologic changes in the thyroid after irradiation for Hodgkin's and non-Hodgkin's lymphoma. Cancer 64:825–829
6. Tronko M, Bogdanova T, Voskoboynyk L et al (2010) Radiation induced thyroid cancer: fundamental and applied aspects. Exp Oncol 32:200–204
7. Bounacer A, Wicker R, Caillou B et al (1997) High prevalence of activating ret proto-oncogene rearrangements, in thyroid tumors from patients who had received external radiation. Oncogene 15:1263–1273
8. Collins BJ, Chiappetta G, Schneider AB et al (2002) RET expression in papillary thyroid cancer from patients irradiated in childhood for benign conditions. J Clin Endocrinol Metab 87:3941–3946
9. Nikiforova MN, Ciampi R, Salvatore G et al (2004) Low prevalence of BRAF mutations in radiation-induced thyroid tumors in contrast to sporadic papillary carcinomas. Cancer Lett 209:1–6
10. Ciampi R, Knauf JA, Kerler R et al (2005) Oncogenic AKAP9-BRAF fusion is a novel mechanism of MAPK pathway activation in thyroid cancer. J Clin Invest 115:94–101
11. Boomsma MJ, Bijl HP, Langendijk JA (2011) Radiation-induced hypothyroidism in head and neck cancer patients: a systematic review. Radiother Oncol 99:1–5
12. Constine LS, Donaldson SS, McDougall IR et al (1984) Thyroid dysfunction after radiotherapy in children with Hodgkin's disease. Cancer 53:878–883
13. Feinmesser R, Lubin E, Segal K et al (1997) Carcinoma of the thyroid in children – a review. J Pediatr Endocrinol Metab 10:561–568
14. Lazar L, Lebenthal Y, Steinmetz A et al (2009) Differentiated thyroid carcinoma in pediatric patients: comparison of presentation and course between prepubertal children and adolescents. J Pediatr 154:708–714
15. Tamura K, Shimaoka K, Friedman M (1981) Thyroid abnormalities associated with treatment of malignant lymphoma. Cancer 47:2704–2711
16. Hancock SL, Cox RS, McDougall IR (1991) Thyroid diseases after treatment of Hodgkin's disease. N Engl J Med 325:599–605
17. Sklar C, Whitton J, Mertens A et al (2000) Abnormalities of the thyroid in survivors of Hodgkin's disease: data from the Childhood Cancer Survivor Study. J Clin Endocrinol Metab 85:3227–3232
18. Illes A, Biro E, Miltenyi Z et al (2003) Hypothyroidism and thyroiditis after therapy for Hodgkin's disease. Acta Haematol 109:11–17
19. Kaplan MM, Garnick MB, Gelber R et al (1983) Risk factors for thyroid abnormalities after neck irradiation for childhood cancer. Am J Med 74:272–280
20. Bolling T, Geisenheiser A, Pape H et al (2011) Hypothyroidism after head-and-neck radiotherapy in children and adolescents: preliminary results of the "Registry for the Evaluation of Side Effects After Radiotherapy in Childhood and Adolescence" (RiSK). Int J Radiat Oncol Biol Phys 81:e787–e791
21. Demirkaya M, Sevinir B, Saglam H et al (2011) Thyroid functions in long-term survivors of pediatric Hodgkin's lymphoma treated with chemotherapy

and radiotherapy. J Clin Res Pediatr Endocrinol 3:89–94

22. Chow EJ, Friedman DL, Stovall M et al (2009) Risk of thyroid dysfunction and subsequent thyroid cancer among survivors of acute lymphoblastic leukemia: a report from the Childhood Cancer Survivor Study. Pediatr Blood Cancer 53:432–437

23. Devney RB, Sklar CA, Nesbit ME Jr et al (1984) Serial thyroid function measurements in children with Hodgkin disease. J Pediatr 105:223–227

24. Sutcliffe SB, Chapman R, Wrigley PF (1981) Cyclical combination chemotherapy and thyroid function in patients with advanced Hodgkin's disease. Med Pediatr Oncol 9:439–448

25. Ogilvy-Stuart AL, Shalet SM, Gattamaneni HR (1991) Thyroid function after treatment of brain tumors in children. J Pediatr 119:733–737

26. Sklar CA, Kim TH, Ramsay NK (1982) Thyroid dysfunction among long-term survivors of bone marrow transplantation. Am J Med 73:688–694

27. Borgstrom B, Bolme P (1994) Thyroid function in children after allogeneic bone marrow transplantation. Bone Marrow Transplant 13:59–64

28. Boulad F, Bromley M, Black P et al (1995) Thyroid dysfunction following bone marrow transplantation using hyperfractionated radiation. Bone Marrow Transplant 15:71–76

29. Hawkins MM, Kingston JE (1988) Malignant thyroid tumours following childhood cancer. Lancet 2:804

30. Socie G, Salooja N, Cohen A et al (2003) Nonmalignant late effects after allogeneic stem cell transplantation. Blood 101:3373–3385

31. Sanders JE, Hoffmeister PA, Woolfrey AE et al (2009) Thyroid function following hematopoietic cell transplantation in children: 30 years' experience. Blood 113:306–308

32. Mazzaferri EL, de los Santos ET, Rofagha-Keyhani S (1988) Solitary thyroid nodule: diagnosis and management. Med Clin N Am 72:1177–1211

33. Acharya S, Sarafoglou K, LaQuaglia M et al (2003) Thyroid neoplasms after therapeutic radiation for malignancies during childhood or adolescence. Cancer 97:2397–2403

34. Metzger ML, Howard SC, Hudson MM et al (2006) Natural history of thyroid nodules in survivors of pediatric Hodgkin lymphoma. Pediatr Blood Cancer 46:314–319

35. Bhatia S, Yasui Y, Robison LL et al (2003) High risk of subsequent neoplasms continues with extended follow-up of childhood Hodgkin's disease: report from the Late Effects Study Group. J Clin Oncol 21:4386–4394

36. Tucker MA, Jones PH, Boice JD Jr et al (1991) Therapeutic radiation at a young age is linked to secondary thyroid cancer. The Late Effects Study Group. Cancer Res 51:2885–2888

37. Metayer C, Lynch CF, Clarke EA et al (2000) Second cancers among long-term survivors of Hodgkin's disease diagnosed in childhood and adolescence. J Clin Oncol 18:2435–2443

38. Neglia JP, Friedman DL, Yasui Y et al (2001) Second malignant neoplasms in five-year survivors of childhood cancer: childhood cancer survivor study. J Natl Cancer Inst 93:618–629

39. Sankila R, Garwicz S, Olsen JH et al (1996) Risk of subsequent malignant neoplasms among 1,641 Hodgkin's disease patients diagnosed in childhood and adolescence: a population-based cohort study in the five Nordic countries. Association of the Nordic Cancer Registries and the Nordic Society of Pediatric Hematology and Oncology. J Clin Oncol 14:1442–1446

40. Svahn-Tapper G, Garwicz S, Anderson H et al (2006) Radiation dose and relapse are predictors for development of second malignant solid tumors after cancer in childhood and adolescence: a population-based case-control study in the five Nordic countries. Acta Oncol 45:438–448

41. Wolden SL, Lamborn KR, Cleary SF et al (1998) Second cancers following pediatric Hodgkin's disease. J Clin Oncol 16:536–544

42. Taylor AJ, Croft AP, Palace AM et al (2009) Risk of thyroid cancer in survivors of childhood cancer: results from the British Childhood Cancer Survivor Study. Int J Cancer 125:2400–2405

43. Schneider AB, Recant W, Pinsky SM et al (1986) Radiation-induced thyroid carcinoma. Clinical course and results of therapy in 296 patients. Ann Intern Med 105:405–412

44. Adams MJ, Shore RE, Dozier A et al (2010) Thyroid cancer risk 40+ years after irradiation for an enlarged thymus: an update of the Hempelmann cohort. Radiat Res 174:753–762

45. Favus MJ, Schneider AB, Stachura ME et al (1976) Thyroid cancer occurring as a late consequence of head-and-neck irradiation. Evaluation of 1,056 patients. N Engl J Med 294:1019–1025

46. Ron E, Lubin JH, Shore RE et al (1995) Thyroid cancer after exposure to external radiation: a pooled analysis of seven studies. Radiat Res 141:259–277

47. DeGroot LJ (1989) Clinical review 2: diagnostic approach and management of patients exposed to irradiation to the thyroid. J Clin Endocrinol Metab 69:925–928

48. McDougall IR, Coleman CN, Burke JS et al (1980) Thyroid carcinoma after high-dose external radiotherapy for Hodgkin's disease: report of three cases. Cancer 45:2056–2060

49. Garwicz S, Anderson H, Olsen JH et al (2000) Second malignant neoplasms after cancer in childhood and adolescence: a population-based case-control study in the 5 Nordic countries. The Nordic Society for Pediatric Hematology and Oncology. The Association of the Nordic Cancer Registries. Int J Cancer 88:672–678

50. Sandhu A, Constine LS, O'Mara RE et al (2000) Subclinical thyroid disease after radiation therapy detected by radionuclide scanning. Int J Radiat Oncol Biol Phys 48:181–188

51. Rose J, Wertheim BC, Guerrero MA (2012) Radiation treatment of patients with primary pediatric malignancies: risk of developing thyroid cancer as a

secondary malignancy. Am J Surg 204:881–886; discussion 886–887

52. Bhatti P, Veiga LH, Ronckers CM et al (2010) Risk of second primary thyroid cancer after radiotherapy for a childhood cancer in a large cohort study: an update from the childhood cancer survivor study. Radiat Res 174:741–752

53. Haddy N, El-Fayech C, Guibout C et al (2012) Thyroid adenomas after solid cancer in childhood. Int J Radiat Oncol Biol Phys 84:e209–e215

54. Sigurdson AJ, Ronckers CM, Mertens AC et al (2005) Primary thyroid cancer after a first tumour in childhood (the Childhood Cancer Survivor Study): a nested case-control study. Lancet 365:2014–2023

55. Veiga LH, Bhatti P, Ronckers CM et al (2012) Chemotherapy and thyroid cancer risk: a report from the childhood cancer survivor study. Cancer Epidemiol Biomarkers Prev 21:92–101

56. Bhatia S, Ramsay NK, Bantle JP et al (1996) Thyroid abnormalities after therapy for Hodgkin's disease in childhood. Oncologist 1:62–67

57. Liao Z, Ha CS, Vlachaki MT et al (2001) Mantle irradiation alone for pathologic stage I and II Hodgkin's disease: long-term follow-up and patterns of failure. Int J Radiat Oncol Biol Phys 50:971–977

58. Constine LS, Tarbell N, Hudson MM et al (2008) Subsequent malignancies in children treated for Hodgkin's disease: association with gender and radiation dose. Int J Radiat Oncol Biol Phys 72:24–33

59. Dores GM, Metayer C, Curtis RE et al (2002) Second malignant neoplasms among long-term survivors of Hodgkin's disease: a population-based evaluation over 25 years. J Clin Oncol 20:3484–3494

60. Green DM, Hyland A, Barcos MP et al (2000) Second malignant neoplasms after treatment for Hodgkin's disease in childhood or adolescence. J Clin Oncol 18:1492–1499

61. Ronckers CM, Sigurdson AJ, Stovall M et al (2006) Thyroid cancer in childhood cancer survivors: a detailed evaluation of radiation dose response and its modifiers. Radiat Res 166:618–628

62. Faraci M, Barra S, Cohen A et al (2005) Very late nonfatal consequences of fractionated TBI in children undergoing bone marrow transplant. Int J Radiat Oncol Biol Phys 63:1568–1575

63. Bucci A, Shore-Freedman E, Gierlowski T et al (2001) Behavior of small thyroid cancers found by screening radiation-exposed individuals. J Clin Endocrinol Metab 86:3711–3716

64. Getaz EP, Shimaoka K, Rao U (1979) Anaplastic carcinoma of the thyroid following external irradiation. Cancer 43:2248–2253

65. Komorowski RA, Hanson GA, Garancis JC (1978) Anaplastic thyroid carcinoma following low-dose irradiation. Am J Clin Pathol 70:303–307

66. Wiest PW, Hartshorne MF, Inskip PD et al (1998) Thyroid palpation versus high-resolution thyroid ultrasonography in the detection of nodules. J Ultrasound Med 17:487–496

67. Eden K, Mahon S, Helfand M (2001) Screening high-risk populations for thyroid cancer. Med Pediatr Oncol 36:583–591

68. Cappelli C, Castellano M, Pirola I et al (2007) The predictive value of ultrasound findings in the management of thyroid nodules. QJM 100:29–35

69. Stewart RR, David CL, Eftekhari F et al (1989) Thyroid gland: US in patients with Hodgkin disease treated with radiation therapy in childhood. Radiology 172:159–163

70. Soberman N, Leonidas JC, Cherrick I et al (1991) Sonographic abnormalities of the thyroid gland in longterm survivors of Hodgkin disease. Pediatr Radiol 21:250–253

71. Cooper DS, Doherty GM, Haugen BR et al (2009) Revised American Thyroid Association management guidelines for patients with thyroid nodules and differentiated thyroid cancer. Thyroid 19: 1167–1214

72. Gharib H, Papini E, Valcavi R et al (2006) American Association of Clinical Endocrinologists and Associazione Medici Endocrinologi medical guidelines for clinical practice for the diagnosis and management of thyroid nodules. Endocr Pract 12:63–102

73. Marcial-Vega VA, Order SE, Lastner G et al (1990) Prevention of hypothyroidism related to mantle irradiation for Hodgkin's disease: preparative phantom study. Int J Radiat Oncol Biol Phys 18:613–618

74. Bantle JP, Lee CK, Levitt SH (1985) Thyroxine administration during radiation therapy to the neck does not prevent subsequent thyroid dysfunction. Int J Radiat Oncol Biol Phys 11:1999–2002

75. Common late effects of childhood cancer by body system: thyroid gland (2008) Last accessed 30 June 2008. Available at: http://www.cancer.gov/cancertopics/pdq/treatment/lateeffects/HealthProfessional/page3#Section_67

76. Sklar CA, Constine LS (1995) Chronic neuroendocrinological sequelae of radiation therapy. Int J Radiat Oncol Biol Phys 31:1113–1121

77. American Association of Clinical Endocrinologists and Associazione Medici Endocrinologi medical guidelines for clinical practice for the diagnosis and management of thyroid nodules (2006) Endocr Pract 12:63–102

78. Cooper DS, Doherty GM, Haugen BR et al (2006) Management guidelines for patients with thyroid nodules and differentiated thyroid cancer. Thyroid 16:109–142

79. Mihailescu DV, Schneider AB (2008) Size, number and distribution of thyroid nodules and their risk of malignancy in radiation-exposed patients who underwent surgery. J Clin Endocrinol Metab. 93(6): 2188–93

80. Samaan NA, Schultz PN, Ordonez NG et al (2008) A comparison of thyroid carcinoma in those who have and have not had head and neck irradiation in childhood. J Clin Endocrinol Metab 93(6): 2188–2193

81. Tillman BN, Elbermani W (2007) eds. Atlas of human anatomy, clinical edition, 1st edn. Mud Puddle Books, Inc. New York

82. Zhang S (1999) An atlas of histology, Springer, New York

# Cardiovascular Effects of Cancer Therapy

# 10

David A. Briston, Thomas R. Cochran,
Peter J. Sambatakos, Stefanie R. Brown,
and Steven E. Lipshultz

## Contents

During the past 40 years, advances in cancer treatment have drastically improved survival rates for children with cancer. Of the 325,000 childhood cancer survivors in the United States, 24 % have survived greater than 30 years from diagnosis [1]. This growing population of survivors brings the wide array of potential late effects of cancer therapy to light [2]. The developing cardiovascular system is particularly vulnerable to cardiotoxic cancer

D.A. Briston MD
Children's Heart Center, The Children's Hospital at Montefiore/Albert Einstein College of Medicine, 3415 Bainbridge Avenue, R-1; Bronx, NY 10467, USA

T.R. Cochran
University of Kansas Medical Center, 3901 Rainbow Boulevard, Kansas City, KS 66160, USA

P.J. Sambatakos MD
Division of Pediatric Cardiology, New York-Presbyterian/Morgan Stanley Children's Hospital, 3959 Broadway #517; New York, NY 10032, USA

S.R. Brown MD
Departments of Internal Medicine and Pediatrics, University of Miami Miller School of Medicine, 1611 NW 12th Avenue C600D, Miami, FL 33136, USA

S.E. Lipshultz MD, FAAP, FAHA (✉)
Medicine (Cardiology), Oncology, Obstetrics and Gynecology, Molecular Biology and Genetics, Family Medicine and Public Health Sciences, and Pharmacology, Wayne State University School of Medicine, Detroit, MI, USA

Center for Urban Responses to Environmental Stressors, Wayne State University School of Medicine, Detroit, MI, USA

Carman and Ann Adams Department of Pediatrics, Children's Research Center of Michigan, Children's Hospital of Michigan, Wayne State University School of Medicine, Detroit, MI, USA

NCI-designated Comprehensive Cancer Center, Karmanos Cancer Institute, 3901 Beaubien Boulevard, 1K40, Detroit, MI 48201-2196, USA
e-mail: slipshultz@med.wayne.edu

© Springer International Publishing 2015
C.L. Schwartz et al. (eds.), *Survivors of Childhood and Adolescent Cancer:
A Multidisciplinary Approach*, Pediatric Oncology, DOI 10.1007/978-3-319-16435-9_10

therapies such as anthracyclines and radiation. These treatment modalities have been found to result in chronic, progressive cardiac dysfunction occurring months to decades after treatment [3–6].

While contemporary treatment protocols seek to balance oncologic efficacy with cardiotoxic risk, via cardioprotective agents, lower cumulative doses of anthracyclines, and reduced dose, field and volume of radiation, long-term survivors of childhood cancer continue to experience the consequence of earlier treatment approaches. For example, a 5-year-old girl treated in the 1970s for acute lymphoblastic leukemia (ALL) with multimodality therapy including 465 mg/m$^2$ cumulative dose of doxorubicin and cranial radiation developed congestive heart failure (CHF) after 34 months of complete remission, and dilated cardiomyopathy at the age of 16. Bouts of CHF were treated with beta-blockers, diuretics, digoxin, angiotensin-converting enzyme (ACE) inhibitors, an implantable cardiac defibrillator, and ultimately a cardiac transplant at age 36. Unfortunately, she discontinued her medications 6 months posttransplant and suffered cardiac death [7]. In this patient and others, the late-occurring effects of childhood cancer treatment include diastolic and systolic dysfunction, conduction abnormalities, cardiomyocyte necrosis, heart failure, heart transplantation, medication noncompliance, depression, and suicide. In addition, even subclinical, treatment-induced changes could predispose to or exacerbate premature onset of hypertension [8, 9], diabetes mellitus [10], obesity [11], and cardiovascular disease (CVD) [3, 12–17].

Early detection and prevention are crucial to reduce the cardiovascular damage of modern treatment modalities. Although the late cytotoxic effects of cancer therapy may not be completely avoidable, continued development of pediatric protocols is crucial to reducing negative treatment outcomes.

## 10.1 Pathophysiology

The heart begins developing at week 3 of gestation and completes primary morphogenesis at the end of week 8. Early in this time period, myocardial cell replication is high and then tapers off as the septum develops [18]. Cell size remains constant with most embryonic growth occurring through hyperplasia instead of hypertrophy [19]. Late prenatal and early postnatal increases in cardiac mass are marked by both hyperplasia and hypertrophy [20]. By 6 months of age, with the adult number of cardiomyocytes nearly present, subsequent increases in cardiac mass occur via hypertrophy. In order to maintain healthy cardiac output after cardiomyocyte necrosis, the surviving cardiomyocytes undergo compensatory hypertrophy [21]. Hypertrophy of the cardiomyocytes is often observed along with easily determined echocardiographic parameters such as reduced wall thickness and interstitial fibrosis [21]. Therefore, late cardiac failure could be a result of the surviving cardiomyocytes' inability to meet the cardiac demands of a growing body.

The pumping action of the heart is accomplished by the synchronized contraction of cardiomyocytes. An action potential is initiated at the sinus node located in the right atrium. The action potential then travels to the atrioventricular node and His-Purkinje system and ultimately onto the cardiomyocytes in the ventricles. In order for the heart to pump optimally, multiple factors must integrate properly. The actin and myosin filaments in the cardiomyocyte must be in their relaxed state when the action potential arrives. This allows for optimal cross bridging and contractility. Also, there must be calcium in the sarcoplasmic reticulum available to catalyze the cross bridging. Finally, the cardiomyocytes must return to their relaxed state before the next action potential arrives. Anthracyclines and radiation are known to impede the myofibrils from returning to their resting state.

## 10.2 Cytotoxic Effects of Therapy

### 10.2.1 Chemotherapy

#### 10.2.1.1 Anthracyclines

Anthracycline-induced acute cardiac damage is characterized by swelling of the sarcoplasmic reticulum, distortion of myofibrils, and necrosis of cardiomyocytes [22]. The exact mechanism involved with myocardial toxicity from anthracyclines has yet to be completely established. However, studies suggest that highly reactive oxygen species (ROS) play a role in damaging cardiomyocytes [23]. Decreasing numbers of functional cardiomyocytes are associated with diastolic and systolic dysfunction found later in the survivors' lives [24].

The antineoplastic effect of anthracyclines depends on several mechanisms involving inhibition of topoisomerase II, high binding affinity to DNA thus blocking synthesis, altered fluidity and ion channels of cellular membranes, the generation of free ROS, and the disruption of mitochondria [25]. Anthracyclines form complexes with intercellular iron and generate ROS, such as hydrogen peroxide, which readily cause lipid peroxidation and subsequently cellular membrane damage [25, 26]. Due to low levels of catalase, cardiomyocytes are especially vulnerable to ROS. Also, cardiolipin found in the inner membrane of cardiac mitochondria has a high affinity for anthracyclines, which allows higher concentrations of anthracycline in cardiomyocytes [27, 28]. Anthracyclines have also been found to suppress antioxidant enzymes, such as myocardial glutathione oxidase, making cardiomyocytes even more susceptible to damage. Increased oxidant stress results in cardiomyocyte apoptosis via mitogen-activated protein kinase pathways [26]. Changes independent of oxidative stress include impaired apoptotic signaling [29], cardiac stem cell depletion [30], altered gene expression [31], and inhibited release of calcium in the sarcoplasmic reticulum [32].

Alteration of mitochondrial structure and function induced by anthracyclines also affects contractility. Mitochondrial membrane permeability alterations cause intra- and extramitochondrial calcium ion concentrations to change [33]. Additionally, anthracyclines decrease the concentration of subunits in the respiratory chain [34–36]. These abnormalities of the respiratory chain could produce more ROS, further damaging the mitochondria ultimately resulting in cardiomyocyte death [36].

### 10.2.1.2 Alkylating Agents

Alkylating drugs such as cyclophosphamide, cisplatin, and ifosfamide have been associated with cardiotoxicity (Table 10.1). Clinical manifestations include intramyocardial edema in conjunction with serosanguinous pericardial effusion [37] and are associated with left ventricular (LV) wall thickness and mass increases.

The proposed mechanism is direct vascular endothelial injury followed by the leaking of toxic metabolites, interstitial hemorrhage, and edema [38]. Cyclophosphamide may also initiate ischemic cardiomyocyte damage through the formation of intracapillary microemboli [39]. Cyclophosphamide can accentuate cardiotoxicity induced by anthracyclines due in part to an associated myopericarditis [40]. Sequential dosing may also cause the cardiomyocytes to become more sensitive to cyclophosphamide [40]. Ifosfamide is another potentially cardiotoxic alkylating agent with a similar structure to cyclophosphamide. High doses of ifosfamide are associated with cardiac dysfunction analogous to that of cyclophosphamide [41]; cardiac damage resulting in CHF and arrhythmias has been reported in adults [42].

### 10.2.1.3 Tyrosine Kinase Inhibitors

Tyrosine kinase inhibitors (TKI), such as imatinib, interfere with targeted pathways in neoplasms on an intracellular level [43]. However, TKIs also inhibit kinase enzymes in cardiac tissue. Cardiac biopsies of mice treated with imatinib revealed abnormalities of mitochondria, vacuoles, and the endoplasmic reticulum [44]. TKIs are a drug class only recently implemented as part of pediatric protocols. One small retrospective strategy found that of 36 pediatric leukemia patients exposed to imatinib, only 2 children developed cardiomyopathy (these 2 patients were also exposed to anthracyclines, cyclophosphamide, or radiation) [45]. Further studies are needed to determine what screening tools should be put in place before and after receiving TKI therapy.

### 10.2.1.4 Other

5-Fluorouracil and paclitaxel are less commonly used in pediatric cancer therapy. Rare case reports of cardiotoxicity, including coronary artery disease (CAD), cardiomyopathy, and myocardial ischemia and infarction, have been attributed to these agents, primarily in adults [46–48].

## 10.2.2 Radiation

Exposure to radiation can have many effects on the heart including, but not limited to, valvular injury, conduction and autonomic defects, CAD, pericarditis, myocarditis, and cardiomyopathy [49]. The extent of damage to the heart is dependent on the techniques used, the radiation dose administered (including the size of the daily fractions), and the volume of the heart that is irradiated, in addition to the concomitant use of cardiotoxic agents such as anthracyclines.

Microcirculatory damage to the myocardium is characterized by diffuse, nonspecific interstitial fibrosis. Lesions are often localized and can be millimeters to several centimeters in size. Fibrosis can differ from one area of the myocardium to the next [50, 51]. The proportion of type I collagen increases compared to type III collagen leading to altered compliance of the myocardium and ultimately diastolic dysfunction [52]. Myocardial cells involved with conduction are also damaged by radiation [53–55]. Injury to the capillary endothelial cells leads to obstructed

**Table 10.1** Potential cardiotoxicity of cancer therapy

| Drug | Toxic dose range | Acute toxicity | Chronic toxicity |
|---|---|---|---|
| Doxorubicin (Adriamycin RDF, Doxil) | >550 mg/m² (total dose) | Arrhythmias, pericarditis-myocarditis syndrome, myocardial infarction, sudden cardiac death | Cardiomyopathy/CHF, conduction abnormalities/arrhythmias |
| Mitoxantrone (Novantrone) | >100–140 mg/m² (total dose) | CHF, decreases in left ventricular ejection fraction, myocardial infarction, ECG changes, arrhythmias | |
| Cyclophosphamide (Cytoxan) | >100–120 mg/kg (over 2 days) | Hemorrhagic cardiac necrosis, reversible systolic dysfunction, ECG changes, CHF | |
| Ifosfamide (Ifex) | | ECG changes, CHF, arrhythmias | |
| Cisplatin (Platinol) | Conventional dose | Myocardial ischemia, Raynaud's phenomenon, ECG changes | |
| Fluorouracil (Adrucil, Efudex) | Conventional dose | Myocardial infarction, angina, cardiogenic shock/sudden death, dilated cardiomyopathy | |
| Trastuzumab (Herceptin) | | Ventricular dysfunction, CHF | Cardiomyopathy |
| Paclitaxel (Taxol) | Conventional dose | Sudden death, bradyarrhythmia, myocardial dysfunction, myocardial infarction | |
| Amsacrine (Amsa-PD) | Conventional dose | Ventricular arrhythmia, ECG changes | Cardiomyopathy |
| Cytarabine (Cytosar-U) | | CHF, pericarditis, arrhythmias | |
| Arsenic trioxide (Trisenox) | | Arrhythmias, pericardial effusion | |
| Interferon alpha-2A (Roferon) | Conventional dose | Exacerbates underlying cardiac disease, hypotension, arrhythmias | Cardiomyopathy |
| Interleukin-2 (Aldesleukin) | Conventional dose | Myocardial injury/myopericarditis, ventricular arrhythmias, hypotension, sudden death | Dilated cardiomyopathy |
| Mitomycin (Mutamycin) | Conventional dose | CHF | Congestive heart failure |
| Vincristine (Oncovin) | Conventional dose | Myocardial infarction, hypotension, cardiovascular autonomic neuropathy | |
| Vinblastine (Velban) | Conventional dose | Myocardial infarction, Raynaud's phenomenon | |
| Busulfan (Busulfex) | Conventional oral daily dose | Endocardial fibrosis, pulmonary fibrosis, pulmonary hypertension, cardiac tamponade | |
| Tyrosine kinase inhibitor (Imatinib) | Conventional dose | CHF | |

capillary lumens, which engenders thrombus formation.

Inflammatory pathways are thought to be important in the pathogenesis of atherosclerosis, ischemic stroke, and myocardial infarction [56]. Exposure to radiation can activate the pathways leading to inflammation [57]; chronic inflammation increases the risk of developing atherosclerosis and can impair the vasculature of the heart which damages the cardiomyocytes and leads to fibrosis [58]. Radiation can also lead to the production of ROS, which cause oxidative damage to cardiomyocytes [59].

Historically, thickening of the pericardium was a significant risk for patients exposed to radiotherapy [60]. Pericardial adipose tissue was replaced with collagen and fibrin. Similar to the myocardium, small blood vessels with increased permeability propagate in the pericardium. Ischemia and fibrosis occurs due to the damage of the vascular system. Dysfunction of the lymphatic and venous systems of the heart then leads to buildup of extracellular fluids [50]. Thickening of the pericardium has become less prevalent with modern day techniques.

Radiation may cause fibrosis in valves with or without calcification [60, 61]. The pathogenesis of valvular damage is not completely understood. The valves of the heart are avascular, and therefore the mechanism cannot be attributed to microvascular damage. Studies have found that the prevalence and severity of damage are higher in valves on the left side of the heart than valves found on the right [61, 62].

Even with few risk factors other than radiotherapy, many patients develop subsequent CAD. The left anterior descending and right coronary arteries are the most commonly affected vessels. However, with a mean radiation dose of $42 \pm 7$ Gy, McEniery et al. demonstrated 8 out of 15 patients developed at least a 50 % stenosis of the left main coronary artery [63]. This could be a result of the older technique of anterior-weighted irradiation (due to lower energies that necessitated high superficial doses in order to deposit sufficient dose at depth). Proximal narrowing of the vessel occurs and frequently includes the coronary ostia [60, 61, 63–65]. The exact mechanism of radiation-associated CAD is unknown and, histologically, may be similar to atherosclerotic-induced CAD. However, radiotherapy-associated CAD appears to have increased media and adventitial destruction as well as more loss of smooth muscle cells [66].

## 10.3 Clinical Manifestations

### 10.3.1 Anthracycline-Induced Cardiomyopathy

Anthracyclines are one of the most well-known classes of chemotherapeutic agents associated with cardiovascular toxicity. Therapy involving anthracyclines has three categories of cardiotoxicity identified by the time signs or symptoms

**Table 10.2** Characteristics of different types of anthracycline cardiotoxicity

| Characteristic | Acute cardiotoxicity | Early-onset chronic progressive cardiotoxicity | Late-onset chronic progressive cardiotoxicity |
|---|---|---|---|
| Onset | Within the first week of anthracycline treatment | <1 year after the completion of anthracycline treatment | ≥1 year after the completion of anthracycline treatment |
| Risk factor dependence | Unknown | Yes | Yes |
| Clinical features in adults | Transient depression of myocardial contractility | Dilated cardiomyopathy | Dilated cardiomyopathy |
| Clinical features in children | Transient depression of myocardial contractility; myocardial necrosis (cTnT elevation); arrhythmia | Restrictive cardiomyopathy and/or dilated cardiomyopathy; arrhythmia | Restrictive cardiomyopathy and/or dilated cardiomyopathy; arrhythmia |
| Course | Usually reversible on discontinuation of anthracycline | Can be progressive | Can be progressive |

become apparent and how quickly CHF symptoms worsen. The categories include acute, early onset, and late onset (Table 10.2). Late-onset cardiotoxicity occurs any time after the first year following treatment and is the focus of this chapter.

Chronic CHF, decreased exercise therapy, and LV dysfunction are all potential indicators of these three cardiotoxicity categories [67]. Signs of acute cardiotoxicity can span from small abnormalities in electrocardiographic or echocardiographic readings to severe CHF. QTc interval prolongation has been noted in the acute phase following doxorubicin administration, but no adverse sequelae are attributed to this [68]. Acute changes are generally transient and are indicated by systolic dysfunction of the LV observed by echocardiography in less than 1 % of patients [16, 69, 70]. Although most patients recover from acute changes, those who received a high cumulative dose may experience permanent damage. Children who experience LV dysfunction during or immediately after anthracycline therapy are at the highest risk for chronic, progressive cardiac abnormalities [3].

Early-onset cardiotoxicity is characterized by LV dysfunction, electrophysiologic changes, decreased exercise capacity, and clinical CHF [16, 67, 69–74]. Late-onset LV dysfunction is more common among survivors of childhood cancer [16, 75]. Late LV dysfunction has been found to occur as far as two decades following completion of treatment. This type of cardiac deterioration most likely stems from damage induced by treatment that was not severe enough to cause observable symptoms during therapy. Progressive LV dilation, LV wall thinning, and decreased LV contractility develop from cardiomyocyte death and/or damage [76]. In order to maintain cardiac output and LV systolic function, the LV dilates, leading to thinning of the ventricular walls. These changes in structure place more stress on the walls of the LV, further compromising its systolic performance. Eventually, dilation of the LV is unable to meet the additional stress and metabolic demands placed on the heart, leading to CHF. Additional stressors on the heart that can exacerbate underlying dysfunction include acute viral infection [77], growth hormone therapy [78], pregnancy, and physical strain such as lifting weights [77, 79, 80].

Abnormalities have been found to increase over time and are often monitored in echocardiographic measurements, such as LV fractional shortening (LVFS), LV end diastolic dimension, LV afterload, LV contractility, and LV diastolic filling phase indices including strain [21, 80, 81]. Electrocardiograms (ECG) and exercise stress tests can also detect cardiac abnormalities [21]. Lipshultz et al. found that a majority of survivors of ALL had abnormal LV afterload indicative of reduced LV contractility after a median of 6 years of follow-up [21]. The findings are suggestive of progressive rather than static cardiotoxicity because 24 of 34 patients had increased LV afterload values on their last study when compared to earlier measurements.

### 10.3.1.1 Drug-Related Risk Factors

Higher cumulative dose of anthracyclines is a well-known risk factor for LV dysfunction (Table 10.3) [21, 81]. In a study of 6,493 patients who received varying cumulative doses of anthracyclines, the prevalence of CHF was 0.15 % with doses of 400 mg/m$^2$ or less, while it was 7 % among those who had cumulative doses of 550 mg/m$^2$ or more [82]. Also, those who received the higher cumulative dose of anthracycline had a relative risk greater than five of clinically apparent cardiotoxicity [83]. In 1991, Lipshultz et al. found that high cumulative dose of anthracycline was the strongest predictor of cardiotoxicity in a cohort of 115 ALL survivors who received doxorubicin [21]. Another cohort was constructed by Steinherz et al. who demonstrated decreased cardiac function using echocardiography over time in patients who had received anthracyclines 4–20 years prior [80]. Similarly, data from the National Wilms' Tumor Study Group found that cumulative dose of doxorubicin increased the patient's relative risk of CHF by a factor of 3.3 for every 100 mg/m$^2$ of doxorubicin [84]. Though increases in dose of doxorubicin lead to increased cardiotoxicity, the relationship is not linear (Fig. 10.1). Notably, LV dysfunction is still reported in patients with total dose less than 300 mg/m$^2$ [85, 86]. As alluded to above, the dose of a cardiotoxic agent is only one determinant in overall cardiac risk assessment, and no dose of anthracycline is absolutely safe [87].

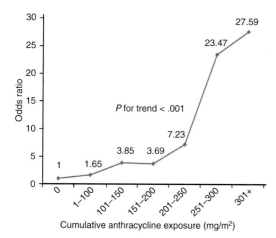

**Fig. 10.1** Dose-response relationship between cumulative anthracycline exposure and risk of cardiomyopathy. Patients with no exposure to anthracyclines served as the reference group. Magnitude of risk is expressed as odds ratio, which was obtained using conditional logistic regression adjusting for age at diagnosis, sex, and chest radiation (Reprinted with permission from the publisher Blanco et al. [247]

Echocardiographic measures of cardiac strain were measured in a cohort of pediatric oncology patients treated with a single dose of anthracycline as compared to another that received at least 228 mg/m² or more [21]. Children who received a single dose had less impaired LV function than those who received more. In this population, LVFS and LV contractility were significantly reduced, reflecting cardiac dysfunction. Left ventricular afterload, which is a direct function of blood pressure, LV dimension, and inversely related to LV wall thickness, was greatly elevated in those who received more anthracycline. This was attributed to a reduced LV wall thickness. LV contractility was also decreased.

### 10.3.1.2 Drug Delivery

Rate of administration has been suggested as another possible segregating factor in determining anthracycline toxicity (Table 10.3). Some studies found that children who received higher anthracycline dose rates experienced cardiotoxicity independent of cumulative dose [88]. Additionally, in adult protocols, continuous infusion of anthracyclines was associated with reduced cardiotoxicity [89]. Despite the lack of evidence on efficacy in the pediatric population, many pediatric protocols incorporated continuous infusion based on adult study findings [90–92]. However, evidence to date does not support a cardioprotective difference between continuous infusions as compared to bolus doses in children. While it was thought that prolonged exposure might reduce the peak dose and help prevent anthracycline-induced cardiomyopathy, this appears not to be so according to echocardiographic measures published in 2002 [91]. Left ventricular structure and function were not significantly different between the two groups who received doxorubicin either as a bolus or as a continuous infusion. Multiple echocardiographic measurements were used in this study to evaluate LV function, and in both cohorts equivalent levels of LV dysfunction were observed. Continued follow-up of this cohort had similar findings after 8 years [92]. Subclinical cardiotoxicity after moderate doses of anthracycline was not mitigated by 6-hour infusions in another study [93], which also suggests that rate of infusion is not an important parameter in determining risk.

### 10.3.1.3 Liposomal Anthracyclines

Clinical trials with doxorubicin began in the 1960s but not until the 1990s was its liposomal form used [94]. By encapsulating doxorubicin within a liposome, the volume of distribution is decreased, thus decreasing toxicity while preserving efficacy (Table 10.3) [95]. Liposomes also appear to localize their encapsulated drug directly at tumor sites by having an affinity for leaky tumor vasculature [95].

No difference in efficacy was noted in patients with metastatic breast cancer when comparing pegylated liposomal to conventional doxorubicin, but the incidence of cardiotoxicity decreased from 19 to 4 % ($p < 0.001$) [96]. The process of pegylating involves attaching polyethylene glycol to the molecule to further decrease immunogenicity and clearance while enhancing therapeutic effects. Additionally, two studies provided evidence that pegylated doxorubicin appears

**Table 10.3** Risk factors for cardiotoxicity

| Risk factor | Comment | References |
|---|---|---|
| Cumulative anthracycline dose | Cumulative doses >500 mg/m² are associated with significantly elevated long-term risk | [3, 21, 70, 81] |
| Time after therapy | Incidence of clinically important cardiotoxicity increases progressively after therapy | [3, 21, 81, 90] |
| Rate of anthracycline administration | Prolonged administration to minimize circulating dose may decrease toxicity; results are mixed | [90, 91] |
| Individual anthracycline dose | Higher individual doses are associated with increased late cardiotoxicity, even when cumulative doses are limited; no dose is risk-free | [3, 81, 90] |
| Type of anthracycline | Liposomal encapsulated preparations may reduce cardiotoxicity. Data on anthracycline analogues and differences in cardiotoxicity are conflicting | [70, 89] |
| Radiation therapy | Cumulative radiation dose >30 Gy; as little as 5 Gy increases the risk; before, after, or concomitant with anthracycline treatment | [67, 69, 90] |
| Concomitant therapy | Trastuzumab, cyclophosphamide, bleomycin, vincristine, amsacrine, and mitoxantrone, among others, may increase susceptibility or toxicity | [69, 70] |
| Preexisting cardiac risk factors | Hypertension; ischemic, myocardial, and valvular heart disease; prior cardiotoxic treatment | [71] |
| Personal health habits | Smoking, alcohol consumption, energy drinks, stimulants, prescription and illicit drugs | [90] |
| Comorbidities | Diabetes, obesity, renal dysfunction, pulmonary disease, endocrinopathies, electrolyte and metabolic abnormalities, sepsis, infection, pregnancy, viruses, elite athletic participation, low vitamin D levels | [71, 90] |
| Age | Both young and advanced age at treatment are associated with elevated risk | [21, 81, 90] |
| Sex | Females are at greater risk than males | [81] |
| Complementary therapies | More information needs to be collected to assess risk | [90] |
| Additional factors | Trisomy 21; African-American ancestry | [70] |

to accumulate in myocardial cells in a reduced amount when compared to doxorubicin [97, 98]. Further evidence of decreased cardiotoxicity is provided when comparing serial left ventricular ejection fraction (LVEF) measurements as cardiomyopathy is decreased at cumulative doses above 500 mg/m² [98]. There are no randomized studies of pegylated doxorubicin in children.

### 10.3.1.4 Novel Anthracycline Analogues

Epirubicin, an epimer of doxorubicin, exhibits less cumulative dose cardiotoxicity than doxorubicin. Epirubicin was associated with cardiotoxicity in 3 % of patients at a cumulative dose of 900 mg/m² and 10 % at 1,000 mg/m². Doxorubicin had a 5 % incidence at 500 mg/m² and 15 % at greater than 600 mg/m², almost double that of epirubicin [99]. One study found similar efficacy rates when comparing non-pegylated liposomal doxorubicin and epirubicin in 160 patients [100].

However, several studies suggest epirubicin may cause subclinical cardiac injury [71]. While no CHF was noted for patients receiving epirubicin at a cumulative dose of 400–500 mg/m$^2$, the LVEF was decreased significantly in one third of patients at a dose of 450 mg/m$^2$ [101]. While clinical cardiotoxicity is decreased in the short term, long-term follow-up is necessary to adequately assess epirubicin toxicity.

Idarubicin is an analogue of doxorubicin that has been shown to exhibit decreased cardiotoxicity when compared to doxorubicin. While providing a decrease in cardiomyopathy (5 % at its target dose of 150–290 mg/m$^2$) [102], subclinical cardiac effects were observed at lower cumulative doses (150 mg/m$^2$) [102]. Similar to epirubicin, idarubicin appears to provide less clinical cardiotoxicity but subclinical effects remain.

Mitoxantrone is part of the anthracenedione family but is structurally similar to anthracycline. This class has antiviral, antibacterial, immunomodulatory, and antitumor properties. While mitoxantrone has been shown to be effective in treating various malignancies, the risk of CHF remains elevated compared to other antineoplastic therapies. The risk of CHF at the upper limit of dosing (140 mg/m$^2$) is 2.6 % (Table 10.1) [103]. However, in evaluating subclinical cardiac function, a decrease in LVEF to less than 50 % was seen in 2 % of patients [103].

Monoclonal antibodies against vascular endothelial growth factor, such as bevacizumab and trastuzumab, are used to treat a variety of solid tumors. These antibodies affect myocardial homeostasis and can lead to changes in cardiomyocytes function and metabolism [104]. One randomized controlled study found that when combined with anthracycline treatment, bevacizumab was associated with heart failure in 3.8 % of these adult patients [105]. It is unknown whether bevacizumab enhances cardiomyopathy in children.

## 10.3.2 Radiation Exposure and Cardiac Toxicity

Radiation-induced CVD is a major cause of morbidity and mortality in pediatric patients receiving mediastinal radiation. Complications can be both acute and chronic and include pericarditis, CAD, cardiomyopathy, valvular defects, veno-occlusive disease, and conduction abnormalities. Methods to prevent these complications include assessing patient risk factors and adjusting dose and size of the radiation portal. Doses greater than 40 Gy have been associated with increased cardiac mortality [106].

The onset of radiation-induced cardiotoxicity typically is 10 or more years following completion of therapy. Thickening of the pericardium due to high doses of mediastinal radiation has become rare with modern day practices. Complications such as restrictive cardiomyopathy and myocardial infarction are more prevalent in children treated with radiation. Nonetheless, the cohort of survivors who received high-dose mediastinal radiation is aging, and data suggest that they will be experiencing the complications outlined herein. Unlike others who have cardiac disease, the clinical symptoms of myocardial infarctions can be harder to detect or even nonexistent in this population [107].

Also, radiotherapy is associated with diastolic dysfunction and anthracyclines with systolic dysfunction. One study evaluated cardiac status of 48 long-term survivors of Hodgkin lymphoma treated with mantle irradiation [108]. At a median follow-up of 14 years, LV systolic dysfunction was found in five (10 %) of the survivors, although three of these five had also been treated with anthracyclines. On the other hand, 18 (37 %) had LV measurements indicating diastolic dysfunction.

Valvular dysfunction is an increasingly common finding in these patients. In the same study previously mentioned, Adams et al. found at least one heart valve abnormality in 20 (43 %) of the survivors [108]. Other studies have found similar echocardiographic findings [109–112]. Valvular heart disease may be progressive and can contribute to CHF [62].

#### 10.3.2.1 Dose Reduction

Historically, radiation doses of 30–40 Gy were used in pediatric Hodgkin lymphoma and were associated with subsequent cardiotoxicity. Current radiation exposure is at or below doses of 25 Gy [113], much less than the aforementioned 40 Gy causing clinical cardiotoxicity. Further studies of cardiotoxic events at this level are necessary, and follow-up of the patients who received the much higher doses of radiotherapy should be closely pursued.

Reduction of the volume of radiation received by the patient has been achieved through the utilization of involved-field radiotherapy as opposed to mantle radiotherapy. This technique reduced the relative risk of cardiac-related death from 5.3 to 1.4 in patients treated for Hodgkin lymphoma [114]. Similar reductions of predicted risk have been reported by others [115, 116]. Subcarinal blocking of the LV has also been found to reduce the incidence of pericarditis [117]. Further reductions in radiation volume are now being tested and include involved site and involved node radiation therapy; both approaches will decrease the dose to the heart [118].

#### 10.3.2.2 Targeted Therapy

Three-dimensional conformal radiation therapy and proton therapy are currently being studied for their ability to reduce dose of radiation received by cardiac structures. Three-dimensional conformal radiation therapy uses CT imaging to gather tissue density and depth information which assists in the calculation of dose distribution, with the radiation fields delivering this dose from multiple angles. Proton therapy uses charged particles as opposed to high-energy photons to deliver therapeutic radiation. These charged particles have reduced exit dose as they leave normal tissue, which may confer reduced toxicity. Further research is required to determine the capability of these contemporary techniques in reducing radiation exposure to cardiac structures.

Respiratory maneuvers during radiation, such as quiet breathing or breath holding, may decrease radiation to the heart and, thus, cardiotoxicity. In one study of breast cancer patients, deep inspiration was performed, which displaces the heart caudally. In 21 % of patients, the heart was displaced out of the radiation field [119].

### 10.4 Detection and Screening

#### 10.4.1 Cardiac Considerations

Assessment of multiple studies has shown that childhood cancer survivors are at increased risk of CVD compared to the general population as early as 1 year after treatment [120] and for at least 45 years after initial diagnosis [121, 122]. Studies comparing long-term survivors to their siblings have shown higher rates of CHF, myocardial infarction, valvular disease [123], and subclinical dysfunction [124]. Death from cardiac disease is the third leading cause of death in long-term survivors [120, 121, 125]. Long-term survivors of childhood cancer who received potentially cardiotoxic therapies should undergo regular, repeated evaluations of cardiac status, even if the patient is asymptomatic. Although screening regimens have been suggested for patients treated with doxorubicin and/or irradiation [49, 126–129], no specific regimen for childhood cancer survivors has ever been tested for efficacy and cost-effectiveness. Nevertheless, serial evaluation recognizes the following: (1) as the survivor grows and matures, demands on the heart increase, which a damaged heart at some point may no longer be able to meet, (2) lifestyle changes may further stress the heart, and (3) cancer therapy-related heart disease may itself be progressive.

Furthermore, survivors need to be screened as they undertake or contemplate changes in their life that increase cardiac stress such as beginning a new exercise program, starting growth hormone therapy, becoming pregnant, or undergoing anesthesia. It has been shown that growth hormone deficiency is seen after radiation to the hypothalamic-pituitary axis, which many long-term survivors have received. The LV wall, which has been shown to be thinned after anthracycline and radiation treatment (Fig. 10.2), is increased in diameter after growth hormone therapy is

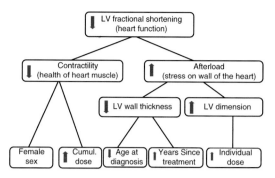

**Fig. 10.2** Marginal (Kaplan-Meier) and (C-E) cause-specific (competing risk) cumulative incidence of cardiac events (CEs) in childhood cancer survivors. Marginal cumulative incidence for all CEs, stratified according to potential cardiotoxic (CTX) therapy or no CTX therapy, log-rank $p<0.001$ (Reprinted with permission from the publisher Wouters et al. [89])

started. However, this change only lasts as long as growth hormone replacement therapy is continued [130]. Clearly, those patients who have had an abnormal finding or study, let alone a symptomatic cardiac event at any time, should have more frequent cardiac screening. The importance of screening all survivors treated with potentially cardiotoxic therapy is underscored by the fact that Lipshultz and colleagues could not find a correlation between patient- or parent-reported symptoms and measures of LV function or exercise tolerance in those treated for ALL with doxorubicin with or without chest irradiation [21].

Longer follow-up is important since it is known that both the prevalence and severity of LV abnormalities increase over time (Fig. 10.3) [81, 131]. Lipshultz et al. demonstrated an increased incidence of LV dysfunction when increasing the length of follow-up of 120 patients [81]. Acute LV dysfunction can be treated with anticongestive therapy and usually shows an initial improvement, but a progressive decline is expected even with appropriate long-term medications. In following pediatric cancer survivors at 6 years after anthracycline administration, it was found that 65 % had silent cardiac dysfunction [21, 69, 81]. Pregnancy, infection, cocaine use, and demanding exercise regimens may not be the only stressors that precipitate CHF. Although one

study found no cases of peripartum cardiomyopathy in following 53 survivors at a mean follow-up of 20 years [132], the study is not adequately powered. Further research on a larger scale should be conducted to investigate stressors and their effects on the heart. Clinically significant cardiotoxicity such as CHF or cardiac rhythm-related symptoms can initially appear either during the third trimester of pregnancy or during the first few months postpartum and may be attributable to intravascular volume increases during pregnancy or to other pregnancy-associated changes. Pregnancy should be considered to be a cardiac stressor for survivors and follow-up as high-risk patients is recommended. Screening protocols should include close serial monitoring with involvement of a multidisciplinary team approach. There is need for continued cardiac monitoring, even in asymptomatic patients, particularly during stressful circumstances [133].

Cardiac evaluation of the survivor should first begin with a thorough annual history and physical examination [126]. Self-reported symptoms without specific questioning do not necessarily correlate well with cardiovascular abnormalities detected by specialized testing; it is essential that information be determined by specific, quantitative parameters (e.g., "Can you walk up two flights of stairs without becoming short of breath?"). Changes in exercise tolerance, dyspnea on exertion, palpitations, and syncope should all be evaluated by specific screening modalities because they may be the manifestations of the late anthracycline-related cardiotoxicity (CHF and arrhythmias). Worrisome findings on physical examination include tachypnea, tachycardia, gallops, rales, hepatomegaly, peripheral edema, and diminished peripheral pulse volume and perfusion, any of which is suggestive of cardiac abnormalities.

The history should not only evaluate risk from therapy but also traditional CVD risk factors such as hypertension, tobacco abuse, diabetes, family history of early CVD, gender, and age. Landy et al. using the traditional scoring systems for CVD risk (the Pathobiological Determinants of Atherosclerosis in Youth (PDAY) and the Framingham Risk Calculator (FRC)) found that long-term survivors had a similar risk profile to their siblings. While a higher proportion of survivors had PDAY odds ratios and FRC risk ratio(s) greater than 4, this was not statistically significant possibly suggesting that the increased risk of CVD is truly due to therapeutic cardiotoxicity [128].

### 10.4.1.1 Assessment of Coronary Artery Disease

All childhood cancer survivors should be screened regularly for CAD risk factors. While those treated with mantle radiation are probably most at risk for CAD, survivors treated with anthracyclines and high-dose cyclophosphamide may also have damaged hearts that can ill afford further compromise from myocardial ischemia or infarction. Patients who received brain irradiation, especially those with proven growth hormone deficiency or other hypothalamic-pituitary axis dysfunction, may also be at higher risk, compared with other survivors. Risk factor for CAD, such as family history, hypertension, tobacco abuse, hyperlipidemia [134], obesity, diabetes mellitus, and a sedentary lifestyle, should be evaluated at each long-term visit. Counseling to reduce such risk factors is extremely important. Signs and symptoms of pericarditis, cardiomyopathy, valvular disease, arrhythmia, and CAD should all raise concern.

As in other children, chest pain is usually due to costochondritis (Tietze's syndrome) in young survivors and is characterized by point tenderness, discomfort with inspiration, and response to nonsteroidal analgesics. However, because of the sharply increased risk of myocardial infarction in survivors treated with mediastinal irradiation, myocardial infarction should be ruled out in any such patient who presents acutely. In a study of 294 survivors of Hodgkin disease who received mediastinal radiation of 35 Gy, 18.4 % (54 of 294) had abnormal stress testing, and on invasive coronary angiography, 22 had coronary stenoses of more than 50 % of the luminal diameter [135]. Although the possibility of myocardial ischemia is strongly suggested by crushing pain (especially with exercise), diaphoresis, dyspnea, and nausea, the absence of these symptoms does not necessarily exclude ischemia because chest irradiation may cause individuals to feel cardiac pain abnormally [136]. Complaints of chest pain, even in young survivors treated with mediastinal irradiation, require additional evaluation.

### Noninvasive Coronary Artery Imaging

In 2008, the American Heart Association published a scientific statement regarding noninvasive coronary artery imaging comparing magnetic resonance angiography and multidetector CT angiography [137]. With regard to detection of coronary atherosclerosis, studies of magnetic resonance angiography at multiple centers show a sensitivity ranging from 65 to 93 % and specificity of 42–100 %. A meta-analysis of 64-slice CT angiography found 6 studies with sensitivity of 93 % and specificity of 96 % and found 19 studies with a sensitivity of 86 % and specificity of 96 %. Each of these two modalities has its benefits and limitations. CT angiography has higher spatial resolution with a shorter examination time and wider availability when compared to magnetic resonance angiography, while magnetic resonance angiography has no exposure to ionizing radiation or iodinated contrast. The summary recommendations state that neither modality should be used for screening asymptomatic patients, but both have potential benefit for symptomatic patients with intermediate coronary risk by standard criteria. Patients with high pretest likelihood for stenosis should undergo invasive angiography as opposed to CT angiography due to likelihood of need for intervention [137].

### Invasive Procedures

In all survivors treated with potentially cardiotoxic therapies, angiography and cardiac catheterization are appropriate for evaluating symptomatic disease (angina and CHF, respectively). They are not appropriate for routine serial screening in the asymptomatic survivor. According to some experts, however, these procedures should be performed if any clinically significant cardiac lesion is found due to the fact that CAD can be asymptomatic and is often present in those who received mediastinal irradiation [138].

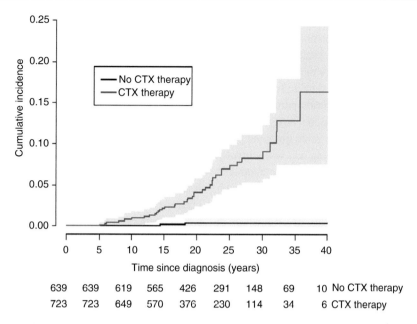

**Fig. 10.3** The relationships between cardiac and noncardiac findings in long-term survivors of childhood malignancy treated with anthracycline therapy (Reprinted with permission from the publisher Van der Pal et al. [248]

### 10.4.1.2   Assessment of Cardiomyopathy and Congestive Heart Failure

**Imaging**

The most common screening methods for anthracycline-associated cardiomyopathy are echocardiograms, radionuclide ventriculography – also commonly referred to as radionuclide angiography (RNA) – and ECGs. These methods are also useful for screening for radiation-associated cardiotoxicity with subtle differences. Echocardiography and RNA are both excellent methods of measuring LV systolic function, but echocardiography has the advantage over RNA of being noninvasive. Echocardiography also has the advantage of being able to evaluate heart structures such as the pericardium and valves. Unfortunately, it can be technically difficult in adults due to body habitus and bone density.

Fractional shortening and ejection fraction are reliable echocardiographic measures of LV systolic function. Fractional shortening is the percentage of change in LV dimension between systole and diastole. Both measurements, however, are dependent on loading conditions, which may vary considerably, particularly during chemotherapy [139, 140]. Load-independent measures of cardiomyocyte health and myocardial function can be provided by measurements of wall stress and contractility, i.e., the relationship between wall stress and the heart rate corrected velocity of circumferential fiber shortening [140]. Additionally, anatomic measurements such as posterior wall thickness and LV dimension are useful. Current monitoring recommendations include obtaining echocardiograms of these measurements at regular intervals after therapy [126, 129]. Several studies show abnormal LVFS in long-term survivors versus controls [24, 141, 142]. The recommended monitoring intervals depend on cumulative anthracyclines dose, other therapies received, the detection of abnormalities, any symptoms the patient may experience, and coexistent stressors such as growth or participation in competitive athletics.

Echocardiographic modalities such as strain and strain rate are used to measure regional myocardial wall motion as well as LV systolic and diastolic function. Adult studies on breast cancer patients have found that strain rate imaging allowed for earlier and better detection of subtle changes in preclinical cardiac function such as longitudinal LV function [74, 143–145]. Although studies have found high positive predictive value for longitudinal strain, this measure depends partially on the prevalence of the condition being studied. Although positive predictive value gives the probability that a positive screening test will correctly identify an outcome of interest, it does not validate a test as cost-effective or practical. Further research is required to elucidate the validity of strain and strain rate as surrogate measures of LV function in childhood cancer survivors [146].

Radionuclide ventriculography determines an ejection fraction that is arguably more accurate than that derived from echocardiography by calculating the change in radioactivity at end diastole to that at end systole. However, this measure is load-dependent, and no load-independent measure of cardiomyocyte health exists for this modality. Although it has been recommended as a baseline study to be repeated every 5 years in anthracycline-treated children (in addition to more frequent echocardiography [109, 126, 127]), further studies are necessary to determine whether RNA is of clinical value for the entire cohort of asymptomatic patients. It is clearly useful for those in whom a good echocardiogram cannot be obtained, which is frequently the case in adults. However, it should be noted that the LVFS on echocardiography and the ejection fraction on RNA are not directly convertible.

Myocardial performance index is a ratio of isovolumic contraction and relaxation times to ejection time and is a newer form of evaluation of cardiac dysfunction using Doppler echocardiography. Changes in myocardial performance index can occur before changes in the echocardiographic measures of LV function suggesting that myocardial performance index may also be a useful tool in evaluation of early asymptomatic cardiac dysfunction [147, 148].

A significant difference in anthracyclines and radiation-associated cardiomyopathy is the type of cardiac dysfunction caused. Although otherwise quite different from other types of dilated cardiomyopathy [13], anthracycline-associated cardiomyopathy resembles dilated cardiomyopathy because it primarily causes diastolic dysfunction. Lipshultz et al. found that survivors of childhood ALL treated with anthracyclines initially developed dilated cardiomyopathy as evidenced by reduced shortening fractions and contractility with LV dilation [3]. As time progressed, they developed signs of restrictive cardiomyopathy such as smaller LV dimensions and decreased wall thickness [73] (Fig. 10.4). Radiation damage differs from that of anthracyclines as it causes restrictive cardiomyopathy, which primarily leads to diastolic dysfunction (i.e., problems with filling the heart). Both conditions, however, can cause CHF in the long term. Therefore, it is important to screen for both with the hope that early intervention can delay or prevent CHF. The problem is that measuring diastolic function noninvasively can only be done through imprecise echocardiographic techniques. In addition to measuring LV wall stress, LVFS, and LV wall thickness, measuring LV mass and LV chamber size is recommended, which, if abnormal, may suggest restrictive cardiomyopathy. Measuring the ratio of peak early filling to peak late filling of the LV (E/A ratio) and other indirect echocardiographic indicators of diastolic function is also recommended. Brouwer et al. showed increasing rates of diastolic dysfunction in a cohort of long-term survivors of bone tumors treated with doxorubicin when evaluated at 9 and 14 years posttreatment [149]. Echocardiography is also useful for following valvular and pericardial status. Recommendations for frequency of monitoring of cardiac function are based on age at time of treatment, anthracycline dosage, and whether combined modalities of therapy are used [126, 129]. Lifetime health care cost of echocardiographic screening using Children's Oncology Group guidelines is approximately $500 million for 100,000 anthracycline-exposed survivors (2010 US dollars) or $5,000 per patient and was predicted to extend quality-adjusted life years by 1.8 months and to delay CHF by 8.4 months [150].

## Biomarkers

Blood cardiac biomarkers are garnering interest for the detection of cardiac dysfunction during

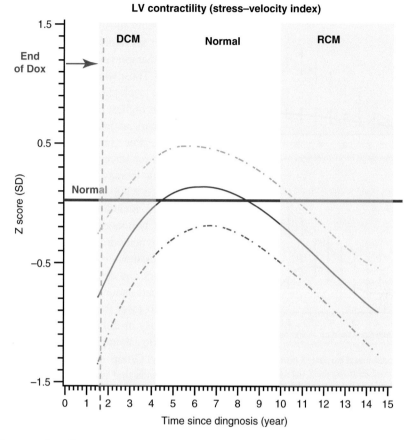

**Fig. 10.4** Z-scores of cardiac measurements from 115 long-term survivors of acute lymphoblastic leukemia treated with doxorubicin, by time since diagnosis (years). The *solid line* is the overall group mean in this model. The *dashed lines* are the *upper* and *lower* 95 % CIs from the predicted mean 2 SEs of the mean. Left ventricular (*LV*) contractility (stress-velocity index) (Reprinted with permission from the publisher Lipshultz [3])

and after therapy, including in long-term survivors. These blood cardiac biomarkers include cardiac troponin T (cTnT) and N-terminal pro-B-type natriuretic peptide (NT-pro-BNP). Lipshultz et al. demonstrated that during and immediately after therapy with doxorubicin with or without dexrazoxane, both cTnT and NT-pro-BNP are elevated in some patients. Dexrazoxane seems to offer protection as a smaller percentage of patients had elevations of either biomarker at all points in the study (Fig. 10.5a, b) [17]. A study of 122 survivors showed no elevations in cTnT. However, 13 % of these patients had abnormal NT-pro-BNP, which correlated with cumulative anthracycline doses. Only 3 % and 7 %, respectively, had a LVFS less than 29 % and LVEF less than 55 % suggesting

that NT-pro-BNP may provide earlier detection of cardiac dysfunction, but at this time study size is a significant limitation to development of recommendations [151].

### 10.4.1.3    Assessment of Dysrhythmias/Conduction Abnormalities

Electrical conduction abnormalities and rhythm disturbances may remain silent until fatal. Serial screening ECGs may identify potentially fatal arrhythmias such as prolonged corrected QT interval, atrioventricular conduction delay, ventricular ectopy, low voltage, second-degree AV block, complete heart block, ST elevation (or depression), and T wave changes. Recommendations

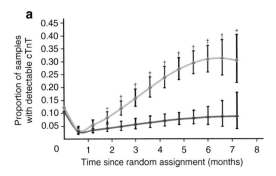

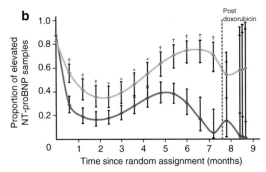

**Fig. 10.5** (**a**) Model-based estimated probability of having an increased cardiac troponin T (*cTnT*) level at each depicted time point in patients treated with doxorubicin, with or without dexrazoxane (Reprinted with permission from the publisher Lipshultz et al. [12]). (**b**) Model-based estimated probability of having an increased N-terminal pro-brain natriuretic peptide (*NT-proBNP*) level at each depicted time point in patients treated with doxorubicin with or without dexrazoxane (Reprinted with permission from the publisher Lipshultz [12])

from the CVD Task Force of the Children's Oncology Group include a baseline ECG at the completion of therapy and, for those with prolonged corrected QT interval, counseling on avoidance of potentially dangerous medications (i.e., tricyclic antidepressants, antifungals, and macrolides) [126].

No study conclusively establishes what screening tool and with what frequency it should be used. Steinherz et al. recommended performing 24-h ECG every 5 years in long-term survivors who had received anthracyclines, and this proposal is commonly followed. No large study has been done that conclusively demonstrates with what frequency screening should be undertaken, although the importance in doing so is clear.

#### 10.4.1.4 Cardiometabolic Screening

Heart-healthy lifestyles should be encouraged in long-term survivors of cancers treated with cardiotoxic therapies even if the patient is asymptomatic [152]. Those who have received anthracyclines, high-dose cyclophosphamide and cardiac radiation are at highest risk of CHF, and cardiac mortality occurs at increased rates within the first decades after cardiotoxic treatments [153]. Protocols for screening those who have survived cardiotoxic therapy have not been tested for efficacy, but a wide scope of monitoring should be considered, including assessment of both modifiable and non-modifiable risk factors. Relevant screening methods include detailed treatment history, assessment of independent cardiovascular risk factors, and detailed review of systems [126]. As the heart endures continued stress, it may not be able to meet the demand. Moreover, cardiac disease may itself be progressive in the setting of cardiotoxic therapies [154]. The Children's Oncology Group consensus statement of 2008 recommends that risk factors should be identified and therapies tailored to the details of the cardiotoxic regimen [126]. When lifestyle changes require an increase in cardiac demand, whether in the form of a physically demanding job or new exercise regimen, screening tests may need to be performed. Moreover, screening is important because symptoms do not consistently correlate with cardiac performance as measured by echocardiographic variables such as LV function [133]. Screening to assess for cardiac dysfunction should be undertaken regularly and aimed at addressing problems earlier rather than later.

#### 10.4.1.5 Exercise Stress Testing

Echocardiography and ECG exercise testing reveal cardiac injury that is not discernible in resting studies [155–158]. Although more research is required to determine the appropriate use of such studies in chemotherapeutic- or radiation-associated CVD [49], it is likely that these tests will be of good predictive value, especially since anthracycline-treated and/or cardiac-irradiated patients appear to decompensate at times of cardiac stress. Cardiopulmonary exercise stress testing also provides the opportunity to measure maximum oxygen consumption, a key prognostic indicator in patients with cardiomyopathy [159]. It is surprisingly low in long-term survivors of childhood cancer treated with anthracyclines and/or mediastinal radiotherapy [108]; long-term survivors without evidence of subclinical cardiac dysfunction using traditional echocardiographic measures had much lower oxygen consumption than sibling controls [160].

Screening tests for measuring the indirect effects on the cardiovascular system should also be performed periodically. In particular, pulmonary and thyroid function tests should be performed for those at risk due to bleomycin or chest irradiation.

### 10.4.1.6  Post-radiation

After chest radiation, early-onset CAD, cardiomyopathy, conduction abnormalities, and pericarditis are believed to be secondary to varying degrees of fibrosis. Fibrotic changes of blood vessels were historically considered to be the mechanism of injury that led to the multiple cardiac pathologies associated with mediastinal radiation [113]. Although vascular damage occurs, the radiation's deleterious effects are not limited to these structures. Valvular, vascular, and myocardial layers are affected, and not only the treatments but also the screening modalities reflect the wide range of damage incurred by mediastinal radiation.

### Early-Onset Coronary Artery Disease

Coronary artery disease is an increasingly common cause of morbidity and mortality in those who receive radiation therapy. Estimates of CAD prevalence suggest that it may be one of the most common complications from mediastinal radiation. In 1992, Boivin et al. demonstrated increased mortality associated with CAD compared to controls at only 10 years of follow-up [161]. Hancock et al. found that survivors of childhood cancer who received radiation therapy experienced excess mortality due to myocardial infarction [114, 162]. The anterior course of the left anterior descending artery has been found to be more susceptible to radiation-induced damage than other arteries in limited studies [163, 164], but the cor-

onary ostia are also susceptible [165]. The right coronary and left main arteries adjacent to their origins at the aorta appear to be damaged with increasing doses of radiation. The course of this damage is still unclear. Theories postulate capillary destruction, epicardial artery damage, and even inflammatory marker upregulation as possible etiologies [106]. While the mechanism remains unclear, the outcome is apparent.

Treatment of CAD in those who have received chest radiation is not different from those who have not. However, should percutaneous coronary interventions fail to be a revascularization option, surgical procedures will be complicated by fibrosis in multiple areas of the mediastinum. The left internal mammary artery, which is commonly used in coronary artery bypass grafting, is more prone to radiation damage given its native anatomical position. Emerging research suggests that delaying radiation and decreasing its dose have minimized CAD prevalence, but even with that improvement, surveillance must be performed [113].

### Valvular Dysfunction

Valvular heart disease is a known complication of mediastinal radiation, and its prevalence is higher than initially thought. Given the avascular nature of cardiac valves, it was suspected that dysfunction would be minimal and would not interfere as significantly with overall function compared with other injuries. However, Wethal et al. found initial valve insufficiency in Hodgkin lymphoma survivors exposed to mediastinal radiotherapy. Later, stenosis may appear [166]. Left-sided heart valves have a higher predilection toward dysfunction after mediastinal radiation. It is suspected to be due to the relatively anterior positioning of the heart valves, which is also considered to be the reason for destruction of the left anterior descending and left internal mammary arteries [167]. Heidenreich et al. published data suggesting that valve insufficiency was more common and that stenosis was rare [168]. Although it is possible the follow-up time accounted for this observation, data remain conflicting regarding the natural history of the valve deterioration. Carlson et al. published a case series that suggests that right-sided heart valvular dysfunction may be more common than previously thought and can be evaluated for with echocardiography in much the same way as left-sided valve dysfunction [62]. An autopsy series was performed in 1996 that demonstrated diffuse heart valvular fibrosis in almost half of patients who received mediastinal radiation [61]. Of the affected heart valves, 79 % were left sided.

Another complication of heart valvular dysfunction involves the increased susceptibility to infection. Recently updated guidelines on antibiotic use for patients with heart disease suggest that patients who have been exposed to mediastinal radiation do not require antibiotics for dental procedures [169]. However, at autopsy, almost one half of patients had significant heart valvular disease in a non-repaired form, which is a potential indication for antibiotic prophylaxis [169]. Further data must be collected to determine if this patient population should use antibiotics before receiving dental care.

Regardless of the affected heart valve, therapy for heart valve dysfunction has traditionally been surgical repair with a median sternotomy. With the advent of percutaneous interventions, this patient population may have an alternative to a surgical procedure marred by possible infection, technical difficulties, and prolonged hospitalization.

### Conduction Abnormalities

A high prevalence of conduction abnormalities following mediastinal radiation has not been proven in a large clinical trial, but fascicular blocks and complete heart block are reported in the immediate post-radiation phase [53, 170]. Some hearts act as if the nervous system has failed altogether with tachycardia mimicking denervation seen in transplantation [108]. Multiple histologic samples have demonstrated neurodegeneration, although supporting data is limited [171].

### Pericarditis

Both acute and delayed pericarditis are sequelae of mediastinal radiation. Increased inflammation coupled to necrosis of tissue likely leads to acute pericarditis although the prevalence of this is lower than previously suspected. Hancock et al. demonstrated that only 8 of 635 patients experienced acute pericarditis and presented with pleuritic chest pain, ST-segment changes, silent pleural effusions, or even as a friction rub on exam [162]. The patients were treated with anti-inflammatory medications and recovered. Delayed pericarditis may present from months to decades after radiation exposure, but usually within 1 year. It is commonly seen as a pericardial effusion on imaging. As a diagnosis of exclusion, multiple other causes should be ruled out. Development of constrictive pericarditis was observed in approximately 7 % of patients who received mediastinal radiation as reported in 1974 [172], but this may overestimate its prevalence in the modern clinical era. Treatment is undertaken rapidly to prevent progression to constrictive pericarditis.

### 10.4.2 Noncardiac Considerations

#### 10.4.2.1 Patient-Related Risk Factors

Younger age at treatment is a risk factor for anthracycline-induced cardiac dysfunction [3, 173]. Children less than age 4 years at time of exposure were at significantly increased risk for development of LV dysfunction [21]. In a study examining the effects of 244–550 mg/m$^2$ of doxorubicin in adult and pediatric survivors of ALL or osteosarcoma, Lipshultz et al. found a younger age of diagnosis to be an independent risk factor for LV dysfunction [81]. Concomitant radiation is also shown to be associated with echocardiographically determined LV dysfunction [120]. While therapy often cannot be delayed due to the acute demands of the oncologic process, the data are convincing that for comparable doses of anthracycline, the younger the age at administration, the worse the LV function over time.

Females appear to be more sensitive to comparable doses of doxorubicin with increased LV dysfunction [174]. The lipophilic properties of anthracyclines may lead to prolonged exposure in individuals with more adipose tissue [81]. Doxorubicin does not distribute well into fat tissue and is metabolized more slowly in the obese [175]. Equivalent doses of anthracyclines may lead to higher dose exposures in the hearts of females since they typically have more body fat than males of the same body surface area. The association between cardiac dysfunction and female sex was stronger in children older than age 12 years, when hormones begin to produce larger differences in fat distribution. Regardless of the mechanism of toxicity, it is known that females have increased sensitivity to similar doses of anthracycline and that the difference appears to be more pronounced in females older than 12 years of age.

Genetic predisposition is a possible factor in determining the risk of anthracycline cardiotoxicity [176–178]. Polymorphisms potentially alter membrane permeability, antioxidant capacity, and metabolism possibly predisposing the patient to cardiac complications. An iron-overload genetic disorder known as hereditary hemochromatosis is of particular interest. As mentioned earlier, anthracycline-induced cardiotoxicity is believed to be in part due to interaction with iron. It is theorized that patients with iron-overload and deficient Hfe gene polymorphisms are associated clinically with hemochromatosis and increased serum iron levels. Patients with Hfe gene polymorphisms and increased serum iron levels are more susceptible to anthracycline-induced cardiotoxicity [179]. Animal studies have found that Hfe deficiency led to mitochondrial degradation and increased mortality when compared to wild-type controls [180]. Findings of greater susceptibility to cardiac damage in individuals with trisomy 21 and black race further support the concept of genetic predisposition [70, 83].

Preexisting conditions also contribute to cardiotoxicity. Underlying pathophysiology should be considered. For instance, those with trisomy 21 are at increased risk of LV dysfunction independent of the iatrogenic effects from the therapies received for leukemia, another condition to which this population has a predisposition.

## 10.4.2.2 Obesity

Obesity has been identified as an important cardiac risk factor [169]. With increased weight comes a litany of other conditions that impair the myocardium and its vascular supply [181, 182]. The cardiometabolic syndrome has become increasing prevalent among people of all ages [183, 184]. Patients who have received cardiotoxic regimens from both chemotherapy and radiation are at increased risk of developing multisystem dysregulation [185]. Data from a small study suggest that not only does increased dose of cardiotoxic therapy portend an increased chance of obesity but also other cardiovascular risk factors such as hyperlipidemia [186]. The increased risk of obesity in pediatric cancer survivors was established in prior studies such as one taken from the NHANES database, which identifies waist circumference and body mass index (BMI) and then calculates total cardiovascular risk factors. This ultimately demonstrates that as many as 17–19 % of otherwise healthy adolescents in the United States are at risk for cardiovascular complications [187]. While this obesity may be iatrogenic in origin, when it is modifiable, it should be addressed promptly to minimize cardiovascular damage.

Studies of pediatric cancer survivors have demonstrated that the CAD displayed is similar regarding the affected vessels and overall pathology as compared to the general population [106]. Given this, obesity should be considered as an equally important modifiable risk factor.

Multiple measures of obesity have been validated, and adiposity is accurately measured with dual-energy X-ray absorptiometry [188]. Not only is information obtained regarding adiposity but also about osteoporosis, which can be a side effect of chemotherapy and radiation [189, 190]. An increase in BMI is a surrogate for obesity and when abnormally increased is accepted as a cardiac risk factor [191]. Multiple measures of obesity have been shown to correlate with worsened outcomes [192]. Irrespective of the manner used to assess obesity, pediatric cancer survivors are at increased risk of early CAD and impaired LV function, so weight control is important to overall cardiac health.

## 10.4.2.3 Diabetes Mellitus

Diabetes mellitus is a family of clinical conditions characterized by hyperglycemia and associated with multiple negative health outcomes.

When the level of hyperglycemia is not so severe as to diagnose diabetes mellitus but is not normal (with normal being defined as having a fasting blood glucose less than 100 mg/dl and a blood hemoglobin A1c measurement less than 5.5 %), a condition known as impaired glucose tolerance (defined as having a 2-h glucose level of 140–199 mg/dl on the 75-g oral glucose tolerance test) exists. It is known to be a harbinger of diabetes mellitus [193]. It is widely accepted that impaired glucose tolerance, colloquially known as pre-diabetes, is reversible. In this way, early identification represents objective risk reduction.

Irrespective of the cause, both micro- and macrovascular complications ensue at increasing rates as time from diagnosis and magnitude of hyperglycemia increases. Prevention of diabetes mellitus is best, but early diagnosis so that proper management may be undertaken is equally important. Renal failure, cardiovascular accidents, and myocardial ischemia are devastating sequelae that occur even with optimal control but can be delayed with treatments.

#### 10.4.2.4 Hypertension

Hypertension is a well-established cardiac risk factor [169]. While data have not conclusively been established in this patient population, given that the CAD profiles are similar with the general adult population, it is reasonable to consider hypertension as an important risk factor [106]. A study of long-term cancer survivors suggests that there is an increased incidence of hypertension in this cohort as compared to age-matched controls, while in another study of 92 survivors, hypertension trended toward being increased ($p = 0.05$) [24, 194]. These studies suggest that there are many comorbid conditions in survivors and that there is a decreased overall quality of life reported [195]. Many antihypertensive medications are available with different mechanisms of action, and when other comorbidities are taken into account, an appropriate medication profile can usually be administered.

Modifiable risk factors are paramount to cardiovascular health. For survivors of pediatric cancers, macrovascular complications occur at an earlier age, so minimization of other risk factors must be undertaken [60, 61]. In general, risky behaviors such as smoking and illicit drug use are to rates in the general population [194], so education should be given to minimize such lifestyle choices. As emphasized in another chapter, preservation of good mental health should be emphasized since it is correlated with fewer risky behaviors [194]. As noted above, obesity is a risk factor and may result from endocrine dysfunction or pharmacotherapy, but it may also stem from lifestyle choices. Alcohol consumption and smoking also contribute to microvascular destruction and independently are known risk factors for macrovascular negative outcomes. In the post-treatment phase of cardiovascular care, screening for modifiable risk factors is imperative.

### 10.5  Management of Established Problems

As signs and symptoms of CHF become evident, therapy clearly becomes compulsory. Many anthracycline- and mediastinal radiotherapy-treated long-term survivors with late CHF may develop restrictive cardiomyopathy. This may result in patients who are more ill than they appear to be, which furthers the need for interventions to be undertaken in a timely manner. When the symptoms are less clear but evidence of abnormal LV afterload, contractility, and/or LVFS remains, the determination of whether or not to implement therapy and, if so, what type becomes more problematic. For instance, ACE inhibitors appear to decrease the heart's normal growth while also causing dry cough unrelated to infection [196]. In the modern era, not only are medications available for treatment but also other interventions including transplantation [197, 198]. The durability of these interventions varies from one case to the next, and the iatrogenic effects may, in some instances, be more burdensome than the benefit they offer [13]. With ACE inhibitors, for instance, the diminished cardiac growth potential associated with their use may be too heavy of a cost to the growing myocardium and may lead to diminished maximal cardiac capacity. In the present day, use of cardiovascular medications and interventions that have been validated for use in other populations is commonplace in children. The type of cardiomyopathy seen in pediatric cancer survivors does not necessarily mimic that seen in ischemic, idiopathic, or postinfectious forms so the use of such pharmacotherapies is not supported by evidence-based data [108]. Outlined below are many of the common therapeutic options for pediatric long-term cancer survivors with cardiomyopathy with evidence obtained predominantly from adult populations.

## 10.5.1 Pharmacologic Management

Therapeutic goals in the treatment of cardiomyopathy include prevention of progression of CVD, and this is often aimed at increasing cardiac output by reducing LV afterload and improving LV contractility. Beta-blockers and ACE inhibitors are cornerstones to this.

ACE inhibitors reduce LV afterload by preventing the conversion of angiotensin I to the vasocontricting agent, angiotensin II. These medications disrupt the hormonal cascade that perpetuates heart failure and also reduce afterload. While ACE inhibitors have been shown to decrease the incidence of CHF and improve survival in patients with ventricular dysfunction, their use in the cancer setting is not as clear. One large study attempted to use ACE inhibitors to slow progression of cardiac dysfunction [199]. While ACE inhibitor-treated patients demonstrated initial improvement in LV dimension, afterload, and LVFS, a 10-year follow-up revealed no differences between the patients who received an ACE inhibitor and those who did not [71, 200]. Another study of adult patients with elevated troponin I levels receiving chemotherapy revealed improvement in LVEF when treated early with enalapril [201], but no long-term follow-up was performed. A prospective study of 18 doxorubicin-treated, long-term survivors of childhood cancer taking enalapril demonstrated improvement that lasted up to 10 years [202], but the results appear to be transient because a decline in function was noted in all patients.

Mechanistically, anthracycline-induced cardiomyopathy appears to be more restrictive, which may explain why ACE inhibitors do not appear to have as much of a benefit as compared its use in other populations [71]. Of note, ACE inhibitors are known to cause cough as a side effect, and the angiotensin receptor blockers are used in their place sometimes; these agents are both teratogenic, and females in their childbearing years must be counseled about their side effect profiles.

Medications that antagonistically bind to beta-adrenergic receptors in the myocardium and thereby have negative chronotropic and inotropic effects are often termed beta-blockers. Decreased mortality is noted in patients of various classification of CHF [203–209]. Multiple studies have shown the varying degrees of benefit associated with beta-blockers with improvements in LVEF noted, and this also is seen in patients who received doxorubicin [209, 210]. A small study was performed on 25 patients prospectively to determine if beta-blockers could dampen the decrease in LVEF, and the placebo group had significant worsening as compared to the study group [211]. More studies are needed in this patient population to investigate the effects of beta-blockers since their benefit is not ubiquitous within this drug class [212–214]. For example, one trial demonstrated that metoprolol tartrate is inferior to carvedilol when examining mortality [209]. Also, one must check for contraindications before starting therapy or escalating dose such as cardiogenic shock or advanced heart block, but the medication class is generally well tolerated even in those with reactive airway disease [215].

Other medication classes also exist for the treatment of heart failure. None of the following treatment modalities have been studied specifically in survivors of pediatric cancer. Aldosterone antagonists have been found to reduce mortality in CHF patients with New York Heart Association stage III or IV symptoms [216]. Aldosterone antagonist use in those with moderate to severe CHF symptoms is considered a class 1B recommendation for treatment in those with preserved renal function and without hyperkalemia who can be serially monitored [191]. Loop diuretics such as furosemide and bumetanide are indicated in treatment of symptomatic fluid retention. Thiazide diuretics such as hydrochlorothiazide, chlorthalidone, and metolazone in general have longer half-lives and are dosed daily for treatment of fluid overload. Potassium-sparing diuretics such as triamterene and amiloride are useful in patients who have persistent hypokalemia. These agents are mainstays of treatment in heart failure patients. The combination of hydralazine and oral nitrates, when used in concert with other appropriate therapies, has been shown to reduce mortality in certain population subsets [217, 218]. Digoxin stimulates the parasympathetic fibers innervating the heart, and its use is associated with fewer hospitalizations related to CHF. However, its use has been shown to have no effect on mortality [219]. The routine use of aspirin is a debated subject. While it is helpful in CAD, which many pediatric cancer survivors have earlier in life, it may be harmful in its blockade of prostaglandins, further worsening hemodynamics. On a case-by-case basis, the determination regarding aspirin use may be made. Other types of medication that might be considered include antimicrobials prior to dental procedures. Given that valvulopathies and other iatrogenic cardiac dysfunction are at significantly increased rates among pediatric cancer survivors, it is worth considering antimicrobials to prevent infective endocarditis, which is a life-threatening infection independently, let alone in the setting of cardiomyopathy. No studies have been performed to date to evaluate this.

## 10.5.2 Cardioprotective Agents

The proposed mechanism of doxorubicin toxicity is related to iron binding to doxorubicin and forming a complex that results in free radical formation. This mechanism is further supported in one study, performed by Miranda et al. which looked at rats with a gene modified to increase iron stored in organs similar to hereditary hemochromatosis [180]. Cardiotoxicity was increased in these rats with increased iron stores when compared to controls. Dexrazoxane decreases superhydroxide free radical formation by binding to intracellular iron and inhibiting the conversion of superoxide anions and hydrogen peroxide [220]. Therefore, dexrazoxane is thought to reduce oxidative stress in the particularly sensitive cardiomyocytes. In addition, preclinical studies show impaired mitochondrial function and ability to replicate in patients treated with doxorubicin. Lipshultz et al. showed increased mitochondrial replication when dexrazoxane was added to doxorubicin therapy [221]. The main side effects of dexrazoxane include myelosuppression and local venous inflammation. The suggested ratio of dexrazoxane to doxorubicin is 10:1 to 20:1 [71].

Studies have shown dexrazoxane along with doxorubicin can decrease acute cardiotoxicity and CHF versus controls [222]. In a study of 534 women with advanced breast cancer, dexrazoxane was shown to prevent marked deterioration of LVEF and the development of CHF [223]. Only 1 of 16 clinical studies showed dexrazoxane may decrease efficacy, necessitating a larger dose of doxorubicin.

Lipshultz et al. performed a study that looked at pediatric patients with ALL treated with doxorubicin and dexrazoxane. The control patients, as compared to those receiving dexrazoxane, were found to have elevated cTnT levels, but without significant decrease in cardiac function. Similarly, as compared to the control group not receiving dexrazoxane, there was no difference in LVFS, incidence of CHF, or incidence of event-free survival (Fig. 10.6) [224, 225].

The 2009 American Society of Clinical Oncology guidelines did not change their 2002 recommendations. Currently, recommendations are for dexrazoxane to not be routinely used during initial doxorubicin therapy. However, they do recommend using dexrazoxane in metastatic breast cancer patients who have received more than 300 mg/m$^2$ as a cumulative dose and who would benefit from further doxorubicin treatment. These recommendations have expanded to include consideration of adding dexrazoxane in other adult malignancies when the cumulative dose of doxorubicin exceeds 300 mg/m$^2$. However, they fail to provide recommendations for pediatric malignancies secondary to insufficient data [226].

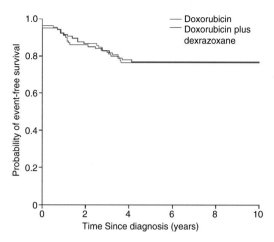

**Fig. 10.6** Event-free survival. All patients randomly assigned treatment ($n = 205$) were eligible for assessment of event-free survival, but by convention, events of induction failure and induction death have been recorded at 0 years (Reprinted with permission from the publisher Lipshultz et al. [90])

Much of our knowledge of the efficacy of amifostine comes from animal models. The proposed mechanism includes decreasing free plasma levels of free radicals by forming disulfides. In addition, amifostine also appears to have direct protective effects on DNA stability [227]. Pretreatment with amifostine has been shown, in rats, to decrease lipid peroxidation and increase protective enzymes including glutathione, which would prevent myocardium destruction.

In vivo studies in rats reveal improvement in cardiac function when amifostine is used along with doxorubicin [228]. In another study of 28 pediatric patients with osteosarcoma, there was no significant difference in response rate when using doxorubicin and amifostine versus placebo [229]. However, while neither group had any CHF symptoms reported, two patients in the placebo group versus zero patients in the amifostine group developed subclinical CHF [229]. This study's power may be too low to fully appreciate a significant difference. There is no clear consensus as to whether or not amifostine improves cardiac outcome in patients treated with doxorubicin. The American Society of Clinical Oncology does not recommend amifostine for use with doxorubicin to prevent cardiotoxicity, but larger studies may be warranted.

### 10.5.3 Nutritional Supplements

Proposed mechanisms for anthracycline toxicity include inhibiting the mitochondrial enzymes, succinic oxidase and NADH oxidase, both of which are dependent on coenzyme Q (CoQ). As expected, an increase in plasma CoQ was noted in patients undergoing treatment with doxorubicin [230]. CoQ is an integral part of mitochondrial membranes and acts as a powerful antioxidant [231]. As one would expect, the concentration of CoQ increases where mitochondria are more numerous. For example, the concentration of CoQ in the heart is 20 times that found in skeletal muscle [232].

In clinical studies, pretreatment with CoQ appeared to decrease acute toxicity. In one study, seven patients receiving doxorubicin without being pretreated with CoQ displayed impairment of cardiac function including increase in heart rate and decreases in LVEF, stroke index, and cardiac index [231]. Another study noted myocardial depression, QRS depression, and QT prolongation with doxorubicin but no such changes in patients pretreated with CoQ [233].

Unfortunately, much of the information involving cardioprotection with selenium is in the form of murine studies. The proposed mechanism of protection involves increasing the activity of glutathione peroxidase, which offers protection against free radical-induced damage [234]. In a 2006 study, researchers found that selenium supplementation in rats increased total antioxidant activity, glutathione concentration, and glutathione peroxidase and catalase activity, thus leading to decreased generation of reactive oxygen metabolites [234]. However, no decrease in mortality was found [235].

### 10.5.4 Non-pharmacologic Management

While the approach to symptomatic chemotherapy-induced cardiomyopathy is aimed at symptom relief and prevention of disease progression, not all of the measures used are pharmacologic. The use of implantable cardiac defibrillators, cardiac resynchronization therapy, ventricular assist devices, and transplantation has made management of CHF more versatile. As with medical therapy, an adequate workup should be undertaken to find reversible causes of cardiac dysfunction. No large study has examined the use of these devices in survivors of pediatric cancers.

Evidence suggests that prophylactic implantable cardiac defibrillators in patients with an LVEF less than or equal to 30 % can decrease mortality from 31 to 22 % at 4 years after device insertion [236]. Current guidelines advocate for the use of implantable cardiac defibrillators as secondary prevention to prolong survival in patients with current or prior CHF symptom with a reduced LVEF and a history of cardiac arrest, ventricular fibrillation, or unstable ventricular tachycardia [191].

Cardiac resynchronization therapy has been shown to improve quality of life, functional status, and exercise capacity with over 4,000 patients enrolled in randomized clinical trials [237]. All-cause mortality decreased by 40 % among those who had cardiac resynchronization therapy compared to those who did not [238]. Current guidelines recommend for the use of cardiac resynchronization therapy in patients with a LVEF less than or equal to 35 %, sinus rhythm, class III–IV New York Heart Association symptoms despite optimal medical therapy who have electrical dyssynchrony (QRS duration greater than 120 ms) unless otherwise contraindicated [191].

Ventricular assist devices are placed both as bridging and destination therapy as they augment cardiac output. One study demonstrates efficacy of ventricular assist devices in patients up to 18 months after insertion [239]. These devices are often used to bridge to cardiac transplantation, a complex therapy marred by a lack of donor organs, high costs of posttransplantation care, and side effects of antirejection medications. Cancer survivors require no significant modification to the immunosuppressive regimen, and their 2-year survival rate is similar to that of other recipients [240]. Pediatric cancer survivors are subjected to the same rigorous screening methods as others with absolute and relative contraindications being reviewed. Having adequate health status to undergo such interventions is important and may not be possible depending on the types of chemical and radiotherapy that the pediatric cancer survivors have been administered.

## 10.5.5 Continuous Infusion

Because dose-dependent toxicity is evident with doxorubicin, continuous infusions were thought to decrease toxicity by decreasing peak drug levels. However, randomized prospective study noted that children with high-risk ALL receiving 48-h infusions with a cumulative dose of 360 mg/$m^2$ did not demonstrate improvement over bolus dosing [91, 92]. Use of different dosing models that contrast bolus and continuous dosing for other malignancies did not demonstrate continuous infusions as superior [241, 242]. Therefore, in addition to the technical difficulties with infusion pumps and constant monitoring, our data suggest that at least for children with high-risk ALL, the standard of care for anthracycline treatment includes bolus dosing rather than continuous infusion.

### Conclusions

Although there is no definitive data on the best preventative cardiac treatment and monitoring strategy, the developing area of cardio-oncology is beginning to provide clinicians with a guide to identifying adverse cardiac effects of anticancer therapy and balancing these issues with the therapy's highly beneficial effect on cancer [69, 243–245]. There must also be caution toward interpreting expert opinion as established guidelines to clinical practice. It is paramount that cardiac treatment and monitoring strategies are based on data-derived certainty. Efficient follow-up care is crucial to the survival of childhood cancer survivors. Progress continues to be made toward the common challenges in transition of care to adult services such as program funding and volume of subspecialty referral [246].

# References

1. Mariotto AB, Rowland JH, Yabroff KR et al (2009) Long-term survivors of childhood cancers in the United States. Cancer Epidemiol Biomarkers Prev 18:1033–1040
2. Meadows AT, D'Angio GJ (1974) Late effects of cancer treatment: methods and techniques for detection. Semin Oncol 1:87–90
3. Lipshultz SE, Lipsitz SR, Sallan SE et al (2005) Chronic progressive cardiac dysfunction years after doxorubicin therapy for childhood acute lymphoblastic leukemia. J Clin Oncol 23:2629–2636
4. Reulen RC, Winter DL, Frobisher C et al (2010) Long-term cause-specific mortality among survivors of childhood cancer. JAMA 304:172–179
5. Tukenova M, Guibout C, Hawkins M et al (2011) Radiation therapy and late mortality from second sarcoma, carcinoma, and hematological malignancies after a solid cancer in childhood. Int J Radiat Oncol Biol Phys 80:339–346
6. Scwartz CL (1999) Long-term survivors of childhood cancer: the late effects of therapy. Oncologist 4:45–54
7. Goldberg JM, Scully RE, Sallan SE et al (2012) Cardiac failure 30 years after treatment containing anthracycline for childhood acute lymphoblastic leukemia. J Pediatr Hematol Oncol 34:395–397
8. Meacham LR, Chow EJ, Ness KK et al (2010) Cardiovascular risk factors in adult survivors of pediatric cancer–a report from the childhood cancer survivor study. Cancer Epidemiol Biomarkers Prev 19:170–181
9. Oeffinger KC, Adams-Huet B, Victor RG et al (2009) Insulin resistance and risk factors for cardiovascular disease in young adult survivors of childhood acute lymphoblastic leukemia. J Clin Oncol 27:3698–3704
10. Meacham LR, Sklar CA, Li S et al (2009) Diabetes mellitus in long-term survivors of childhood cancer. Increased risk associated with radiation therapy: a report for the childhood cancer survivor study. Arch Intern Med 169:1381–1388
11. Garmey EG, Liu Q, Sklar CA et al (2008) Longitudinal changes in obesity and body mass index among adult survivors of childhood acute lymphoblastic leukemia: a report from the Childhood Cancer Survivor Study. J Clin Oncol 26:4639–4645
12. Lipshultz SE, Sallan SE (1993) Cardiovascular abnormalities in long-term survivors of childhood malignancy. J Clin Oncol 11:1199–1203
13. Lipshultz SE, Colan SD (2004) Cardiovascular trials in long-term survivors of childhood cancer. J Clin Oncol 22:769–773
14. Lipshultz SE (2006) Exposure to anthracyclines during childhood causes cardiac injury. Semin Oncol 33:S8–S14
15. Lipshultz SE (2007) Heart failure in childhood cancer survivors. Nat Clin Pract Oncol 4:334–335
16. Lipshultz SE, Alvarez JA, Scully RE (2008) Anthracycline associated cardiotoxicity in survivors of childhood cancer. Heart 94:525–533
17. Lipshultz SE, Miller TL, Scully RE et al (2012) Changes in cardiac biomarkers during doxorubicin treatment of pediatric patients with high-risk acute lymphoblastic leukemia: associations with long-term echocardiographic outcomes. J Clin Oncol 30:1042–1049
18. Clark EB (1990) Growth, morphogenesis, and function: the dynamics of heart development. In: Moller JH, Neal WA, Lock JE (eds) Fetal, neonatal, and infant heart disease. Appleton-Century-Crofts, New York
19. Clark EB, Hu N, Frommelt P et al (1989) Effect of increased pressure on ventricular growth in stage 21 chick embryos. Am J Physiol 257:H55–H61
20. Fishman NH, Hof RB, Rudolph AM et al (1978) Models of congenital heart disease in fetal lambs. Circulation 58:354–364
21. Lipshultz SE, Colan SD, Gelber RD et al (1991) Late cardiac effects of doxorubicin therapy for acute lymphoblastic leukemia in childhood. N Engl J Med 324:808–815
22. Billingham ME (1991) Role of endomyocardial biopsy in diagnosis and treatment of heart disease. In: Silver MD (ed) Cardiovascular pathology. Churchill Livingstone, New York
23. Tokarska-Schlattner M, Zaugg M, Zuppinger C et al (2006) New insights into doxorubicin-induced cardiotoxicity: the critical role of cellular energetics. J Mol Cell Cardiol 41:389–405
24. Brouwer CA, Postma A, Vonk JM et al (2011) Systolic and diastolic dysfunction in long-term adult survivors of childhood cancer. Eur J Cancer 47:2453–2462
25. Minotti G, Menna P, Salvatorelli E et al (2004) Anthracyclines: molecular advances and pharmacologic developments in antitumor activity and cardiotoxicity. Pharmacol Rev 56:185–229
26. Senkus E, Jassem J (2011) Cardiovascular effects of systemic cancer treatment. Cancer Treat Rev 37:300–311
27. Nicolay K, van der Neut R, Fok JJ et al (1985) Effects of adriamycin on lipid polymorphism in cardiolipin-containing model and mitochondrial membranes. Biochim Biophys Acta 819:55–65
28. Leonard RC, Williams S, Tulpule A et al (2009) Improving the therapeutic index of anthracycline chemotherapy: focus on liposomal doxorubicin (Myocet). Breast 18:218–224
29. Kalyanaraman B, Joseph J, Kalivendi S et al (2002) Doxorubicin-induced apoptosis: implications in cardiotoxicity. Mol Cell Biochem 234–235:119–124
30. De Angelis A, Piegari E, Cappetta D et al (2010) Anthracycline cardiomyopathy is mediated by depletion of the cardiac stem cell pool and is rescued by restoration of progenitor cell function. Circulation 121:276–292

31. Thompson KL, Rosenzweig BA, Zhang J et al (2010) Early alterations in heart gene expression profiles associated with doxorubicin cardiotoxicity in rats. Cancer Chemother Pharmacol 66:303–314

32. Olson RD, Li X, Palade P et al (2000) Sarcoplasmic reticulum calcium release is stimulated and inhibited by daunorubicin and daunorubicinol. Toxicol Appl Pharmacol 169:168–176

33. Outomuro D, Grana DR, Azzato F et al (2007) Adriamycin-induced myocardial toxicity: new solutions for an old problem? Int J Cardiol 117:6–15

34. Goormaghtigh E, Huart P, Praet M et al (1990) Structure of the adriamycin-cardiolipin complex. Role in mitochondrial toxicity. Biophys Chem 35:247–257

35. Adachi K, Fujiura Y, Mayumi F et al (1993) A deletion of mitochondrial DNA in murine doxorubicin-induced cardiotoxicity. Biochem Biophys Res Commun 195:945–951

36. Lebrecht D, Walker UA (2007) Role of mtDNA lesions in anthracycline cardiotoxicity. Cardiovasc Toxicol 7:108–113

37. Braverman AC, Antin JH, Plappert MT et al (1991) Cyclophosphamide cardiotoxicity in bone marrow transplantation: a prospective evaluation of new dosing regimens. J Clin Oncol 9:1215–1223

38. Kupari M, Volin L, Suokas A et al (1990) Cardiac involvement in bone marrow transplantation: electrocardiographic changes, arrhythmias, heart failure and autopsy findings. Bone Marrow Transplant 5:91–98

39. Gottdiener JS, Appelbaum FR, Ferrans VJ et al (1981) Cardiotoxicity associated with high-dose cyclophosphamide therapy. Arch Intern Med 141:758–763

40. Friedman HS, Colvin OM, Aisaka K et al (1990) Glutathione protects cardiac and skeletal muscle from cyclophosphamide-induced toxicity. Cancer Res 50:2455–2462

41. Quezado ZM, Wilson WH, Cunnion RE et al (1993) High-dose ifosfamide is associated with severe, reversible cardiac dysfunction. Ann Intern Med 118:31–36

42. Kandylis K, Vassilomanolakis M, Tsoussis S et al (1989) Ifosfamide cardiotoxicity in humans. Cancer Chemother Pharmacol 24:395–396

43. Schlessinger J (2000) Cell signaling by receptor tyrosine kinases. Cell 103:211–225

44. Kerkela R, Grazette L, Yacobi R et al (2006) Cardiotoxicity of the cancer therapeutic agent imatinib mesylate. Nat Med 12:908–916

45. Daves M, Dixit A, Sankaran H et al (2011) No increased risk of cardiotoxicity in pediatric patients with leukemia imatinib therapy. Pediatr Blood Cancer 56:925

46. Yeh ET, Bickford CL (2009) Cardiovascular complications of cancer therapy: incidence, pathogenesis, diagnosis, and management. J Am Coll Cardiol 53:2231–2247

47. Floyd JD, Nguyen DT, Lobins RL et al (2005) Cardiotoxicity of cancer therapy. J Clin Oncol 23:7685–7696

48. Rowinsky EK, McGuire WP, Guarnieri T et al (1991) Cardiac disturbances during the administration of taxol. J Clin Oncol 9:1704–1712

49. Adams MJ, Hardenbergh PH, Constine LS et al (2003) Radiation-associated cardiovascular disease. Crit Rev Oncol Hematol 45:55–75

50. Stewart JR, Fajardo LF (1984) Radiation-induced heart disease: an update. Prog Cardiovasc Dis 27:173–194

51. Fajardo LF, Stewart JR, Cohn KE (1968) Morphology of radiation-induced heart disease. Arch Pathol 86:512–519

52. Chello M, Mastroroberto P, Romano R et al (1996) Changes in the proportion of types I and III collagen in the left ventricular wall of patients with post-irradiative pericarditis. Cardiovasc Surg 4:222–226

53. Orzan F, Brusca A, Gaita F et al (1993) Associated cardiac lesions in patients with radiation-induced complete heart block. Int J Cardiol 39:151–156

54. Cohen SI, Bharati S, Glass J et al (1981) Radiotherapy as a cause of complete atrioventricular block in Hodgkin's disease. An electrophysiological-pathological correlation. Arch Intern Med 141:676–679

55. La Vecchia L (1996) Physiologic dual chamber pacing in radiation-induced atrioventricular block. Chest 110:580–581

56. Pearson TA, Mensah GA, Alexander RW et al (2003) Markers of inflammation and cardiovascular disease: application to clinical and public health practice: a statement for healthcare professionals from the Centers for Disease Control and Prevention and the American Heart Association. Circulation 107:499–511

57. Schultz-Hector S, Trott KR (2007) Radiation-induced cardiovascular diseases: is the epidemiologic evidence compatible with the radiobiologic data? Int J Radiat Oncol Biol Phys 67:10–18

58. Little MP, Tawn EJ, Tzoulaki I et al (2008) A systematic review of epidemiological associations between low and moderate doses of ionizing radiation and late cardiovascular effects, and their possible mechanisms. Radiat Res 169:99–109

59. Robbins ME, Zhao W (2004) Chronic oxidative stress and radiation-induced late normal tissue injury: a review. Int J Radiat Biol 80:251–259

60. Brosius FC 3rd, Waller BF, Roberts WC (1981) Radiation heart disease. Analysis of 16 young (aged 15 to 33 years) necropsy patients who received over 3,500 rads to the heart. Am J Med 70:519–530

61. Veinot JP, Edwards WD (1996) Pathology of radiation-induced heart disease: a surgical and autopsy study of 27 cases. Hum Pathol 27:766–773

62. Carlson RG, Mayfield WR, Normann S et al (1991) Radiation-associated valvular disease. Chest 99:538–545

63. McEniery PT, Dorosti K, Schiavone WA et al (1987) Clinical and angiographic features of coronary artery disease after chest irradiation. Am J Cardiol 60:1020–1024

64. King V, Constine LS, Clark D et al (1996) Symptomatic coronary artery disease after mantle irradiation for Hodgkin's disease. Int J Radiat Oncol Biol Phys 36:881–889

65. Joensuu H (1993) Myocardial infarction after irradiation in Hodgkin's disease: a review. Recent Results Cancer Res 130:157–173

66. Yusuf SW, Sami S, Daher IN (2011) Radiation-induced heart disease: a clinical update. Cardiol Res Pract 2011:317659

67. Adams MJ, Lipshultz SE (2005) Pathophysiology of anthracycline- and radiation-associated cardiomyopathies: implications for screening and prevention. Pediatr Blood Cancer 44:600–606

68. Nousiainen T, Vanninen E, Rantala A et al (1999) QT dispersion and late potentials during doxorubicin therapy for non-Hodgkin's lymphoma. J Intern Med 245:359–364

69. Giantris A, Abdurrahman L, Hinkle A et al (1998) Anthracycline-induced cardiotoxicity in children and young adults. Crit Rev Oncol Hematol 27:53–68

70. Krischer JP, Epstein S, Cuthbertson DD et al (1997) Clinical cardiotoxicity following anthracycline treatment for childhood cancer: the Pediatric Oncology Group experience. J Clin Oncol 15:1544–1552

71. Barry E, Alvarez JA, Scully RE et al (2007) Anthracycline-induced cardiotoxicity: course, pathophysiology, prevention and management. Expert Opin Pharmacother 8:1039–1058

72. Grenier MA, Lipshultz SE (1998) Epidemiology of anthracycline cardiotoxicity in children and adults. Semin Oncol 25:72–85

73. Diamond MB, Franco VI, Miller TL et al (2012) Preventing and treating anthracycline-related cardiotoxicity in survivors of childhood cancer. Curr Cancer Ther Rev 8:141–151

74. Suter TM, Ewer MS (2013) Cancer drugs and the heart: importance and management. Eur Heart J 34:1102–1111

75. Curigliano G, Mayer EL, Burstein HJ et al (2010) Cardiac toxicity from systemic cancer therapy: a comprehensive review. Prog Cardiovasc Dis 53:94–104

76. Kim DH, Landry AB 3rd, Lee YS et al (1989) Doxorubicin-induced calcium release from cardiac sarcoplasmic reticulum vesicles. J Mol Cell Cardiol 21:433–436

77. Ali MK, Ewer MS, Gibbs HR et al (1994) Late doxorubicin-associated cardiotoxicity in children. The possible role of intercurrent viral infection. Cancer 74:182–188

78. Lipshultz SE, Colan SD, Sanders SP et al (1989) Cardiac mechanics after growth hormone therapy in pediatric adriamycin recipients. Pediatr Res 25:153A

79. Steinherz LJ, Steinherz PG, Tan C (1995) Cardiac failure and dysrhythmias 6–19 years after anthracycline therapy: a series of 15 patients. Med Pediatr Oncol 24:352–361

80. Steinherz LJ, Steinherz PG, Tan CT et al (1991) Cardiac toxicity 4 to 20 years after completing anthracycline therapy. JAMA 266:1672–1677

81. Lipshultz SE, Lipsitz SR, Mone SM et al (1995) Female sex and drug dose as risk factors for late cardiotoxic effects of doxorubicin therapy for childhood cancer. N Engl J Med 332:1738–1743

82. Von Hoff DD, Layard MW, Basa P et al (1979) Risk factors for doxorubicin-induced congestive heart failure. Ann Intern Med 91:710–717

83. Krischer JP, Cuthbertson DD, Epstein S et al (1997) Risk Factors for early anthracycline clinical cardiotoxicity in children: the pediatric oncology group experience. Prog Pediatr Cardiol 8:83–90

84. Green DM, Grigoriev YA, Nan B et al (2001) Congestive heart failure after treatment for Wilms' tumor: a report from the National Wilms' Tumor Study group. J Clin Oncol 19:1926–1934

85. Bristow MR, Mason JW, Billingham ME et al (1978) Doxorubicin cardiomyopathy: evaluation by phonocardiography, endomyocardial biopsy, and cardiac catheterization. Ann Intern Med 88:168–175

86. Cortes EP, Lutman G, Wanka J et al (1975) Adriamycin (NSC-123127) cardiotoxicity: a clinicopathologic correlation. Cancer Chemother Rep 6:215–225

87. Trachtenberg BH, Landy DC, Franco VI et al (2011) Anthracycline-associated cardiotoxicity in survivors of childhood cancer. Pediatr Cardiol 32:342–353

88. Gupta M, Steinherz PG, Cheung NK et al (2003) Late cardiotoxicity after bolus versus infusion anthracycline therapy for childhood cancers. Med Pediatr Oncol 40:343–347

89. Wouters KA, Kremer LC, Miller TL et al (2005) Protecting against anthracycline-induced myocardial damage: a review of the most promising strategies. Br J Haematol 131:561–578

90. Lipshultz SE, Miller TL, Lipsitz SR et al (2010) Late cardiac status in long-term survivors of childhood high-risk all 8 years after continuous or bolus infusion of doxorubicin: the DFCI childhood ALL 91-01 randomized trial. J Clin Oncol 28(9513):2010

91. Lipshultz SE, Giantris AL, Lipsitz SR et al (2002) Doxorubicin administration by continuous infusion is not cardioprotective: the Dana-Farber 91-01 acute lymphoblastic leukemia protocol. J Clin Oncol 20:1677–1682

92. Lipshultz SE, Miller TL, Lipsitz SR et al (2012) Continuous versus bolus infusion of doxorubicin in children with ALL: long-term cardiac outcomes. Pediatrics 130:1003–1011

93. Levitt GA, Dorup I, Sorensen K et al (2004) Does anthracycline administration by infusion in children affect late cardiotoxicity? Br J Haematol 124:463–468

94. Cattel L, Ceruti M, Dosio F (2003) From conventional to stealth liposomes: a new frontier in cancer chemotherapy. Tumori 89:237–249

95. Gabizon A, Martin F (1997) Polyethylene glycolcoated (pegylated) liposomal doxorubicin. Rationale for use in solid tumours. Drugs 54(Suppl 4):15–21

96. O'Brien ME, Wigler N, Inbar M et al (2004) Reduced cardiotoxicity and comparable efficacy in a phase III trial of pegylated liposomal doxorubicin HCl (CAELYX/Doxil) versus conventional doxorubicin for first-line treatment of metastatic breast cancer. Ann Oncol 15:440–449

97. Berry G, Billingham M, Alderman E et al (1998) The use of cardiac biopsy to demonstrate reduced cardiotoxicity in AIDS Kaposi's sarcoma patients treated with pegylated liposomal doxorubicin. Ann Oncol 9:711–716

98. Safra T, Muggia F, Jeffers S et al (2000) Pegylated liposomal doxorubicin (doxil): reduced clinical cardiotoxicity in patients reaching or exceeding cumulative doses of 500 mg/m2. Ann Oncol 11:1029–1033

99. Trudeau M, Pagani O (2001) Epirubicin in combination with the taxanes. Semin Oncol 28:41–50

100. Chan S, Davidson N, Juozaityte E et al (2004) Phase III trial of liposomal doxorubicin and cyclophosphamide compared with epirubicin and cyclophosphamide as first-line therapy for metastatic breast cancer. Ann Oncol 15:1527–1534

101. Lahtinen R, Kuikka J, Nousiainen T et al (1991) Cardiotoxicity of epirubicin and doxorubicin: a double-blind randomized study. Eur J Haematol 46:301–305

102. Anderlini P, Benjamin RS, Wong FC et al (1995) Idarubicin cardiotoxicity: a retrospective study in acute myeloid leukemia and myelodysplasia. J Clin Oncol 13:2827–2834

103. Cohen BA, Mikol DD (2004) Mitoxantrone treatment of multiple sclerosis: safety considerations. Neurology 63:S28–S32

104. Chen T, Zhou G, Zhu Q et al (2010) Overexpression of vascular endothelial growth factor 165 (VGEF165) protects cardiomyocytes against doxorubicin-induced apoptosis. J Chemother 22:402–406

105. Miller K, Wang M, Gralow J et al (2007) Paclitaxel plus bevacizumab versus paclitaxel alone for metastatic breast cancer. N Engl J Med 357:2666–2676

106. Filopei J, Frishman W (2012) Radiation-induced heart disease. Cardiol Rev 20:184–188

107. Sorensen K, Levitt GA, Bull C et al (2003) Late anthracycline cardiotoxicity after childhood cancer: a prospective longitudinal study. Cancer 97:1991–1998

108. Adams MJ, Lipsitz SR, Colan SD et al (2004) Cardiovascular status in long-term survivors of Hodgkin's disease treated with chest radiotherapy. J Clin Oncol 22:3139–3148

109. Glanzmann C, Huguenin P, Lutolf UM et al (1994) Cardiac lesions after mediastinal irradiation for Hodgkin's disease. Radiother Oncol 30:43–54

110. Kreuser ED, Voller H, Behles C et al (1993) Evaluation of late cardiotoxicity with pulsed Doppler echocardiography in patients treated for Hodgkin's disease. Br J Haematol 84:615–622

111. Gustavsson A, Eskilsson J, Landberg T et al (1990) Late cardiac effects after mantle radiotherapy in patients with Hodgkin's disease. Ann Oncol 1:355–363

112. Lund MB, Ihlen H, Voss BM et al (1996) Increased risk of heart valve regurgitation after mediastinal radiation for Hodgkin's disease: an echocardiographic study. Heart 75:591–595

113. Darby SC, Cutter DJ, Boerma M et al (2010) Radiation-related heart disease: current knowledge and future prospects. Int J Radiat Oncol Biol Phys 76:656–665

114. Hancock SL, Tucker MA, Hoppe RT (1993) Factors affecting late mortality from heart disease after treatment of Hodgkin's disease. JAMA 270:1949–1955

115. Weber DC, Peguret N, Dipasquale G et al (2009) Involved-node and involved-field volumetric modulated arc vs. fixed beam intensity-modulated radiotherapy for female patients with early-stage supra-diaphragmatic Hodgkin lymphoma: a comparative planning study. Int J Radiat Oncol Biol Phys 75:1578–1586

116. Maraldo MV, Brodin NP, Vogelius IR et al (2012) Risk of developing cardiovascular disease after involved node radiotherapy versus mantle field for Hodgkin lymphoma. Int J Radiat Oncol Biol Phys 83:1232–1237

117. Carmel RJ, Kaplan HS (1976) Mantle irradiation in Hodgkin's disease. An analysis of technique, tumor eradication, and complications. Cancer 37:2813–2825

118. Specht L, Yahalom J, Illidge T et al (2014) Modern radiation therapy for Hodgkin lymphoma: field and dose guidelines from the international lymphoma radiation oncology group (ILROG). Int J Radiat Oncol Biol Phys 89:854–862

119. Chen MH, Cash EP, Danias PG et al (2002) Respiratory maneuvers decrease irradiated cardiac volume in patients with left-sided breast cancer. J Cardiovasc Magn Reson 4:265–27

120. Abosoudah I, Greenberg ML, Ness KK et al (2011) Echocardiographic surveillance for asymptomatic late-onset anthracycline cardiomyopathy in childhood cancer survivors. Pediatr Blood Cancer 57:467–472

121. Mertens AC, Liu Q, Neglia JP et al (2008) Cause-specific late mortality among 5-year survivors of childhood cancer: the Childhood Cancer Survivor Study. J Natl Cancer Inst 100:1368–1379

122. Landy DC, Miller TL, Lopez-Mitnik G et al (2012) Aggregating traditional cardiovascular disease risk factors to assess the cardiometabolic health of childhood cancer survivors: an analysis from the Cardiac Risk Factors in Childhood Cancer Survivors Study. Am Heart J 163:295–301.e292

123. Mulrooney DA, Yeazel MW, Kawashima T et al (2009) Cardiac outcomes in a cohort of adult survivors of childhood and adolescent cancer: retrospective analysis of the Childhood Cancer Survivor Study cohort. BMJ 339:b4606

124. Mavinkurve-Groothuis AM, Groot-Loonen J, Marcus KA et al (2010) Myocardial strain and strain rate in monitoring subclinical heart failure in asymptomatic long-term survivors of childhood cancer. Ultrasound Med Biol 36:1783–1791

125. Lawless SC, Verma P, Green DM et al (2007) Mortality experiences among 15+ year survivors of childhood and adolescent cancers. Pediatr Blood Cancer 48:333–338

126. Shankar SM, Marina N, Hudson MM et al (2008) Monitoring for cardiovascular disease in survivors of childhood cancer: report from the Cardiovascular Disease Task Force of the Children's Oncology Group. Pediatrics 121:e387–e396

127. Steinherz LJ, Graham T, Hurwitz R et al (1992) Guidelines for cardiac monitoring of children during and after anthracycline therapy: report of the Cardiology Committee of the Childrens Cancer Study Group. Pediatrics 89:942–949

128. Adams MJ, Lipshultz SE, Schwartz C et al (2003) Radiation-associated cardiovascular disease: manifestations and management. Semin Radiat Oncol 13:346–356

129. Children's Oncology Group (2012) Long-term follow-up guidelines for survivors of childhood, adolescent, and young adult cancers. www.survivorshipguidelines.org. Accessed 20 Apr 2012

130. Lipshultz SE, Vlach SA, Lipsitz SR et al (2005) Cardiac changes associated with growth hormone therapy among children treated with anthracyclines. Pediatrics 115:1613–1622

131. Postma A, Bink-Boelkens MT, Beaufort-Krol GC et al (1996) Late cardiotoxicity after treatment for a malignant bone tumor. Med Pediatr Oncol 26:230–237

132. van Dalen EC, van der Pal HJ, van den Bos C et al (2006) Clinical heart failure during pregnancy and delivery in a cohort of female childhood cancer survivors treated with anthracyclines. Eur J Cancer 42:2549–2553

133. Lipshultz SE, Sanders SP, Goorin AM et al (1994) Monitoring for anthracycline cardiotoxicity. Pediatrics 93:433–437

134. Lipshultz SE, Schaechter J, Carrillo A et al (2012) Can the consequences of universal cholesterol screening during childhood prevent cardiovascular disease and thus reduce long-term health care costs? Pediatr Endocrinol Rev 9:698–705

135. Heidenreich PA, Schnittger I, Strauss HW et al (2007) Screening for coronary artery disease after mediastinal irradiation for Hodgkin's disease. J Clin Oncol 25:43–49

136. Hancock SL (1998) Cardiac toxicity after cancer therapy. Research issues in Cancer Survivorship Meeting. National Cancer Institute, Bethesda

137. Bluemke DA, Achenbach S, Budoff M et al (2008) Noninvasive coronary artery imaging: magnetic resonance angiography and multidetector computed tomography angiography: a scientific statement from the american heart association committee on cardiovascular imaging and intervention of the council on cardiovascular radiology and intervention, and the councils on clinical cardiology and cardiovascular disease in the young. Circulation 118:586–606

138. Orzan F, Brusca A, Conte MR et al (1993) Severe coronary artery disease after radiation therapy of the chest and mediastinum: clinical presentation and treatment. Br Heart J 69:496–500

139. Lipshultz SE, Colan SD (1993) The use of echocardiography and Holter monitoring in the assessment of anthracycline-treated patients. In: Bricker JT, Green DM, D'Angio GJ (eds) Cardiac toxicity after treatment for childhood cancer. Wiley-Liss, New York

140. Colan SD, Borow KM, Neumann A (1984) Left ventricular end-systolic wall stress-velocity of fiber shortening relation: a load-independent index of myocardial contractility. J Am Coll Cardiol 4:715–724

141. van der Pal HJ, van Dalen EC, Hauptmann M et al (2010) Cardiac function in 5-year survivors of childhood cancer: a long-term follow-up study. Arch Intern Med 170:1247–1255

142. Sieswerda E, Kremer LC, Vidmar S et al (2010) Exercise echocardiography in asymptomatic survivors of childhood cancer treated with anthracyclines: a prospective follow-up study. Pediatr Blood Cancer 54:579–584

143. Jurcut R, Wildiers H, Ganame J et al (2008) Strain rate imaging detects early cardiac effects of pegylated liposomal Doxorubicin as adjuvant therapy in elderly patients with breast cancer. J Am Soc Echocardiogr 21:1283–1289

144. Hare JL, Brown JK, Leano R et al (2009) Use of myocardial deformation imaging to detect preclinical myocardial dysfunction before conventional measures in patients undergoing breast cancer treatment with trastuzumab. Am Heart J 158:294–301

145. Sawaya H, Sebag IA, Plana JC et al (2011) Early detection and prediction of cardiotoxicity in chemotherapy-treated patients. Am J Cardiol 107:1375–1380

146. Lipshultz SE, Cochran TR, Wilkinson JD (2012) Screening for long-term cardiac status during cancer treatment. Circ Cardiovasc Imaging 5:555–558

147. Karakurt C, Kocak G, Ozgen U (2008) Evaluation of the left ventricular function with tissue tracking and tissue Doppler echocardiography in pediatric malignancy survivors after anthracycline therapy. Echocardiography 25:880–887

148. Iarussi D, Pisacane C, Indolfi P et al (2005) Evaluation of left ventricular function in long-term survivors of childhood Hodgkin disease. Pediatr Blood Cancer 45:700–705

149. Brouwer CA, Gietema JA, van den Berg MP et al (2006) Long-term cardiac follow-up in survivors of a malignant bone tumour. Ann Oncol 17:1586–1591

150. Wong FL, Bhatia S, Kurian S et al (2012) Cost-effectiveness of the Children's Oncology Group (COG) Long-term Follow-up (LTFU) guidelines in reducing the risk of Congestive Heart Failure (CHF) in long-term Childhood Cancer Survivors (CSS). ASCO annual meeting, Chicago

151. Mavinkurve-Groothuis AM, Groot-Loonen J, Bellersen L et al (2009) Abnormal NT-pro-BNP levels in asymptomatic long-term survivors of childhood cancer treated with anthracyclines. Pediatr Blood Cancer 52:631–636

152. Simbre VC, Duffy SA, Dadlani GH et al (2005) Cardiotoxicity of cancer chemotherapy: implications for children. Paediatr Drugs 7:187–202

153. Oeffinger KC, Mertens AC, Sklar CA et al (2006) Chronic health conditions in adult survivors of childhood cancer. N Engl J Med 355:1572–1582

154. Lipshultz SE, Landy DC, Lopez-Mitnik G et al (2012) Cardiovascular status of childhood cancer survivors exposed and unexposed to cardiotoxic therapy. J Clin Oncol 30:1050–1057

155. Larsen RL, Barber G, Heise CT et al (1992) Exercise assessment of cardiac function in children and young adults before and after bone marrow transplantation. Pediatrics 89:722–729

156. Schwartz CL, Hobbie WL, Truesdell S et al (1993) Corrected QT interval prolongation in anthracycline-treated survivors of childhood cancer. J Clin Oncol 11:1906–1910

157. Weesner KM, Bledsoe M, Chauvenet A et al (1991) Exercise echocardiography in the detection of anthracycline cardiotoxicity. Cancer 68:435–438

158. Correa CR, Litt HI, Hwang WT et al (2007) Coronary artery findings after left-sided compared with right-sided radiation treatment for early-stage breast cancer. J Clin Oncol 25:3031–3037

159. Mancini DM, Eisen H, Kussmaul W et al (1991) Value of peak exercise oxygen consumption for optimal timing of cardiac transplantation in ambulatory patients with heart failure. Circulation 83:778–786

160. De Caro E, Smeraldi A, Trocchio G et al (2011) Subclinical cardiac dysfunction and exercise performance in childhood cancer survivors. Pediatr Blood Cancer 56:122–126

161. Boivin JF, Hutchison GB, Lubin JH et al (1992) Coronary artery disease mortality in patients treated for Hodgkin's disease. Cancer 69:1241–1247

162. Hancock SL, Donaldson SS, Hoppe RT (1993) Cardiac disease following treatment of Hodgkin's disease in children and adolescents. J Clin Oncol 11:1208–1215

163. Campbell J, King SBI, Douglas JSJ et al (1985) Prevalence and distribution of disease in patients catheterized for suspected coronary disease. McGraw-Hill, New York

164. Lind PA, Pagnanelli R, Marks LB et al (2003) Myocardial perfusion changes in patients irradiated for left-sided breast cancer and correlation with coronary artery distribution. Int J Radiat Oncol Biol Phys 55:914–920

165. Waller BF (2011) Non-atherosclerotic coronary heart disease. McGraw-Hill, York New

166. Wethal T, Lund MB, Edvardsen T et al (2009) Valvular dysfunction and left ventricular changes in Hodgkin's lymphoma survivors. A longitudinal study. Br J Cancer 101:575–581

167. Schultz-Hector S, Balz K (1994) Radiation-induced loss of endothelial alkaline phosphatase activity and development of myocardial degeneration. An ultrastructural study. Lab Invest 71:252–260

168. Heidenreich PA, Hancock SL, Lee BK et al (2003) Asymptomatic cardiac disease following mediastinal irradiation. J Am Coll Cardiol 42:743–749

169. Nishimura RA, Carabello BA, Faxon DP et al (2008) ACC/AHA 2008 guideline update on valvular heart disease: focused update on infective endocarditis: a report of the American College of Cardiology/ American Heart Association Task Force on Practice Guidelines endorsed by the Society of Cardiovascular Anesthesiologists, Society for Cardiovascular Angiography and Interventions, and Society of Thoracic Surgeons. J Am Coll Cardiol 52:676–685

170. Lee PJ, Mallik R (2005) Cardiovascular effects of radiation therapy: practical approach to radiation therapy-induced heart disease. Cardiol Rev 13:80–86

171. Smith AL, Book WM (2011) Effect of noncardiac drugs, electricity, poison and radiation on the heart. In: Fuster V, Walsh RA, Harrington RA (eds) Hurst's the heart, 13th edn. McGraw Hill, New York

172. Greenwood RD, Rosenthal A, Cassady R et al (1974) Constrictive pericarditis in childhood due to mediastinal irradiation. Circulation 50:1033–1039

173. Swain SM, Whaley FS, Ewer MS (2003) Congestive heart failure in patients treated with doxorubicin: a retrospective analysis of three trials. Cancer 97:2869–2879

174. Silber JH, Jakacki RI, Larsen RL et al (1993) Increased risk of cardiac dysfunction after anthracyclines in girls. Med Pediatr Oncol 21:477–479

175. Rodvold KA, Rushing DA, Tewksbury DA (1988) Doxorubicin clearance in the obese. J Clin Oncol 6:1321–1327

176. Wang L, Weinshilboum R (2006) Thiopurine S-methyltransferase pharmacogenetics: insights, challenges and future directions. Oncogene 25:1629–1638

177. Deng S, Wojnowski L (2007) Genotyping the risk of anthracycline-induced cardiotoxicity. Cardiovasc Toxicol 7:129–134

178. Blanco JG, Leisenring WM, Gonzalez-Covarrubias VM et al (2008) Genetic polymorphisms in the carbonyl reductase 3 gene CBR3 and the NAD(P) H:quinone oxidoreductase 1 gene NQO1 in patients

who developed anthracycline-related congestive heart failure after childhood cancer. Cancer 112:2789–2795

179. Lipshultz SE, Lipsitz SR, Kutok JL et al (2013) Impact of hemochromatosis gene mutations on cardiac status in doxorubicin-treated survivors of childhood high-risk leukemia. Cancer 119:3555–3562

180. Miranda CJ, Makui H, Soares RJ et al (2003) Hfe deficiency increases susceptibility to cardiotoxicity and exacerbates changes in iron metabolism induced by doxorubicin. Blood 102:2574–2580

181. Qureshi MY, Wilkinson JD, Lipshultz SE (2012) The relationship of childhood obesity with cardiomyopathy and heart failure. In: Lipshultz SE, Miller TL, Messiah SE (eds) Pediatric metabolic syndrome: comprehensive clinical review and related health issues. Springer Verlag London Ltd, London; acting in cooperation with Springer-Verlag GmbH Berlin Heidelberg, Spring Science and Business Media LLC New York and Springer Japan KK

182. Brown SR, Lipshultz SE (2012) Childhood metabolic syndrome and cancer risk. In: Lipshultz SE, Miller TL, Messiah SE (eds) Pediatric metabolic syndrome: comprehensive clinical review and related health issues. Springer Verlag London Ltd, London; acting in cooperation with Springer-Verlag GmbH Berlin Heidelberg, Spring Science and Business Media LLC New York and Springer Japan KK

183. Franks PW, Hanson RL, Knowler WC et al (2010) Childhood obesity, other cardiovascular risk factors, and premature death. N Engl J Med 362:485–493

184. Sumner AD, Khalil YK, Reed JF 3rd (2012) The relationship of peripheral arterial disease and metabolic syndrome prevalence in asymptomatic US adults 40 years and older: results from the National Health and Nutrition Examination Survey (1999–2004). J Clin Hypertens (Greenwich) 14:144–148

185. Siviero-Miachon AA, Monteiro CM, Pires LV et al (2011) Early traits of metabolic syndrome in pediatric post-cancer survivors: outcomes in adolescents and young adults treated for childhood medulloblastoma. Arq Bras Endocrinol Metabol 55:653–660

186. Sohn YB, Kim SJ, Park SW et al (2011) The metabolic syndrome and body composition in childhood cancer survivors. Korean J Pediatr 54:253–259

187. Lipshultz SE, Wilkinson JD, Messiah SE et al (2009) Clinical research directions in pediatric cardiology. Curr Opin Pediatr 21:585–593

188. Wasilewski-Masker K, Kaste SC, Hudson MM et al (2008) Bone mineral density deficits in survivors of childhood cancer: long-term follow-up guidelines and review of the literature. Pediatrics 121:e705–e713

189. Hudson MM, Mertens AC, Yasui Y et al (2003) Health status of adult long-term survivors of childhood cancer: a report from the Childhood Cancer Survivor Study. JAMA 290:1583–1592

190. Mattano LA Jr, Sather HN, Trigg ME et al (2000) Osteonecrosis as a complication of treating acute lymphoblastic leukemia in children: a report from the Children's Cancer Group. J Clin Oncol 18:3262–3272

191. Hunt SA, Abraham WT, Chin MH et al (2009) 2009 Focused update incorporated into the ACC/AHA 2005 guidelines for the diagnosis and management of heart failure in adults A report of the American College of Cardiology Foundation/American Heart Association Task Force on Practice Guidelines Developed in Collaboration With the International Society for Heart and Lung Transplantation. J Am Coll Cardiol 53:e1–e90

192. Miller TL, Lipsitz SR, Lopez-Mitnik G et al (2010) Characteristics and determinants of adiposity in pediatric cancer survivors. Cancer Epidemiol Biomarkers Prev 19:2013–2022

193. Cosson E, Hamo-Tchatchouang E, Banu I et al (2010) A large proportion of prediabetes and diabetes goes undiagnosed when only fasting plasma glucose and/or HbA1c are measured in overweight or obese patients. Diabetes Metab 36: 312–318

194. Klosky JL, Howell CR, Li Z et al (2012) Risky health behavior among adolescents in the childhood cancer survivor study cohort. J Pediatr Psychol 37:634–646

195. Kenney LB, Nancarrow CM, Najita J et al (2010) Health status of the oldest adult survivors of cancer during childhood. Cancer 116:497–505

196. Lipshultz SE, Lipsitz SR, Sallan SE (2003) Treatment for asymptomatic anthracycline-induced cardiac dysfunction in childhood cancer survivors: the need for evidence: in reply (letter). J Clin Oncol 21:3377–3378

197. Levit G, Bunch K, Rogers CA et al (1996) Cardiac transplantation in childhood cancer survivors in Great Britain. Eur J Cancer 32A:826–830

198. Levitt G, Anazodo A, Burch M et al (2009) Cardiac or cardiopulmonary transplantation in childhood cancer survivors: an increasing need? Eur J Cancer 45:3027–3034

199. Silber JH, Cnaan A, Clark BJ et al (2004) Enalapril to prevent cardiac function decline in long-term survivors of pediatric cancer exposed to anthracyclines. J Clin Oncol 22:820–828

200. Effect of enalapril on survival in patients with reduced left ventricular ejection fractions and congestive heart failure. The SOLVD Investigators (1991) N Engl J Med 325:293–302

201. Cardinale D, Colombo A, Sandri MT et al (2006) Prevention of high-dose chemotherapy-induced cardiotoxicity in high-risk patients by angiotensin-converting enzyme inhibition. Circulation 114:2474–2481

202. Lipshultz SE, Lipsitz SR, Sallan SE et al (2002) Long-term enalapril therapy for left ventricular dysfunction in doxorubicin-treated survivors of childhood cancer. J Clin Oncol 20:4517–4522

203. Dargie HJ (2001) Effect of carvedilol on outcome after myocardial infarction in patients with left-ventricular

dysfunction: the CAPRICORN randomised trial. Lancet 357:1385–1390

204. Effect of metoprolol CR/XL in chronic heart failure: Metoprolol CR/XL Randomised Intervention Trial in Congestive Heart Failure (MERIT-HF) (1999) Lancet 353:2001–2007

205. The Cardiac Insufficiency Bisoprolol Study II (CIBIS-II): a randomised trial (1999) Lancet 353:9–13

206. Colucci WS, Packer M, Bristow MR et al (1996) Carvedilol inhibits clinical progression in patients with mild symptoms of heart failure. US Carvedilol Heart Failure Study Group. Circulation 94:2800–2806

207. Eichhorn EJ, Bristow MR (2001) The carvedilol prospective randomized cumulative survival (COPERNICUS) trial. Curr Control Trials Cardiovasc Med 2:20–23

208. Packer M, Fowler MB, Roecker EB et al (2002) Effect of carvedilol on the morbidity of patients with severe chronic heart failure: results of the carvedilol prospective randomized cumulative survival (COPERNICUS) study. Circulation 106:2194–2199

209. Poole-Wilson PA, Swedberg K, Cleland JG et al (2003) Comparison of carvedilol and metoprolol on clinical outcomes in patients with chronic heart failure in the Carvedilol Or Metoprolol European Trial (COMET): randomised controlled trial. Lancet 362:7–13

210. Noori P, Hou SM (2001) Mutational spectrum induced by acetaldehyde in the HPRT gene of human T lymphocytes resembles that in the p53 gene of esophageal cancers. Carcinogenesis 22:1825–1830

211. Kalay N, Basar E, Ozdogru I et al (2006) Protective effects of carvedilol against anthracycline-induced cardiomyopathy. J Am Coll Cardiol 48:2258–2262

212. Domanski MJ, Borkowf CB, Campeau L et al (2000) Prognostic factors for atherosclerosis progression in saphenous vein grafts: the postcoronary artery bypass graft (Post-CABG) trial. Post-CABG Trial Investigators. J Am Coll Cardiol 36:1877–1883

213. Flather MD, Shibata MC, Coats AJ et al (2005) Randomized trial to determine the effect of nebivolol on mortality and cardiovascular hospital admission in elderly patients with heart failure (SENIORS). Eur Heart J 26:215–225

214. A trial of the beta-blocker bucindolol in patients with advanced chronic heart failure (2001) N Engl J Med 344:1659–1667

215. Albouaini K, Andron M, Alahmar A et al (2007) Beta-blockers use in patients with chronic obstructive pulmonary disease and concomitant cardiovascular conditions. Int J Chron Obstruct Pulmon Dis 2:535–540

216. Pitt B, Zannad F, Remme WJ et al (1999) The effect of spironolactone on morbidity and mortality in patients with severe heart failure. Randomized Aldactone Evaluation Study Investigators. N Engl J Med 341:709–717

217. Carson P, Ziesche S, Johnson G et al (1999) Racial differences in response to therapy for heart failure:

analysis of the vasodilator-heart failure trials. Vasodilator-Heart Failure Trial Study Group. J Card Fail 5:178–187

218. Taylor AL, Ziesche S, Yancy C et al (2004) Combination of isosorbide dinitrate and hydralazine in blacks with heart failure. N Engl J Med 351:2049–2057

219. The effect of digoxin on mortality and morbidity in patients with heart failure. The Digitalis Investigation Group (1997) N Engl J Med 336:525–533

220. Pai VB, Nahata MC (2000) Cardiotoxicity of chemotherapeutic agents: incidence, treatment and prevention. Drug Saf 22:263–302

221. Lipshultz SE, Miller TL, Gerschenson M et al (2012) Impaired mitochondrial structure and function which is abrogated by dexrazoxane in doxorubicin-treated childhood ALL survivors. ASCO Annual meeting, Chicago

222. Davidson N (2011) Preserving cardiac health in the breast cancer patient treated with anthracyclines. In: Olver IN (ed) The MASCC textbook of cancer supportive care and survivorship. Springer, New York/London

223. Swain SM, Whaley FS, Gerber MC et al (1997) Cardioprotection with dexrazoxane for doxorubicin-containing therapy in advanced breast cancer. J Clin Oncol 15:1318–1332

224. Lipshultz SE, Rifai N, Dalton VM et al (2004) The effect of dexrazoxane on myocardial injury in doxorubicin-treated children with acute lymphoblastic leukemia. N Engl J Med 351:145–153

225. Asselin B, Devidas M, Zhou T et al (2012) Cardioprotection and safety of dexrazoxane (DRZ) in children treated for newly diagnosed T-cell acute lymphoblastic leukemia (T-ALL) or advanced stage lymphoblastic leukemia (T-LL). ASCO annual meeting, Chicago

226. Hensley ML, Hagerty KL, Kewalramani T et al (2009) American Society of Clinical Oncology 2008 clinical practice guideline update: use of chemotherapy and radiation therapy protectants. J Clin Oncol 27:127–145

227. Grdina DJ, Kataoka Y, Murley JS (2000) Amifostine: mechanisms of action underlying cytoprotection and chemoprevention. Drug Metabol Drug Interact 16:237–279

228. Nazeyrollas P, Frances C, Prevost A et al (2003) Efficiency of amifostine as a protection against doxorubicin toxicity in rats during a 12-day treatment. Anticancer Res 23:405–409

229. Gallegos-Castorena S, Martinez-Avalos A, Mohar-Betancourt A et al (2007) Toxicity prevention with amifostine in pediatric osteosarcoma patients treated with cisplatin and doxorubicin. Pediatr Hematol Oncol 24:403–408

230. Eaton S, Skinner R, Hale JP et al (2000) Plasma coenzyme Q(10) in children and adolescents undergoing doxorubicin therapy. Clin Chim Acta 302:1–9

231. Conklin KA (2005) Coenzyme Q10 for prevention of anthracycline-induced cardiotoxicity. Integr Cancer Ther 4:110–130

232. Ranasarma T, Slavik M, Muggia FM (1985) Natural occurrence distribution of coenzyme Q. Wiley, Chichester

233. Okuma K, Ota K (1986) The effect of coenzyme Q10 on ECG changes induced by doxorubicin (Adiramycin). Elsevier/North-Holland Biomedical Press, Amsterdam

234. Danesi F, Malaguti M, Nunzio MD et al (2006) Counteraction of adriamycin-induced oxidative damage in rat heart by selenium dietary supplementation. J Agric Food Chem 54:1203–1208

235. Bjelakovic G, Nikolova D, Gluud LL et al (2007) Mortality in randomized trials of antioxidant supplements for primary and secondary prevention: systematic review and meta-analysis. JAMA 297:842–857

236. Moss AJ, Zareba W, Hall WJ et al (2002) Prophylactic implantation of a defibrillator in patients with myocardial infarction and reduced ejection fraction. N Engl J Med 346:877–883

237. Abraham WT, Hayes DL (2003) Cardiac resynchronization therapy for heart failure. Circulation 108:2596–2603

238. Cleland JG, Daubert JC, Erdmann E et al (2005) The effect of cardiac resynchronization on morbidity and mortality in heart failure. N Engl J Med 352:1539–1549

239. Pagani FD, Miller LW, Russell SD et al (2009) Extended mechanical circulatory support with a continuous-flow rotary left ventricular assist device. J Am Coll Cardiol 54:312–321

240. Dillon TA, Sullivan M, Schatzlein MH et al (1991) Cardiac transplantation in patients with preexisting malignancies. Transplantation 52:82–85

241. Ewer MS, Jaffe N, Ried H et al (1998) Doxorubicin cardiotoxicity in children: comparison of a consecutive divided daily dose administration schedule with single dose (rapid) infusion administration. Med Pediatr Oncol 31:512–515

242. Casper ES, Gaynor JJ, Hajdu SI et al (1991) A prospective randomized trial of adjuvant chemotherapy with bolus versus continuous infusion of doxorubicin in patients with high-grade extremity soft tissue sarcoma and an analysis of prognostic factors. Cancer 68:1221–1229

243. Lipshultz SE, Adams MJ (2010) Cardiotoxicity after childhood cancer: beginning with the end in mind. J Clin Oncol 28:1276–1281

244. Lipshultz SE, Cochran TR, Franco VI, Miller TL (2013) Treatment-related cardiotoxicity in survivors of childhood cancer. Nat Rev Clin Oncol 10:697–710

245. Lipshultz SE, Adams MJ, Colan SD et al (2013) Long-term cardiovascular toxicity in children, adolescents, and young adults Who receive cancer therapy: pathophysiology, course, monitoring, management, prevention, and research directions: a scientific statement from the American Heart Association. Circulation 128:1927–1995

246. Kenney LB, Bradeen H, Kadan-Lottick NS et al (2011) The current status of follow-up services for childhood cancer survivors, are we meeting goals and expectations: a report from the Consortium of New England Childhood Cancer Survivors. Pediatr Blood Cancer 57:1062–1066

247. Blanco JG, Sun CL, Landier W et al (2012) Anthracycline-related cardiomyopathy after childhood cancer: role of polymorphisms in carbonyl reductase genes--a report from the Children's Oncology Group. J Clin Oncol 30:1415–1421

248. van der Pal HJ, van Dalen EC, van Delden E et al (2012) High risk of symptomatic cardiac events in childhood cancer survivors. J Clin Oncol 30:1429–1437

# Pulmonary Effects of Antineoplastic Therapy

**11**

Sughosh Dhakal, Daniel Weiner, Cindy Schwartz, and Louis S. Constine

## Contents

S. Dhakal, MD
Department of Radiation Oncology, University of Rochester Medical Center, 601 Elmwood Ave Box 647, Rochester, NY 14642, USA
e-mail: sughosh_dhakal@urmc.rochester.edu

D. Weiner, MD (✉)
Division of Pediatric Pulmonology, Children's Hospital of Pittsburgh, 4401 Penn Avenue, Floor 3, Pittsburg, PA 19224, USA
e-mail: Daniel.weiner@chp.edu

C. Schwartz, MD
Department of Pediatrics, MD Anderson Cancer Center, 1515 Holcombe Blvd Box 87, Houston, TX 77030, USA
e-mail: clschwartz@mdanderson.org

L.S. Constine, MD
Departments of Radiation Oncology and Pediatrics, University of Rochester Medical Center, 601 Elmwood Ave Box 647, Rochester, NY 14642, USA
e-mail: louis_constine@urmc.rochester.edu

© Springer International Publishing 2015
C.L. Schwartz et al. (eds.), *Survivors of Childhood and Adolescent Cancer: A Multidisciplinary Approach*, Pediatric Oncology, DOI 10.1007/978-3-319-16435-9_11

Pulmonary toxicity is common after cancer therapy and can result from all therapeutic modalities. The consequential decrease in lung function ranges in severity from subclinical to life-threatening or even fatal and can manifest in the acute setting or many years after completion of therapy. Radiation effects are due to direct insult to the pulmonary parenchyma and, for younger children, impaired thoracic musculoskeletal development. Radiation pneumonitis can occur in the acute/subacute setting, as well as fibrosis with comprised gas exchange as a late effect of direct lung irradiation; thoracic wall malformation can cause restriction of function as a chronic sequela. The pulmonary effects of cytotoxic drugs usually present as acute effects, but there is the potential for significant late morbidity and mortality. Of course, surgical interventions can also cause both acute and/or late pulmonary effects as well, depending on the specific procedure. Although treatment approaches for the management of pediatric cancers are continually adapted to provide optimal therapy while minimizing toxicities, to a varying degree all therapies have the potential for both acute and late pulmonary toxicity. Of note, the cumulative incidence of pulmonary complications rises with increasing time since diagnosis, which suggests that adult survivors of childhood cancer require lifelong monitoring and management of potential new-onset pulmonary morbidity as they age. Knowledge of cytotoxic therapies and an understanding of lung physiology and how it may be altered by therapy facilitate appropriate clinical care and monitoring of long-term survivors.

## 11.1 Pathophysiology

### 11.1.1 Development of the Lung

An understanding of the pathophysiology of lung toxicity due to cancer therapies requires an understanding of the development of the lungs.

Lung development is a complex process [105] that begins on day 26 of gestation and continues for at least several years postnatal. During the embryonic period, the primitive lung bud arises from the foregut, elongates caudally, and branches to form the major airways. The pseudoglandular phase follows; the process of

branching continues and the smaller airways are formed. Fetal breathing movements are identified as early as 8 weeks, and by the end of this phase, the two lobes of the left lung and three lobes of the right lung can be identified. Cartilage and smooth muscle cells are present, and about half of the epithelial cell types that will eventually comprise the mature lung are identifiable. The airway branching is completed, the interstitial tissue decreases, and prospective gas exchange regions begin to appear during the canalicular phase. A differentiation process occurs in the cuboidal epithelial cells, and Type I and II pneumocytes appear. Type I pneumocytes are the functional exchange unit of the lung, while Type II pneumocytes produce surfactant, a phospholipid substance that serves to decrease surface tension within the Type I cell and prevent it from collapsing. Vascularization of the lung occurs throughout development, and, at this point, the capillaries can be found in close proximity to the pneumocytes. The saccular phase of development extends from 24 weeks through 38 weeks gestation. During this time, there is continued thinning of the connective tissue between the potential air spaces, further maturation of the Type II pneumocytes, and increased surfactant production. Primitive alveoli, lined by both Type I and Type II pneumocytes, can now be identified as pouches in the walls of the saccules and respiratory bronchioles (Table 11.1).

The alveoli phase of development extends from 36 weeks gestation through about 3 years of age. At birth, there are few alveoli present, but potential airspaces are identifiable as smooth-walled ducts and saccules with thickened septa. Inflation of the saccules occurs at birth. The septa become thin and grow into air spaces, forming partitions within the pouches. Within a few months the infant's alveoli resemble those of the adult, with greatly increased surface area available for gas exchange. Completion of the vascularization process during this time results in single capillary networks associated with each area of gas exchange [118, 150]. After birth, minor structural changes continue to occur. The alveolar surfaces become more complex, and the alveoli become more numerous with the increase in body size.

**Table 11.1** Prenatal and Early Childhood lung development

| Stage | Weeks | Major developments |
|---|---|---|
| Embryonic | 4–9 | Formation of major airways |
| Pseudoglandular | 5–17 | Formation of bronchial tree and portions of respiratory parenchyma |
| | | Birth of the acinus |
| Canalicular | 16–27 | Last generations of the lung periphery formed |
| | | Epithelial differentiation |
| | | Air–blood barrier formed |
| Saccular | 24–38 | Expansion of air spaces |
| | | Surfactant detectable in amniotic fluid |
| Alveolar | 36–3 years | Secondary septation |

The most rapid phase of pulmonary growth occurs within the first few years of life, followed at 4–6 years of age by a slow growth phase. According to autopsy studies [99], the maximum numbers of alveoli are achieved by approximately 8 years of age. After this point it is believed that alveolar surface volume increases without an increase in alveolar number [149]. However, recent studies have suggested that formation of new alveoli may continue into adolescence [99]. In regard to musculoskeletal development, radiographic measurement of lung diameters demonstrates linear growth during childhood and a spurt at puberty [142].

## 11.1.2 Pathophysiologic Changes Induced by Cytotoxic Therapy

Primary lung malignancies are very rare in children; however, the lung is a common site for metastases, sometimes even years after the completion of definitive therapy. Therapy-related pulmonary toxicity is due to either local therapies (radiation or surgery) directed at the lung parenchyma and chest wall or chemotherapy that is administered systemically but likewise negatively affects these organs and structures. Of course, many patients receive multimodality treatment that potentially compounds acute and late toxicity.

The pathogenesis of pulmonary toxicity secondary to cytotoxic therapy is largely based on animal experimentation. However, it is believed to occur through one of four mechanisms of injury: (1) DNA damage from the drug or radiation itself, (2) damage inflicted by free radical generation, (3) allergic response to the cytotoxic agent, and (4) subsequent injury induced by the inflammatory response to the primary damage itself. Pulmonary fibrosis, which mediates many of the long-term effects, can arise from collagen deposits that occur after cellular damage. In addition, the breakdown of actual lung tissue can trigger an inflammatory reaction that activates increased production of elastin by actin-expressing smooth muscle cells. This also results in pulmonary fibrosis. While there are several postulated means of injury to the pulmonary tissue, the common finding in all is diffuse alveolar damage. The cytotoxic changes start as endothelial blebs in the alveolar capillaries and lead to capillary leak syndrome. These are then associated with interstitial edema. There is destruction and a resulting decrease in number of Type I pneumocytes, as well as reactive changes and proliferation of Type II pneumocytes. More recently, progress has been made in understanding the molecular and cellular events after radiation lung injury, leading to clinically and histologically recognizable changes. The process appears to be dynamic and to involve proinflammatory cytokines, profibrotic cytokines, chemokines, and adhesion molecules in modulating and recruiting immune cells to the sites of radiation lung injury [24]. Long-term effects on the lungs are the result of this complex process.

### 11.1.2.1 Pathophysiology of Chemotherapy-Induced Disease

Drug-related pulmonary disease may be the result of toxicity, allergy, or idiosyncrasy [39]. Toxicity, with a dose–response, has been shown for bleomycin, chlorambucil, and the nitrosoureas. Pulmonary damage, likely mediated through allergic mechanisms, is caused by cyclo-phosphamide, methotrexate, procarbazine, and bleomycin. Pulmonary disease has also been associated with mitomycin, cytosine arabinoside, the vinca alkaloids, and alkylating agents.

Bleomycin may be the most commonly recognized cause of pulmonary toxicity; the pathogenesis of bleomycin injury has been studied extensively [29, 58, 71]. Lung injury following low-dose bleomycin may be idiosyncratic, possibly attributable to genetically impaired drug metabolism. Having inherently low levels of bleomycin hydrolase [76], an enzyme that inactivates bleomycin, the lung is particularly vulnerable to bleomycin injury. Mouse data demonstrate that strain sensitivity to bleomycin is related to different levels of bleomycin hydrolase activity [62]. Hence, individual variations in bleomycin sensitivity may be explained at least in part by genetically determined levels of bleomycin hydrolase activity. Free radical formation and oxidative damage also play a role in bleomycin-induced lung injury. Fibrosis after bleomycin therapy develops under the influence of immune processes that include activation of effector cells, including alveolar macrophages, and release of cytokines. Tumor necrosis factor may play a pivotal role [82, 106]. Pathology demonstrates endothelial and Type I cell necrosis with Type II hyperplasia and hyaline membranes. Bleomycin-induced pulmonary effects usually occur during or within a year of treatment.

Alkylating agents, such as the nitrosoureas, are known to cause late-onset pulmonary fibrosis. The fibrosis noted after nitrosourea therapy demonstrates less inflammation than bleomycin-induced fibrosis, but consistency in Type I depletion and Type II hyperplasia with excess collagen deposition. The formation of free radicals and lipid peroxidation of phospholipid membranes may also be the mechanism by which cyclophosphamide and mitomycin damage the capillary endothelium [28]. Permeability increases, resulting in interstitial edema. Hyaline membranes form as plasma proteins, and fluid enters the alveoli through the denuded epithelium. Type I pneumocytes swell, become necrotic, and are replaced by cuboidal cells. Proliferation of fibroblasts then occurs. This process may evolve slowly, with fibrosis increasing over a period of years. Interstitial pneumonitis (either the desquamative type that appears to be an earlier stage or the usual type with fibrinous exudation, hyaline membranes, and interstitial fibrosis) is also seen with alkylating agents. This pneumonitis may lead to the development of chronic pulmonary fibrosis that is characterized by the enhanced production and deposition of collagen and other matrix components. Pulmonary veno-occlusive disease, with vasculitis and intimal fibrosis resulting in pulmonary hypertension, has been reported after either bleomycin or mitomycin [34].

## 11.1.2.2 Pathophysiology of Radiation-Induced Disease

Similar histopathologic changes and resultant physiologic abnormalities are found in the lung following radiotherapy and chemotherapy. Subclinical injuries resulting from radiation to the lung are most likely present in all patients, even after very small doses of radiation. Studies of the immunological regulation of inflammation after radiation in animals have revealed a complex interaction between local tissues, resident cells, and circulating immune cells, mediated through chemokines, adhesion molecules, inflammatory cytokines, and fibrotic cytokines. Chemokine monocyte chemotactic protein-1 (MCP1) [66], adhesion molecules (intercellular adhesion molecule-1 [ICAM-1]) [56, 69], and interferon-inducible protein-10 (IP-10) [66] appear to be involved in initiating radiation lung injury [24, 54, 56, 66, 124, 128, 148]. Afterward, there appears to be a cascade of proinflammatory cytokines and fibrotic cytokines (Fig. 11.1) [129].

In the first few days to weeks after irradiation, ultrastructural alterations in the capillary endothelial lining become evident. The cells become pleomorphic and vacuolated and may slough, thereby producing areas of denuded basement membrane and occlusion of the capillary lumen by debris and thrombi [51, 79, 86, 116]. There is exudation of proteinaceous material into the alveoli, leading to impairment of gas exchange. Studies have shown that radiation-induced lung injury is characterized by alveolar infiltrates of mononuclear cells, primarily CD4+ T cells and

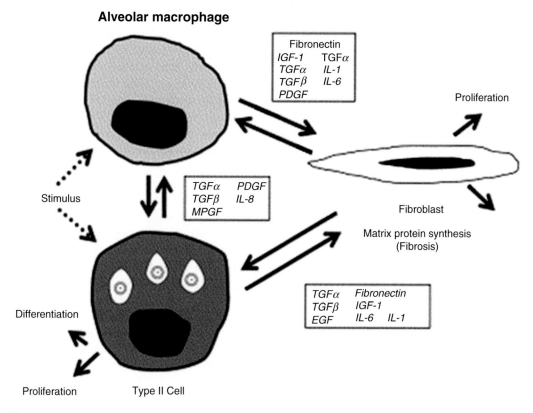

**Alveolar macrophage**

Fibronectin
IGF-1    TGFα
TGFα    IL-1
TGFβ    IL-6
PDGF

Proliferation

Stimulus

TGFα    PDGF
TGFβ    IL-8
MPGF

Fibroblast

Matrix protein synthesis
(Fibrosis)

Differentiation

TGFα    Fibronectin
TGFβ    IGF-1
EGF      IL-6    IL-1

Proliferation          Type II Cell

**Fig. 11.1** Cell–cell interaction and control of gene expression by growth factors in lung injury (With permission from Rubin et al. [129])

macrophages/monocytes (mononuclear alveolitis), and that there is a relative scarcity of neutrophils [40, 43], a common marker for infectious processes. Lavage fluids obtained from bronchoscopy have confirmed this finding in patients with active pneumonitis [84, 98, 124]. In a few weeks the interstitial edema organizes into collagen fibrils, which eventually leads to thickening of the alveolar septa. These exudative changes may resolve in a few weeks to a few months. However, depending on the volume of lung parenchyma irradiated, the total dose, and the dose per fraction, the changes can result in an acute radiation pneumonitis.

Although no specific lesion is entirely characteristic of pneumonitis, current evidence suggests that damage to the Type II pneumocyte and to the endothelial cell is closely linked to the pneumonitic process [21, 113, 151, 152]. The type II pneumocyte, which produces surfactant and maintains patent alveoli, has been well studied.

After radiation exposure a rapid decrease in the content of cytoplasmic surfactant-containing lamellar bodies occurs, followed by the ultimate sloughing of some of the cells into the alveolar lumen [111, 112]. Changes in the surfactant system that lead to alterations in alveolar surface tension and low compliance are most likely a direct result of the radiation [113, 130, 131], although it has been postulated that the changes indirectly result from exudation of plasma proteins [52]. Endothelial cell damage results in changes in perfusion and permeability of the vessel wall. Endothelial leakage and increased permeability allow immune cells to undergo transendothelial migration and extravasation from the vascular compartment into the alveolar space.

Late lung injury is characterized by progressive fibrosis of the alveolar septa, which become thickened by bundles of elastic fibers. The alveoli collapse and are obliterated by connective tissue. The mechanisms of chronic injury may be related to the effects of radiation on the pulmonary vasculature (endothelial cells) or somatic cells. The nature of the triggering event in the pathogenesis of radiation-related lung fibrosis is complex. The classic hypothesis that fibrosis is a connective tissue replacement process following parenchymal cell death has been challenged, and the exact mechanisms of early injuries leading to the late effects are not entirely understood. Cytokine-mediated multicellular interactions that initiate and sustain the fibrogenic process take place within hours to days after radiation in animal research models. Experimental data suggest that the progression of the initial lung injury to the pneumonitic phase may be the result of a cytokine and cellular interaction, which subsequently regulates the fibrotic phase of the presentation [24, 127–129]. In addition, it has been recently hypothesized that chronic hypoxia, and the perpetual injury to normal tissue through reactive oxygen species, may also be a contributing mechanism to chronic and progressive fibrosis [158]. Studies in animals have confirmed the protective effect of fractionated radiation therapy, which is several small doses of radiation as compared to a comparable dose delivered in a single large treatment, indicating a significant degree of recovery of lung tissue between fractions [141, 160].

### 11.1.2.3 Categorization of Pulmonary Disease

Lung disease may be categorized as follows: interstitial, obstructive, restrictive, or a combination. Most long-term toxicity is the result of interstitial disease, which involves inflammation and fibrosis of the alveolar walls and changes in the capillary endothelium and alveolar epithelial lining cells, as described below. The histologic hallmarks of interstitial lung disease are proliferation of fibroblasts and excessive deposition of collagen [135]. Interstitial lung disease also may impact the small airways. As alveolar–capillary membrane destruction is an integral part of interstitial disease, pulmonary function tests demonstrate a decrease in the measured diffusing capacity [135].

Pulmonary disease after chemotherapy or radiation therapy may also have an obstructive component. Obstructive diseases result from airway narrowing. This may be due to bronchospasm, mucus, or luminal narrowing as a result of edema and inflammation or scarring [97]. Airway narrowing due to disease can be detected as a decrease in expiratory airflow. Pulmonary function tests demonstrate a decrease in the ratio of the volume exhaled in 1 s (FEV1) to the total exhaled forced vital capacity (FVC).

Restrictive lung diseases occur as a result of alterations in the elasticity of the pulmonary system [42], which may be due to parenchymal disease originating in the lung or from structural anomalies of the chest wall. In the healthy lung, collagen and elastin fibers contribute to the formation of an organized web, which has a significant ability to stretch and recoil [42]. Disruption of this organization from inflammation and fibrosis occurs as a result of injury and response to cytotoxic therapy, thereby decreasing the elasticity of the lung and resulting in restrictive disease. Additionally, in the child, cytotoxic therapy may impair the proliferation and maturation of alveoli, leading to inadequate alveoli number and lung growth and resulting in chronic respiratory insufficiency.

Restrictive lung disease may also occur as a result of growth impairment of the lung or musculoskeletal structures, which is predominantly a consequence of radiation therapy. Inhibition of growth of the thoracic cage (i.e., muscle, cartilage, and bone) can limit chest wall compliance, with resultant restrictive problems. Naturally, younger children are more vulnerable to chronic respiratory damage from impairment of the normal growth and development of the lungs and the thoracic cage.

In restrictive respiratory disease, pulmonary function testing demonstrates an increased FEV1/FVC ratio with an increased maximal expiratory airflow. With more advanced restrictive disease, total lung capacity, vital capacity, and lung volumes are decreased, with evidence of uneven distribution of ventilation [97]. Please refer to Sect. 11.3.1 for a detailed discussion of pulmonary function tests.

## 11.2 Clinical Manifestations

### 11.2.1 Long-Term Effect in Pediatric Population

Potential pulmonary complications of therapy leading to a range of respiratory manifestations have been reported by the Childhood Cancer Survivor Study. Study participants were asked whether they had ever been told by a physician, or other healthcare professional, that they have or had a particular diagnosis, such as pulmonary fibrosis. This self-report study demonstrated that long-term survivors described a statistically significant increased relative risk of lung fibrosis, recurrent pneumonia, chronic cough, pleurisy, use of supplemental oxygen, abnormal chest wall, exercise-induced SOB, bronchitis, recurrent sinus infection, and tonsillitis for all time periods, including during therapy, from the completion of therapy to 5 years off therapy and >5 years after therapy. Significant associations existed between the development of fibrosis and treatment with radiation therapy and between the use of supplemental oxygen, recurrent pneumonia, chronic cough, and pleurisy and treatment with radiation therapy and/or multiple chemotherapy agents [92]. In regard to mortality, a large retrospective study of greater than 20,000 5-year survivors of childhood cancer reported a significant excess rate of deaths largely due to treatment-related causes rather than progression or recurrence of the primary disease; furthermore, pulmonary causes accounted for excess mortality risk (standard mortality ratio, 8.8) second only to death from secondary malignancy (standard mortality ratio, 15.2) [7].

Pulmonary toxicity is frequently reported in survivors of Hodgkin lymphoma, but it also complicates the cure of survivors of germ cell tumors, rhabdomyosarcoma, neuroblastoma, bone tumors, and acute lymphoblastic leukemia (ALL) [16, 55, 61, 67, 72, 94, 101, 102]. Although many of the patients that have been studied received radiation therapy, the intensified use of chemotherapy accounts for some or all of the toxicity in subsets of survivors. In fact, pulmonary complications are

a major cause of morbidity and mortality following hematopoietic stem cell transplant [145], which is now an established treatment approach for many pediatric malignancies.

Studies with long-term follow-up suggest that the cumulative incidence of pulmonary complications increases with increasing time since treatment [63]. This appears to be far in excess of decreases in lung function with normal aging, suggesting that the effects of early lung injury from cancer therapy compound expected decreases and that survivors should be monitored indefinitely for new-onset pulmonary morbidity as they age.

### 11.2.2 Radiotherapy: Clinical Presentations

Pneumonitis and pulmonary fibrosis are the two most important consequences of irradiation of the lung. Pulmonary fibrosis occurs in almost 100 % of patients receiving high doses of radiation, but it may not be of clinical significance if the volume is small. The clinically significant presentation of pulmonary toxicity is usually pneumonitis, due to its prevalence and potential morbid outcome. The presentation varies with the type of lung injury present. Often there are complaints of a nonproductive cough, fever, and dyspnea. However, the presentation can also be quite acute with respiratory insufficiency and acute respiratory distress syndrome (ARDS). Other presentations include bronchospasm, pleural effusion, bronchiolitis obliterans, pulmonary veno-occlusive disease, sarcoidosis, pulmonary alveolar proteinosis, pneumothorax, and pulmonary hemorrhage.

When radiation therapy is the only modality used, radiation pneumonitis follows the completion of the definitive course of treatment. Cough, pink sputum, dyspnea, and pleuritis are common complaints during the subacute pneumonitic phase, which generally occurs 1–3 months after completion of radiation. When chemotherapy is administered in conjunction with radiation, as in total body irradiation (TBI) and BMT-conditioning regimens, reactions can occur during treatment. The fibrotic phase of radiation injury starts 3–6 months after completion of radiation and is progressive. The clinical manifestations of fibrosis are worsening dyspnea, increasing probability of oxygen dependence, and declining pulmonary function test results.

### 11.2.2.1 Subacute Radiation Pneumonitis

Subacute pneumonitis is a pneumonopathy that usually occurs 1–3 months after the completion of radiation. It is well described in the adult literature after the treatment of lung cancer [5, 6, 122], but little of the data from such studies are relevant to modern pediatric cancer therapies. Pneumonitis can occur unexpectedly, with little or no warning. Because of this, many attempts have been made to identify clinical risk factors. The factors that influence risk include total lung radiation dose, irradiated lung volume exceeding 20 Gy vs 25 Gy vs 30 Gy, mean lung dose, fractionation of radiotherapy, daily fraction size, performance status, pre-treatment pulmonary function, gender, low pre-treatment blood oxygen, and high C-reactive protein [49, 59, 64, 74, 123, 125, 136].

Symptoms of subacute pneumonitis syndrome include low-grade fever and nonspecific respiratory symptoms such as congestion, cough, and fullness in the chest. In more severe cases, dyspnea, pleuritic chest pain, and nonproductive cough may be present. Later, small amounts of sputum, sometimes bloodstained, may be produced. Physical signs in the chest are usually absent, although a pleural friction rub or pleural fluid may be detected. Evidence of alveolar infiltrates or consolidation is sometimes found in the region corresponding to pneumonitis. This results from an acute exudative edema that is initially faint but may progress to homogenous or patchy air space consolidation. Frequently there is an associated volume loss in the affected portion of the lung.

CT studies of the lung have been used to evaluate lung density in this situation. Because of its sensitivity to increased lung density, CT has been favored for radiographic detection of pulmonary damage in humans [81, 85, 155]. CT findings demonstrate a well-defined, dose–response relationship [85]. Four patterns of radiation-induced changes have been defined in lung on CT: homogenous (slight increase in radiodensity), patchy consolidation, discrete consolidation, and solid consolidation [81]. These patterns, corresponding to both pneumonitic and fibrotic phases, have varying timetables and may appear weeks to years after radiotherapy.

### 11.2.2.2 Radiation Fibrosis

In contrast to the acute reaction, clinically apparent chronic effects of cytotoxic therapy may be observed from a few months to years following treatment, even though histologic and biochemical changes are evident sooner. Pulmonary fibrosis develops insidiously in the previously irradiated field and stabilizes after 1–2 years.

The clinical symptomatology related to the radiographic changes is proportional to the extent of the lung parenchyma involved and preexisting pulmonary reserve. After thoracic radiation, restrictive changes gradually develop and progress with time [51]. Gas exchange abnormalities occur approximately at the same time as the changes in lung volumes. These abnormalities consist of a fall in diffusion capacity, mild arterial hypoxemia that may manifest only with exercise, and a low or normal $PaCO_2$ level. The changes appear to be consistent with a parenchymal lung defect and ventilation–perfusion inequality that results in a component of effective shunt [52]. Radionuclide evaluations have demonstrated that underperfusion, rather than underventilation, is the cause of these inequalities, reflecting radiation injury to the microvasculature [119, 120, 157]. Larger doses of irradiation cause reductions in lung compliance that start at the time of pneumonitis and persist thereafter [117]. The compliance of the chest wall is usually much less affected in adults and adolescents than in young children, in whom interference with growth of both lung and chest wall leads to marked reductions in mean total lung volumes and diffusion capacity (DLCO) [165]. Whole-lung irradiation in doses of 11–14 Gy has resulted in restrictive changes in the lungs of children treated for various malignancies [10, 83, 93]. Consequently, RT in younger children, particularly those younger than 3 years old, results in increased chronic toxicity [93]. One to 2 years after radiation, clinical symptoms stabilize and are often minimal if fibrosis is limited to less than 50 % of one lung [134]. A mild deterioration in pulmonary function may be demonstrated as fibrosis develops. There is a reduction in maximum breathing capacity that is particularly evident in patients with bilateral radiation fibrosis. Tidal volume usually decreases, and breathing frequency tends to increase, resulting in an overall moderate increase in minute ventilation [139]. Most studies have found these changes to persist indefinitely, with little recovery unless there are concurrent improvements in pulmonary function with lung tumor response [41, 45, 50]. Functional compensation by adjacent lung regions [100] limits the effect of radiation on pulmonary function tests when small volumes of lung are irradiated. Dyspnea and progressive chronic cor pulmonale leading to right heart failure may occur when >50 % of a lung is irradiated.

Radiologic changes consistent with fibrosis are seen in most patients who have received lung irradiation, even if they do not develop acute pneumonitis. Chest radiographs have linear streaking, radiating from the area of previous pneumonitis and sometimes extending outside the irradiated region, with concomitant regional contraction, pleural thickening, and tenting of the diaphragm. The hilum or mediastinum may be retracted with a densely contracted lung segment, resulting in compensatory hyperinflation of the adjacent or contralateral lung tissue. This is usually seen 12 months to 2 years after radiation. When chronic fibrosis occurs in the absence of an earlier clinically evident pneumonitic phase [113, 126, 140], chest radiography generally reveals scarring that corresponds to the shape of the radiation portal. Eventually, dense fibrosis can develop, especially in the area of a previous tumor [127]. CT is currently favored to image regions subjected to RT [81, 85, 155]. Magnetic resonance imaging (MRI) is being explored and may have promise in accurately distinguishing radiation fibrosis from recurrent tumor. Although radiation tolerance doses

may be exceeded, not all patients will develop complications, given that the sensitivity to radiation varies from patient to patient.

### 11.2.2.3 Radiation Tolerance Doses and Tolerance Volumes

Radiation-associated sequelae are dependent on radiation dose and fractionation, as well as volume of lung exposed. With high doses exceeding clinical thresholds (8.0–12.0 Gy, single dose), pulmonary reactions clinically express themselves as a pneumonitic process 1–3 months after the completion of thoracic irradiation. Lethality can occur if both lungs are irradiated to high doses (approximately 8–10 Gy, single dose, or greater than 20–25 Gy in a fractionated schedule) or if threshold doses of drugs are exceeded. Recovery from pneumonitis usually occurs, however, and is followed almost immediately by the second phase, which is progressive fibrosis. The clinical pathologic course is biphasic and again dependent upon the dose and volume of lung exposed. Lower doses of lung irradiation (approximately 7 Gy, single dose, or 15–18 Gy in a fractionated schedule) produce subclinical pathologic effects that can be expressed by added insult, such as infection or drugs.

**Single Dose, Whole Lung Volume** Total body irradiation (TBI) in the setting of bone marrow transplantation (BMT) and half-body irradiation (HBI) initially used single doses of 8.0–10.0 Gy, without lung correction factors for lung density [44, 45, 47, 50–53, 57, 58, 68, 69, 71]. Death resulting from interstitial pneumonitis was often attributed to secondary opportunistic infection after BMT for leukemia. Pulmonary failure 1–3 months later was mistaken for lymphangitic carcinomatosis after HBI. At autopsy, radiation pneumonopathy became evident. Studies of fatal pneumonitis following TBI and HBI conducted by Keane et al. [71] and Fryer et al. [44] provided precise dose–response curves for injury, both with and without lung inhomogeneity correction. The threshold dose for fatal pneumonitis was 7.0 Gy with the TD5 (tolerance dose for 5 % probability of death) at 8.2 Gy, the TD50 at 9.3 Gy, and the TD90 at 11.0 Gy, corrected for pulmonary transmission. The dose–response is so sharp that a difference of 2.0 Gy could change zero mortality to 50 % lethality.

**Fractionated Dose, Whole Lung Volume** The tolerance of the whole lung to fractionated doses of radiation is well described, particularly in Wilms' tumor patients [10, 15, 83, 93, 115, 165]. In the absence of chemotherapy and with daily doses of 1.3–1.5 Gy, the TD5 is 26.5 Gy and the TD50 is 30.5 Gy. Young children experience more chronic toxicity at lower doses than older children and adults because of interference with lung and chest wall development, in addition to fibrosis and volume loss [96]. After 20 Gy, mean total lung volumes and DLCO are reduced to 60 % of predicted values [165]. Even within the dose range currently used for whole lung irradiation (11–14 Gy), restrictive changes occur [10, 83, 93].

**Whole Lung Volume, Dose Rate** Dose rate has a profound impact on lung damage, with a decrease in the incidence of injury from 90 % to 50 % with decrease in dose rate from 0.5 to 0.1 Gy per minute [44, 71].

**Fractionated Dose, Partial Lung Volume** Clinical tolerance of partial lung volumes to fractionated radiation is not well quantified. There are, however, some relevant data from Mah and colleagues [85]. They showed that, using an increase in lung density within the irradiated volume on CT in the posttreatment period as an endpoint, each 5 % increase in effective dose was associated with a 12 % increase in the incidence of pneumonitis. Doses above 30 Gy over a period of 10–15 days, and 45–50 Gy over a period of 25–30 days, caused radiographic changes in 30–90 % of patients. The need for a clinical guideline in estimating radiation injury prompted the collaborative work by a task force to address the normal tissue tolerance in the standard, fractionated radiation setting. Information was obtained from a diverse group of patients afflicted with various diseases of the thoracic region, but mostly from patients with Hodgkin's disease, lung cancer, or a disease requiring large-volume

**Table 11.2** Lung tolerance dose (TD) in fractionated radiotherapy

| Lung volume | TD 5/5[a] | TD 50/5[b] |
| --- | --- | --- |
| 1/3 | 4,500 cGy | 6,500 cGy |
| 2/3 | 3,000 cGy | 4,000 cGy |
| 3/3 (whole lung) | 1,750 cGy | 2,450 cGy |

[a]The probability of 5 % complication within 5 years of treatment
[b]The probability of 50 % complication within 5 years of treatment

irradiation (hemibody or total body radiation) [37]. The doses agreed on by the physicians in the taskforce are shown in Table 11.2. It is important to note that these values were defined for adult, not pediatric, patients.

More recently, as part of the Quantitative Analysis of Normal Tissue Effects in the Clinic (QUANTEC) effort, a logistic regression fitted to radiation pneumonitis vs mean lung dose was created from data from all published studies, again, predominantly involving adult patients, of a significant size that had extractable complication rates binned by mean dose (Fig. 11.2). The authors note that some of the variation around the fitted curve is possibly explained by differences in patient selection, as well as differences in the grade of RP reported in the various studies; however, there is a relatively small 68 % confidence interval (stippled lines). Of importance is the gradual increase in dose–response, which suggests that there is no absolute "safe" mean lung dose below which pneumonitis is certain not to develop.

An international effort similar to the above QUANTEC analysis is currently underway specific to the pediatric population.

## 11.2.3 Chemotherapy: Clinical Manifestations

As increasing numbers of patients are cured with chemotherapy, reports of agents responsible for acute, and possibly chronic, pulmonary toxicity are expanding. Drug-related lung injury is most commonly an acute phenomenon, occurring during or shortly after the chemotherapeutic agent(s) is administered [28].

**Fig. 11.2** Rate of radiation pneumonitis after fractionated partial lung radiotherapy (*RT*) related to (**a**) mean lung dose and (**b**) different values of Vx. Confidence intervals shown are _1 standard deviation (With permission from Marks et al. [87])

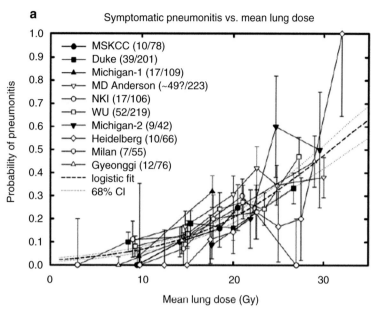

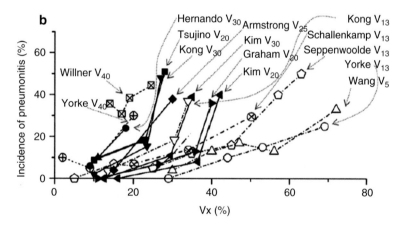

### 11.2.3.1 Patterns of Toxicity

Three typical patterns of pulmonary toxicity have been described: acute hypersensitivity (or inflammatory interstitial pneumonitis), noncardiogenic pulmonary edema, and pneumonitis or fibrosis.

Hypersensitivity reactions are rare but can be induced by such agents as methotrexate, procarbazine, bleomycin, BCNU, and paclitaxel. Cough, dyspnea, low-grade fever, eosinophilia, "crackles" on exam, and interstitial or alveolar infiltrates are noted. These reactions occur during therapy and usually resolve with discontinuation of the offending drug and, potentially, corticosteroid use.

Noncardiogenic pulmonary edema, characterized by endothelial inflammation and vascular leak, may arise upon initiation of treatment with methotrexate, cytosine arabinoside, ifosfamide, cyclophosphamide, and interleukin-2 [28, 77, 146]. All-trans retinoic acid (ATRA) syndrome, a potentially fatal cytokine release syndrome, occurs in 23–28 % of patients receiving ATRA. Pulmonary edema has also been described in patients treated with bleomycin who are exposed to supplemental oxygen. These acute reactions generally have a good prognosis. Hypersensitivity reactions and noncardiogenic pulmonary edema are unlikely to result in late-onset pulmonary toxicity.

Drug-induced pneumonitis or fibrosis has a similar clinical presentation to that described after

RT. Bleomycin, the nitrosoureas, and cyclophosphamide are most commonly the etiologic agents, although methotrexate and vinca alkaloids have also been implicated [28]. This syndrome is particularly worrisome because symptoms may not be detectable until months after a critical cumulative dose has already been reached or exceeded. In addition, persistent subclinical findings may indicate a potential for late decompensation.

### 11.2.3.2 Specific Agents

**Bleomycin** The incidence of bleomycin pulmonary toxicity is 6–10 %, with a mortality of 1–2 %. One study in children with rhabdomyosarcoma exposed to bleomycin demonstrated an incidence of toxicity of 70 % based on decreased DLCO [67]. A risk factor for bleomycin-induced pulmonary toxicity is the cumulative dose with a 10 % risk at doses of 400–500 IU/m$^2$ [14, 132] although injury may occur at doses as low as 20 IU/m$^2$. The elderly [14] and children or adolescents [44] may be more sensitive, especially when bleomycin is administered in conjunction with RT. Of children treated for Hodgkin's disease with 70–120 IU/m$^2$ of bleomycin [44], 9 % had grade 3 or 4 pulmonary toxicity, according to DLCO. Three patients (5 %) had clinical symptomatology, and one patient died. Only one patient had received RT. Although pediatric trials now use a significantly lower maximal dose than many adult studies, 80 % of the drug is excreted by the kidney, which can result in an increased risk of toxicity due to renal insufficiency [114, 143]. Other chemotherapeutic agents such as cisplatin, cyclophosphamide, doxorubicin, methotrexate, and vincristine [8, 121] may also increase risk. Exposure to high levels of oxygen or to pulmonary infection, especially within a year of treatment, is associated with a risk for immediate progressive respiratory failure [47]. Risks associated with surgery after treatment with bleomycin may be due to fluid overload [35]. These risks may persist for longer periods of time. There may be a potential increase in pulmonary toxicity with the use of granulocyte colony stimulating factor (G-CSF), which is mediated via the increased numbers of neutrophils [30].

Patients with acute bleomycin toxicity most commonly present with dyspnea and a dry cough. Fine bibasilar rates may progress to coarse rales involving the entire lung. Radiographs reveal an interstitial pneumonitis with a bibasilar reticular pattern or fine nodular infiltrates. In advanced cases, widespread infiltrates are seen, occasionally with lobar consolidation [132]; however, the consolidation may involve only the upper lobes. Large nodules may mimic metastatic cancer [89]. Loss of lung volume may occur. Pulmonary function testing reveals a restrictive ventilatory defect with hypoxia, hypocapnia, and chronic respiratory alkalosis due to impaired diffusion and hyperventilation [154]. The DLCO is thought by some to be the most sensitive screening tool for bleomycin toxicity [154]. In patients who develop mild toxicity, discontinuation of bleomycin may lead to a reversal of the abnormalities [32], but some patients will have persistent radiographic or pulmonary function abnormalities [9, 107, 164].

**Nitrosoureas** The risk of nitrosourea pulmonary toxicity is age and dose dependent with patients who have received higher doses of nitrosoureas (e.g., greater than 1,500 mg/m$^2$ in adults and 750 mg/m$^2$ in children) more likely to present with an interstitial pneumonitis identical to that seen after bleomycin therapy [1]. Fibrosis may be early onset or late onset. Radiation therapy also increases risk, as does underlying pulmonary abnormality, such as chronic obstructive pulmonary disease, although this is rarely a factor in children. Bone marrow transplant patients may develop pulmonary fibrosis with BCNU as one of the contributing etiologies [103]. As part of a preparative regimen including etoposide and melphalan, BCNU at 600 mg/m$^2$ was associated with unacceptable pulmonary toxicity, but doses of 450 mg/m$^2$ were tolerated in the acute period [2]. Chemotherapy prior to bone marrow transplant may induce inflammatory changes that render the lung more susceptible to further, potentially irreversible, injury with high-dose therapy [12]. Although pulmonary fibrosis has been most commonly associated with BCNU, it has been described after other nitrosoureas as well [13, 33]. Bibasilar rales with a bibasilar reticular pattern may be seen on chest radiograph, and restrictive ventilatory defects are seen as well. Abnormalities may be restricted to the upper lobes. A decreased diffusion capacity may precede all other signs [137]. Discontinuation of therapy may alter the course of BCNU-induced pulmonary disease. However, once pulmonary infiltrates are noted, the disease may be irreversible [162]. In a documented study, 47 % of survivors of childhood brain tumors treated with BCNU and radiation died of lung fibrosis, 12 % within 3 years of treatment, and the remainder 6–17 years posttreatment. Additional patients were known to have pulmonary fibrosis and remained at risk for late decompensation. In this study, age was a risk factor. The median age of the patients who died was 2.5 years, while the median age of survivors was 10 years. In fact, all patients treated under the age of 5 years had died [104].

**Cyclophosphamide** Fibrosis after treatment with cyclophosphamide is rare, with a reported incidence less than 1 %. However, one study [72] found that 4 of 15 children treated with high-dose cyclophosphamide without mediastinal RT had significantly decreased forced vital capacities; 2 of these children also had a decreased FEV1. In addition, one of the children had pulmonary fibrosis and a chest wall deformity. Two children who received more than 50 g/m$^2$ of cyclophosphamide had delayed (greater than 7 years) fatal pulmonary fibrosis, with severe restrictive lung disease. Severely decreased anteroposterior chest dimensions in these patients were attributed to inability of the lung to grow in accordance with body growth. Fibrosis may also develop late after prolonged treatment with relatively low doses of cyclophosphamide. Although there may be recovery if symptoms occur during therapy and the drug is discontinued with administration of corticosteroids, the course may be one of progressive fibrosis nonetheless.

**Hematopoietic Stem Cell Transplant (HSCT)** Patients who are treated with HSCT are at risk of pulmonary toxicity because of multiple potential factors, such as preexisting pulmonary dysfunction; the preparative conditioning regimen, which may include cyclophosphamide, busulfan, carmustine, and total body irradiation (TBI); and the presence of graft-vs-host disease [21, 78, 134, 162]. Although most transplant survivors are not clinically compromised, restrictive lung disease may occur. Obstructive disease is less common, as is the recently described late-onset pulmonary syndrome, which includes the spectrum of restrictive and obstructive disease. Bronchiolitis obliterans, with or without organizing pneumonia, diffuse alveolar damage, and interstitial pneumonia, may occur as a component of this syndrome, generally 6–12 months after transplant. Cough, dyspnea, or wheezing may occur with either normal chest radiograph or diffuse or patchy infiltrates; however, most patients are symptom-free [78, 162]. Cerveri et al. [21] evaluated pulmonary function tests in survivors of pediatric HSCT at baseline and at 3–6, 12, and 24 months after transplant. Before transplant, at 3–6 months after transplant, and at 24 months after transplant, 44 %, 85 %, and 62 % of children, respectively, had abnormal pulmonary function tests. A restrictive abnormality was most common at 3–6 months after transplant.

**Other Agents** Acute pulmonary effects have occurred with cytosine arabinoside (noncardiogenic pulmonary edema) [3, 57] and vinca alkaloids in association with mitomycin (bronchospasm or interstitial pneumonitis) [29, 53], but delayed pulmonary toxicity has not been described. Hypersensitivity reactions to the antimetabolites (methotrexate, mercaptopurine, and azathioprine) may cause either a desquamative interstitial pneumonitis or an eosinophilic pneumonitis [77, 155, 159]. Recovery usually occurs within 10–45 days after methotrexate-induced pulmonary toxicity [144].

However, long-term follow-up of 26 childhood leukemia survivors revealed that 17 (65 %) patients had one or more abnormalities of vital capacity, total lung capacity, reserve volume, or diffusion capacity [138]. All children with these deficiencies were diagnosed and treated before age 8. The findings have also been attributed to an impairment of lung growth, which normally proceeds exponentially by cell division during the first 8 years of life. Other studies have also demonstrated long-term changes in pulmonary function in survivors of ALL treated without spinal radiation or bone marrow transplant [102].

Busulfan can result in late pulmonary fibrosis, with no consistently identified risk factors. Unlike many other agents, the risk does not appear to be dose related. The clinical and pathologic picture is like that of bleomycin-induced fibrosis. The mortality from busulfan fibrosis is high [1]. Although reports of pulmonary toxicity with other agents are rare, pneumonitis and fibrosis should be considered in the differential of patients presenting with respiratory symptoms. New agents may also present a risk for late pulmonary toxicity. See Table 11.2 [1, 90].

## 11.2.4   Thoracic Surgery

Lung resections are performed in children for a number of reasons, including congenital malformations, infections, bronchiectasis, and metastatic malignancies. Interestingly, the majority of children who undergo lung resection do well with mild sequelae, if any, in adulthood [80]. A large study of 230 patients who were evaluated on average 33 years after pneumonectomy provides interesting data on the long-term compensatory potential and possible mechanisms of recovery in young children and adults following surgery [75]. The study found that children who underwent surgery before the age of 5 years had ventilatory capacity close to what would be predicted for two lungs, which the authors argue suggests that compensatory growth by way of hyperplasia might have been the most important adaptive mechanism in this group. Perhaps more surprisingly, even in the patients who underwent surgery between the ages of 6 and 20 years, a significant difference was still found as compared to the group of patients operated on at an older age, which indicates that in this period compensatory growth, possibly simple hypertrophy, still played an important but gradually decreasing role.

Unfortunately, few studies have investigated pulmonary toxicity specifically in the context of pediatric cancer therapy.

## 11.2.5   Treatment and Clinical or Environmental Interactions

### 11.2.5.1 Chemotherapy: Chemotherapy Interactions

In considering the risk of pulmonary toxicity from chemotherapy, the potential for chemotherapy – chemotherapy interactions – must be taken into account. Toxicity is seen at much lower doses than expected with drug combinations such as nitrosoureas and cyclophosphamide [147], bleomycin and cisplatin, or vincristine, doxorubicin, and cyclophosphamide [8, 77, 121]. Vinca alkaloids appear to cause pulmonary toxicity only in the presence of mitomycin [29, 77].

### 11.2.5.2 Radiation and Chemotherapy Combinations: Interaction and Tolerance

Many antineoplastic agents potentiate the damaging effects of radiation on the lung. Phillips [116] and Wara [160] demonstrated that dactinomycin administration lowered the radiation dose threshold for pneumonitis. Testing the effects of commonly used chemotherapeutic agents, Phillips and colleagues [116] reported that the administration of dactinomycin, cyclophosphamide, and, to a lesser extent, vincristine enhanced the lethal potential of thoracic irradiation. The effect of dactinomycin was seen when given as long as 30 days before irradiation, but it was not seen when given 30 days after the irradiation. The administration of bleomycin and lung irradiation together produces lung toxicity that is more common and severe than when either agent is given alone. Catane [20] found pulmonary toxicity in 19 % of patients, and it was fatal in 10 %. This toxicity appears to be maximal when bleomycin is given concurrently with radiation [36]. Although 500 IU of bleomycin without RT can be lethal in 1–2 % of patients, as little as 30 IU can be fatal when given with RT. The effects of RT are also potentiated by doxorubicin. In addition to the enhanced toxicity observed in skin, intestines, and heart, the lung also appears to be very sensitive to this combination [18, 22]. Of 24 patients with lung cancer treated with low-dose doxorubicin and RT, 13 developed pneumonitis [156].

### 11.2.5.3 Other Interactions

Although not as well defined, surgical interventions and other factors, such as repeat or chronic infections and toxic environment exposures such as cigarette smoke, can decrease the threshold for development of late pulmonary effects from therapy.

## 11.3 Detection and Screening

Pulmonary disease occurring in patients treated for cancer can present a diagnostic problem because of the multiplicity of possible etiologies. Progressive cancer, infections, emboli, allergy, irradiation, or drugs (and their interaction) can be causative. Clinical findings, radiologic studies, and pulmonary function tests can be nonspecific; however, these factors represent measurable endpoints to quantify toxicity.

### 11.3.1 Measurable Endpoints

**Symptoms** Fever, cough, and shortness of breath are the most common symptoms of radiation-induced pneumonopathy. Temperature, respiratory rate, oxyhemoglobin saturation, frequency of cough, and the nature of sputum produced should all be recorded. Varying degrees of dyspnea, as well as orthopnea, can be present depending on the severity of pulmonary damage. To standardize grading in the literature, the grading criteria in Common Terminology Criteria for Adverse Events (CTCAE), published by the National Cancer Institute and National Institute of Health [27], have been expanded to be useful for the long-term survivor.

**Signs** The principal signs of both acute and delayed pneumonopathy are the increase in respi-

ratory rate, dullness to percussion of the chest, auscultation of crackles, and, in severe cases, cyanosis.

**Radiography** Plain anteroposterior (AP) and lateral chest films are useful when the disease involves a large volume of lung. The acute pneumonitic phase manifests as a fluffy infiltrate, and the late fibrotic phase can follow the intermediate phase of contraction. However, routine chest radiography has a low level of reliability in detecting small volumes of pneumonopathy, particularly if they are located close to the chest wall. Chest radiography also lacks the ability to quantify the volume of affected lung vs the total lung volume.

When chronic fibrosis occurs, chest radiography generally reveals scarring that corresponds to the shape of the radiation portal. CT scans have the capability of presenting three-dimensional images and calculating three-dimensional volumes of functional lung in a defined range of Hounsfield units. One can also detect small infiltrates that may be adjacent to the chest wall, for example, in the case of tangential field RT, where infiltrates are calculated as a percentage of the total lung volume. Mah [85] has shown a quantitative relationship between the volume of abnormality on CT and RT dose (converted to a single dose equivalent). Radiographic changes after chemotherapy are often bibasilar fibrosis. Fibrosis confined to the upper lobes has also been described after treatment with BCNU [110] and bleomycin [88].

**Pulmonary Function Tests (PFTs)** Pulmonary function testing (PFT) is a broad term that encompasses a variety of techniques and tests. The indications for pulmonary function testing include (a) documenting the presence of obstructive or restrictive abnormalities in the course of establishing a diagnosis, (b) monitoring the course of a known pulmonary disease (e.g., cystic fibrosis, asthma, etc.), (c) monitoring for pulmonary toxicity of treatment (e.g., amiodarone, radiation, chemotherapy), (d) monitoring response to therapy, and (e) describing normal and abnormal lung growth.

The values measured in the laboratory are usually normalized with the use of reference equations, most commonly utilizing the subject's height and gender and sometimes modifying for ethnicity and age. With these equations, a predicted value can be calculated for each parameter, and the measured flows can be reported as a percentage of the predicted value or as a standardized deviation score (Z-score). It should be noted that comparing test results between pulmonary function laboratories must be done with caution if different reference equations are used.

Ideally, patients can serve as their own control for the effects of chemotherapy or radiotherapy if measurements are obtained prior to treatment. Abnormal PFTs prior to treatment may also alert the practitioner to patients at higher risk for pulmonary toxicity. Indeed, abnormal lung function has been shown to predict early pulmonary complications [70] and higher mortality following stem cell transplantation in both adults [109] and children [48]. In addition, PFT abnormalities may be present in the absence of clinical symptoms and may herald the development of clinical disease.

### 11.3.1.1 Spirometry

Spirometry is the measurement of airflow during a maximally forced exhalation. The subject breathes through a mouthpiece connected to a pneumotachometer while wearing noseclips. After inhalation to total lung capacity, the subject is coached to exhale rapidly and forcefully until the lungs have emptied. The test does require the ability to cooperate with the technician. This is commonly expected after age 6, although children as young as 4 have been able to perform spirometry with practice and normative data does exist even for very young children [11].

The test is informative because airflow rates are inversely proportional to the fourth power of the radius of the airway; therefore, even minimally obstructed airways result in greatly reduced airflow rates. Indeed, the hallmark of obstructive lung diseases (such as asthma, obliterative bronchiolitis, and chronic GVHD [108]) is reduced airflows. Properly performed tests are very reproducible within subjects, making them useful for assessing response to treatment over time.

Several parameters can be calculated from these maneuvers. First, the total exhaled volume is termed the forced vital capacity (FVC). The volume exhaled in the first second is termed the $FEV_1$. The airflow rate between 25 % of the exhaled volume and 75 % of the exhaled volume is termed the $FEF_{25-75\%}$. The pattern of these parameters can suggest an obstructive defect or a restrictive defect. Specifically, a reduced $FEV_1$ and $FEV_1$/FVC ratio may suggest an obstructive defect, while a reduced FVC and normal $FEV_1$/FVC ratio may suggest a restrictive defect. However, measurement of lung volumes is required to accurately diagnose restrictive disease. To complicate matters, some patients can have both obstructive and restrictive defects.

If an obstructive defect is documented, reversibility can also be assessed utilizing spirometry. Following administration of the bronchodilator (e.g., albuterol), testing is repeated after 15–20 min. Commonly, a 12 % increase in the $FEV_1$ is considered indicative of a significant response.

### 11.3.1.2 Lung Volumes

Disease states that affect lung growth would be expected to alter lung volume in addition to airway caliber. These diseases include pulmonary hypoplasia or space-occupying lesions (e.g., lymphoma), bronchopulmonary dysplasia, and, specifically to children and young adults, conditions that alter the growth of the rib cage (thoracic dystrophies and radiation to the chest wall).

Restrictive lung disease is defined by the presence of reduced lung volume, which can be measured utilizing a dilution technique and, more commonly, plethysmography (Fig. 11.3). Both techniques are typically used to measure resting lung volume or functional residual capacity (FRC). A lung capacity is the sum of two or more lung volumes; in the case of FRC, it is the sum of residual volume (RV, the amount of gas remaining in the lung after a maximal exhalation) and expiratory reserve volume (ERV, the amount of gas exhaled from resting lung volume until the lung is empty). In combination with spirometry,

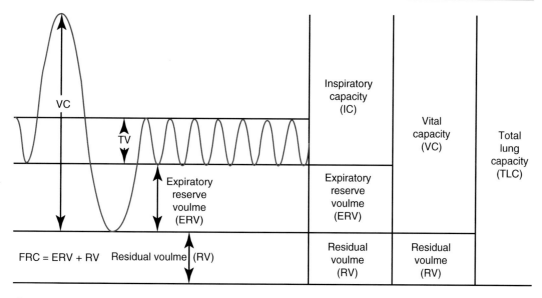

**Fig. 11.3** Lung volumes (From Gibson [46])

other lung volumes and capacities can be calculated: total lung capacity (TLC) = RV + FVC.

Plethysmography utilizes the principle of Boyle's Law, i.e., in a closed system, pressure and volume change inversely when temperature is constant. With the subject sitting in a fixed volume chamber ("body box") and breathing on a mouthpiece, a shutter is closed in the inspiratory limb of the breathing circuit. The subject makes continued respiratory efforts, resulting in small changes in the volume of the lung and corresponding inverse volume changes in the box. Pressures in the box and at the mouth are measured, and this allows for calculation of the lung volume at which the panting efforts began. The subject usually begins the maneuvers at the end of a breath, and this "resting" lung volume is termed FRC. Younger children may have difficulty with the maneuver.

The pattern of lung volumes can also assist in diagnosis. Typically, patients with obstructive diseases (including obliterative bronchiolitis) will have an increased RV, especially as a fraction of total lung capacity (RV/TLC). The TLC may be normal or elevated. In contrast, low lung volumes are the hallmark of restrictive lung disease, and these patients will have a reduced TLC and RV.

### 11.3.1.3 Diffusing Capacity

The diffusing capacity for carbon monoxide $(D_LCO)$ is an integrative measurement that describes the transfer of carbon monoxide (as a surrogate for oxygen) from the alveolus into the red blood cell. This transfer is proportional to the surface area of the alveolar/capillary membrane and the pressure gradient for oxygen between the alveolus and the blood and inversely proportional to the thickness of the alveolar–capillary membrane. The measurement depends on the fact that CO is more soluble in blood than in lung tissue because it binds much more rapidly and tightly to hemoglobin in the blood. Thus, the partial pressure of CO in the blood remains very low, which maintains a diffusion gradient for the gas.

In the single-breath technique for measurement of $D_LCO$, the patient exhales completely to residual volume and inhales to total lung capacity a gas mixture 0.3 % carbon monoxide and an inert gas (usually helium or methane). The subject holds their breath for 10 s during which CO diffuses into the blood. The uptake of CO (in ml/min) is divided by the partial pressure gradient for CO (between alveolus and pulmonary capillary) to calculate $D_LCO$ (ml/mmHg/min). Alveolar ventilation is calculated from the inspired and expired concentrations of the inert gas, and this is used to calculate a dilutional factor for the inspired CO concentration and to normalize the $D_LCO$ according to lung volume in which the CO is diluted ($D_LCO/VA$ in ml/mmHg/min/L). The measurement should be adjusted for the patient's hemoglobin and, if present in significant amounts, carboxyhemoglobin. The measurement assumes a negligible concentration of carboxyhemoglobin, which may not be true in the presence of hemolysis [100]. Younger children, and subjects with significant restriction or dyspnea, may have difficulty cooperating with this testing. In these patients, oxyhemoglobin desaturation with activity or exercise would be suggestive of diffusion impairment.

Diseases that decrease the surface area for diffusion (emphysema, pulmonary emboli, resection of lung tissue) or diseases that increase the thickness of the alveolar–capillary membrane (fibrosis, pulmonary edema, proteinosis) would both decrease the diffusing capacity of the lung. Increased $D_LCO$ is much less common but can be seen in patients with alveolar hemorrhage (hemoglobin in the airspace appears to make uptake of CO very high), polycythemia, or during exercise (via recruitment of more pulmonary capillaries). This test may be useful in evaluating patients with diffuse lung diseases or assessment of patients with pulmonary vascular obstruction.

### 11.3.1.4 Musculoskeletal Strength

The respiratory muscles (including the diaphragm, intercostals muscles, and others) contract intermittently 24 h per day to perform the work of ventilation. Many diseases can affect the strength of these muscles, putting patients at risk for hypoventilation, impaired airway clearance of secretions, and respiratory insufficiency. These conditions include primary muscular disorders, conditions affecting nerve transmission to the muscles (neuropathies, including vincristine toxicity), malnutrition, and stretch of the muscles beyond their optimal length–tension relationship (which can occur in hyperinflation). Additionally, bone development is critically important. As noted previously, radiation to the chest wall and certain systemic agents can likewise affect pulmonary function.

Typically, maximal expiratory pressure (MEP, $P_Emax$) is measured by having the subject inhale maximally to TLC and blow out as hard as possible into a mouthpiece connected to a pressure transducer and with an occluded distal end. Similarly, maximal inspiratory pressure (MIP, $P_Imax$) is measured by having the subject exhale completely to RV and inhale rapidly against the occluded tube. Usually several repeated maneuvers are required to elicit the maximal effort.

### 11.3.1.5 Pulmonary Function Tests in Infants

Most of the tests described above have been adapted to infants, with the obvious challenge being that maximal efforts cannot be elicited voluntarily. Infants and toddlers are usually sedated and placed supine with a mask over mouth and nose to measure airflow and pressure at the mouth. These techniques require specialized equipment and expertise not available in all pulmonary function laboratories.

The raised volume rapid thoracic compression technique is one method that has been used to generate maximal expiratory flow by applying a positive pressure externally to the chest. This involves a plastic jacket that encircles the chest and abdomen of the sedated, supine infant and a face mask over the mouth and nose to measure flow. The infant's lung is first inflated to a predetermined pressure (typically 30 cm $H_2O$), resulting in an end-inspiratory lung volume close to total lung capacity. From this raised lung volume, the jacket encompassing the chest is rapidly inflated from a pressure reservoir, generating a full expiratory flow–volume curve.

Another technique, which is less commonly available, is the forced deflation technique. This involves using a negative pressure (vacuum) to deflate the lungs after an inflation to total lung capacity. This technique is only used in anesthetized, intubated patients. It is a relatively quick and reproducible test that can be accomplished at the time of other operative procedures (central line placement, bone marrow aspiration, etc.).

Lung volumes can also be measured by plethysmographic methods. The infant is placed within a rigid, airtight, plexiglass plethysmograph. The infant breathes through a face mask connected to an airway pressure gauge and a pneumotach to measure flow and volume.

A shutter within the face mask can briefly occlude the infant's airway; continued respiratory efforts alternately compress and rarify the gas within the lung, and Boyle's Law is used to calculate FRC as it is in older children.

Tests to measure diffusing capacity have been adapted to infants [19], although no commercially available equipment is available for this purpose. This is unfortunate, as these measures might be the most sensitive tests to detect early, primarily interstitial, pulmonary toxicity that would precede development of restrictive disease.

**Nuclear Medicine Tests** To evaluate therapy-induced pneumonopathy, qualitative and quantitative radionuclide studies, consisting of perfusion studies, ventilation studies, gallium scans, and quantitative ventilation/perfusion scintigraphy, have been utilized in some institutions. These nuclear studies have been primarily for research interests and have not been routinely applied to the clinical management of patients.

**Laboratory Tests of Serum or Blood** Erythrocyte sedimentation rate (ESR) has been evaluated as a potential early marker of pulmonary toxicity from bleomycin [60]. The nonspecific nature of this value may make clinical application difficult, as increases in ESR would also be expected in infection or recurrent disease. Despite the identification of these clinical contributing factors, research has tended to focus on the development of a reliable and simple diagnostic laboratory test that could predict the risk of post-radiation pneumonitis and, in particular, could be administered prior to the start of therapy.

There is a need for early biochemical markers of normal tissue damage that would predict late effects and that would allow the radiation oncologist and medical oncologist to determine whether their treatment is exceeding normal tissue tolerance [126]. If biochemical markers of tissue damage could be detected in the subclinical phase, prior to the accumulation of significant injury, one could terminate therapy or institute treatment to prevent or attenuate later lesions. An ideal marker would be a simple, reproducible, biochemical test. In the recent years, some circulating cytokine markers have been independently found to be potential predictors of radiation pneumonitis. These include proinflammatory cytokines interleukin-1α (IL-1α) and interleukin-6 (IL-6) [25, 26], fibrotic cytokine-transforming growth factor β (TGF-β) [4], and ICAM [65]. Chen and colleagues tested the ability of IL-1α and IL-6 measurements to predict radiation pneumonitis [23]. The predictive power of IL-1α and IL-6 appeared to be strongest for the blood samples collected prior to radiotherapy than during RT. While both inflammatory cytokines can serve as diagnostic testing tools, IL-6 was found to be a more powerful predictor than IL-1α of radiation pneumonitis. The specificity and positive predictive value of IL-6 were as high as 80 % for the blood samples collected prior to RT. The application of these cytokine markers in the predictive diagnosis of radiation pneumonitis may prove to have clinical utility in the near future and deserves further investigation.

In addition to cytokines, the release of many substances into the circulation could reflect and may also predict the degree of RT and chemotherapy injury to the lung. These include the surfactant apoprotein, procollagen type 3 angiotensin-converting enzyme, blood plasminogen-activating factor, and prostacyclin. These various substances have been correlated with either acute or delayed radiation-induced pneumonopathy. Significant additional work is required to evaluate the usefulness of such blood level measurements.

## 11.4 Management of Established Pulmonary Toxicity Induced by Cytotoxic Therapy

Hopefully in the future, pulmonary toxicity will be prevented rather than managed. Strict attention should be paid to drug doses and cumulative drug–dose restrictions. When RT is given, volumes and doses should be minimized and given in accordance with accepted tolerance. During drug therapy, monitoring of symptoms and signs, PFTs, and chest radiographs can aid in detecting problems early, and the causative agent can be withdrawn. After bleomycin withdrawal, early stages of bleomycin-induced pneumonitis have clinically and radiographically reversed [89].

## 11.4.1 Precautions for Minimizing Potential Complications

Assessing baseline pulmonary function prior to therapy is important and especially so for patients with underlying pulmonary pathology such as lung disease of prematurity, chronic obstructive pulmonary disease, and idiopathic lung fibrosis. The detection of abnormalities may allow for better anticipatory guidance and counseling. Counseling on the risks of smoking and environmental tobacco smoke exposure is imperative for these patients, even in the absence of symptoms or abnormalities on evaluation. Patients should also be aware of the potential risks of general anesthesia and notify physicians of their treatment history if they are to undergo anesthesia. For those with compromised lung condition, therapy should be tailored to minimize injury from cytotoxic agents and radiation damage. When following survivors of cancer, vigilant evaluation of symptoms of respiratory compromise is necessary and should be anticipated when thoracic RT or drugs with known pulmonary toxicity have been used. Depending on the findings and other circumstances, lung biopsy may be considered to confirm fibrosis or exclude the recurrence of cancer. Chronic cough, dyspnea, or change in exercise should be further evaluated with chest radiography and PFTs. This is also imperative in patients scheduled for general anesthesia. In the absence of symptoms, chest radiographs and lung function testing are recommended every 2–5 years. The number of potential pulmonary toxic agents, the cumulative doses, and the radiation dose and field size are all factors to be considered in setting follow-up intervals.

## 11.4.2 Preventative Therapy

The difficult issue in screening is that there is no definitive therapy. Before therapy, the prophylactic administration of steroids has no proven benefit and may present potential risks. A study of inhaled fluticasone propionate, however, demonstrated some potential benefit with reduction of acute pneumonitis in patients treated for breast cancer [91]. Confirmation of this benefit and whether like interventions can reduce long-term pulmonary sequelae requires further study. The role of amifostine as a radioprotector in preventing lung toxicity has been investigated. Amifostine is a sulfhydryl compound that was originally developed as an agent to protect against ionizing radiation in the event of nuclear war [31, 133]. It was also found to protect normal tissues from toxicities of radiotherapy for head and neck tumors [17], alkylating agents, and cisplatin [161, 166]. Recent clinical studies have shown a reduction in pneumonitis using amifostine in chemoradiation treatments for lung cancer [5, 73]; however, further investigation is required until its use becomes standard clinical practice.

There is a lack of studies quantifying the impact of smoking after exposure to chemotherapy and radiation therapy, but it very likely increases the risk of lung damage. In the Childhood Cancer Survivors Study (CCSS), survivors smoked at lower rates than the general population, but more than a quarter reported a history of having ever smoked, and 17 % reported currently smoking [39]. Smokers who responded to the study expressed a higher desire to quit than the general population. Interventions have been developed and studied to decrease smoking and improve smoking cessation in long-term survivors [38, 153]. Similarly, parents and caregivers of children with cancer should be encouraged to avoid exposing their children to environmental tobacco smoke.

Viral respiratory infections can cause significant morbidity in patients with established lung disease. Hand hygiene can help decrease the spread of viral pathogens, and influenza vaccination should be encouraged in non-immunosuppressed patients. Passive immunoprophylaxis against respiratory syncytial virus (with palivizumab) is also available for young children at high risk of pulmonary complications with this infection.

### 11.4.3 Therapy for Established Toxicity

Corticosteroids play a useful role in the relief of symptoms from pneumonitis caused by a variety of drugs and RT. Severe symptoms necessitating treatment can be relieved markedly and rapidly by corticosteroids in half of affected patients [95, 163, 164]; however, prevention or reversal of the fibrotic phase does not occur. Supportive care with bronchodilators, expectorants, antibiotics, bed rest, and oxygen can be beneficial for relief of symptoms in pneumonitis and fibrosis. In cases of radiation or chemotherapy-induced pneumonitis in which corticosteroids have been used, it is important to withdraw steroids very slowly to avoid reactivation. Patients with very significant restriction (vital capacity <30 % predicted) or diffusion impairment are at increased risk for hypoxemia and may require supplemental oxygen. In addition, they may demonstrate evidence of hypoventilation and in some cases may benefit from noninvasive ventilation.

### 11.5 Future Studies

We have come to appreciate the complexity of interstitial pneumonitis from cancer therapy, now seen as a process involving an active communication and interaction between resident cell types of the lung parenchyma and circulatory immune and inflammatory cells. There is increasing evidence of immune cells augmenting pneumonitis through complex autocrine, paracrine, and systemic regulatory mechanisms critically orchestrated by cytokines [24, 129].

Further investigation of the molecular mechanisms involved in pneumonitis and fibrosis will allow for timely intervention and proper protection. Interferons and other cytokines that oppose or inhibit fibrosis-promoting growth factors potentially may be used during therapy, resulting in the desired enhanced therapeutic ratio. Chemoprotective agents are being investigated for their ability to reduce the toxicity of chemotherapy, including lung injury. It is essential, of course, that they do not disturb the efficacy of the treatment. Improvement of radiotherapy targeting and normal tissue sparing, such as three-dimensional conformal radiotherapy and intensity-modulated radiotherapy (IMRT), will minimize radiation to nontarget normal lung tissue. Novel interventions, such as mechanisms to increase the level of bleomycin hydrolase in susceptible patients or viral-mediated transfer of a bleomycin resistance gene, may hold promise for future applications in clinical treatment. What may prove to be the most important is the recognition of those at enhanced risk for long-term pulmonary toxicity as a result of their genotype. Understanding of such risk factors could lead to therapy tailored to an individual risk profile.

## References

1. Abid S, Malhotra V, Perry M (2001) Radiation induced and chemotherapy induced pulmonary injury. Curr Opin Oncol 13:1–16
2. Ager S, Mahendra P, Richards EM et al (1996) High-dose carmustine, etoposide and melphalan (BEM) with autologous stem cell transplantation: a dose-toxicity study. Bone Marrow Transplant 17:335–340
3. Anderson BS, Cogan BM, Keating MJ (1984) Subacute pulmonary failure complicating therapy with high dose ara-C in acute leukemia. Cancer 56:2181–2184
4. Anscher MS, Kong FM, Andrews K et al (1998) Plasma transforming growth factor beta1 as a predictor of radiation pneumonitis. Int J Radiat Oncol Biol Phys 41:1029–1035
5. Antonadou D, Throuvalas N, Petridis A (2003) Effect of amifostine on toxicities associated with radiochemotherapy in patients with locally advanced non-small cell lung cancer. Int J Radiat Oncol Biol Phys 57:402–408
6. Antonia SJ, Wagner H, Williams C (1995) Concurrent paclitaxel/cisplatin with thoracic radiation in patients with stage III A/B non-small cell carcinoma of the lung. Semin Oncol 22:34–37
7. Armstrong GT, Liu Q, Yasui Y et al (2009) Late mortality among 5-year survivors of childhood cancer: a summary from the Childhood Cancer Survivor Study. J Clin Oncol 27:2328–2338
8. Bauer KA, Skarin AT, Balikian JP (1983) Pulmonary complications associated with combination chemotherapy programs containing bleomycin. Am J Med 74:557–563
9. Bellamy EZ, Husband JE, Blaquiere RM (1985) Bleomycin related lung damage: CT evidence. Radiology 156:155–158

10. Benoist MR, Lemerle J, Jean R et al (1982) Effects on pulmonary function of whole lung irradiation for Wilms' tumor in children. Thorax 37:175–180

11. Beydon N, Davis SD, Lombardi E et al (2007) An official American Thoracic Society/European Respiratory Society statement: pulmonary function testing in preschool children. Am J Respir Crit Care Med 175:1304–1345

12. Bhalla KS, Wilczynski SW, Abushamaa AM, Petros WP (2000) Pulmonary toxicity of induction chemotherapy prior to standard or high-dose chemotherapy with autologous hematopoietic support. Am J Respir Crit Care Med 161:17–25

13. Block M, Lachowiez RM, Rios C (1990) Pulmonary fibrosis associated with low-dose adjuvant methyl-CCNU. Med Pediatr Oncol 18:256–260

14. Blum RH, Carter SK, Agre K (1973) A clinical review of bleomycin – a new antineoplastic agent. Cancer 31:903–914

15. Bölling T, Schuck A, Paulussen M, Dirksen U, Ranft A, Könemann S, Dunst J, Willich N, Jürgens H (2008) Whole lung irradiation in patients with exclusively pulmonary metastases of Ewing tumors. Toxicity analysis and treatment results of the EICESS-92 trial. Strahlenther Onkol 184(4):193–7

16. Bossi G, Cerveri I, Volpini E et al (1997) Long-term pulmonary sequelae after treatment of childhood Hodgkin's disease. Ann Oncol 8(Suppl 1):19–24

17. Brizel DM, Wasserman TH, Henke M et al (2000) Phase III randomized trial of amifostine as a radioprotector in head and neck cancer. J Clin Oncol 18:3339–3345

18. Cassady JR, Richter MP, Piro AJ (1975) Radiation-Adriamycin interactions: preliminary clinical observations. Cancer 36:946–949

19. Castillo A, Llapur CJ, Martinez T et al (2006) Measurement of single breath-hold carbon monoxide diffusing capacity in healthy infants and toddlers. Pediatr Pulmonol 41:544–550

20. Catane R, Schwade JG, Turrisi AT (1979) Pulmonary toxicity after radiation and bleomycin: a review. Int J Radiat Oncol Biol Phys 5:1513–1518

21. Cerveri I, Fulgoni P, Giorgiani G (2001) Lung function abnormalities after bone marrow transplantation in children: has the trend recently changed? Chest 120:1900–1906

22. Chan PYM, Kagan AR, Byfteld JE (1979) Pulmonary complications of combined chemotherapy and radiotherapy in lung cancer. Front Radiat Ther Oncol 13:136–144

23. Chen Y, Hyrien O, Williams J et al (2005) Interleukin (IL)-1A and IL-6: applications to the predictive diagnostic testing of radiation pneumonitis. Int J Radiat Oncol Biol Phys 62:260–266

24. Chen Y, Okunieff P, Ahrendt SA (2003) Translational research in lung cancer. Semin Surg Oncol 21:205–219

25. Chen Y, Rubin P, Williams J et al (2001) Circulating IL-6 as a predictor of radiation pneumonitis. Int J Radiat Oncol Biol Phys 49:641–648

26. Chen Y, Williams J, Ding I et al (2002) Radiation pneumonitis and early circulatory cytokine markers. Semin Radiat Oncol 12(1 Suppl 1):26–33

27. Common Terminology Criteria for Adverse Events (CTCAE) (2003) Version 3.0. US Department of Health and Human Services. National Institutes of Health, National Cancer Institute

28. Cooper JAD, DA W, Matthay RA (1986) Drug induced pulmonary disease, part I. Cyto-toxic drugs. Am Rev Respir Dis 133:321–340

29. Cooper JA, Zitnik R, Matthay RA (1988) Mechanisms of drug-induced pulmonary disease. Ann Rev Med 39:395–404

30. Couderc LJ, Stelianides S, Frachon I et al (1999) Pulmonary toxicity of chemotherapy and G/GM-CSF: a report of five cases. Respir Med 93:65–68

31. Davidson DE, Grenan MM, Sweeney TR (1980) Biological characteristics of some improved radio-protectors. In: Brady LW (ed) Radiation sensitizers. Masson, New York, pp 309–320

32. DeLana M, Guzzon A, Monfardini S (1972) Clinical radiologic and histopathologic studies on pulmonary toxicity induced by treatment with bleomycin. Cancer Chemother Rep 56:343–355

33. Dent RG (1982) Fatal pulmonary toxic effects of lomustine. Thorax 37:627–629

34. Doll DC, Ringenberg Q, Yarbo JW (1986) Vascular toxicity associated with antineoplastic agents. J Clin Oncol 4:1405–1417

35. Donat SM, Levy DA (1998) Bleomycin associated pulmonary toxicity: is perioperative oxygen restriction necessary? J Urol 160:1347–1352

36. Einhorn L, Krause M, Hornback N, Furnas B (1976) Enhanced pulmonary toxicity with bleomycin and radiotherapy in oat cell lung cancer. Cancer 37:2414–2416

37. Emami B, Lyman J, Brown A et al (1991) Tolerance of normal tissue to therapeutic irradiation. Int J Radiat Oncol Biol Phys 21:109–122

38. Emmons KM, Butterfield RM, Puleo E et al (2003) Smoking among participants in the childhood cancer survivors cohort: the Partnership for Health Study. J Clin Oncol 21:189–196

39. Emmons K, Li FP, Whitton J et al (2002) Predictors of smoking initiation and cessation among childhood cancer survivors: a report from the childhood cancer survivor study. J Clin Oncol 20:1608–1616

40. Engelstad RB (1940) Pulmonary lesions after roentgen and radium irradiation. Am J Roentgenol 43:676–681

41. Evans RF, Sagerman RH, Ringrose TL (1974) Pulmonary function following mantle field irradiation for Hodgkin's disease. Radiology 111:729–731

42. Fontán JP, Haddad GG (2004) St Louis respiratory pathophysiology. In: Behrman RE, Kliegman RM, Jenson H (eds) Nelson textbook of pediatrics. Elsevier, Amsterdam, pp 1362–1370

43. Fryer CJH, Fitzpatrick PJ, Rider WD (1978) Radiation pneumonitis: experience following a large single dose of radiation. Int J Radiat Oncol Biol Phys 4:931–936

44. Fryer CJ, Hutchinson RJ, Krailo M (1990) Efficacy and toxicity of 12 courses of ABVD chemotherapy followed by lowdose regional radiation in advanced Hodgkin's disease in children: a report from the children cancer study group. J Clin Oncol 8:1971–1980

45. Germon PA, Brady LW (1968) Physiologic changes before and after radiation treatment for carcinoma of the lung. JAMA 206:809–814

46. Gibson CM (ed) Lung volumes. http://www.wikidoc.org/index.php.Lung_volumes. Accessed 30 Oct 2013

47. Gilson AJ, Sahn SA (1985) Reactivation of bleomycin lung toxicity following oxygen administration. Chest 88:304–306

48. Ginsberg JP, Aplenc R, McDonough J et al (2010) Pre-transplant lung function is predictive of survival following pediatric bone marrow transplantation. Pediatr Blood Cancer 54:454–460

49. Graham MV, Burdy JA, Emami B (1999) Clinical dose-volume histogram analysis for pneumonitis after 3D treatment for non-small cell lung cancer. Int J Radiat Oncol Biol Phys 45:323–329

50. Gross NJ (1977) Pulmonary effects of radiation therapy. Ann Intern Med 86:81–92

51. Gross NJ (1980) Experimental radiation pneumonitis IV. Leakage of circulatory proteins onto the alveolar surface. J Lab Clin Med 95:19–31

52. Gross NJ (1981) The pathogenesis of radiation-induced lung damage. Lung 159:115–125

53. Gunstream SR, Seidenfeld JJ, Sobonya RE (1983) Mitomycin associated lung disease. Cancer Treat Rep 67:301–304

54. Hakenjos L, Bamberg M, Rodemann HP (2000) TGF-β1mediated alterations of rat lung fibroblast differentiation resulting in the radiation-induced fibrotic phenotype. Int J Radiat Biol 76:503–509

55. Hale GA, Marina NM, Jones-Wallace D, Greenwald CA (1999) Late effects of treatment for germ cell tumors during childhood and adolescence. J Pediatr Hematol Oncol 21:115–122

56. Hallahan DF, Virudachlam S (1997) Intercellular adhesion molecule –1 knockout abrogates radiation induced pulmonary inflammation. Proc Natl Acad Sci U S A 94:6432–6437

57. Haupt HM, Hutchins GM, Moore GW (1981) Ara-C lung: non-cardiogenic pulmonary edema complicating cytosine-arabinoside therapy of leukemia. Am J Med 70:256–261

58. Hay J, Shahriar S, Laurent G (1991) Mechanisms of bleomycin-induced lung damage. Arch Toxicol 65:81–94

59. Hernando ML, Marks LB, Bentel GC (2001) Radiation-induced pulmonary toxicity: a dose-volume histogram analysis in 201 patients with lung cancer. Int J Radiat Oncol Biol Phys 51:650–659

60. Higa GM, AlKhouri N, Auber ML (1997) Elevation of the erythrocyte sedimentation rate precedes exacerbation of bleomycin-induced pulmonary toxicity: report of two cases and review of literature. Pharmacotherapy 17:1315–1321

61. Hirsch A, Vander Els N, Straus DJ, Gomez EG, Leung D, Portlock CS, Yahalom J (1996) Effect of ABVD chemotherapy with and without mantle or mediastinal irradiation on pulmonary function and symptoms in early-stage Hodgkin's disease. J Clin Oncol 14:1297–1305

62. Hoyt DG, Lazo JS (1992) Murine strain differences in acute lung injury and activation of poly(ADP-ribose) polymerase by in vitro exposure of lung slices to bleomycin. Am J Respir Ces Mol Biol 7:645–651

63. Hudson MM, Mulrooney DA, Bowers DC et al (2009) High-risk populations identified in Childhood Cancer Survivor Study investigations: implications for risk-based surveillance. J Clin Oncol 27:2405–2414

64. Inoue A, Kunitoh H, Sekine I (2001) Radiation pneumonitis in lung cancer patients: a retrospective study of risk factors and the long-term prognosis. Int J Radiat Oncol Biol Phys 49:649–655

65. Ishii Y, Kitamura S (1999) Soluble intercellular adhesion molecule-1 as an early detection marker for radiation pneumonitis. Eur Respir J 13:733–738

66. Johnston CJ, Wright TW, Rubin P, Finkelstein JN (1998) Alterations in the expression of chemokine mRNA levels in fibrosis-resistant and -sensitive mice after thoracic irradiation. Exp Lung Res 4:321–337

67. Kaplan E, Sklar C, Wilmott R et al (1996) Pulmonary function in children treated for rhabdomyosarcoma. Med Pediatr Oncol 27:79–84

68. Kataoka M, Kawamura M, Itoh H, Hamamoto K (1992) Ga-67 citrate scintigraphy for the early detection of radiation pneumonitis. Clin Nucl Med 17:27–31

69. Kawana A, Shioya S, Katoh H et al (1997) Expression of intercellular adhesion molecule-1 and lymphocyte function-associated antigen-1 on alveolar macrophages in the acute stage of radiation-induced lung injury in rats. Radiat Res 147:431–436

70. Kaya Z, Weiner DJ, Yilmaz D et al (2009) Lung function, pulmonary complications, and mortality after allogeneic blood and marrow transplantation in children. Biol Blood Marrow Transpl 15:817–826

71. Keane TJ, van Dyk J, Rider WD (1981) Idiopathic interstitial pneumonia following bone marrow transplantation: the relationship with total body irradiation. Int J Radiat Oncol Bio Phys 7:1365–1370

72. Kharasch VS, Lipsitz S, Santis W et al (1996) Long-term pulmonary toxicity of multiagent chemotherapy including bleomycin and cyclophosphamide in osteosarcoma survivors. Med Pediatr 27:85–91

73. Komaki R, Lee JS, Kaplan B et al (2002) Randomized phase III study of chemoradiation with or without amifostine for patients with favorable performance status inoperable stage II-III non-small cell lung cancer: preliminary results. Semin Radiat Oncol 12(1 Suppl 1):46–49

74. Kwa SLS, Lebesque JV, Theuws JCM (1998) Radiation pneumonitis as a function of mean lung dose: an analysis of pooled data of 540 patients. Int J Radiat Oncol Biol Phys 42:1–9

75. Laros CD, Westermann CJ (1987) Dilatation, compensatory growth, or both after pneumonectomy during childhood and adolescence. A thirty-year follow-up study. J Thorac Cardiovasc Surg 93:570–576

76. Lazo JS, Merrill WW, Pham ET (1984) Bleomycin hydrolase activity in pulmonary cells. J Pharmacol Exp Ther 231:583–588

77. Lehne G, Lote K (1990) Pulmonary toxicity of cytotoxic and immunosuppressive agents. A review. Acta Oncol 29:113–124

78. Leiper AD (2002) Non-endocrine late complications of bone marrow trans-plantation in childhood: part II. Br J Haematol 118:23–43

79. Leroy EP, Liebner EJ, Jensick RJ (1966) The ultrastructure of canine alveoli after supervoltage irradiation of the thorax. Lab Invest 15:1544–1558

80. Lezama-del Valle Valle P, Blakely ML, Lobe TE (1999) Physiologic consequences of pneumonectomy. Long-term consequences of pneumonectomy done in children. Chest Surg Clin N Am 9: 485–495

81. Libshitz HI, Shuman LS (1984) Radiation induced pulmonary change: CT findings. J Comput Assist Tomogr 8:15–19

82. Libura J, Bettens F, Radkowski A et al (2002) Risk of chemotherapy-induced pulmonary fibrosis is associated with polymorphic tumour necrosis factor-a2 gene. Eur Respir J 19:912–918

83. Littman P, Meadows AT, Polgar G (1976) Pulmonary function in survivors of Wilms' tumor: patterns of impairment. Cancer 37:2773–2776

84. Maasilta P, Hallman M, Taskinen E (1993) Bronchoalveolar lavage fluid findings following radiotherapy for non-small cell lung cancer. Int J Radiat Oncol Biol Phys 26:117–123

85. Mah K, Poon PY, van Dyk J (1986) Assessment of acute radiation-induced pulmonary changes using computed tomography. J Comput Assist Tomogr 10:736–743

86. Maisin JR (1974) The influence of radiation on blood vessels and circulation. HI. Ultrastructure of the vessel wall. Curr Top Radiat Res Q 10:29–57

87. Marks LB, Bentzen SM, Deasy JO et al (2010) Radiation dose-volume effects in the lung. Int J Radiat Oncol Biol Phys 76:S70–S76

88. Marruchella A, Franco C, Garavaldi G et al (2002) Bleomycin-induced upper lobe fibrosis: a case report. Tumori 88:414–416

89. McCrea ES, Diaconis JJN, Wade C (1981) Bleomycin toxicity simulating metastatic nodules to the lungs. Cancer 48:1096–1100

90. McDonald S, Rubin P, Phillips TL, Marks LB (1995) Injury to the lung from cancer therapy: clinical syndromes, measurable endpoints, and potential scoring systems. Int J Radiat Oncol Biol Phys 31:1187–1203

91. McGaughey DS, Nikcevich DA, Long GD et al (2001) Inhaled steroids as prophylaxis for delayed pulmonary toxicity syndrome in breast cancer patients undergoing high-dose chemotherapy and autologous stem cell transplantation. Biol Blood Marrow Transpl 7:274–278

92. Mertens AC, Yasua Y, Liu Y, Stovall M (2002) Pulmonary complications in survivors of childhood and adolescent cancer. A report from the childhood cancer survivor study. Cancer 95:2431–2441

93. Miller RW, Fusner JE, Fink R (1986) Pulmonary function abnormalities in long term survivors of childhood cancer. Med Pediatr Oncol 14:202–207

94. Mosher RB, McCarthy BJ (1998) Late effects in survivors of bone tumors. J Pediatr Oncol Nurs 15:72–84

95. Moss W, Haddy F, Sweany S (1960) Some factors altering the severity of acute radiation pneumonitis: variation with cortisone, heparin and antibiotics. Radiology 75:50–54

96. Motosue MS, Zhu L, Srivastava K et al (2012) Pulmonary function after whole lung irradiation in pediatric patients with solid malignancies. Cancer 118:1450–1456

97. Nadel J (2000) General principles and diagnostic approach. In: Murray JF, Nadel JA (eds) Textbook of respiratory medicine. Saunders, St Louis, pp 1173–1182

98. Nakayama Y, Makino S, Fukuda Y (1996) Activation of lavage lymphocytes in lung injuries caused by radiotherapy for lung cancer. Int J Radiat Oncol Biol Phys 34:459–467

99. Narayanan M, Owers-Bradley J, Beardsmore CS et al (2012) Alveolarization continues during childhood and adolescence: new evidence from helium-3 magnetic resonance. Am J Respir Crit Care Med 185:186–191

100. Needleman JP, Franco ME, Varlotta L et al (1999) Mechanisms of nocturnal oxyhemoglobin desaturation in children and adolescents with sickle cell disease. Pediatr Pulmonol 28:418–422

101. Neve V, Foot AB, Michon J et al (1999) Longitudinal clinical and functional pulmonary follow-up after

megatherapy, fractionated total body irradiation, and autologous bone marrow transplantation for metastatic neuroblastoma. Med Pediatr Oncol 32:170–176

102. Nysom K, Holm K, Olsen JH et al (1998) Pulmonary function after treatment for acute lymphoblastic leukaemia in childhood. Br J Can 78:21–27

103. O'Driscoll BR, Hasleton PS, Taylor PM (1990) Active lung fibrosis up to 17 years after chemotherapy with carmustine (BCNU) in childhood. N Engl J Med 323:378–382

104. O'Driscoll BR, Kalra S, Gattamaneni HR, Woodcock AA (1995) Late carmustine fibrosis. Age ate treatment may influence severity and survival. Chest 107:1355–1357

105. Ochs M (2012) The structural and physiologic basis of respiratory disease. In: Wilmott R, Boat T, Chernick V et al (eds) Kendig and Chernick's disorders of the respiratory tract in children, 8th edn. Saunders, Philadelphia, pp 35–74

106. Ortiz LA, Lasky JA, Hamilton R (1998) Expression of TNF and the necessity for TNF receptors in bleomycin-induced lung injury in mice. Exp Lung Res 24:721–743

107. Osanto S, Bukman A, van Hoek F (1992) Long term effects of chemotherapy in patients with testicular cancer. J Clin Oncol 10:574–579

108. Palmas A, Tefferi A, Myers JL et al (1998) Late-onset noninfectious pulmonary complications after allogeneic bone marrow transplantation. Br J Haematol 100:680–687

109. Parimon T, Madtes DK, Au DH et al (2005) Pretransplant lung function, respiratory failure, and mortality after stem cell transplantation. Am J Respir Crit Care Med 172:384–390

110. Parish JM, Muhm JR, Leslie KO (2003) Upper lobe pulmonary fibrosis associated with high-dose chemotherapy containing BCNU for bone marrow transplantation. Mayo Clin Proc 78:630–634

111. Penney DP, Rubin P (1977) Specific early fine structural changes in the lung following irradiation. Int J Radiat Oncol Biol Phys 2:1123–1132

112. Penney DP, Shapiro DL, Rubin P (1981) Effects of radiation on the mouse lung and potential induction of radiation pneumonitis. Virchows Arch B Cell Pathol 37:327–336

113. Penney DP, Siemann DW, Rubin P (1982) Morphologic changes reflecting early and late effects of irradiation of the distal lung of the mouse review. Scanning Microsc 1:413–4255

114. Perry DJ, Weiss RB, Taylor HG (1982) Enhanced bleomycin toxicity during acute renal failure. Cancer Treat Rep 66:592–593

115. Phillips T (1981) Pulmonary section-cardiorespiratory workshops. Cancer Clin Trial 4(Suppl):45–52

116. Phillips TL, Wharam MD, Margolis LW (1975) Modification of radiation injury to normal tissues by chemotherapeutic agents. Cancer 35:1678–1684

117. Phillips TL, Wyatt JP (1980) Radiation fibrosis. In: Fishman AP (ed) Pulmonary diseases and disorders, vol 1. McGraw-Hill, New York

118. Post M, Copland I (2002) Overview of lung development. Acta Pharmacol Sin 23(Suppl):4–7

119. Prato FS, Kurdyak R, Saibil EA (1977) Physiological and radiographic assessment during the development of pulmonary radiation fibrosis. Radiology 122:389–397

120. Prato FS, Kurdyak R, Saibil EA (1977) Regional and total lung function in patients following pulmonary irradiation. Invest Radiol 12:224–237

121. Rabinowitz M, Souhami L, Gil RA (1990) Increased pulmonary toxicity with bleomycin and cisplatin chemotherapy combinations. Am J Clin Oncol 13:132–138

122. Reckzeh B, Merte H, Pfluger K-H (1996) Severe lymphocytopenia and interstitial pneumonia in patients treated with paclitaxel and simultaneous radiotherapy for nonsmall cell lung cancer. J Clin Oncol 14:1071–1076

123. Roach M, Gandara D, You H-S (1995) Radiation pneumonitis following combined modality therapy for lung cancer: analysis of prognostic factors. J Clin Oncol 13:2606–2612

124. Roberts CM, Foulcher E, Zaunders JJ (1993) Radiation pneumonitis: a possible lymphocyte-mediated hypersensitivity reaction. Ann Intern Med 118:696–700

125. Robnett TJ, Machtay M, Vines EF (2000) Factors predicting severe radiation pneumonitis in patients receiving definitive chemoradiation for lung cancer. Int J Radiat Oncol Biol Phys 48:89–94

126. Rubin P (1977) Radiation toxicity: quantitative radiation pathology for predicting effects. Cancer 39(Suppl 2):729–736

127. Rubin P, Finkelstein J, McDonald S (1991) The identification of new early molecular mechanisms in the pathogenesis of radiation induced pulmonary fibrosis. Int J Radiat Oncol Biol Phys 21(Suppl I):163, abstract

128. Rubin P, Finkelstien J, Shapiro D (1992) Molecular biology mechanisms in the radiation induction of pulmonary injury syndromes: interrelationship between the alveolar macrophage and the septal fibroblast. Int J Radiat Oncol Biol Phys 24:93–101

129. Rubin P, Johnston CJ, Williams JP (1995) A perpetual cascade of cytokines post-irradiation leads to pulmonary fibrosis. Int J Radiat Oncol Biol Phys 33:99–109

130. Rubin P, Shapiro DL, Finkelstein JN (1980) The early release of surfactant following lung irradiation of alveolar type II cells. Int J Radiat Oncol Biol Phys 6:75–77

131. Rubin P, Siemann DW, Shapiro DL (1983) Surfactant release as an early measure of radiation pneumonitis. Int J Radiat Oncol Biol Phys 9:1669–1673

132. Samuels ML, Douglas EJ, Holoye PV (1976) Large dose bleomycin therapy and pulmonary toxicity. JAMA 235:1117–1120

133. Schuchter L, Glick J (1993) The current status of WR-2721 (amifostine): a chemotherapy and radiation therapy protector. Biol Ther Cancer Update 1:1–10

134. Schultz KR, Green GJ, Wensley D et al (1994) Obstructive lung disease in children after allogeneic bone marrow transplantation. Blood 84: 3212–3220

135. Schwarz MI, King TE, Cherniack RM (2000) Principles of and approach to the patient with interstitial lung disease. In: Murray JF, Nadel JA (eds) Textbook of respiratory medicine. Saunders, St Louis, pp 1649–1670

136. Segawa Y, Takigawa N, Kataoka M (1997) Risk factors for development of radiation pneumonitis following radiation therapy with or without chemotherapy for lung cancer. Int J Radiat Oncol Biol Phys 39:91–98

137. Selker RG, Jacobs SA, Moore PB (1980) 1,3-Bis (2-chloroethyl)-l-nitrosourea (BCNU)-induced pulmonary fibrosis. Neurosurgery 7:560–565

138. Shaw NJ, Tweedale PM, Eden OB (1989) Pulmonary function in childhood leukemia survivors. Med Pediatr Oncol 17:149–154

139. Shrivastava PN, Hans L, Concannon JP (1974) Changes in pulmonary compliance and production of fibrosis in x-irradiated lungs of rats. Radiology 112:439–440

140. Siemann DW, Hill RP, Penney DP (1982) Early and late pulmonary toxicity in mice evaluated 180 and 420 days following localized lung irradiation. Radiat Res 89:396–407

141. Siemann DW, Rubin P, Penney DP (1986) Pulmonary toxicity following multi-fraction radiotherapy. Br J Cancer 53:365–367

142. Simon G, Reid L, Tanner JM et al (1972) Growth of radiologically determined heart diameter, lung width, and lung length from 5–19 years, with standards for clinical use. Arch Dis Child 47:373–381

143. Sleijfer S, van der Mark TW, Schraffordt Koops H, Mulder NH (1996) Enhanced effects of bleomycin on pulmonary function disturbances in patients with decreased renal function due to cisplatin. Eur J Cancer 32A:550–552

144. Sostman HD, Matthay RA, Puinam CE (1976) Methotrexate induced pneumonitis. Medicine 55:371–389

145. Soubani AO, Miller KB, Hassoun PM (1996) Pulmonary complications of bone marrow transplantation. Chest 109:1066–1077

146. Spector I, Zimbler H, Ross S (1979) Early-onset cyclophosphamide induced interstitial pneumonitis. JAMA 242:2852–2854

147. Stewart P, Buckner CD, Thomas ED (1983) Intensive chemotherapy with autologous marrow transplantation for small cell carcinoma of the lung. Cancer Treat Rep 7:1055–1059

148. Theise ND, Henegariu O, Grove J et al (2002) Radiation pneumonitis in mice: a severe injury model for pneumocyte engraftment from bone marrow. Exp Hematol 30:1333–1338

149. Thurlbeck WM (1975) Postnatal growth and development of the lung. Am Rev Respir Dis 111:803–844

150. Thurlbeck WM (1988) In: Murray JF, Nadel JA (eds) Textbook of respiratory medicine. Saunders, Philadelphia

151. Travis EL (1980) Early indicators of radiation injury on the lung: are they useful predictors for late changes? Int J Radiat Oncol Biol Phys 6:1267–1269

152. Travis EL, Hanley RA, Fenn JO (1977) Pathologic changes in the lung following single and multifraction irradiation. Int J Radiat Oncol Biol Phys 2:475–490

153. Tyc VL, Rai SN, Lensing S et al (2003) Intervention to reduce intentions to use tobacco among pediatric cancer survivors. J Clin Oncol 21:1366–1372

154. Van Barneveld PWC, Veenstra G, Sleifer DT (1985) Changes in pulmonary function during and after bleomycin treatment in patients with testicular carcinoma. Cancer Chemother Pharmacol 14:168–171

155. Van Dyk J, Hill RP (1983) Postirradiation lung density changes measured by computerized tomography. Int J Radiat Oncol Biol Phys 9:847–852

156. Verschoore J, Lagrange JL, Boublil JL et al (1987) Pulmonary toxicity of a combination of low-dose doxorubicin and irradiation for inoperable lung cancer. Radiother Oncol 9:281–288

157. Vieras F, Bradley EW, Alderson PO (1983) Regional pulmonary function after irradiation of the canine lung: radionuclide evaluation. Radiology 147:839–844

158. Vujaskovic Z, Anscher MS, Feng QF et al (2001) Radiation induced hypoxia may perpetuate late normal tissue injury. Int J Radiat Oncol Biol Phys 50:851–855

159. Wall MA, Wohl MEB, Jaffe N (1979) Lung function in adolescents receiving high dose methotrexate. Pediatrics 63:741–746

160. Wara WM, Phillips TL, Margolis LW (1973) Radiation pneumonitis: a new approach to the derivation of timedose factors. Cancer 32:547–552

161. Wasserman TH, Phillips TL, Ross G, Kane LJ (1981) Differential protection against cytotoxic chemotherapeutic effects on bone marrow CFUs by Wr-2721. Cancer Clin Trials 4:3–6

162. Watkins TR, Chien JW, Crawford SW (2005) Graft versus host-associated pulmonary disease and other idiopathic pulmonary complications after hematopoietic stem cell transplant. Semin Respir Crit Care Med 26:482–489

163. Weinstein AS, Diener-West M, Nelson DF, Pakuris E (1986) Pulmonary toxicity of carmustine in patients treated for malignant glioma. Cancer Treat Rep 70:943–946

164. White DA, Stover DE (1984) Severe bleomycin induced pneumonitis. Clinical features and response to corticosteroids. Chest 86:723–728

165. Wohl ME, Griscom NT, Traggis DG, Jaffe N (1975) Effects of therapeutic irradiation delivered in early childhood upon subsequent lung function. Pediatrics 55:507–516

166. Yuhas JM, Spellman JM, Jordan SW et al (1980) Treatment of tumours with the combination of WR-2721 and cis-dichlorodiammineplatinum (II) or cyclophosphamide. Br J Cancer 42:574–585

# Late Gastrointestinal and Hepatic Effects

# 12

Sharon M. Castellino and Melissa M. Hudson

## Contents

S.M. Castellino, MD, MSC (✉)
Wake Forest School of Medicine, Department of
Pediatrics; Section Hematology/Oncology,
Winston-Salem, NC 27157, USA
e-mail: scastell@wakehealth.edu

M.M. Hudson, MD
St. Jude Children's Research Hospital,
Memphis, TN, USA

## 12.1 Introduction

Radiation and specific chemotherapeutic agents often produce acute transient gastrointestinal (GI) or hepatic toxicity, but latent and persistent adverse events are less commonly reported. However, these relatively uncommon late gastrointestinal and hepatic complications are potentially life threatening and capable of severely compromising quality of life. Although the most common malignancies that can be complicated by GI and hepatic injury are abdominal sarcomas (rhabdomyosarcoma and other soft tissue sarcomas), a limited number of reports describe GI complications in pediatric patients with genitourinary solid tumors or in those with lymphoma who underwent staging laparotomy [1–6]. Children at risk for GI complications following treatment for childhood cancer represent a minority as indicated by data from the Childhood Cancer Survivor Study (CCSS) in which 12 % of participating survivors had an abdominal primary tumor and 30 % had sustained abdominal surgery and/or radiation treatment to fields exposing gastrointestinal organs [7]. The severity of GI tract and hepatic toxicity among at-risk survivors is related to the specific treatment modality and intensity employed and to the time since therapy exposure; multimodal therapy confers additive risks. Other comorbid conditions, for example, transfusion-acquired hepatitis or graft-versus-host disease (GVHD), may enhance risk [8–12].

© Springer International Publishing 2015
C.L. Schwartz et al. (eds.), *Survivors of Childhood and Adolescent Cancer:*
*A Multidisciplinary Approach*, Pediatric Oncology, DOI 10.1007/978-3-319-16435-9_12

Many reports describe complications resulting from now outdated treatment modalities. While there is a paucity of literature about long-term gastrointestinal outcomes, the CCSS estimates a cumulative incidence of any self-reported GI condition of 38 % at 20 years from the childhood cancer diagnosis [7]. Compared to siblings, survivors reported an increased number of late complications of the upper and lower GI tract and of the liver. The relative risk (RR) of any GI complication was 1.7, and there was a substantial risk of survivors reporting two or more liver problems (RR 12.2, 95 % CI 4.8–30.7) [7]. Long-term outcomes after venoocclusive disease, chronic graft-versus-host disease, and transfusion-acquired hepatitis remain to be established as these conditions have been associated with subclinical liver dysfunction that may predispose to clinically significant liver disease in aging childhood cancer survivors [13–16]. This chapter summarizes complications involving the GI tract and hepatobiliary system observed following treatment for childhood cancer in the context of normal organ pathophysiology. These sequelae may develop after a variety of therapeutic interventions, for example, radiation, chemotherapy, surgery, or bone marrow transplantation, or from supportive therapies such as blood product transfusion. Guidelines for after completion of therapy monitoring of predisposed childhood cancer survivors and recommendations for health protective risk reducing counseling will also be provided.

## 12.2 Upper and Lower Gastrointestinal Tract

### 12.2.1 Pathophysiology

#### 12.2.1.1 Normal Anatomy and Physiology

The upper GI tract extends from the oropharynx to the ileocecal valve and includes the esophagus, stomach, and small intestine. The esophagus is a distensible tube lined by an inner mucosa of squamous epithelium that is surrounded by a submucosa, a muscularis externa composed of both striated and smooth muscles, and an outermost connective tissue layer. The neurovascular supply and mucous glands, which are located primarily in the submucosa, open into the lumen of the esophagus. The lower esophageal sphincter prevents esophageal injury from reflux of gastric contents, while the epithelium and mucous glands protect against peptic injury. Salivation and esophageal peristalsis also protect the esophageal mucosa by facilitating acid clearance.

Located inferior to the left hemidiaphragm, the stomach is anatomically divided into the cardia, fundus, body, and antrum. A thick muscular walled pylorus forms a sphincter that connects the gastric antrum to the duodenum. The stomach is lined by an inner mucosa of columnar epithelium that is surrounded by a submucosa and an outer muscularis comprised of longitudinal and circular smooth muscle. Gastric mucosal glands secrete mucus, hydrochloric acid, or hormones that regulate gastric secretions and motility. The gastric fundus mucosa secretes an intrinsic factor required for absorption of vitamin $B_{12}$ by the small intestine.

The small intestine contains mucosal, submucosal, and muscularis layers similar to that of the stomach. The mucosal layer of the small intestine is composed of rapidly proliferating epithelium arranged in villi that increase the absorptive and digestive surface area. The columnar cells forming the villi are arranged in microvilli that form the brush border of the small intestine luminal surface. The digestive enzymes, disaccharidases and peptidases, are located on the surface of the microvilli. Several ligaments fix the duodenum into a C-shaped configuration in the retroperitoneum. The superior mesenteric artery (SMA) arises from the aorta at the level of L1 vertebral body and is normally encased in the mesenteric fat pad, with the duodenum traversing the fat pad space between the SMA and the aorta. The head of the pancreas lies in the concavity. Suspended by the mesentery, the jejunum and most of the ileum are usually freely mobile within the abdominal cavity. The ileocecal valve functions as a sphincter that prevents bacterial contamination of the small bowel.

Originating in the right lower quadrant, the colon ascends to the hepatic flexure, traverses the abdomen to the splenic flexure, and then descends in a tortuous fashion to the anus. The splenic flexure and rectosigmoid region are two "watershed" areas of arterial blood flow to the colon predisposed to ischemic injury. Similar to the small bowel, the colon is lined with columnar epithelium, but there are no villi. Transport of electrolytes and water occurs in the microvilli located on the luminal surface of the epithelial cells. Copious goblet cells secrete mucus onto the luminal surface of the colon.

### 12.2.1.2   Organ Damage Induced by Cytotoxic Therapy

Acute GI toxicity develops frequently following radiation and a variety of chemotherapeutic agents and is characterized by recovery without sequelae in the majority of individuals. The most common gastrointestinal tract complications observed in long-term childhood cancer survivors typically result from chronic mucosal inflammation that interferes with absorption and digestion of nutrients (enteritis) or predisposes to scarring (fibrosis) of intra-abdominal tissues. Persistent or chronic GI effects are most often observed in long-term survivors treated with radiation [17], although specific chemotherapeutic agents may enhance the risk of chronic injury. Combined modality therapy and other treatment complications may have additive adverse effects. For example, chronic infections or graft-versus-host disease (GVHD) may exacerbate radiation-induced enterocolitis. Similarly, extensive bowel resection may contribute to malabsorption associated with chronic enteritis.

Complications related to fibrosis are the most commonly observed late GI effect in childhood cancer survivors. Fibrosis may involve any site within the GI tract as well as extraintestinal structures. Pathologically, fibrosis developing within the wall of the upper GI tract may produce thickening of the serosa, muscularis, and submucosa (Fig. 12.1) leading to an increased risk of stricture formation. Because of its rapid cell turnover, the submucosa is especially prone to the development of fibrosis. Fibrosis of extraintestinal tissues predisposes to formation of adhesions [1, 18]. Enteritis, or inflammation of the mucosa or

lamina propria, ulceration, and villous atrophy may occur in association with or independent of fibrosis (Fig. 12.1). Focal vascular changes associated with chronic ischemia in the submucosa and mesentery may be responsible for these lesions. Chronic GVHD involving the GI tract of survivors treated with bone marrow transplantation is characterized by mononuclear infiltration of the lamina propria, mucosal ulceration, and reepithelialization [19]. Less commonly observed GI tract sequelae are related to the anatomic revisions undertaken during intra-abdominal exoneration and bowel resections, GI tract dysmotility associated with neuronal toxicity, and esophageal varices from portal hypertension. Secondary malignancies of the GI tract have been observed with increasing frequency in aging long-term childhood cancer survivors. The risk of gastrointestinal SMNs was 4.6-fold higher in the CCSS than in the general population, and the standardized incidence ratio for colorectal cancer specifically was 4.2 (95 % CI, 3.8–6.3). Adenocarcinoma is the predominant histology [20–22]. Radiation has been implicated as the primary contributor to GI tract carcinogenesis. Alkylating agent chemotherapies, specifically procarbazine and platinum drugs, appear to enhance this risk [20–23]. The reader should refer to Chap. 19 for a more detailed description of the second malignancy after childhood cancer.

### 12.2.2  Clinical Manifestations

Clinical signs and symptoms of GI tract toxicity are related to the specific tissues involved and to the severity of injury. Mild injury to GI tract tissues may be asymptomatic and noted as an incidental finding at the time of a diagnostic imaging procedure, surgery, or autopsy. More severe injury produces chronic or persistent symptoms associated with inflammation and fibrosis of specific tissues. Upper GI symptoms are most common, with a cumulative incidence of 26 %, and lower GI complications are reported with an incidence of 15 % [7]. Common constitutional symptoms referable to the GI tract include dysphagia, odynophagia,

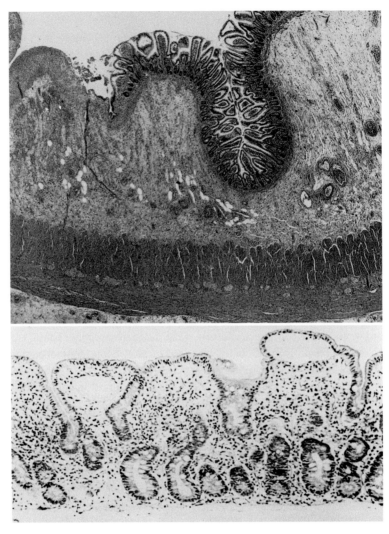

**Fig. 12.1** *Top*, delayed radiation injury in the wall of the ileum, approximately 10 years after exposure to undetermined (kilorad) dose of external radiation for adjacent intra-abdominal neoplasm (hematoxylin and eosin stain, ×21). Note chronic ulceration (*left third*) and extensive fibrosis of submucosa and subserosa. Villous atrophy is slight in this case (From Fajardo [18]). *Bottom*, histologic picture of the small bowel at the time of obstruction, demonstrating severe villous blunting, distended lymphatics, and an abnormally dense mucosal round cell infiltrate. The normal columnar epithelium is lost, with only low cuboidal cells present. Villi are shortened (hematoxylin and eosin stain, ×10) (From Donaldson et al. [1])

indigestion/heartburn, vomiting, abdominal pain (which may be focal or generalized), colic, constipation/obstipation, diarrhea, and GI bleeding with or without anemia. The clinical sequelae of fibrosis include partial or complete bowel obstruction from strictures or adhesions. Chronic enteritis and bowel resection may result in malabsorption, bowel ulceration/perforation, or fistula formation.

Nonspecific symptoms of anorexia, fatigue, and wasting may also be observed. Individuals with chronic hyperchloremic metabolic acidosis resulting from excess GI bicarbonate loss may present with obtundation and confusion. This complication is rare, but can develop following ureterosigmoidostomy or ileal or jejunal loop procedures. A young child with upper GI tract obstruction and reflux may present with aspiration pneumonia. Older age at diagnosis, intensified therapy, abdominal radiation, and abdominal surgery increase the risk of certain GI complications [7].

### 12.2.2.1 Radiation

Radiation injury of the GI tract has been the most extensively studied cause of fibrosis and enteritis. According to data from cohorts of adults treated with radiation for abdominopelvic tumors, radiation complications typically develop within 5 years after treatment in individuals who experienced acute GI toxicity [24]. However, primary presentations of strictures or inflammatory lesions may occur as late as 20 years after radiation [17, 25]. The risk of radiation injury to the GI tract is related to the cumulative radiation dose, daily fraction dose, and extent of treatment volume [26, 27]. Fixed loops of the duodenum and terminal ileum are more prone to radiation injury than the esophagus or other intestinal sites [6, 25]. The incidence of small bowel fibrosis is about 5 % after 40–50 Gy and rises to 40 % when doses exceed 60 Gy [26, 28]. Chronic GI tract injury is uncommon after treatment doses below 42 Gy given over 4–4.5 weeks.

Limited studies are available describing the chronic effects of GI radiation therapy in children [17]. Many of the data on the risk of bowel adhesions and obstruction in this population are confounded by the fact that most of the cancer survivors had prior abdominal surgery as a risk factor for late gastrointestinal effects [17]. Donaldson et al. comprehensively evaluated intestinal symptoms in 44 children with Wilms tumor, teratoma, or lymphoma (including Hodgkin lymphoma) treated with whole abdominal (10–40 Gy) and involved field (25–40 Gy) radiation [1]. Additional interventions predisposing to GI tract toxicity in the group included abdominal laparotomy in 43(98 %) and chemotherapy in 25 (57 %). Late small bowel obstruction was observed in 36 % of patients surviving 19 months to 7 years, which was uniformly preceded by small bowel toxicity during therapy. Infants and children younger than 2 years appeared to experience more acute and chronic GI toxicity following intensive radiation or com-

bined modality therapy compared to older children.

Several reports document GI toxicity in long-term survivors of genitourinary rhabdomyosarcoma [2, 3, 29]. Investigators from the Intergroup Rhabdomyosarcoma Study evaluated late effects in long-term survivors of paratesticular and bladder/prostate rhabdomyosarcoma [5]. Radiation-related complications occurred in approximately 10 % of patients and included intraperitoneal adhesions with bowel obstruction, chronic diarrhea, and stricture or enteric fistula formation. Similar findings were observed in another small cohort of survivors of paratesticular rhabdomyosarcoma treated at a single institution [29]. A report on long-term survivors of germ cell tumors reported up to 25 % had gastrointestinal dysfunction in patients who had received 25–30 Gy to the abdomen and pelvis. The late effects included chronic diarrhea or constipation, stool incontinence, bowel obstruction, rectal prolapse, strictures, or fistula formation [30]. The small number of patients and GI events reported in these studies precluded correlation of host and treatment factors predicting GI toxicity.

Radiation can enhance the risk of late postsurgical small bowel obstruction in long-term childhood survivors, but this complication has been rarely observed with contemporary techniques and doses. Donaldson reported only one case of late bowel obstruction in 79 surgically staged pediatric patients with Hodgkin lymphoma treated with radiation (35–44 Gy) [31]. Similarly, high-dose radiation used in earlier protocols for Hodgkin lymphoma in adolescents and young adults has been associated with a 1 % incidence of late onset nonspecific abdominal pain attributable to retroperitoneal fibrosis involving the genitourinary tract rather than the GI tract [32]. However, children irradiated at lower doses for Wilms tumor less commonly develop chronic small bowel obstruction [17].

Thoracic radiation, particularly when administered to young children at high cumulative doses (40 Gy or more), predisposes to the development of esophageal strictures [4, 33]. The frequency of stricture formation after mediastinal radiation has ranged from 17 % to 42 % in older series [34–36]. This complication is uncommonly observed following contemporary treatment for pediatric tumors which have reduced or eliminated radiation in many frontline therapies. Acute radiation esophagitis developing during radiation administration is likely the nidus for stricture formation or tracheoesophageal fistulas; fungal esophagitis may also enhance the risk of this complication [33, 37]. Subacute or chronic candidal esophagitis may predispose to stricture formation that usually involves the upper third of the esophagus [37, 38] (Figure 12.2). Strictures developing in individuals with chronic candidal esophagitis have been seen in association with intramucosal pseudodiverticulitis, an inflammatory disorder characterized by digitation of excretory ducts of the submucosal glands. Another characteristic histopathology includes the development of mucosal bridges that may result in webs. Similarly, the administration of radiation-enhancing chemotherapeutic agents like doxorubicin may augment the risk of stricture formation by inducing recurrent episodes of esophagitis through a "recall" phenomenon [39–41]. This premise concurs with the increased frequency of strictures observed in patients treated with combined modality therapy including radiation and radiomimetic chemotherapy.

### 12.2.2.2 Chemotherapy

In general, chemotherapy plays a less prominent role in the development of chronic enteritis. Multiple chemotherapeutic agents produce acute GI toxicity and typically manifest as mucositis; complete resolution of symptoms after completion of therapy is the usual clinical course. Anthracyclines and dactinomycin have potent radiomimetic effects that enhance acute GI toxicity and likely contribute to late onset radiation-related GI toxicity [40–42]. Rapid chemotherapy-induced tumor lysis has been associated with intestinal necrosis and fistula formation [43]. Both alkylating agents and anthracyclines were associated with dose-dependent risk of upper GI and liver complications in the CCSS cohort. Vincristine exposure is associated with late liver and lower GI complications [7].

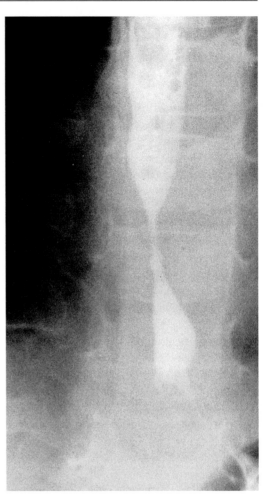

**Fig. 12.2** Barium study showing distal esophageal stricture in a 5-year-old girl previously treated for ALL. The distal location of the stricture and its endoscopic appearance suggest that gastroesophageal reflux and chronic esophagitis may have played a role in the pathogenesis of the stricture (Courtesy of Dr. S. Kocoshis)

### 12.2.2.3 Surgery

Abdominal surgery is associated with a lifelong risk of developing adhesive and obstructive complications involving the GI tract. Numerous pediatric studies describe adhesive or obstructive complications that most commonly develop within the acute or subacute postoperative period [44–46]. In contrast, information about very late onset adhesive and obstructive complications in childhood cancer survivors are more likely to be found in manuscripts describing global long-term outcome after pediatric sarcomas, in which the incidence of complications related to adhesions and obstructions is approximately 10 % [3, 5, 29]. Notably, in addition to laparotomy, risk factors for postoperative complications included intensive combination chemotherapy including radiomimetic agents and radiation therapy. Investigators from the National Wilms Tumor Study Group observed small bowel obstruction in 7 % of patients; however, the incidence of late onset obstruction (more than 1 year from laparotomy) occurred in fewer than 2 % of patients, with events rarely reported more than 5 years postoperatively [44]. Jockovich et al. evaluated long-term complications of laparotomy in a cohort of 133 pediatric and adult patients who had undergone staging laparotomy with splenectomy before treatment of Hodgkin lymphoma [45]. At a median follow up of 15.7 years (range, 2.5–28 years) after laparotomy, the most frequent surgical complication was small bowel obstruction, which occurred in 9.8 % and required surgical intervention in 6.8 %. Patients younger than 15 years of age at the time of laparotomy had a higher risk of small bowel obstruction compared to older patients, perhaps related to the increased intensity of the pediatric surgical staging protocols. An increased frequency of obstructive complications is also anticipated in survivors who have undergone multiple laparotomies for staging and assessment of tumor response [31, 42].

Rarely, a temporary or permanent enterostomy is required for the management of cancer-related GI toxicity, for example, after resection of ischemic bowel, for a refractory GI tract stricture or fistula, or for chronic fecal incontinence. Affected survivors must cope with physical and psychological issues related to stoma maintenance. Finally, excess gastrointestinal bicarbonate loss associated with ureterosigmoidostomy or ileal or jejunal loop procedures predisposes to hyperchloremic metabolic acidosis [47]. These individuals are also at increased risk of developing adenocarcinoma of the large bowel [48].

#### 12.2.2.4 Hematopoietic Stem Cell Transplant (HSCT)

The incidence and severity of delayed GI tract toxicity following allogeneic hematopoietic stem cell transplantation are related to the cumulative radiation dose used in the conditioning regimen, the presence of GVHD, or a combination of both. Whereas GI tract toxicity is frequent in the acute transplant setting, chronic late problems affecting GI tissues are relatively uncommon. Xerostomia may result from sclerodermatous changes of the mucous membranes and salivary glands and predispose to accelerated tooth decay and periodontal disease [49]. Esophageal stricture formation is the most common form of delayed GI toxicity and may require dilation procedures to maintain satisfactory oral intake [50, 51]. Affected tissues show characteristic weblike intraluminal membranes that form strictures; some patients also demonstrate perimuscular fibrosis similar to that seen in scleroderma [50, 51]. GVHD of the small bowel may result in chronic diarrhea from malabsorption (Fig. 12.3). Steatorrhea and diarrhea may also signal the presence of bacterial overgrowth with stasis syndrome. As a result, many individuals with chronic GVHD involving the GI tract are anorexic and undernourished. Endoscopic evaluation with biopsy is generally required to identify the specific GI pathology and provide appropriate therapeutic interventions.

### 12.2.3  Detection and Screening

Assessment of cancer-related GI tract sequelae should begin with a thorough history with close attention to symptoms referable to GI tract pathology including dysphagia, odynophagia, vomiting, chronic abdominal pain, chronic constipation or diarrhea, hematochezia, or melena (Tables 12.1 and 12.2). Anorexia, intolerance to certain foods, fatigue, and impaired weight gain or growth may be secondary nonspecific complaints. Physical examination should assess nutritional status, which can be inferred by height and weight, and abdominal findings suggesting GI pathology like distension and pain. Although not routinely used in pediatric assessments, a digital rectal exam and fecal occult blood test should be performed on children presenting with signs and symptoms of GI tract pathology.

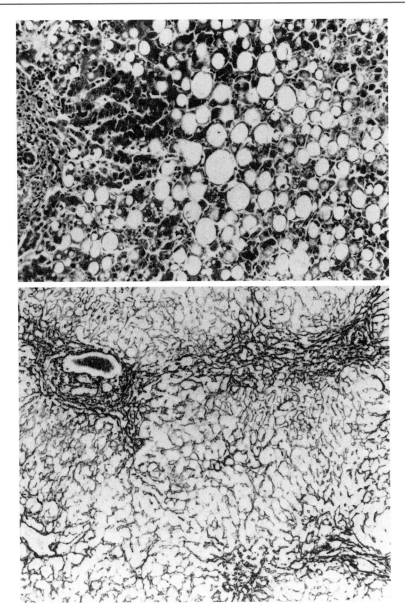

**Fig. 12.3** Colonic mucosa in graft-versus-host disease. Glands show architectural disruption with infiltration of lymphocytes accompanied by epithelial cell necrosis and dropout. Hematoxylin and eosin stain, 20× original magnification (Courtesy of Dr. J. Jenkins)

Aside from screening levels of vitamin $B_{12}$ and folate, laboratory studies are largely obtained to assess secondary effects of GI tract pathology. Anemia and microcytosis may reflect iron deficiency from GI tract blood loss or from malabsorption. Macrocytic anemia may result from vitamin $B_{12}$ or folate deficiency associated with chronic malabsorption or resection of the terminal ileum. Albumin and serum protein are useful to assess protein stores in patients with chronic diarrhea or fistulas and should be monitored periodically in individuals with chronic malabsorption. A hemoglobin and hematocrit provides useful information in patients who present with hematochezia, but

**Table 12.1** Chemotherapy-associated gastrointestinal and hepatic late effects

| Therapeutic agent | Potential late effects | Modifying factors | Health screening and management |
|---|---|---|---|
| Dactinomycin | No known late effects Dactinomycin has been associated with acute venoocclusive disease, from which the majority of patients recover without sequelae | Treatment: abdominal radiation | History and physical exam annually Laboratory: ALT, AST, bilirubin, baseline at entry into long-term follow-up, then as clinically indicated Screen for viral hepatitis in patients with persistently abnormal liver function |
| Mercaptopurine Thioguanine | Hepatic dysfunction[a] Sinusoidal obstruction syndrome/VOD[b] | Medical conditions: viral hepatitis, VOD, thiopurine S-methyltransferase, deficiency, iron overload | Hepatitis A and B immunizations for patients lacking immunity Gastroenterology/hepatology consultation as clinically indicated |
| Methotrexate | Hepatic dysfunction[a] | Treatment: abdominal radiation Medical conditions: viral hepatitis | |

[a]Acute toxicities including elevations in liver transaminase (ALT, AST) predominate from which the majority of patients recover without sequelae
[b]VOD – venoocclusive disease of the liver, now termed sinusoidal obstruction syndrome

further radiographic and endoscopic evaluation is typically needed to identify the site and specific pathological lesion. Gastroenterology or surgical consultation may be required to establish the diagnosis or provide remedial interventions.

In the absence of abdominopelvic radiation fields, the preferred screening evaluations for GI tract malignancies are the same as for the asymptomatic general population: beginning at age 50, patients should initiate screening with tests that can detect cancer (e.g., guaiac-based fecal occult blood test, immunochemical fecal occult blood test, or stool for exfoliated DNA) and advanced lesions (e.g., flexible sigmoidoscopy, colonoscopy, double-contrast barium enema, computed tomography colonography) (Table 12.3) [52]. Several studies have described an excess risk of gastrointestinal malignancies in childhood cancer survivors treated with abdominal/pelvic radiation [20–22]. Since the median reported age of onset and time since primary cancer of this complication is 33 years age (range 9.7–59 years) and 23 years (range 2–49 years), respectively, it seems prudent to consider an earlier onset of screening colonoscopy in at-risk childhood cancer survivors or in survivors with risk who are symptomatic. The current Children's Oncology Group Guideline

recommends monitoring for occult colorectal malignancies to begin 10 years after radiation or at age 35 years (whichever occurs last) in asymptomatic survivors (Table 12.3) [53]. While the efficacy of this approach has not been validated in longitudinal trials, this represents a conservative strategy that would increase the likelihood of early detection of an occult GI malignancy of the lower GI tract.

There are currently no screening recommendations for upper GI complications. However, reports of Barrett esophagus [54] and the recognized incidence of SMN in the esophagus, stomach, and hepatobiliary tree should motivate prompt evaluation of symptomatic survivors with this condition [20, 22].

### 12.2.4 Management of Established Problems

Optimal management of cancer-related GI complications requires cooperation between the survivor's primary physician, gastroenterologist, and surgeon. Conditions requiring intervention most often result from primary or secondary consequences of chronic inflammation or fibrosis of GI tissues. Esophagitis and gastritis are usually

**Table 12.2** Radiation-associated gastrointestinal and hepatic late effects

| Treatment fields | Potential late effects | Modifying factors | Health screening and management |
|---|---|---|---|
| Spinal (cervical, thoracic, whole) Chest (mediastinal, mantle, whole lung) Abdomen (upper quadrant, flank, whole) Total body irradiation Total lymphoid irradiation | Esophageal stricture | Treatment: higher radiation dose, radiomimetic chemotherapy (e.g., doxorubicin, actinomycin) Medical conditions: gastroesophageal reflux disease, severe/chronic candidal esophagitis, chronic graft-versus-host disease | History and physical exam annually Gastroenterology consultation as clinically indicated |
| All abdominal (upper quadrant, flank, whole) and pelvic Spinal (thoracic, lumbar, sacral, whole) Total body irradiation Total lymphoid irradiation | Bowel obstruction | Treatment: higher radiation dose to bowel, especially dose $\geq$45 Gy, abdominal surgery | History and physical exam annually KUB and surgical consultation as clinically indicated |
| | Chronic enterocolitis Fistula, strictures | Treatment: higher radiation dose to bowel, especially dose $\geq$ 45 Gy, abdominal surgery | History and physical exam annually Laboratory: serum protein, albumin annually in patients with chronic diarrhea or fistula Gastroenterology and surgical consultation as clinically indicated |
| | Cholelithiasis | Treatment: abdominal radiation, abdominal surgery, ileal conduit, total parenteral nutrition, hematopoietic stem cell transplant for marrow failure syndrome Medical conditions: obesity | History and physical exam annually Gallbladder ultrasound and surgical consultation as clinically indicated |
| | Gastrointestinal and hepatobiliary malignancy | Treatment: higher radiation dose to bowel, especially dose $\geq$30 Gy, higher daily fraction dose, alkylating agent chemotherapy | History and physical exam annually Oncology and surgical consultation as clinically indicated See Table 12.3 for colorectal cancer screening guidelines |
| Whole abdomen Hepatic Total body irradiation | Hepatic fibrosis Cirrhosis | Treatment: radiation dose $\geq$40 Gy to at least 1/3 of liver volume or 20–30 Gy to entire liver Medical conditions: chronic hepatitis, iron overload Health behaviors: alcohol use | History and physical exam annually Laboratory: ALT, AST, bilirubin baseline at entry into long-term follow-up Screen for viral hepatitis in patients with persistently abnormal liver function Hepatitis A and B immunizations for patients lacking immunity Gastroenterology/hepatology consultation as clinically indicated |

managed by dietary modification and a variety of pharmacologic agents, including $H_2$ antagonists and proton pump inhibitors, which eliminate or reduce acid production by the parietal cells. Prokinetic agents are also helpful if acid reflux is contributing to chronic esophagitis. Adjunctive agents like Carafate, which binds to the proteins of denuded mucosa, may also be used as a physical barrier to mucosal irritation.

Upper GI tract strictures are best evaluated by barium swallow (Fig. 12.2) followed by endoscopy. Repeated endoscopy and dilation procedures may be required for long-term management of esophageal strictures. Concurrent evaluation

**Table 12.3**  Colorectal cancer (CRC) screening in childhood cancer survivors

| CRC risk groups | Risk group definition | Recommended surveillance |
|---|---|---|
| Average risk related to cancer treatment | Survivor without high-risk cancer treatment exposures, familial or hereditary risk, or history of inflammatory bowel disease | Beginning at age 50 years[a]: Annual high-sensitivity guaiac-based fecal occult blood test or immunochemical fecal occult blood test combined with one of the following: Flexible sigmoidoscopy every 5 years or Colonoscopy every 10 years or Double-contrast barium enema every 5 years or Computed tomography colonography every 5 years |
| High risk related to family history or genetic syndrome | Family history of CRC or adenomatous polyps in first-degree relative before age 60 or in 2 or more first-degree relatives at any age  Known or suspected presence of familial adenomatous polyposis (FAP) or hereditary nonpolyposis colorectal cancer (HNPCC) | Early and heightened surveillance with colonoscopy based on specific condition[b]: Beginning at age 40 or 10 years before the youngest case of first-degree relative with CRC or adenomatous polyps Beginning at age 10–12 years for FAP Beginning at age 20–25 years or 10 years before the youngest case in the family for HNPCC |
| High risk related to inflammatory bowel disease | History of chronic ulcerative colitis or Crohn's disease | Early and heightened surveillance with colonoscopy every 1–2 years: Beginning 8 years after the onset of pancolitis or 12–15 years after the onset of left-sided colitis |
| High risk related to cancer treatment | Treatment with radiation fields involving the colon and rectum: all abdominal (e.g., upper quadrant, flank, whole) and pelvic fields, spinal (thoracic, lumbar, sacral, whole), total body irradiation,[c] total lymphoid irradiation | Beginning at age 35 years or 10 years postradiation therapy (whichever occurs last)[c]: Colonoscopy every 5 years |

[a]Adapted from the American Cancer Society (ACS) guidelines
[b]Adapted from the Children's Oncology Group Guidelines (www.survivorshipguidelines.org)
[c]Risk related to total body irradiation alone is not established; therefore, screening in this group should be determined on individual basis

and treatment of peptic esophagitis is important to reduce the risk of further mucosal injury. Surgical procedures that reduce or prevent reflux may also be undertaken to minimize the risk of recurrent stricture formation. Patients who have unrevealing barium swallow study or upper endoscopy may have dysphagia resulting from abnormal motility associated with neuronal injury; this can be identified through manometric studies. Chronic constipation and obstipation may be predisposed by more severe motility abnormalities. Aggressive treatment with laxatives and enemas is required for individuals who develop stool impaction. Regular treatment with stool softeners and peristaltic stimulants reduces the risk of this complication.

Chronic enteritis may be associated with malabsorption. Affected patients present with chronic diarrhea, abdominal distension, failure to thrive, and other signs of protein deficiency. In cases with malabsorption, contrast studies are used to determine the site of pathology and small bowel biopsies to define the histologic features. Individual tests of absorption, including the D-xylose absorption test, lactose breath hydrogen test, 72-h fecal fat determinations, serum $B_{12}$ and folate levels, measurement of stool pH and reducing substances, and the Schilling test, are used to define the defect. Bacterial contamination of the small bowel may also predispose to malabsorption; strictures and blind loops may also contribute to this complication. Intubation and quantitative bacterial cultures of the small bowel may be required to confirm the diagnosis, especially in the absence of the ileocecal valve or in the presence of small bowel stasis. Bacterial overgrowth responds to appropriate antimicrobial therapy like tetracycline or metronidazole. Chronic diarrhea associated with bile salt malabsorption after ileal resection may improve with cholestyramine. Refractory malabsorption associated with villous atrophy may require enteral or parenteral nutritional support.

While the management of acute GI bleeding is generally easily accomplished in the primary care setting, evaluation and treatment of chronic GI blood loss associated with chronic enterocolitis or proctitis usually requires more extensive evaluation by subspecialists to localize the site of bleeding. Following contrast diagnostic imaging studies, endoscopic evaluation is used to confirm inflammation, ulceration, or less commonly malignancy. Biopsy will determine the etiology of mucosal lesions. Only rarely are more aggressive interventions, for example, enterolysis, tagged red blood cell study, or exploratory laparotomy, needed to localize the site of GI tract bleeding.

Patients presenting with signs and symptoms of bowel obstruction should be promptly evaluated with abdominal radiographs, decompression (if clinically indicated), and the appropriate contrast imaging. Chronic or refractory intestinal obstruction associated with strictures or adhesions may eventually require surgical intervention for definitive correction.

## 12.3 Hepatobiliary Tree

### 12.3.1 Pathophysiology

#### 12.3.1.1 Normal Anatomy and Physiology

The liver is the largest organ in the body and consists of right and left lobes joined posteroinferiorly at the porta hepatis. The gallbladder lies under the visceral surface of the liver. The hepatic lobule, which contains a central vein that is a tributary of the hepatic vein, is the basic ultrastructural unit of the liver. The central vein of each hepatic lobule drains into the inferior vena cava. Columns of hepatocytes radiate from the center of each lobule and are separated by sinusoids. Hepatic sinusoids are lined with reticuloendothelial or Kupffer cells. The hepatic lobule is divided into three functional zones that each receives blood of varying nutrient and oxygen content. Zone 3, which receives the least oxygen and nutrients, is the most vulnerable to injury. Hepatic arterioles, portal vein radicles, and branches of the left and right hepatic ducts are located in portal triads between the hepatic lobules. The left and right hepatic ducts fuse at the porta hepatis to form the common hepatic duct. The cystic duct, which drains the gallbladder, joins the hepatic duct to form the common bile duct that drains into the duodenum.

Liver function is diverse and includes synthesis of enzymes, albumin, coagulation proteins, urea, and steroids such as cholesterol and primary bile acids, conjugation of bilirubin, detoxification of drugs, and storage of fat-soluble vitamins. Hepatocytes are also responsible for gluconeogenesis and glycolysis. The Kupffer cells, which engage in phagocytosis and secrete cytokines, play a role in immune regulation.

#### 12.3.1.2 Changes Induced by Cytotoxic Therapy

Fibrosis, which is generally periportal and concentric (Fig. 12.4), is the most frequently described long-term complication of antineoplastic therapy observed in the liver [56]. Hepatic fibrosis may be associated with fatty infiltration, focal necrosis, nodular regeneration or cirrhosis, and portal hypertension. Chronic hepatitis, regardless of its etiology, is characterized by portal-periportal lymphoplasmacytic infiltration with varying degrees of fibrosis and piecemeal necrosis. The histopathology of sinusoidal obstruction syndrome (SOS) [formerly termed venoocclusive disease, VOD] demonstrates endothelial injury, fibrin deposition, and microthrombi in hepatic sinusoids; if progressive, fibrous obliteration of central veins, centrilobular necrosis, and hepatic outflow obstruction ensue. GVHD is

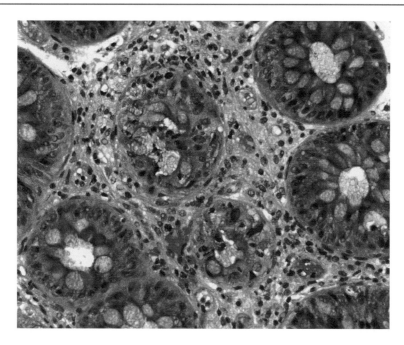

**Fig. 12.4** Chronic methotrexate liver damage. There is fatty change together with chronic portal inflammation and fibrosis. Hematoxylin and eosin stain, ×180. Reprinted with the kind permission of Dr. R.S. Patrick and Chapman Hall, Ltd.)

associated with hepatocellular necroinflammatory changes suggestive of chronic active hepatitis, a paucity of interlobular bile ducts, and intrahepatic cholestasis (Fig. 12.5) [14, 19]. Cell-mediated immune dysregulation is implicated in the pathophysiology of chronic GVHD in most studies. However, findings of deposits of immunoglobulin and complement along the dermal-epidermal junction in 85 % of individuals with chronic GVHD suggest that humoral mechanism may play a role as well [57]. Hepatocellular carcinoma has been rarely reported in patients treated with chemotherapy and radiation therapy for Wilms tumor and in long-term survivors of childhood leukemia with chronic hepatitis C infection [58–60].

## 12.3.2 Clinical Manifestations

Liver injury related to treatment for childhood cancer is most often subclinical and may develop without a history of prior acute toxicity. Asymptomatic abnormalities of serum transaminases (alanine aminotransferase and aspartate aminotransferase) are most commonly observed.

In the setting of chronic GVHD, alkaline phosphatase and bilirubin may also be elevated. However, bilirubin elevation is variable and does not correlate with clinical outcome. Patients with chronic liver dysfunction frequently report constitutional complaints like pruritus, fatigue, and weight loss. In contrast, hepatic sinusoidal obstruction syndrome (or venoocclusive disease) is characterized by the acute onset of jaundice, right upper quadrant pain, hepatomegaly, ascites, liver dysfunction, and thrombocytopenia. The clinical course of sinusoidal obstruction syndrome varies from mild and reversible to life threatening with progressive hepatic failure. The impact of acute sinusoidal obstruction syndrome on long-term hepatic function has not been established. Chronic progressive hepatic fibrosis associated with cirrhosis may cause portal hypertension and resulting sequelae like hypersplenism and variceal bleeding. If cirrhosis leads to liver decompensation, clinical signs and symptoms of hepatic synthetic dysfunction appear including ascites and coagulopathy. As hepatic failure ensues, affected individuals manifest progressive metabolic derangements and encephalopathy.

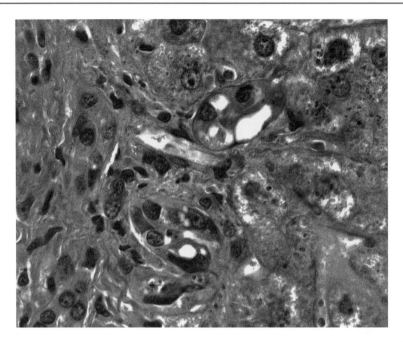

**Fig. 12.5** Hepatic portal triad in graft-versus-host disease. Bile ducts show epithelial damage in the form of irregular cellular and nuclear size and spacing around the duct lumen with some epithelial cells completely missing. Epithelial cell cytoplasm is vacuolated and shows variable eosinophilia. In this example a paucity of lymphocytes is noted. Hematoxylin and eosin stain, 60× original magnification (Courtesy of Dr. J. Jenkins)

### 12.3.2.1 Radiation

The majority of reports describing acute radiation hepatopathy in pediatric patients involve obsolete radiation technology and treatment approaches. Radiation-induced liver disease (RILD) typically presents in the first 12 weeks after completion of radiation and histologically demonstrates endothelial cell injury [61]. Persistent or late onset radiation hepatopathy after contemporary treatment is uncommon in the absence of other predisposing conditions, for example, viral hepatitis. The low frequency of hepatopathy after contemporary radiation suggests that the liver has the potential for complete resolution of acute hepatic injury, but this has not been confirmed in prospective studies in pediatrics.

In a Dutch cohort of long-term survivors of childhood cancer, radiotherapy involving the liver was an independent risk for increased ALT and GGT levels at a median of 12 years from therapy [62]. RILD has been studied in children with Wilms tumor, neuroblastoma, and rhabdomyosar-

coma [42, 55, 63–66]. The risk of injury increases with radiation dose, hepatic volume, younger age at treatment, prior partial hepatectomy, and concomitant receipt of radiomimetic chemotherapy like dactinomycin or doxorubicin. Extrapolating from adult data, the whole liver generally has good tolerance to radiation doses up to 30–35 Gy, delivered using conventional fractionation. Survivors who received $\geq 40$ Gy to at least one third liver volume, $\geq 30$ Gy to the whole abdomen, or an upper abdominal field involving the entire liver are at greatest risk for hepatic dysfunction [61]. However, smaller volumes of the liver may be safely irradiated to higher doses, accounting for the radiosensitizing effects of specific chemotherapies. While contemporary three-dimensional planning permits more accurate delivery of high-dose radiation to liver tumors with a promise of normal liver sparing, long-term liver function outcomes are not yet available.

Among survivors of HSCT, 75 % of children receiving 7–12 Gy total body irradiation (TBI) develop liver dysfunction and up to 25 % show signs of hepatic venoocclusive disease acutely. The relationship of acute injury to long-term liver toxicity is unclear as many HSCT patients do not survive severe acute liver toxicity. Given the many contributing factors to liver disease in transplant survivors, the contribution of TBI specifically is confounded.

### 12.3.2.2 Chemotherapy

Several chemotherapeutic agents used in the treatment of pediatric malignancies are associated with acute or subacute hepatotoxicity [67–69]. Unless there is an exacerbating condition like chronic hepatitis or GVHD, most children usually recover completely from acute hepatic injury related to chemotherapy [70–72].

The clinical features of acute methotrexate-induced hepatotoxicity are well described [73] and the transient elevations of serum transaminases, alkaline phosphatase, or lactate dehydrogenase; biochemical changes do not correlate with the severity or persistence of hepatic injury [74–77]. The incidence of long-term chemotherapy-associated hepatotoxicity appears to be low. Estimating prevalence is also confounded by varied means of defining hepatic dysfunction, ranging from various cutoffs on liver enzymes to inclusion of measure synthetic function [71]. The risk of fibrosis or cirrhosis after daily oral methotrexate is more than twofold the incidence observed after intermittent parenteral administration (less than 5 %) [78, 79]. As a consequence, this method of administering methotrexate has not been used in leukemia therapy for over 30 years. Studies evaluating hepatic histology in children treated with methotrexate demonstrated mild structural changes and a low incidence of portal fibrosis [74–76]. Delayed hepatotoxicity is not reported in osteosarcoma survivors, who receive shorter duration high-dose methotrexate, despite their elevated transaminases during therapy. These findings suggest that methotrexate-induced fibrosis regresses or stabilizes after discontinuation of the agent and rarely produces end-stage liver disease [76, 77].

The antimetabolites, 6-thioguanine and 6-mercaptopurine, are associated with subacute hepatocellular and cholestatic injury [80].

Genetic polymorphisms leading to deficiency in the enzyme thiopurine S-methyltransferase (TPMT) are associated with a rare complication of venoocclusive disease in children with leukemia on 6-thioguanine [81, 82]. While the majority of children with this complication recover clinically, a subset has progressive fibrosis and evolution to portal hypertension. Late liver dysfunction manifests as persistent hepatosplenomegaly and thrombocytopenia [81, 83–85].

The tyrosine kinase inhibitors and other targeted biologic agents (i.e., gemtuzumab ozogamicin, imatinib) have been associated with acute hepatic dysfunction; long-term data on liver outcomes in survivors is not yet available.

### 12.3.2.3 Hepatic Sinusoidal Obstruction Syndrome

Hepatic radiation and a variety of chemotherapeutic agents have been implicated in the causation of sinusoidal obstruction syndrome [SOS, formerly termed venoocclusive disease (VOD)]. Initially, SOS was attributed to the concomitant administration of hepatic radiation and radiosensitizing drugs like dactinomycin and doxorubicin [64, 86]. Subsequent investigations demonstrated that treatment with dactinomycin and vincristine chemotherapy alone could produce SOS [66, 87, 88]. In fact, several chemotherapeutic agents used in conventional dosing regimens have been associated with the development of SOS including dactinomycin, cytosine arabinoside, dacarbazine, 6-mercaptopurine, and 6-thioguanine. Myeloablative chemotherapy used in conditioning regimens before hematopoietic stem cell transplantation may also cause SOS. The most common agents in these cases are cyclophosphamide, carmustine, and busulfan. Whatever the cause, the clinical course described in most chemotherapy series is consistent with full recovery for the majority of children. In contrast, transplant-associated SOS has a high acute mortality, and information is lacking about long-term outcomes in that group.

### 12.3.2.4 Hematopoietic Stem Cell Transplant (HSCT)

Liver disease in long-term survivors of childhood cancer treated with bone marrow transplantation may result from chronic GVHD, chronic infection, sinusoidal obstruction syndrome, nodular regenerative hyperplasia from cytoreductive therapy, iron overload, or drug-related liver injury [14, 89]. Chronic GVHD is the most frequent late complication after allogeneic hematopoietic stem cell transplantation [90]. Approximately 80 % of individuals with chronic GVHD have liver involvement [91, 92]. Drug toxicity from immunosuppressive agents, antibiotics, antifungal and antiviral drugs, sedatives, antiemetics, and antipyretics may exacerbate chronic GVHD [14, 90]. Chronic infections, most commonly hepatitis C, may also accelerate the course of liver injury and result in cirrhosis (Fig. 12.6) [8, 16]. Siderosis, noted in approximately 90 % of long-term survivors of HSCT, may exacerbate the course of viral hepatitis [14, 93]. Reports documenting deaths from cirrhosis and hepatic failure suggest that chronic liver disease may predispose to early mortality in long-term survivors treated with allogeneic HSCT [8, 94].

### 12.3.2.5  Transfusion-Acquired Chronic Hepatitis

Childhood cancer survivors transfused before the introduction of effective screening measures for hepatitis B and C represent a significant population at risk for transfusion-acquired infectious hepatitis. Hepatitis B screening was implemented in 1971 in the United States. Hepatitis C screening by the first-generation enzyme immunoassay (EIA) was initiated in 1990; a more sensitive second-generation EIA became available in 1992. Transfusion-acquired viral hepatitis remains a significant risk in long-term survivors who received transfusions before donor screening was available. Although hepatitis B is characterized by an aggressive acute clinical course and a low rate of chronic infection ($\leq$10 %), the more mild and often asymptomatic acute infection with hepatitis C is associated with a high risk of chronic infection (approximates 80 %) (Fig. 12.6) [95]. Regardless of the etiology, survivors with chronic hepatitis experience significant morbidity and mortality related to cirrhosis, end-stage liver disease, and

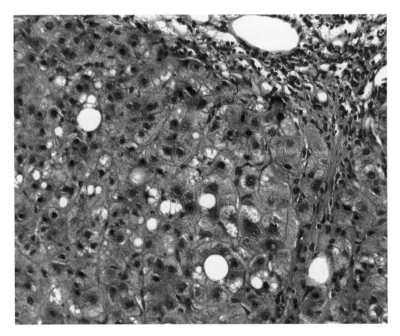

**Fig. 12.6** Regenerative liver nodule and portal triad in hepatitis C disease. Narrow bands of connective tissue separate small nodules of regenerative liver which shows fatty metamorphosis of some individual hepatocytes. The portal triad contains a dense lymphocytic infiltrate that in some cases may contain germinal centers. Hematoxylin and eosin stain, 20× original magnification (Courtesy of Dr. J. Jenkins)

hepatocellular carcinoma [10, 15, 58, 96, 97]. Coinfection with hepatitis B and C appears to accelerate the progression of liver disease as does the immunosuppression or hepatotoxicity associated with allogeneic HSCT [58, 74, 97, 98].

The prevalence of transfusion-related HCV infection (positive EIA or PCR) has ranged from 5 % to almost 50 % depending on the geographic location of the center [10, 15, 96, 97]. Among these, chronic infection is common, as evidenced by PCR detection of viral RNA ranging from 70 % to 100 % in cohorts studied [15, 99–101]. Most patients are asymptomatic, but laboratory evaluations of ALT are abnormal in 29–79 %. Chronically infected survivors of childhood cancer develop progressive fibrosis and cirrhosis at rates similar to adult cohorts with transfusion-acquired HCV cohorts or hemophiliacs coinfected with HIV and HBV [15, 102–104]. More aggressive chronic infection has also been observed in survivors coinfected with hepatitis B, on concomitant immunosuppression, or with hematopoietic stem cell transplantation-associated hepatotoxicity. Further longitudinal follow-up may more accurately define the long-term sequelae of transfusion-associated hepatitis C acquired during treatment of childhood cancer.

### 12.3.2.6   Other Late Hepatobiliary Complications

Less commonly reported hepatobiliary complications include cholelithiasis, focal nodular hyperplasia (FNH), nodular regenerative hyperplasia, and hepatic microvesicular fatty change and siderosis. The CCSS noted an almost twofold excess risk of gallbladder disease among survivors compared to sibs (1.9 95 % 1.7–2.2) [7]. In a single institution study including 6,050 childhood cancer patients, Mahmoud et al. reported a higher risk of biliary calculi in childhood cancer patients (median age, 12.4 years) without underlying chronic hemolytic anemia or preexisting history of gallstones before treatment compared to rates observed in the general population [105]. The cumulative risk of cholelithiasis was 0.42 % at 10 years and 1.03 % at 18 years after diagnosis. Treatment factors associated with an increased risk of cholelithiasis included a history of ileal

conduit (RR 61.6; 27.9–135.9), parenteral nutrition (RR 23.0; 9.8–54.1), abdominal surgery (RR 15.1; 7.1–32.2), and abdominal radiation (RR 7.4; 3.2–17.0). HSCT has also been associated with cholelithiasis [106]. The frequency of conventional predisposing factors like family history, obesity, oral contraceptive use, and pregnancy was not higher among study patients compared to rates observed in the general population.

Focal nodular hyperplasia (FNH) is often an incidental finding on imaging in childhood cancer survivors. Reports of FNH indicate presentation at 5–14 years from initial cancer diagnosis. FNH in childhood cancer survivors sometimes differs from that in the general population in presenting with multifocal smaller lesions, lacking the characteristic central scar [107, 108]. Recent reports of FNH include survivors of neuroblastoma and survivors with hepatic radiation exposure [109–112]. The pathogenesis of FNH is poorly understood, but is thought to be a reaction to a localized vascular anomaly. Others have speculated that FNH results from vascular injuries such as thrombosis, intimal hyperplasia, high sinusoidal pressures, or increased flow [113, 114]. High doses of alkylating agents (e.g., busulfan or melphalan), sinusoidal obstruction syndrome, and hepatic radiation may produce vascular injury and the subsequent localized circulatory disturbances. While FNH can mimic relapse of primary tumor or a subsequent malignant neoplasm, providers and survivors should be educated that FNH lesions rarely need intervention. The lesion is usually characterized noninvasively with specificity by MRI (Fig. 12.7) [115]. FNH is associated with infrequent complications and the absence of malignant transformation; hence, only close follow-up is recommended [108, 111, 116, 117].

Nodular regenerative hyperplasia (NRH) is a rare condition characterized by the development of multiple monoacinar regenerative hepatic nodules. The presence of mild fibrosis distinguishes NRH from FNH and cirrhosis. Like FNH, the pathogenesis of NRH is not well established, but may represent a nonspecific tissue adaptation to heterogeneous hepatic blood flow [118]. NRH

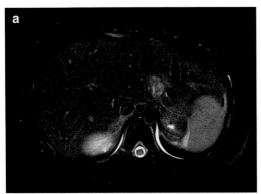

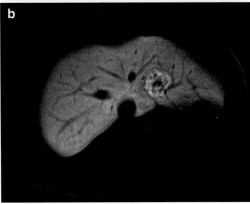

**Fig. 12.7** Focal nodular hyperplasia (FNH) in an 18-year-old patient treated with surgery, chemotherapy, 21.6 Gy to the left upper abdominal cavity, and autologous stem cell transplant for neuroblastoma at age 2 years. (**a**) Axial T2-weighted magnetic resonance imaging (MRI) with fat saturation shows the hyperintense mass in the left lobe of the liver. (**b**) On delayed phase imaging (obtained 30 min following the hepatobiliary MR contrast agent, gadoxetic acid disodium (Gd-EOB-DTPA)), the lesion retains contrast which is a specific sign for liver FNH (Courtesy of Dr. L. Golding)

has rarely been observed in survivors of childhood cancer treated with chemotherapy, with or without liver radiotherapy [119, 120]. Biopsy may be required to distinguish NRH from malignancy.

In a study of childhood leukemia, Finnish investigators described the results of liver biopsy in 27 patients who had recently completed intensified therapy for acute lymphoblastic leukemia. Fatty infiltration was detected in 93 % and siderosis in 70 % of patients; 52 % exhibited both histologic abnormalities [120, 121]. Fibrosis developed in 11 % and was associated with higher levels of serum LDL cholesterol.

Prospective studies are needed to show whether acute post-therapy liver fatty change after childhood leukemia contributes to the development of steatohepatitis or the metabolic syndrome characterized by obesity, glucose intolerance, and dyslipidemia and whether siderosis predisposes to more severe liver histopathology.

## 12.3.3 Detection and Screening

Screening of childhood cancer survivors treated with hepatotoxic chemotherapy and radiation therapy should begin with a thorough physical examination and history of health behaviors (Tables 12.1, 12.2, and 12.4) [69]. Physical findings suggesting liver dysfunction, e.g., spider angioma, palmar erythema, hepatomegaly, splenomegaly, icterus, or ascites, may be observed in individuals with long-standing liver dysfunction associated with significant hepatic fibrosis. Patients transfused with any blood product before implementation of blood donor testing for hepatitis B (1972) or C (1993) should been screened for viral hepatitis; PCR can establish the diagnosis of chronic infection (Table 12.4). COG Guidelines recommend screening based on year of diagnosis rather than transfusion history since transfusion status may be difficult to ascertain [122].

Since most childhood cancer survivors with hepatic dysfunction are asymptomatic, baseline screening of liver function with ALT, AST, and bilirubin should be performed beginning at 2 years after completion of therapy. Serum ferritin should also be checked in survivors of HSCT. Persistent liver dysfunction should prompt referral for GI/hepatic evaluation with liver biopsy. Individuals with abnormal screening or established chronic liver disease should undergo annual evaluations of hepatic synthetic function with a prothrombin time and albumin. Anemia and thrombocytopenia may be associated with complications related to portal hypertension including hypersplenism and variceal bleeding. Esophagogastroduodenoscopy is recommended to screen for varices in individuals with chronic liver dysfunction. A yearly serum

**Table 12.4** Transfusion-associated hepatic late effects

| Cancer treatment period | Late effect | Health screening and management[a] |
|---|---|---|
| Diagnosis prior to 1972[b] | Chronic hepatitis B infection | Hepatitis B surface antigen (HBsAg) Hepatitis B core antibody (anti-HBc or HBcAb) Gastroenterology or hepatic consultation for antiviral therapy |
| Diagnosis prior to 1993[b] | Chronic hepatitis C infection | Hepatitis C antibody Hepatitis C PCR (to establish chronic disease in patients with positive hepatitis C antibody or in immunosuppressed patient with negative hepatitis C antibody) Gastroenterology or hepatic consultation for antiviral therapy |
| High-volume transfusion history (e.g., hematopoietic stem cell transplant recipient) during any period | Iron overload | AST, ALT, bilirubin, ferritin baseline at entry into long-term follow-up, then as clinically indicated MRI or liver biopsy for liver iron quantification for those with persistently abnormal liver function Phlebotomy or chelation therapy |

[a]All patients with risk by means of exposure to hepatotoxins should be counseled with regard to receiving the hepatitis A and B vaccine

[b]The Children's Oncology Group Guidelines recommend screening based on year of diagnosis rather than transfusion history since a high proportion of survivors and non-oncology providers are unaware of transfusion status

alpha fetoprotein level and hepatic ultrasound should be obtained in patients with established cirrhosis to monitor for neoplastic complications (e.g., adenoma or hepatocellular carcinoma).

### 12.3.4 Management

Therapy is not available to reverse hepatic fibrosis induced by antineoplastic therapy or chronic viral infection. Enhancing health literacy to minimize further hepatic injury is therefore critical for childhood cancer survivors, most of whom were exposed to hepatotoxic therapy. Mulder et al. found that higher BMI z-score and alcohol intake of >14 units per week were independent risks for persistent elevation of transaminases and/or GGT [62]. Standard recommendations should include abstinence or minimal alcohol use, particularly the avoidance of binge drinking. Avoidance of obesity is recommended, as it is a known risk factor for nonalcoholic steatohepatitis (NASH). Immunization against hepatitis A

and B should be encouraged in patients who have not established immunity to these hepatotropic viruses (Tables 12.2 and 12.4). Careful attention of survivors and providers should be directed to prescription and nonprescription drugs and herbal and supplement use that may exacerbate liver injury (http://www.hepfi.org/living). Survivors should also receive counseling about precautions to reduce viral transmission to household and sexual contacts. Patients with persistent liver dysfunction associated with chronic viral hepatitis may benefit from antiviral therapy. Consultation with GI/hepatology subspecialists will facilitate access to optimal antiviral therapies. Treatment is standardly preceded by a liver biopsy to define the etiology and histopathological features of the liver injury.

Treatment of established fibrosis is largely symptomatic. Patients with cirrhosis may remain asymptomatic for many years. Portal hypertension and GI bleeding from varices may herald the onset of decompensated cirrhosis. Treatment with beta-blockers may significantly reduce the incidence of variceal bleeding [123,

124]. Eventually, hepatic failure is manifest as jaundice, hepatic encephalopathy, hypoproteinemia, progressive ascites, and coagulopathy. Supportive care in end-stage liver disease includes a low-protein diet with lactulose and neomycin to minimize urea production, blood and plasma products to replete albumin and coagulation proteins, salt restriction and diuretics to prevent ascites formation, and sclerotherapy or vascular shunting to reduce portal pressure and prohibit variceal bleeding. Liver transplantation is the only definite and lifesaving treatment for patients with presenting with decompensated cirrhosis.

# References

1. Donaldson SS, Jundt S, Ricour C et al (1975) Radiation enteritis in children. A retrospective review, clinicopathologic correlation, and dietary management. Cancer 35:1167–1178
2. Spunt SL, Sweeney TA, Hudson MM et al (2005) Late effects of pelvic rhabdomyosarcoma and its treatment in female survivors. J Clin Oncol 23:7143–7151
3. Heyn R, Raney RB Jr, Hays DM et al (1992) Late effects of therapy in patients with paratesticular rhabdomyosarcoma. Intergroup Rhabdomyosarcoma Study Committee. J Clin Oncol 10:614–623
4. Mahboubi S, Silber JH (1997) Radiation-induced esophageal strictures in children with cancer. Eur Radiol 7:119–122
5. Raney B Jr, Heyn R, Hays DM et al (1993) Sequelae of treatment in 109 patients followed for 5 to 15 years after diagnosis of sarcoma of the bladder and prostate. A report from the Intergroup Rhabdomyosarcoma Study Committee. Cancer 71:2387–2394
6. Papazian A, Capron JP, Ducroix JP et al (1983) Mucosal bridges of the upper esophagus after radiotherapy for Hodgkin's disease. Gastroenterology 84:1028–1031
7. Goldsby R, Chen Y, Raber S et al (2011) Survivors of childhood cancer have increased risk of gastrointestinal complications later in life. Gastroenterology 140:1464–1471.e1
8. Socie G, Stone JV, Wingard JR et al (1999) Long-term survival and late deaths after allogeneic bone marrow transplantation. Late Effects Working Committee of the International Bone Marrow Transplant Registry. N Engl J Med 341:14–21
9. Strickland DK, Riely CA, Patrick CC et al (2000) Hepatitis C infection among survivors of childhood cancer. Blood 95:3065–3070
10. Cesaro S, Bortolotti F, Petris MG et al (2010) An updated follow-up of chronic hepatitis C after three decades of observation in pediatric patients cured of malignancy. Pediatr Blood Cancer 55:108–112
11. Locasciulli A, Testa M, Valsecchi MG et al (1997) Morbidity and mortality due to liver disease in children undergoing allogeneic bone marrow transplantation: a 10-year prospective study. Blood 90:3799–3805
12. Locasciulli A, Bacigalupo A, Van Lint MT et al (1990) Hepatitis B virus (HBV) infection and liver disease after allogeneic bone marrow transplantation: a report of 30 cases. Bone Marrow Transplant 6:25–29
13. Knapp AB, Crawford J, Rappeport JM, Gollan JL (1987) Cirrhosis as a consequence of graft versus host disease. Gastroenterology 92:513–519
14. McDonald GB (2010) Hepatobiliary complications of hematopoietic cell transplantation, 40 years on. Hepatology 51:1450–1460
15. Castellino S, Lensing S, Riely C et al (2004) The epidemiology of chronic hepatitis C infection in survivors of childhood cancer: an update of the St Jude Children's Research Hospital hepatitis C seropositive cohort. Blood 103:2460–2466
16. Strasser SI, Sullivan KM, Myerson D et al (1999) Cirrhosis of the liver in long-term marrow transplant survivors. Blood 93:3259–3266
17. Bolling T, Willich N, Ernst I (2010) Late effects of abdominal irradiation in children: a review of the literature. Anticancer Res 30:227–231
18. Fajardo L (1989) Radiation-induced pathology of the alimentary tract. In: Whitehead R (ed) Gastrointestinal and oesophageal pathology. Churchill Livingstone, Edinburgh
19. Shulman H (1990) Pathology of chronic graft-vs.-host disease. In: Burakoff S (ed) Graft-vs-host disease immunology, pathophysiology and treatment. Marcel Dekker, New York
20. Henderson TO, Oeffinger KC, Whitton J et al (2012) Secondary gastrointestinal cancer in childhood cancer survivors: a cohort study. Ann Intern Med 156:757–766, W-260
21. Nottage K, McFarlane J, Krasin MJ et al (2012) Secondary colorectal carcinoma after childhood cancer. J Clin Oncol 30:2552–2558
22. Tukenova M, Diallo I, Anderson H et al (2012) Second malignant neoplasms in digestive organs after childhood cancer: a cohort-nested case-control study. Int J Radiat Oncol Biol Phys 82:e383–e390
23. Bhatia S, Yasui Y, Robison LL et al (2003) High risk of subsequent neoplasms continues with extended follow-up of childhood Hodgkin's disease: report from the Late Effects Study Group. J Clin Oncol 21:4386–4394
24. Roswit B (1974) Complications of radiation therapy: the alimentary tract. Semin Roentgenol 9:51–63
25. Berthrong M, Fajardo LF (1981) Radiation injury in surgical pathology. Part II. Alimentary tract. Am J Surg Pathol 5:153–178
26. Kavanagh BD, Pan CC, Dawson LA et al (2010) Radiation dose-volume effects in the stomach and

small bowel. Int J Radiat Oncol Biol Phys 76:S101–S107

27. Rodriguez ML, Martin MM, Padellano LC et al (2010) Gastrointestinal toxicity associated to radiation therapy. Clin Transl Oncol 12:554–561

28. Emami B, Lyman J, Brown A et al (1991) Tolerance of normal tissue to therapeutic irradiation. Int J Radiat Oncol Biol Phys 21:109–122

29. Hughes LL, Baruzzi MJ, Ribeiro RC et al (1994) Paratesticular rhabdomyosarcoma: delayed effects of multimodality therapy and implications for current management. Cancer 73:476–482

30. Hale GA, Marina NM, Jones-Wallace D et al (1999) Late effects of treatment for germ cell tumors during childhood and adolescence. J Pediatr Hematol Oncol 21:115–122

31. Donaldson SS, Glatstein E, Rosenberg SA et al (1976) Pediatric Hodgkin's disease. II. Results of therapy. Cancer 37:2436–2447

32. Chao N, Levine J, Horning SJ (1987) Retroperitoneal fibrosis following treatment for Hodgkin's disease. J Clin Oncol 5:231–232

33. Lal DR, Foroutan HR, Su WT et al (2006) The management of treatment-related esophageal complications in children and adolescents with cancer. J Pediatr Surg 41:495–499

34. Seaman WB, Ackerman LV (1957) The effect of radiation on the esophagus; a clinical and histologic study of the effects produced by the betatron. Radiology 68:534–541

35. Lepke RA, Libshitz HI (1983) Radiation-induced injury of the esophagus. Radiology 148:375–378

36. Goldstein HM, Rogers LF, Fletcher GH et al (1975) Radiological manifestations of radiation-induced injury to the normal upper gastrointestinal tract. Radiology 117:135–140

37. Simson JN, Kinder RB, Isaacs PE et al (1985) Mucosal bridges of the oesophagus in Candida oesophagitis. Br J Surg 72:209–210

38. Kelly K, Storey L, O' Sullivan L et al (2010) Esophageal strictures during treatment for acute lymphoblastic leukemia. J Pediatr Hematol Oncol 32:124–127

39. Horwich A, Lokich JJ, Bloomer WD (1975) Doxorubicin, radiotherapy, and oesophageal stricture. Lancet 2:561–562

40. Newburger PE, Cassady JR, Jaffe N (1978) Esophagitis due to adriamycin and radiation therapy for childhood malignancy. Cancer 42:417–423

41. Boal DK, Newburger PE, Teele RL (1979) Esophagitis induced by combined radiation and adriamycin. AJR Am J Roentgenol 132:567–570

42. Tefft M, Lattin PB, Jereb B et al (1976) Acute and late effects on normal tissues following combined chemo- and radiotherapy for childhood rhabdomyosarcoma and Ewing's sarcoma. Cancer 37:1201–1217

43. Meyers PA, Potter VP, Wollner N et al (1985) Bowel perforation during initial treatment for childhood non-Hodgkin's lymphoma. Cancer 56:259–261

44. Ritchey ML, Kelalis PP, Breslow N et al (1992) Surgical complications after nephrectomy for Wilms' tumor. Surg Gynecol Obstet 175:507–514

45. Jockovich M, Mendenhall NP, Sombeck MD et al (1994) Long-term complications of laparotomy in Hodgkin's disease. Ann Surg 219:615–621; discussion 621–624

46. Hays DM, Ternberg JL, Chen TT et al (1984) Complications related to 234 staging laparotomies performed in the Intergroup Hodgkin's Disease in Childhood study. Surgery 96:471–478

47. Zinchke H, Segura JW (1975) Ureterosigmoidostomy: critical review of 173 cases. J Urol 113:324–327

48. Gittes RF (1986) Carcinogenesis in ureterosigmoidostomy. Urol Clin North Am 13:201–205

49. Deeg HJ, Storb R, Thomas ED (1984) Bone marrow transplantation: a review of delayed complications. Br J Haematol 57:185–208

50. McDonald GB, Sullivan KM, Plumley TF (1984) Radiographic features of esophageal involvement in chronic graft-vs.-host disease. AJR Am J Roentgenol 142:501–506

51. McDonald GB, Sullivan KM, Schuffler MD et al (1981) Esophageal abnormalities in chronic graft-versus-host disease in humans. Gastroenterology 80:914–921

52. Smith RA, Brooks D, Cokkinides V et al (2013) Cancer screening in the United States, 2013: a review of current American Cancer Society guidelines, current issues in cancer screening, and new guidance on cervical cancer screening and lung cancer screening. CA Cancer J Clin 63:88–105

53. Landier W, Bhatia S, Eshelman DA et al (2004) Development of risk-based guidelines for pediatric cancer survivors: the Children's Oncology Group Long-Term Follow-Up Guidelines from the Children's Oncology Group Late Effects Committee and Nursing Discipline. J Clin Oncol 22:4979–4990

54. Schiavetti A, Di Nardo G, Ingrosso A et al (2011) Barrett esophagus in long-term survivors of childhood solid tumors. J Pediatr Hematol Oncol 33:559–561

55. Jirtle RL, Anscher M, Alati T (1990) Radiation sensitivity of the liver. Adv Radiat Biol 14:269–311

56. Patrick RS, McGee JOD (1980) Biopsy pathology of the liver. Chapman Hall, Ltd, London

57. Tsoi MS, Storb R, Jones E et al (1978) Deposition of IgM and complement at the dermoepidermal junction in acute and chronic cutaneous graft-vs-host disease in man. J Immunol 120:1485–1492

58. Strickland DK, Jenkins JJ, Hudson MM (2001) Hepatitis C infection and hepatocellular carcinoma after treatment of childhood cancer. J Pediatr Hematol Oncol 23:527–529

59. Blatt J, Olshan A, Gula MJ et al (1992) Second malignancies in very-long-term survivors of childhood cancer. Am J Med 93:57–60

60. Bassal M, Mertens AC, Taylor L et al (2006) Risk of selected subsequent carcinomas in survivors of

childhood cancer: a report from the Childhood
Cancer Survivor Study. J Clin Oncol 24:476–483

61. Pan CC, Kavanagh BD, Dawson LA et al (2010)
Radiation-associated liver injury. Int J Radiat Oncol
Biol Phys 76:S94–S100

62. Mulder RL, Kremer LC, Koot BG et al (2013)
Surveillance of hepatic late adverse effects in a large
cohort of long-term survivors of childhood cancer:
prevalence and risk factors. Eur J Cancer
49:185–193

63. Tefft M (1977) Radiation related toxicities in
National Wilms' Tumor Study number 1. Int J Radiat
Oncol Biol Phys 2:455–463

64. Kun LE, Camitta BM (1978) Hepatopathy following
irradiation and adriamycin. Cancer 42:81–84

65. Bhanot P, Cushing B, Philippart A et al (1979)
Hepatic irradiation and adriamycin cardiotoxicity. J
Pediatr 95:561–563

66. Flentje M, Weirich A, Potter R et al (1994)
Hepatotoxicity in irradiated nephroblastoma patients
during postoperative treatment according to SIOP9/
GPOH. Radiother Oncol 31:222–228

67. Field KM, Michael M (2008) Part II: liver function
in oncology: towards safer chemotherapy use.
Lancet Oncol 9:1181–1190

68. Perry M (1992) Chemotherapeutic agents and hepatotoxicity. Semin Oncol 19:551–565

69. Castellino S, Muir A, Shah A et al (2010) Hepatobiliary late effects in survivors of childhood and adolescent cancer: a report from the Children's
Oncology Group. Pediatr Blood Cancer 54:663–669

70. Locasciulli A, Vergani GM, Uderzo C et al (1983)
Chronic liver disease in children with leukemia in
long-term remission. Cancer 52:1080–1087

71. Mulder RL, van Dalen EC, Van den Hof M et al
(2011) Hepatic late adverse effects after antineoplastic treatment for childhood cancer. Cochrane
Database Syst Rev (7):CD008205

72. Bessho F, Kinumaki H, Yokota S et al (1994) Liver
function studies in children with acute lymphocytic
leukemia after cessation of therapy. Med Pediatr
Oncol 23:111–115

73. Nesbit M, Krivit W, Heyn R et al (1976) Acute and
chronic effects of methotrexate on hepatic, pulmonary, and skeletal systems. Cancer 37:1048–1057

74. Parker D, Bate CM, Craft AW et al (1980) Liver
damage in children with acute leukaemia and non-
Hodgkin's lymphoma on oral maintenance chemotherapy. Cancer Chemother Pharmacol 4:121–127

75. McIntosh S, Davidson D, O'Brien RT, Pearson HA
(1977) Methotrexate hepatotoxicity in children with
leukemia. J Pediatr 90:1019–1021

76. Topley JM, Benson J, Squier MV, Chessells JM
(1979) Hepatotoxicity in the treatment of acute lymphoblastic leukemia. Med Pediatr Oncol 7:393–399

77. Locasciulli A, Mura R, Fraschini D et al (1992)
High-dose methotrexate administration and acute
liver damage in children treated for acute lymphoblastic leukemia. A prospective study. Haematologica
77:49–53

78. Hutter RVP, Shipkey F, Tan CTC, Murphy ML,
Chowdhury M (1960) Hepatic fibrosis in children
with acute leukemia: a complication of therapy.
Cancer 13:288–307

79. Colsky J, Greenspan E, Warren TN (1955) Hepatic
fibrosis in children with acute leukemia after therapy
with folic acid antagonists. Arch Pathol Lab Med
59:198–206

80. Stork LC, Matloub Y, Broxson E et al (2010) Oral
6-mercaptopurine versus oral 6-thioguanine and
veno-occlusive disease in children with standard-
risk acute lymphoblastic leukemia: report of the
Children's Oncology Group CCG-1952 clinical trial.
Blood 115:2740–2748

81. De Bruyne R, Portmann B, Samyn M et al (2006)
Chronic liver disease related to 6-thioguanine in
children with acute lymphoblastic leukaemia. J
Hepatol 44:407–410, Epub 2005

82. Lennard L, Richards S, Cartwright CS et al (2006)
The thiopurine methyltransferase genetic polymorphism is associated with thioguanine-related
veno-occlusive disease of the liver in children with
acute lymphoblastic leukemia. Clin Pharmacol
Ther 80:375–383

83. Broxson EH, Dole M, Wong R et al (2005) Portal
hypertension develops in a subset of children with
standard risk acute lymphoblastic leukemia treated
with oral 6-thioguanine during maintenance therapy.
Pediatr Blood Cancer 44:226–231

84. Piel B, Vaidya S, Lancaster D et al (2004) Chronic
hepatotoxicity following 6-thioguanine therapy for
childhood acute lymphoblastic leukaemia. Br J
Haematol 125:410–411; author reply 412

85. Rawat D, Gillett PM, Devadason D et al (2011)
Long-term follow-up of children with
6-thioguanine-related chronic hepatoxicity following treatment for acute lymphoblastic leukaemia. J
Pediatr Gastroenterol Nutr 53:478–479

86. Johnson FL, Balis F (1982) Hepatopathy following
irradiation and chemotherapy for Wilms' tumor. Am
J Pediatr Hematol Oncol 4:217–221

87. Green DM, Norkool P, Breslow NE et al (1990)
Severe hepatic toxicity after treatment with vincristine and dactinomycin using single-dose or divided-
dose schedules: a report from the National Wilms'
Tumor Study. J Clin Oncol 8:1525–1530

88. Raine J, Bowman A, Wallendszus K et al (1991)
Hepatopathy-thrombocytopenia syndrome–a complication of dactinomycin therapy for Wilms' tumor:
a report from the United Kingdom Childrens Cancer
Study Group. J Clin Oncol 9:268–273

89. Farthing MJG, Clark M, Sloane JP (1982) Liver disease after bone marrow transplantation. Gut
23:465–474

90. Zecca M, Prete A, Rondelli R et al (2002) Chronic graft-
versus-host disease in children: incidence, risk factors,
and impact on outcome. Blood 100:1192–1200

91. Fisher VL (1999) Long-term follow-up in hematopoietic stem-cell transplant patients. Pediatr
Transplant 3(Suppl 1):122–129

92. Sullivan KM, Agura E, Anasetti C et al (1991) Chronic graft-versus-host disease and other late complications of bone marrow transplantation. Semin Hematol 28:250–259

93. McKay PJ, Murphy JA, Cameron S et al (1996) Iron overload and liver dysfunction after allogeneic or autologous bone marrow transplantation. Bone Marrow Transplant 17:63–66

94. Yau JC, Zander AR, Srigley JR et al (1986) Chronic graft-versus-host disease complicated by micronodular cirrhosis and esophageal varices. Transplantation 41:129–130

95. Centers for Disease Control and Prevention (1998) Recommendations for prevention and control of hepatitis C virus (HCV) infection and HCV-related chronic disease. MMWR 47(19):1–39

96. Locasciulli A, Testa M, Pontisso P et al (1997) Prevalence and natural history of hepatitis C infection in patients cured of childhood leukemia. Blood 90:4628–4633

97. Paul IM, Sanders J, Ruggiero F et al (1999) Chronic hepatitis C virus infections in leukemia survivors: prevalence, viral load, and severity of liver disease. Blood 93:3672–3677

98. Locasciulli A, Bacigalupo A, Vanlint MT et al (1991) Hepatitis C virus infection in patients undergoing allogeneic bone marrow transplantation. Transplantation 52:315–318

99. Fink FM, Hocker-Schulz S, Mor W et al (1993) Association of hepatitis C virus infection with chronic liver disease in paediatric cancer patients. Eur J Pediatr 152:490–492

100. Arico M, Maggiore G, Silini E et al (1994) Hepatitis C virus infection in children treated for acute lymphoblastic leukemia. Blood 84:2919–2922

101. Cesaro S, Petris MG, Rossetti F et al (1997) Chronic hepatitis C virus infection after treatment for pediatric malignancy. Blood 90:1315–1320

102. Goedert JJ, Eyster ME, Lederman MM et al (2002) End-stage liver disease in persons with hemophilia and transfusion-associated infections. Blood 100:1584–1589

103. Franchini M, Rossetti G, Tagliaferri A et al (2001) The natural history of chronic hepatitis C in a cohort of HIV-negative Italian patients with hereditary bleeding disorders. Blood 98:1836–1841

104. Liang TJ, Rehermann B, Seeff LB et al (2000) Pathogenesis, natural history, treatment, and prevention of hepatitis C. Ann Intern Med 132:296–305

105. Mahmoud H, Schell M, Pui CH (1991) Cholelithiasis after treatment for childhood cancer. Cancer 67:1439–1442

106. Safford SD, Safford KM, Martin P et al (2001) Management of cholelithiasis in pediatric patients who undergo bone marrow transplantation. J Pediatr Surg 36:86–90

107. Do RK, Shaylor SD, Shia J et al (2011) Variable MR imaging appearances of focal nodular hyperplasia in pediatric cancer patients. Pediatr Radiol 41:335–340

108. Gobbi D, Dall'Igna P, Messina C et al (2010) Focal nodular hyperplasia in pediatric patients with and without oncologic history. Pediatr Blood Cancer 55:1420–1422

109. Benz-Bohm G, Hero B, Gossmann A et al (2010) Focal nodular hyperplasia of the liver in longterm survivors of neuroblastoma: how much diagnostic imaging is necessary? Eur J Radiol 74:e1–e5

110. Towbin AJ, Luo GG, Yin H et al (2011) Focal nodular hyperplasia in children, adolescents, and young adults. Pediatr Radiol 41:341–349

111. Sugito K, Uekusa S, Kawashima H et al (2011) The clinical course in pediatric solid tumor patients with focal nodular hyperplasia of the liver. Int J Clin Oncol 16:482–487

112. Bouyn CI, Leclere J, Raimondo G et al (2003) Hepatic focal nodular hyperplasia in children previously treated for a solid tumor. Incidence, risk factors, and outcome. Cancer 97:3107–3113

113. Kumagai H, Masuda T, Oikawa H et al (2000) Focal nodular hyperplasia of the liver: direct evidence of circulatory disturbances. J Gastroenterol Hepatol 15:1344–1347

114. Wanless IR, Albrecht S, Bilbao J et al (1989) Multiple focal nodular hyperplasia of the liver associated with vascular malformations of various organs and neoplasia of the brain: a new syndrome. Mod Pathol 2:456–462

115. Choi JY, Lee HC, Yim JH et al (2011) Focal nodular hyperplasia or focal nodular hyperplasia-like lesions of the liver: a special emphasis on diagnosis. J Gastroenterol Hepatol 26:1004–1009

116. Grazioli L, Bondioni MP, Haradome H et al (2012) Hepatocellular adenoma and focal nodular hyperplasia: value of gadoxetic acid-enhanced MR imaging in differential diagnosis. Radiology 262:520–529

117. Masetti R, Biagi C, Kleinschmidt K et al (2011) Focal nodular hyperplasia of the liver after intensive treatment for pediatric cancer: is hematopoietic stem cell transplantation a risk factor? Eur J Pediatr 170:807–812

118. Wanless IR (1990) Micronodular transformation (nodular regenerative hyperplasia) of the liver: a report of 64 cases among 2,500 autopsies and a new classification of benign hepatocellular nodules. Hepatology 11:787–797

119. Chu WC, Roebuck DJ (2003) Nodular regenerative hyperplasia of the liver simulating metastases following treatment for bilateral Wilms tumor. Med Pediatr Oncol 41:85–87

120. Halonen P, Mattila J, Ruuska T et al (2003) Liver histology after current intensified therapy for childhood acute lymphoblastic leukemia: microvesicular fatty change and siderosis are the main findings. Med Pediatr Oncol 40:148–154

121. Halonen P, Mattila J, Suominen P et al (2003) Iron overload in children who are treated for acute lymphoblastic leukemia estimated by liver siderosis and serum iron parameters. Pediatrics 111:91–96

122. Lansdale M, Castellino S, Marina N et al (2010) Knowledge of hepatitis C virus screening in long-term pediatric cancer survivors: a report from the Childhood Cancer Survivor Study. Cancer 116:974–982

123. Bernard B, Lebrec D, Mathurin P et al (1997) Propranolol and sclerotherapy in the prevention of gastrointestinal rebleeding in patients with cirrhosis: a meta-analysis. J Hepatol 26:312–324

124. Bernard B, Lebrec D, Mathurin P et al (1997) Beta-adrenergic antagonists in the prevention of gastrointestinal rebleeding in patients with cirrhosis: a meta-analysis. Hepatology 25:63–70

# The Ovary

# 13

Debra L. Friedman

## Contents

D.L. Friedman, MD
Division of Pediatric Hematology/Oncology,
Vanderbilt University School of Medicine,
2220 Pierce Avenue 397 PRB, Nashville, TN
37232-6310, USA
e-mail: debra.l.friedman@vanderbilt.edu

## 13.1 Pathophysiology

### 13.1.1 Normal Organ Development

Hormonal function and potential for fertility are synchronous in females, as the ovary both produces oocytes and secretes steroid hormones. Prepubertal females possess their lifetime supply of oocytes with no new oogonia formed after birth. Active mitosis of oogonia occurs during fetal life, reaching a peak of six to seven million by 20 weeks of gestation and then rapidly declining to one to two million at birth. At the onset of puberty, only 300,000 remain [1]. The cortices of the ovaries harbor the follicles within connective tissue. These follicles arise from the germinal epithelium, which covers the free surface of the ovary. Through involution, atresia, and, to a much lesser extent, ovulation, the follicles disappear entirely at menopause.

At initiation of puberty, there is a surge in the production of gonadotropin-releasing hormone (GnRH) by the hypothalamus. GnRH then stimulates release of the gonadotropins by the pituitary gland: follicle-stimulating hormone (FSH), responsible for follicular maturation, and luteinizing hormone (LH), responsible for ovarian luteinization. With menarche, the menstrual cycle occurs approximately every 28 days. Each cycle is marked by an estrogen-dependent mid-cycle surge of FSH and LH. After ovulation, the corpus luteum forms and produces progesterone,

© Springer International Publishing 2015
C.L. Schwartz et al. (eds.), *Survivors of Childhood and Adolescent Cancer:
A Multidisciplinary Approach*, Pediatric Oncology, DOI 10.1007/978-3-319-16435-9_13

estradiol, and 17-hydroxyprogesterone, as well as the endometrial changes required for implantation of a fetus. In the absence of fertilization, there is no chorionic gonadotropin from a conceptus; the corpus luteum becomes exhausted and progesterone and estrogen falls. At this time, FSH increases and the endometrium sloughs, resulting in menstruation. The normal premenopausal ovary contains degenerating ova and follicles in varying stages of maturity. Another ovarian hormone now being investigated in the field of reproductive endocrinology is anti-Mullerian hormone (AMH) thought to be the most sensitive indicator of ovarian reserve [2].

Ovarian hormones also have critical physiologic effects on other organs and bodily processes, including the stimulation of libido, the maturation and function of the breasts and vagina, bone mineralization, and the integrity of the cardiovascular system. With depletion of oocytes by radiotherapy, chemotherapy, or normal senescence, the ovaries undergo atresia. As a result, menstruation and estrogen production cease, and menopause ensues.

## 13.1.2 Organ Damage Induced by Cytotoxic Therapy

Radiotherapy and chemotherapy each may cause transitory or permanent effects on hormonal function, reproductive capacity, and sexual function. Primary ovarian failure, impaired development of secondary sexual characteristics, menstrual irregularities, including oligomenorrhea and amenorrhea, or premature menopause may occur. The menopausal state, when it occurs prematurely, is associated with the same physical symptoms as are seen with normal aging, including hot flashes, loss of libido, and osteoporosis [3, 4]. Such effects are not simply physically bothersome to survivors, but adversely impact their quality of life [5]. The specific effects are dependent on the ovarian dose of radiation and the chemotherapeutic

agents and their doses. They also depend on the developmental status of the patient at the age of treatment.

## 13.1.3 Cytotoxic Effects of Radiotherapy

Radiation causes a decrease in the number of ovarian follicles, impaired follicular maturation, cortical fibrosis and atrophy, generalized hypoplasia, and hyalinization of the capsule. Females treated prior to puberty have a greater number of ova than do older women. Thus, ovarian function is more likely to be preserved after radiotherapy in prepubertal females, compared with postpubertal females [6]. The dose of radiation that will ablate ovarian function depends on the patient's age and, by implication, stage of sexual development, but overall modeling suggests that the dose of radiation required to destroy 50 % of immature oocytes is <2 Gy [7].

Several investigators have provided information regarding the dose of radiotherapy that results in sterility in women of varying ages. Wallace and colleagues reported on 19 adult females treated in childhood with whole abdominal radiotherapy to a total dose of 30 Gy. Using the assumption that the number of oocytes within the ovary declines exponentially by atresia from approximately 2,000,000 at birth to approximately 2,000 at menopause, they were able to estimate that the LD50 (radiation causing ablation in 50 % of patients) for the human oocyte is not greater than 4 Gy [8]. Ash's summary of clinical information on radiation to the human ovary is shown in Table 13.1. Menopause was induced by a dose of 12–15 Gy in women under 40 years of age, whereas women over 40 years of age required only 4–7 Gy for the same clinical effect. Permanent sterility occurred in 60 % of females 15–40 years of age receiving 5–6 Gy [9]. When one considers doses to the ovary after single fractions, temporary sterility can occur with ovarian doses of 1.7–6.4 Gy and permanent sterility after doses of 3.2–10 Gy [10]. Whole

**Table 13.1** Effect of fractionated ovarian X-irradiation on ovarian function in women of reproductive age irradiated for malignant or nonmalignant disease

| Minimum ovarian dose (GY) | Effect |
|---|---|
| 0.6 | None |
| 1.5 | No deleterious effect in most young women. Some risk of sterilization especially in women aged >40 |
| 2.5–5.0 | Variable. Aged 15–40 years: about 60 % sterilized permanently, some with temporary amenorrhea. Aged >40: usually 100 % permanently sterile |
| 5–8 | Variable. Aged 15–40 years: about 70 % sterilized permanently; of the remainder, some temporary amenorrhea |
| >8 | 100 % permanently sterilized |

Modified from [7]

No attempt has been made to allow for variation in mode of fractionation

abdomen doses of 20–30 Gy are associated with primary or premature secondary ovarian failure in young females [8, 11].

## 13.1.4  Cytotoxic Effects of Chemotherapy

The effects of chemotherapy on ovarian function are both agent- and dose-dependent, and this effect may be additive to that resulting from abdominopelvic radiotherapy. Alkylating agents affect the resting oocyte in a dose-dependent, cell cycle-independent manner. Thecal cells and ova are depleted, as are the primordial follicles, resulting in arrest of follicular maturation and decreased estrogen secretion. Again, as was the case with radiotherapy, the effects are more pronounced in postpubertal as compared with prepubertal females, due to the fact that postpubertal females have fewer remaining viable oocytes. The effects worsen with age, as the normal aging process is accompanied by an ongoing depletion of oocytes. Risks of menstrual irregularity,

ovarian failure, and infertility increase with age at treatments. Conversely, younger females can tolerate higher doses of alkylating agents without impairment of fertility, compared with adult females [12–17].

## 13.2  Clinical Manifestations

### 13.2.1  Effects of Radiotherapy on Ovarian Function

The clinical relationship between ovarian failure and the dose of radiation to the ovary is well illustrated by Stillman's study of 182 girls treated at less than 17 years of age with 12–15 Gy of abdominal radiotherapy. Overall, primary ovarian failure occurred in 22 girls (12 %). However, ovarian failure was noted in 68 % of the girls whose ovaries received the full irradiation dose, but in only 14 % of those who had at least one ovary at the edge of the abdominal treatment volume (estimated dose 0.9–10 Gy, with a mean of 2.9 Gy). Conversely, none of 34 girls who received an estimated ovarian dose of 0.5–1.5 Gy (mean: 0.54 Gy) to at least one ovary outside the direct treatment volume had ovarian failure. Covariate and multivariate revealed that the location of the ovaries relative to radiation treatment fields was the only risk factor for ovarian failure [18].

In considering the risk of ovarian failure related to radiotherapy, other fields than the abdomen and pelvis must be considered. Direct or scattered irradiation from the spinal component of craniospinal radiotherapy may also produce ovarian damage [8, 19]. With the expanded use of hematopoietic stem cell transplantation in pediatric oncology, it is important to recall that total body irradiation (TBI) utilized in the conditioning regimen is commonly associated with primary ovarian failure or premature menopause, with prevalence rates as high as 90–100 %. Fraction size is of importance as well as the age of the patient at the time of radiotherapy [20–24].

## 13.2.2 Effects of Chemotherapy on Ovarian Function

The dose–response relationship of alkylating agents, and the effect of age, is a recurring theme in studies of fertility following chemotherapy. Amenorrhea and ovarian failure occur more commonly in adult women treated with cyclophosphamide and other alkylating agents than with adolescents, with prepubertal females tolerating cumulative cyclophosphamide doses as high as 25 g/m$^2$ [13, 25]. In examining protocols with common chemotherapy, 86 % of women >24–30 years have been shown to have ovarian failure, compared with 28–31 % of younger women [3, 25].

It is clear that the sterilizing effects of all alkylating agents are not equal. Mechlorethamine and procarbazine together are perhaps the most damaging of the alkylating agents. These chemotherapy agents were used in the past together for the treatment of Hodgkin lymphoma, often in combination with radiotherapy, resulting in impaired fertility, among other adverse long-term effects [26]. Newer risk-adapted protocols for Hodgkin lymphoma have been developed to avoid mechlorethamine or procarbazine and to limit cumulative doses of other gonadotoxic alkylating agents, without negatively impacting the efficacy of the chemotherapy regimens [27–30].

Newer studies have also been designed to collect long-term follow-up data, and investigators are starting to collect data on the impact of these changes.

In recent years, ifosfamide, a congener of cyclophosphamide, has been used for a variety of solid tumors and lymphoma. The effects of ifosfamide on reproductive function are only beginning to be evaluated. A case report of successful pregnancies in two young women treated with high-dose ifosfamide and cyclophosphamide at Memorial Sloan Kettering was reported in 2001 [31]. In 2008, a small case series, which included 13 females treated for sarcoma with ifosfamide as the only alkylating agent, there was no primary ovarian failure reported. However, AMH levels were lower than an age-matched reference group, suggesting risk for early menopause [32].

Due to improved survivorship from childhood cancer noted as early as the 1970s–1980s, large cohorts of female survivors have reached the third and fourth decades of life, where the risk for infertility and premature menopause has been examined. In this era of treatment for these cohorts, the use of both radiotherapy and chemotherapy together was common, and thus it is not possible to fully separate the effects of the two modalities of therapy.

Two large studies of these survivors demonstrated elevated risks for infertility and premature menopause [11, 33]. A study of 2,498 female survivors, treated between 1945 and 1975, showed a 7 % deficit in fertility, compared with siblings. Between ages 21 and 25 years, survivors had a risk of premature menopause four times greater than that of siblings. Treatment-related risk factors included radiotherapy alone (RR = 3.7), alkylating agents alone (RR = 9.2), or a combination of both (RR = 27). By age 31, 42 % of these women had reached menopause, compared with 5 % of siblings [11]. In a study of 719 survivors treated between 1964 and 1988, 15.5 % of women were unable to conceive. Women treated with abdominopelvic radiotherapy alone had a fertility deficit of 23 %, compared with those treated with surgery. As with the previous study, the risk of infertility and premature menopause increased with increasing dose of abdominopelvic radiotherapy and amount of alkylating agent [33].

Several studies have been conducted within the Childhood Cancer Survivor Study (CCSS), a cohort of survivors treated between 1970 and 1987. In an analysis of 3,390 female survivors, acute ovarian failure was self-reported in 215 (6.3 %). Risk factors in multivariate analysis included increased dose of ovarian radiation, exposure to cyclophosphamide in those 13–20 years of age, and any exposure to procarbazine [34]. Premature menopause was also noted in 8 % of participants studied compared to 0.8 % in a sibling cohort. Risk factors for premature menopause were higher-attained age, increased dose of radiotherapy to the ovaries, increased alkylating agent exposure as determined by the alkylating agent score, and a diagnosis of Hodgkin lymphoma [35]. In another CCSS analysis of 5,149 female participants and 1,441 female siblings, the relative risk for survivors ever being pregnant was 0.81 compared to the siblings. Risk factors in multivariate analysis included ovarian/uterine radiation dose of >5 Gy, hypothalamic/pituitary dose of ≥30 Gy, and alkylating agent dose score of 3 or 4 [36].

Similar to what has been done with conventional chemoradiotherapy protocols, transplant conditioning protocols without TBI are being utilized to avoid some of the associated adverse long-term sequelae. The use of high-dose cyclophosphamide without TBI or other alkylating agents is associated with a lower risk of ovarian failure than conditioning regimens with TBI or multiple alkylating agents. In a study by Sanders, 100 % of women ($n = 15$) younger than age 26 and three of nine older than age 26 who were treated with 200 mg/kg cyclophosphamide recovered normal gonadotropin levels and menstruation posttransplantation [37]. However, many transplant protocols use high doses of alkylating agents together, most commonly busulfan and cyclophosphamide, which are associated with similar degrees of ovarian failure in females as protocols containing TBI [38].

## 13.2.3 Effects of Radiotherapy and Chemotherapy on Reproductive Outcomes

Many survivors of childhood cancer previously treated with cytotoxic therapy will remain fertile, and, therefore, pregnancy outcomes and the risk of cancer or genetic disease in offspring must be addressed. Young women who have been exposed to radiotherapy below the diaphragm are also at risk of impaired uterine development, which can adversely affect pregnancy outcomes, often resulting in premature labor and low-birth-weight infants. The magnitude of the risk is related to the radiotherapy field, total dose, and fractionation schedule. Female long-term survivors treated with total body irradiation and marrow transplantation are at risk for impaired uterine growth and blood flow, and, if pregnancy is achieved, for early pregnancy loss and premature labor. Despite standard hormone replacement, the uterus of the childhood cancer survivor may be impaired in its development and measure only 40 % of normal adult size, the

ultimate uterine volume correlating with the age at which radiotherapy was received [7, 20].

With more childhood cancer survivors retaining fertility, pregnancy outcome data is now available. Of 4,029 pregnancies occurring among 1,915 women followed in the Childhood Cancer Survivor Study (CCSS), there were 63 % live births, 1 % stillbirths, 15 % miscarriages, 17 % abortions, and 3 % unknown or in gestation. Risk of miscarriage was 3.6-fold higher in women treated with craniospinal radiotherapy and 1.7-fold higher in those treated with pelvic radiotherapy. Chemotherapy exposure alone did not increase the risk of miscarriage. Compared with siblings, however, survivors were less likely to have live births and more likely to have medical abortions and low-birth-weight babies [39]. In an updated analysis of this cohort, it was noted that offspring of women who receive uterine radiation doses of >5 Gy were more likely to be small for gestational age [35]. In another analysis from the CCSS, Signorello also found that uterine and ovarian radiation doses of >10 Gy increased risk of stillbirth or neonatal death, and furthermore, for girls treated prior to menarche, uterine or ovarian doses as low as 1.0–2.49 Gy increased the risk of stillbirth or neonatal death [40].

In a Danish population-based cohort, in analysis of 34,000 pregnancies, which included 1,479 pregnancies of childhood cancer survivors, there were no significant differences noted in the proportions of live births, stillbirths, or all kinds of abortions combined between survivors and women without cancer. However, survivors had a 23 % increased risk for spontaneous abortion, with ovarian and uterine radiotherapy as the major significant risk factor [41].

In a Finish population-based cohort, in an analysis of 3,501 and 16,908 children of female cancer patients and siblings, respectively, the risk of stillbirth or early neonatal death was not significantly increased among offspring of cancer survivors as compared to offspring of siblings [42]. In a case-cohort study conducted involving 472 Danish survivors of childhood and adolescent cancer and their 1,037 pregnancies, no statistically significant associations were found between genetic disease in children and parental treatment with alkylating drugs or preconception radiation doses to the testes in male and ovaries in female cancer survivors. A statistically significant association between abdominopelvic irradiation and malformations, stillbirths, and neonatal deaths was not seen in the children of female survivors overall or in the children of mothers receiving high uterine doses [43].

In the National Wilms Tumor Study, records were obtained for 427 pregnancies of >20 weeks duration. In this group, there were 409 single and 12 twin live births. Early or threatened labor, malposition of the fetus, lower-birth-weight (<2,500 g), and premature delivery (<36 weeks) were more frequent among women who had received flank radiotherapy, in a dose-dependent manner [44].

Preservation of fertility and successful pregnancies may occur following HSCT. Sanders and colleagues evaluated pregnancy outcomes in a group of females treated with bone marrow transplant. Among 116 treated before puberty and 23 treated after the onset of puberty who retained ovarian function, 32 (28 %) and 9 (30 %), respectively, became pregnant. Of the 32 pregnancies in those treated with TBI, 16 resulted in early termination, compared with a 21 % prevalence of early termination in those treated with cyclophosphamide alone. There were no pregnancies among the women treated with busulfan and cyclophosphamide [37].

For childhood cancer survivors who have offspring, there is the concern about congenital anomalies, genetic disease, or risk of cancer in the offspring. In the report from the National Wilms Tumor Group, congenital anomalies were marginally increased in the offspring of females who had received flank radiotherapy [44]. However, this risk was not observed in a study of 247 offspring of 148 cancer survivors treated at a single institution [45] or in several larger cohort studies. In a study that compared a group of 2,198 offspring from adult survivors treated for childhood cancer between 1945 and 1975 with a group of 4,544 offspring from sibling controls, there were no differences in the proportion of offspring with cytogenetic syndromes, single-gene defects, or simple malformations. There was no association of type of childhood cancer treatment used and the occurrence of genetic disease in the off-

spring [46]. In the CCSS, among the 1,915 female survivors who reported 4,029 pregnancies, there was no increased risk of offspring with simple malformations, cytogenetic syndromes, single-gene defects, or congenital malformations [35]. In a subsequent analysis from the CCSS, among children of 1,627 female cancer survivors, there was no increased risk for congenital anomalies and no increase conferred from ovarian radiation or alkylating exposure [47].

Similar results were reported in a study of 5,847 offspring of survivors of childhood cancers treated in five Scandinavian countries. In the absence of a hereditary cancer syndrome (such as hereditary retinoblastoma), there was no increased risk of cancer [48]. In an updated analysis from Finland among 26,331 children of pediatric and young adult cancer survivors and 58,155 children of siblings, there was no increased risk of cancer in the offspring of the cancer survivors in the absence of a known cancer predisposition syndrome [49].

Further follow-ups are needed to determine whether patterns of cancer or genetic disease in offspring change with changes in cancer treatments, further elapsed time, and studies of greater numbers of offspring.

## 13.3 Detection and Screening

All prepubertal females who are treated with potentially gonadal toxic radiotherapy or chemotherapy should be rigorously assessed for appropriate progression through puberty. The average age for menarche is 12.7 years ± 1.0 year [50]. An evaluation should include a complete history, a physical examination that includes an assessment of sexual development and pubertal milestones (Tables 13.2 and 13.3) and selected laboratory studies (Table 13.4), as summarized in Table 13.5. Reduced ovarian volume and low inhibin B and anti-Mullerian hormone concentrations in survivors with regular menses may be markers of incipient ovarian failure [2, 7]. In conjunction with the evaluation of gonadal effects, attention must be paid to growth. Cranial radiotherapy confers significant risk for growth hormone deficiency. Once

**Table 13.2** Tanner staging (pubertal milestones) for breast development [40]

| Stage | Age (mean ± SD, years) |
|---|---|
| I. Preadolescent. Only papilla is elevated | |
| II. Breast and papilla are elevated as small mound. Areolar diameter is enlarged | 10.0 ± 1.0 |
| III. Areola and papilla project to form a secondary mound above the level of the breast | 11.9 ± 1.0 |
| IV. There is projection only of papilla because of recession of the areola to the general contour of the breast | 12.9 ± 1.2 |

**Table 13.3** Tanner staging (pubertal milestones) for pubic hair growth [40]

| Stage | Age (mean ± SD, years) |
|---|---|
| I. Preadolescent vellus over pubis is no further developed than that over anterior abdominal wall (i.e., no pubic hair) | |
| II. There is sparse growth of long, slightly pigmented, downy hair, straight or only slightly curled, appearing chiefly along the labia | 11.2 ± 1.1 |
| III. Hair is considerably darker, coarser, and more curled. Hair spreads sparsely over pubic junction | 11.9 ± 1.1 |
| IV. Hair is now adult in type but area covered by it is still considerably smaller than in most adults. There is no spread to medial surface of the thighs | 12.6 ± 1.1 |

**Table 13.4** Laboratory assessment for ovarian function

| Testing | Treatment exposure | Time and frequency of evaluations |
|---|---|---|
| LH, FSH, estradiol | Alkylating agents | Baseline at 11 years of age or older, and then yearly |
| | Abdominopelvic, cranial, or total body radiotherapy | Assessment also of whether the following are present: delayed puberty, irregular menses or amenorrhea, clinical signs or symptoms of estrogen deficiency |
| Free T4, TSH | Neck, cranial, or total body radiotherapy | Yearly |
| | | Assessment also of presence of signs or symptoms of thyroid dysfunction |

Also see Sect. 13.2

patients have reached full sexual maturity, linear growth will stop. Linear and sexual development must, therefore, be monitored simultaneously (see the chapter on "Neuroendocrine Late Effects" for further details). Patients who received radiotherapy to the central nervous system or the neck are also at risk for thyroid dysfunction that can negatively impact gonadal function and linear growth. Even after successful progression through puberty, it is important to monitor the frequency and characteristics of menstrual periods, due to risk for premature menopause. Females with ovarian failure, either primary or secondary, should undergo assessments for impaired bone mineral density. Calcium intake, weight-bearing exercise, a history of fractures, and a family history of osteopenia/osteoporosis should be evaluated. The determination of bone mineral density, using dual-energy X-ray absorptiometry (DXA) scan, and comparison of results with the well-established adult normative values, is indicated for all adult females. Screening in children is less defined. Several different measurement techniques and standards have been applied, but none has been well validated in large pediatric populations (much less in pediatric oncology patients). However, some monitoring is indicated, and trends over time may be of greater value than a single DXA scan. The Children's Oncology Group has published guidelines (www.survivorshipguidelines.org) [51] that are helping in determining surveillance for adverse long-term ovarian or ovarian-associated outcomes, as reviewed by Metzger and colleagues [52].

Pediatric endocrinologists and reproductive endocrinologists/gynecologists are essential consultants in the monitoring, prevention, and management of ovarian late effects in childhood cancer survivors.

**Table 13.5** Pertinent history and physical examination

| History | Physical examination |
|---|---|
| Doses and types of chemotherapy agents received | Height, weight, and height velocity |
| Doses and fields of radiotherapy | Complete examination of all organ systems, with particular attention to pubertal status and thyroid gland |
| Surgical history, especially for patients with CNS and GU tumors | Gynecologic examination in postpubertal females as indicated by treatment history, sexual activity, and overall developmental status |
| Patient and maternal history of menarche and thelarche | |
| Menstrual periods – timing and tempo | |
| Symptoms of estrogen deficiency (hot flashes, dry skin, leg cramps, reduced libido) | |
| Parental heights | |
| Family history of infertility, pregnancy, labor complications, assisted fertilization | |

## 13.4 Management of Established Problems

### 13.4.1 Prevention Strategies

Reduction in the dose or use of alkylating agents and abdominopelvic radiotherapy is the most effective means of preserving ovarian function and promoting positive reproductive outcomes. There are, however, many instances where cytotoxic and gonadal toxic chemotherapy and radiotherapy are still required for long-term cure. As a result, additional strategies need to be employed to minimize adverse long-term outcomes. To shield the ovaries from direct irradiation during abdominal or pelvic radiotherapy, an oophoropexy may be performed if it is possible to move the ovaries to a location that can be safely shielded without jeopardizing the patient for tumor recurrence. Typically, with abdominal radiotherapy for Hodgkin lymphoma that targets lymph nodes, the ovaries are moved to a midline

position in front of or behind the uterus. For pelvic radiotherapy, they may be moved laterally to the iliac wings. This may also be helpful for young girls or adolescents undergoing cranial spinal radiotherapy for brain tumors using historic radiation techniques, though current approaches with intensity modulation allow ovarian sparing. However, if such techniques are not possible, then the ovaries should be marked by the surgeon with clips that can later by identified by a simulator film. Central pelvic blocking at the time of "inverted Y" field will prevent direct irradiation, although scatter dose and transmitted dose will be inevitable. Medial or lateral transposition of the ovaries results in ovarian doses of 8–10 % and 4–5 %, respectively, of the pelvic dose [53]. For most patients, this will be compatible with the preservation of fertility, although there may be temporary amenorrhea.

Because dividing cells are more sensitive to the cytotoxic effects of alkylating agents than are cells at rest, it has been hypothesized that inhibition of the pituitary–gonadal axis by gonadotropin-releasing hormone (GnRH) agonists may protect the ovarian germinal epithelium from the cytotoxic effects of chemotherapy. In a mixed teenage and young adult group of women treated for lymphoma, leukemia, or autoimmune disease, Blumenfeld and colleagues [54, 55] reported a significant benefit in the concomitant use of GnRH agonist treatment with cytotoxic chemotherapy. Pereya and colleagues evaluated the role of GnRH analogs with respect to the prevention of early-onset ovarian insufficiency following chemotherapy in adolescent females. Their study compared prepubertal females treated with GnRH analogs prior to chemotherapy with a control group of prepubertal patients who were not given GnRH analogs. Pereya and colleagues found that GnRH analog treatment before and during chemotherapy might enhance ovarian function and preserve adolescent fertility [56]. However, as reviewed in the literature, and in two randomized prospective studies, it is not clear that there is a benefit, and thus, this is currently not considered a standard of care [57–60].

Progress in reproductive endocrinology has resulted in the availability of several potential options for preserving or permitting fertility in females about to receive potentially toxic chemotherapy or radiotherapy. In pre- and postpubertal females, cryopreservation of ovarian cortical tissue and enzymatically extracted follicles, with the in vitro maturation of prenatal follicles, is of potential clinical use. There is now feasibility of doing this at time of diagnosis in young females diagnosed with cancer, and thus, this is an area of ongoing important research [61–68]. Another option available to the postpubertal female is the stimulation of ovaries with exogenous gonadotropins and the retrieval of mature oocytes for cryopreservation and later in vitro fertilization. These interventions, however, may not be readily available to the pediatric and adolescent patient, and the necessary delay in cancer therapy for ovarian stimulation may then be impractical. Oocyte cryopreservation may be useful in the survivorship population where there is concern over decreasing ovarian reserve. All such approaches harbor the risk that malignant cells will be present in the specimen and reintroduced in the patient at a later date. Those with hematologic or gonadal tumors would be at greatest risk for this eventuality. However, success rates are increasing with newer technologies and further research is ongoing [68]. Standards for best practice in the cryopreservation of gonadal tissue remain to be defined. Should offspring result as a consequence of these assisted fertility techniques, it would be imperative to evaluate the risk of chromosomal and other congenital disorders, which have been reported following assisted reproductive techniques [69, 70].

A critical component to prevention is health counseling for females at risk. For females treated during the prepubertal period, parents should be counseled regarding the risk of primary ovarian failure. Normal gonadal development should be reviewed with recommendations for monitoring of growth and development. Reproductive counseling should be made cautiously and preferably, in conjunction with a specialist in reproductive endocrinology. The effects on the female gonadal system from radiotherapy

and chemotherapy may demonstrate significant interindividual variation, even with identical exposures at identical ages. Postpubertal females who have normal menstrual function should be counseled about appropriate contraception should they currently not wish to conceive a child, and they should also be made aware of their potential risk for premature menopause. Not inconsequential for young adults is the impact of ovarian failure or impending failure in sexual drive or libido, an effect that may be treatable if addressed. Risks for osteopenia and osteoporosis also must be addressed. Appropriate calcium intake, avoidance of substances that interfere with bone deposition and appropriate weight-bearing exercise should be encouraged to maintain skeletal health.

### 13.4.2 Management of Delayed Puberty

Female patients exposed to gonadal toxic therapies during the prepubertal period and who are not progressing appropriately through puberty should be promptly referred to a pediatric endocrinologist for further evaluation and treatment. The use of hormonal replacement therapy for induction and progression of puberty must be closely monitored together with skeletal growth, as the two processes are closely linked. Generally, the recommendation will be to initiate a regimen of hormone replacement such as estrogen, which is now available in a variety of doses and modes of administration. Gonadotropins, gonadotropin agonists or antagonists, progesterone, and growth hormone may also be part of the treatment regimen.

### 13.4.3 Management of Infertility

Postpubertal patients at risk for infertility should be referred to a reproductive endocrinologist to discuss assisted fertility techniques that may be appropriate. These specialists can also monitor fertility status and assist survivors with reproductive decisions.

### 13.4.4 Management of Pregnancy and Delivery

While many childhood cancer survivors may have no prenatal or perinatal complications, others may be at risk and should be managed appropriately by obstetricians and perinatologists. Patients treated with abdominopelvic radiotherapy are at risk for spontaneous abortion, premature labor and delivery, and, compared with controls, small for gestational stage neonates. Those treated with anthracyclines at doses >300 mg/m² or at lower doses, when combined with thoracic radiotherapy, or those women treated with high doses of thoracic radiotherapy (>35 Gy) without anthracyclines, may be at risk for cardiac complications, which may manifest during pregnancy (especially during the third trimester and during delivery). Similarly, women previously treated with bleomycin, carmustine, or busulfan, with higher doses of thoracic radiotherapy, may be at risk for pulmonary fibrosis or decreased diffusing capacity, and this may result in complications during pregnancy and delivery (see the chapters on "Heart and Lung Late Effects" for further details).

### 13.4.5 Management of Premature Menopause

Female survivors who develop premature menopause should be referred to a gynecologist for management and consideration for hormone replacement therapy. The decision to proceed with hormone replacement therapy, and the form that it should take, involves a careful evaluation of many competing healthcare factors, a subject that is beyond the scope of this chapter. However, it is imperative that patients be managed by a team of physicians who are well versed in this area and can assist in carefully weighing the risks and benefits of various hormonal replacement strategies.

### Summary

Both chemotherapy and radiotherapy can affect ovarian function in female survivors of childhood cancer. The effects are varied and dependent on the chemotherapeutic agents and doses, radiotherapy doses, techniques, volumes and fields, and the age and pubertal status of the female. There is also considerable individual variation, the reasons for which remain largely unknown. Problems may include primary ovarian failure, reduced libido, pregnancy complications, and premature menopause. Preventive strategies remain limited. Avoidance or reduction in the dose of gonadal toxic therapies should be attempted where possible. Where this is not possible, advances in reproductive medicine may ultimately allow for ovarian cryopreservation and similar techniques. Survivors should receive health counseling about risks, annual physical examinations with attention paid to endocrine and reproductive function, close monitoring of gonadal function, and referral to pediatric endocrinologists, reproductive endocrinologists, gynecologists, and perinatologists as indicated. In survivors who do become pregnant, the majority will have favorable pregnancy outcomes with healthy offspring, and it does not appear that the offspring will have an increased risk of cancer (in the absence of a known heritable syndrome or congenital anomalies).

Much of what we have learned about gonadal function in female childhood cancer survivors is based on patients treated in the 1960s through the middle 1980s. During the past 20 years, there has been increased awareness of the adverse gonadal effects, and where possible, therapies have been altered to limit these effects. This period has also resulted in the increased use of more dose-intensive chemotherapy regimens and greater use of myeloablative hematopoietic stem cell transplants. Survivorship has increased and, as a result, there are now large cohorts of adult young women treated with more contemporary therapy who will require close follow-up of their gonadal status. It is only with continued follow-up that we will be able to fully appreciate the impact of relatively recent changes in therapy. Challenges still face young females being treated for cancer today with respect to gonadal function. Therefore, it is incumbent upon pediatric oncologists and reproductive specialists to develop better preventive strategies. In addition, there is more to be learned about the interindividual differences in gonadal effects that are seen, despite very similar treatment exposures. The role of genetic predisposition and inherent chemotherapy (or radiotherapy) sensitivity has yet to be studied with respect to most adverse long-term outcomes (including ovarian function) for childhood cancer survivors.

## References

1. Palter S, Olive D (2002) Reproductive physiology. In: Berek J, Adams Hillard P, Adashi E (eds) Novak's gynecology. Lippincott Williams and Wilkins, Philadelphia, pp 163–164
2. Lie Fong S, Laven JS, Hakvoort-Cammel FG, Schipper I, Visser JA, Themmen AP, de Jong FH, van den Heuvel-Eibrink MM (2009) Assessment of ovarian reserve in adult childhood cancer survivors using anti-Mullerian hormone. Hum Reprod 24(4):982–990
3. Chapman RM, Sutcliffe SB, Malpas JS (1979) Cytotoxic induced ovarian failure in women with Hodgkin's disease. JAMA 242:1877–1881
4. Shalet SM (1996) Endocrine sequelae of cancer therapy. Eur J Endocrinol 135:135–143
5. Zebrack BJ, Casillas J, Nohr L, Adams H, Zeltzer LK (2004) Fertility issues for young adult survivors of childhood cancer. Psychooncology 13(10):689–699
6. Friedman DL, Constine LS (2011) Late effects of cancer treatment. In: Haperin EC, Constine LS, Tarbell NJ, Kun LE (eds) Pediatric radiation oncology. Lippincott Williams and Wilkins, Philadelphia, pp 353–396
7. Critchley HO, Wallace WH (2005) Impact of cancer treatment on uterine function. J Natl Cancer Inst Monogr 34:64–68
8. Wallace WH, Shalet SM, Hendry JH, Morris-Jones PH, Gattamaneni HR (1989) Ovarian failure following abdominal irradiation in childhood: the radiosensitivity of the human oocyte. Br J Radiol 62:995–998
9. Ash P (1980) The influence of radiation on fertility in man. Br J Radiol 53:271–278
10. Lushbaugh CC, Casarett GW (1976) The effects of gonadal irradiation in clinical radiation therapy: a review. Cancer 37(Suppl 2):1111–1125
11. Byrne J, Mulvihill JJ, Myers MH, Connelly RR, Naughton MD, Krauss MR, Steinhorn SC, Hassinger DD, Austin DF, Bragg K (1987) Effects of treatment on fertility in long-term survivors of childhood or adolescent cancer. N Engl J Med 317:1315–1321
12. Nicosia SV, Matus-Ridley M, Meadows AT (1985) Gonadal effects of cancer therapy in girls. Cancer 55:2364–2372
13. Damewood MD, Grochow LB (1986) Prospects for fertility after chemotherapy or radiation for neoplastic disease. Fertil Steril 45:443–459
14. Bath LE, Hamish W, Wallace B, Critchley HO (2002) Late effects of the treatment of childhood cancer on the female reproductive system and the potential for fertility preservation. BJOG Int J Obstet Gynaecol 109:107–114
15. Hill M, Milan S, Cunningham D, Mansi J, Smith I, Catovsky D, Gore M, Zulian G, Selby P, Horwich A et al (1995) Evaluation of the efficacy of the VEEP regimen in adult Hodgkin's disease with assessment of gonadal and cardiac toxicity. J Clin Oncol 13:387–395, (see comments). Comment in: J Clin Oncol 1995,13:1283–1284
16. Mayer EI, Dopfer RE, Klingebiel T, Scheel-Walter H, Ranke MB, Niethammer D (1999) Longitudinal gonadal function after bone marrow transplantation for acute lymphoblastic leukemia during childhood. Pediatr Transplant 3:38–44
17. Thomson AB, Critchley HO, Kelnar CJ, Wallace WH (2002) Late reproductive sequelae following treatment of childhood cancer and options for fertility preservation. Best Pract Res Clin Endocrinol Metab 16:311–334
18. Stillman RJ, Schinfeld JS, Schiff I, Gelber RD, Greenberger J, Larson M, Jaffe N, Li FP (1981) Ovarian failure in long-term survivors of childhood malignancy. Am J Obstet Gynecol 139:62–66
19. Halperin EC (1993) Concerning the inferior portion of the spinal radiotherapy field for malignancies that disseminate via the cerebrospinal fluid. Int J Radiat Oncol Biol Phys 26:357–362
20. Critchley HO, Bath LE, Wallace WH (2002) Radiation damage to the uterus – review of the effects of treatment of childhood cancer. Hum Fertil (Camb) 5:61–66
21. Sklar C, Boulad F, Small T, Kernan N (2001) Endocrine complications of pediatric stem cell transplantation. Front Biosci 6:G17–G22
22. Ogilvy-Stuart AL, Clark DJ, Wallace WH, Gibson BE, Stevens RF, Shalet SM, Donaldson MD (1992) Endocrine deficit after fractionated total body irradiation. Arch Dis Child 67:1107–1110
23. Sklar CA (1991) Growth and pubertal development in survivors of childhood cancer. Pediatrician 18:53–60
24. Howell S, Shalet S (1998) Gonadal damage from chemotherapy and radiotherapy. Endocrinol Metab Clin N Am 27:927–943
25. Kreuser ED, Xiros N, Hetzel WD, Heimpel H (1987) Reproductive and endocrine gonadal capacity in patients treated with COPP chemotherapy for Hodgkin's disease. J Cancer Res Clin Oncol 113:260–266
26. Friedman DL, Constine LS (2006) Late effects of treatment for Hodgkin lymphoma. J Natl Compr Cancer Netw 4(3):249–257
27. Schwartz CL, Constine LS, Villaluna D, London WB, Hutchison RE, Sposto R, Lipshultz SE, Turner CS, de Alarcon PA, Chauvenet A (2009) A risk-adapted, response-based approach using ABVE-PC for children and adolescents with intermediate- and high-risk Hodgkin lymphoma: the results of P9425. Blood 114(10):2051–2059, PMCID: 2744567

28. Mauz-Korholz C, Hasenclever D, Dorffel W, Ruschke K, Pelz T, Voigt A, Stiefel M, Winkler M, Vilser C, Dieckmann K, Karlen J, Bergstrasser E, Fossa A, Mann G, Hummel M, Klapper W, Stein H, Vordermark D, Kluge R, Korholz D (2010) Procarbazine-free OEPA-COPDAC chemotherapy in boys and standard OPPA-COPP in girls have comparable effectiveness in pediatric Hodgkin's lymphoma: the GPOH-HD-2002 study. J Clin Oncol 28(23): 3680–3686

29. Metzger ML, Weinstein HJ, Hudson MM, Billett AL, Larsen EC, Friedmann A, Howard SC, Donaldson SS, Krasin MJ, Kun LE, Marcus KJ, Yock TI, Tarbell N, Billups CA, Wu J, Link MP (2012) Association between radiotherapy vs no radiotherapy based on early response to VAMP chemotherapy and survival among children with favorable-risk Hodgkin lymphoma. JAMA 307(24):2609–2616, PMCID: 3526806

30. Wolden SL, Chen L, Kelly KM, Herzog P, Gilchrist GS, Thomson J, Sposto R, Kadin ME, Hutchinson RJ, Nachman J (2012) Long-term results of CCG 5942: a randomized comparison of chemotherapy with and without radiotherapy for children with Hodgkin's lymphoma – a report from the Children's Oncology Group. J Clin Oncol 30(26):3174–3180, PMCID: 3434976

31. Sharon N, Neumann Y, Kenet G, Schachter J, Rechavi G, Toren A (2001) Successful pregnancy after high-dose cyclophosphamide and ifosfamide treatment in two postpubertal women. Pediatr Hematol Oncol 18(4):247–252

32. Williams D, Crofton PM, Levitt G (2008) Does ifosfamide affect gonadal function? Pediatr Blood Cancer 50(2):347–351

33. Chiarelli AM, Marrett LD, Darlington G (1999) Early menopause and infertility in females after treatment for childhood cancer diagnosed in 1964–1988 in Ontario, Canada. Am J Epidemiol 150:245–254

34. Chemaitilly W, Mertens AC, Mitby P, Whitton J, Stovall M, Yasui Y, Robison LL, Sklar CA (2006) Acute ovarian failure in the childhood cancer survivor study. J Clin Endocrinol Metab 91(5):1723–1728

35. Green DM, Sklar CA, Boice JD Jr, Mulvihill JJ, Whitton JA, Stovall M, Yasui Y (2009) Ovarian failure and reproductive outcomes after childhood cancer treatment: results from the Childhood Cancer Survivor Study. J Clin Oncol 27(14):2374–2381, PMCID: 2677923

36. Green DM, Kawashima T, Stovall M, Leisenring W, Sklar CA, Mertens AC, Donaldson SS, Byrne J, Robison LL (2009) Fertility of female survivors of childhood cancer: a report from the childhood cancer survivor study. J Clin Oncol 27(16):2677–2685, PMCID: 2690392

37. Sanders JE, Buckner CD, Leonard JM, Sullivan KM, Witherspoon RP, Deeg HJ, Storb R, Thomas ED (1983) Late effects on gonadal function of cyclophosphamide, total-body irradiation, and marrow transplantation. Transplantation 36:252–255

38. Sanders JE, Hawley J, Levy W, Gooley T, Buckner CD, Deeg HJ, Doney K, Storb R, Sullivan K, Witherspoon R, Appelbaum FR (1996) Pregnancies following high-dose cyclophosphamide with or without high-dose busulfan or total-body irradiation and bone marrow transplantation. Blood 87:3045–3052

39. Green DM, Whitton JA, Stovall M, Mertens AC, Donaldson SS, Ruymann FB, Pendergrass TW, Robison LL (2002) Pregnancy outcome of female survivors of childhood cancer: a report from the Childhood Cancer Survivor Study. Am J Obstet Gynecol 187:1070–1080

40. Signorello LB, Mulvihill JJ, Green DM, Munro HM, Stovall M, Weathers RE, Mertens AC, Whitton JA, Robison LL, Boice JD Jr (2010) Stillbirth and neonatal death in relation to radiation exposure before conception: a retrospective cohort study. Lancet 376(9741):624–630, PMCID: 3008402

41. Winther JF, Boice JD Jr, Svendsen AL, Frederiksen K, Stovall M, Olsen JH (2008) Spontaneous abortion in a Danish population-based cohort of childhood cancer survivors. J Clin Oncol 26(26):4340–4346, PMCID: 2653117

42. Madanat-Harjuoja LM, Lahteenmaki PM, Dyba T, Gissler M, Boice JD Jr, Malila N (2013) Stillbirth, early death and neonatal morbidity among offspring of female cancer survivors. Acta Oncol 52(6):1152–1159

43. Winther JF, Olsen JH, Wu H, Shyr Y, Mulvihill JJ, Stovall M, Nielsen A, Schmiegelow M, Boice JD Jr (2012) Genetic disease in the children of Danish survivors of childhood and adolescent cancer. J Clin Oncol 30(1):27–33, PMCID: 3255559

44. Green DM, Peabody EM, Nan B, Peterson S, Kalapurakal JA, Breslow NE (2002) Pregnancy outcome after treatment for Wilms' tumor: a report from the National Wilms' Tumor Study Group. J Clin Oncol 20:2506–2513

45. Green DM, Fiorello A, Zevon MA, Hall B, Seigelstein N (1997) Birth defects and childhood cancer in offspring of survivors of childhood cancer. Arch Pediatr Adolesc Med 151:379–383

46. Byrne J, Rasmussen SA, Steinhorn SC, Connelly RR, Myers MH, Lynch CF, Flannery J, Austin DF, Holmes FF, Holmes GE, Strong LC, Mulvihill JJ (1998) Genetic disease in offspring of long-term survivors of childhood and adolescent cancer (comment). Am J Hum Genet 62:45–52

47. Signorello LB, Mulvihill JJ, Green DM, Munro HM, Stovall M, Weathers RE, Mertens AC, Whitton JA, Robison LL, Boice JD Jr (2012) Congenital anomalies in the children of cancer survivors: a report from the childhood cancer survivor study. J Clin Oncol 30(3):239–245, PMCID: 3269950

48. Sankila R, Olsen JH, Anderson H, Garwicz S, Glattre E, Hertz H, Langmark F, Lanning M, Moller T, Tulinius H (1998) Risk of cancer among offspring of childhood-cancer survivors. Association of the Nordic Cancer Registries and the Nordic Society of Paediatric

Haematology and Oncology. N Engl J Med 338: 1339–1344

49. Madanat-Harjuoja LM, Malila N, Lahteenmaki P, Pukkala E, Mulvihill JJ, Boice JD Jr, Sankila R (2010) Risk of cancer among children of cancer patients – a nationwide study in Finland. Int J Cancer 126(5):1196–1205, PMCID: 2801768

50. Rosenfield RL (2002) Puberty in the female. In: Sperling MA (ed) Pediatric endocrinology. Saunders, Philadelphia

51. Children's Oncology Group (2008) Long-term follow-up guidelines for survivors of childhood, adolescent and young adult cancers, version 3.0. Children's Oncology Group, Arcadia, Available on-line: www.survivorshipguidelines.org

52. Metzger ML, Meacham LR, Patterson B, Casillas JS, Constine LS, Hijiya N, Kenney LB, Leonard M, Lockart BA, Likes W, Green DM (2013) Female reproductive health after childhood, adolescent, and young adult cancers: guidelines for the assessment and management of female reproductive complications. J Clin Oncol 31(9):1239–1247

53. Haie-Meder C, Mlika-Cabanne N, Michel G, Briot E, Gerbaulet A, Lhomme C, Cosset JM, Sarrazin D, Flamant F, Hayat M (1993) Radiotherapy after ovarian transposition: ovarian function and fertility preservation. Int J Radiat Oncol Biol Phys 25: 419–424

54. Blumenfeld Z, Dann E, Avivi I, Epelbaum R, Rowe JM (2002) Fertility after treatment for Hodgkin's disease. Ann Oncol 13(Suppl 1):138–147

55. Blumenfeld Z, Avivi I, Linn S, Epelbaum R, Ben-Shahar M, Haim N (1996) Prevention of irreversible chemotherapy-induced ovarian damage in young women with lymphoma by a gonadotrophin-releasing hormone agonist in parallel to chemotherapy. Hum Reprod 11:1620–1626

56. Pereyra Pacheco B, Mendez Ribas JM, Milone G, Fernandez I, Kvicala R, Mila T, di Noto A, Contreras Ortiz O, Pavlovsky S (2001) Use of GnRH analogs for functional protection of the ovary and preservation of fertility during cancer treatment in adolescents: a preliminary report. Gynecol Oncol 81:391–397

57. Oktay K, Oktem O (2009) Fertility preservation medicine: a new field in the care of young cancer survivors. Pediatr Blood Cancer 53(2):267–273

58. Oktem O, Oktay K (2007) Quantitative assessment of the impact of chemotherapy on ovarian follicle reserve and stromal function. Cancer 110(10):2222–2229

59. Oktay K, Sonmezer M, Oktem O, Fox K, Emons G, Bang H (2007) Absence of conclusive evidence for the safety and efficacy of gonadotropin-releasing hormone analogue treatment in protecting against chemotherapy-induced gonadal injury. Oncologist 12(9):1055–1066

60. Waxman JH, Ahmed R, Smith D, Wrigley PF, Gregory W, Shalet S, Crowther D, Rees LH, Besser GM, Malpas JS et al (1987) Failure to preserve fertility in patients with Hodgkin's disease. Cancer Chemother Pharmacol 19(2):159–162

61. Gracia CR, Chang J, Kondapalli L, Prewitt M, Carlson CA, Mattei P, Jeffers S, Ginsberg JP (2012) Ovarian tissue cryopreservation for fertility preservation in cancer patients: successful establishment and feasibility of a multidisciplinary collaboration. J Assist Reprod Genet 29(6):495–502. doi:10.1007/s10815-012-9753-7. Epub 2012

62. Donnez J, Dolmans MM, Pellicer A et al (2013) Restoration of ovarian activity and pregnancy after transplantation of cryopreserved ovarian tissue: a review of 60 cases of reimplantation. Fertil Steril 99(6):p15031513

63. Newton H (1998) The cryopreservation of ovarian tissue as a strategy for preserving the fertility of cancer patients. Hum Reprod Update 4:237–247

64. Oktay K, Karlikaya G (2000) Ovarian function after transplantation of frozen, banked autologous ovarian tissue. N Engl J Med 342(25):1919

65. Donnez J, Dolmans MM, Demylle D, Jadoul P, Pirard C, Squifflet J, Martinez-Madrid B, van Langendonckt A (2004) Livebirth after orthotopic transplantation of cryopreserved ovarian tissue. Lancet 364(9443): 1405–1410

66. Oktay K, Buyuk E, Veeck L, Zaninovic N, Xu K, Takeuchi T, Opsahl M, Rosenwaks Z (2004) Embryo development after heterotopic transplantation of cryopreserved ovarian tissue. Lancet 363(9412):837–840

67. Meirow D, Levron J, Eldar-Geva T, Hardan I, Fridman E, Zalel Y, Schiff E, Dor J (2005) Pregnancy after transplantation of cryopreserved ovarian tissue in a patient with ovarian failure after chemotherapy. N Engl J Med 353(3):318–321

68. Oktay K, Cil AP, Bang H (2006) Efficiency of oocyte cryopreservation: a meta-analysis. Fertil Steril 86(1): 70–80

69. Davies MJ, Moore VM, Willson KJ, Van Essen P, Priest K, Scott H, Haan EA, Chan A (2012) Reproductive technologies and the risk of birth defects. N Engl J Med 366(19):1803–1813

70. Farhi A, Reichman B, Boyko V, Mashiach S, Hourvitz A, Margalioth EJ, Levran D, Calderon I, Orvieto R, Ellenbogen A, Meyerovitch J, Ron-El R, Lerner-Geva L (2013) Congenital malformations in infants conceived following assisted reproductive technology in comparison with spontaneously conceived infants. J Matern Fetal Neonatal 26(12):1171–1179

# The Testes

Jill P. Ginsberg

# 14

## Contents

J.P. Ginsberg
Cancer Survivorship, Childern's Hospital of
Philadelphia, Perelman School of Medicine at the
University of Pennsylania
e-mail: ginsbergji@email.chop.edu

The testes are extremely sensitive to chemotherapy, radiation, and surgical interventions. Cancer therapy can interfere with reproductive ability and libido in men. The differential sensitivity of spermatozoa-producing Sertoli cells, however, compared to the testosterone-producing Leydig cells allows for greater effects on the reproductive capacity of men than effects on their sexual function. In this chapter, we review the pathophysiology of the testes and clinical manifestations of the testicular injury in response to gonadotoxic therapies. Furthermore, we will outline methods for screening males for gonadotoxicity and suggest potential fertility preservation methods that can be used in certain instances.

## 14.1 Pathophysiology

### 14.1.1 Overview of Normal Gonadal Development

Although the chromosomal and genetic sex of an embryo is determined at fertilization, male and female morphological sexual characteristics do not differ until the seventh week of gestation [49]. This initial period of early genital development is referred to as the indifferent stage of sexual development. During the fifth week, proliferation of the mesothelial cells and of the underlying mesenchyme produces a bulge on the medial side of the mesonephros, known as the

© Springer International Publishing 2015
C.L. Schwartz et al. (eds.), *Survivors of Childhood and Adolescent Cancer:
A Multidisciplinary Approach*, Pediatric Oncology, DOI 10.1007/978-3-319-16435-9_14

gonadal ridge. Fingerlike epithelial cords then grow into the underlying mesenchyme. The indifferent gonad now consists of an outer cortex and inner medulla [49]. During the sixth week, the primordial germ cells enter the underlying mesenchyme and incorporate into the primary sex cords. In embryos with an XY sex chromosome complex, testis-organizing factor (H-Y antigen) regulated by the Y chromosome determines testicular differentiation; the medulla differentiates into a testis and the cortex regresses. The gonads can be recognized as testes 7–9 weeks postfertilization [49].

The first stage of testis differentiation is the formation of testicular cords consisting of Sertoli precursor cells packed tightly around germ cells. The diploid germ cells undergo meiosis in the fetal testis and remain in meiotic arrest until puberty. Sertoli cells, which provide a location for support and proliferation of spermatogonia are derived from the mesonephros and proliferate only during fetal life and in the neonatal period [77]. After the eighth week of fetal life, the Leydig cell of the fetal testis secretes testosterone. Luteinizing hormone (LH) release is suppressed, and masculinization of the external genitalia and urogenital sinus of the fetus results. By the third month, the penis and prostate form [14]. Normal testes descend by the seventh month of gestation.

### 14.1.2 Anatomy of Normal Testis

The adult testis is an oblong, approximately 4.5 cm long organ weighing 34–45 g [76]. The testis is composed of three principal cell types: germ cells that develop into sperm, Sertoli cells that support and nurture developing germ cells and are also the site of production of the glycoprotein hormone inhibin, and Leydig cells that are responsible for testosterone synthesis [70]. Seminiferous tubules, the sites of spermatogenesis, are formed by germ cells and Sertoli cells. The Leydig cells that are responsible for the production of testosterone lie near the basal compartment of the seminiferous tubules, enabling them to deliver high concentrations of testosterone necessary for normal spermatogenesis and male secondary sexual characteristics [70].

The seminiferous tubules are embedded in a connective tissue matrix containing interspersed Leydig cells, blood vessels, and lymphatics and are surrounded by a basement membrane (tunica propria) upon which the seminiferous epithelium rests. Spermatogenesis takes place in the seminiferous epithelium. The least differentiated germ cells, the spermatogonia, divide to form spermatocytes that immediately undergo meiosis. The haploid spermatids that are formed develop into flagellate motile spermatozoa. This process requires up to 74 days [73]. Since spermatozoa are continuously produced in adult men, a constant supply of germ cell precursors is necessary. The newly formed spermatozoa are transported through the lumen of the seminiferous tubules into the epididymis where they are stored.

### 14.1.3 Hypothalamic-Pituitary-Testicular Axis

The primary regulators of testicular function are the anterior pituitary hormones, luteinizing hormone (LH) and follicle-stimulating hormone (FSH), both of which are released in response to the hypothalamic releasing factor, GnRH. GnRH is secreted from the median eminence into the hypophyseal portal system in a pulsatile manner and acts on the gonadotropes of the pituitary gland to stimulate secretion of LH and FSH [49]. LH regulates Leydig cell function by binding to specific LH receptors on the plasma membrane of Leydig cells. This leads to the formation of the cAMP that drives testosterone biosynthesis via a complex cascade starting with cholesterol [49]. Testosterone is transported from Leydig cells to the seminiferous tubules, where it acts to enhance spermatogenesis. Testosterone is also a prohormone for two different and metabolically active hormones, dihydrotestosterone (DHT) and estradiol. DHT mediates male sexual differentiation and virilization, whereas estradiol mediates bone maturation, mineralization, and epiphyseal fusion [72]. Testosterone controls pituitary LH secretion by a negative feedback mechanism; LH levels will rise when the Leydig cells are unable to produce testosterone.

Sertoli cells are the only cell type of the testis that possess FSH receptors [70]. FSH is delivered to the interstitial area of the testis by way of the arterial system. It then passes through the basement membrane of the seminiferous tubule to reach the Sertoli cells that line this membrane. FSH binds to the FSH receptors of the Sertoli cell and then mediates the synthesis of a variety of proteins and enzymes including the inhibins. Inhibin is a major feedback regulator of FSH and may thus be useful as a marker of spermatogenesis [66, 80]. The production of androgen transport protein by Sertoli cells can be induced and maintained by FSH.

FSH triggers an event in the immature testis that is essential for the completion of spermiogenesis. Thereafter, spermatogenesis will proceed continuously as long as an adequate and uninterrupted supply of testosterone is available. The lack of negative feedback from germinal epithelium results in an elevated FSH level.

### 14.1.4 Normal Developmental Stages

A neonatal surge in testosterone secretion is caused by high LH and FSH concentrations that occur during the first few months of life. From the age of about 3 months until the onset of puberty, plasma concentrations of LH and FSH are quite low and the testes are relatively quiescent [70]. At the onset of puberty, pulsatile secretion of LH (and to a lesser extent, FSH) occurs during sleep that is associated with increased nighttime plasma concentrations of testosterone. As puberty progresses, the increased pulsatile release of gonadotropins and the high concentrations of testosterone are maintained throughout the day and night [70].

In a normal male, the first sign of puberty is enlargement of the testis to larger than 2.5 cm [77]. This is due to seminiferous tubule growth, although Leydig cell enlargement contributes as well. Androgens synthesized in the testes are the driving force behind secondary sexual development,

although adrenal androgens also play a role in normal puberty. The range of onset of normal male puberty extends from 9 to 14 years of age. Boys complete pubertal development in 2–4.5 years (mean 3.2 years) [77]. The development of the external genitalia and pubic hair has been described in stages by Marshall and Tanner (Table 14.1) [47]. The first appearance of spermatozoa in early morning urinary specimens (spermarche) occurs at a mean age of 13.4 years, at gonadal stages 3 and 4 simultaneous with the pubertal growth spurt.

## 14.2 Cytotoxic Effects of Therapy

### 14.2.1 Cytotoxic Effects of Chemotherapy

Testicular dysfunction is among the most common long-term side effects of chemotherapy in men. The germinal epithelium is particularly susceptible to injury by cytotoxic drugs secondary to a high mitotic rate [30]. Leydig cells in contrast appear relatively resistant to the effects of chemotherapy [79]. In 1948, azoospermia after an alkylating agent (nitrogen mustard) was described in 27 of 30 men treated for lymphoma [75]. Subsequently, it has become apparent that all alkylating agents are gonadotoxic [26, 46, 55]. Antimetabolite therapy in general (e.g., methotrexate, mercaptopurine) does not have an adverse impact on male fertility. Cisplatin-based regimens result in temporary impairment of spermatogenesis in all patients but with recovery in a significant percentage [23]. The agents most commonly gonadotoxic in males are listed in Table 14.2.

Initial reports, based upon histological studies and normal basal FSH levels from small numbers of patients, suggested that the immature testis was relatively resistant to chemotherapy. More recently, however, it has become apparent that both the prepubertal and pubertal testes are vulnerable to cytotoxic drugs [6, 30]. Impairment of spermatogenesis may be irreversible in the months to years following chemotherapy. However, late recovery of spermatogenesis up to 14 years following chemotherapy has been

**Table 14.1** Genital development stages [47]

| Stage | Description | Mean age at onset (year) range 95 % |
|---|---|---|
| 1 | Preadolescent. Testes, scrotum, and penis are about same size and proportion as in early childhood. No pubic hair | |
| 2 | Scrotum and testes have enlarged; change in texture and some reddening of the scrotal skin. Testicular length >2 cm <3.2 cm. Sparse growth of long, slightly pigmented downy pubic hair, straight or only slightly curled appearing chiefly at base of penis | 11.6 9.5–13.8 |
| 3 | Growth of penis has occurred, at first mainly in length but some increase in breadth; further growth of testes and scrotum. Testicular length >3.3 cm <4.0 cm. Pubic hair is considerably darker, coarser, and curlier and spreads sparsely | 12.9 10.8–14.9 |
| 4 | Penis further enlarged in length and breadth with development of glans. Testes and scrotum are further enlarged. Scrotal skin has darkened. Testicular length >4.1 cm <4.9 cm. Pubic hair is now adult in type, but the area it covers is still smaller than most adults. There is no spread to medial surface of the thighs | 13.8 11.7–15.8 |
| 5 | Genitalia are adult in size and shape. No further enlargement takes place after stage 5 is reached. Testicular length >5 cm. Pubic hair is adult in quantity and type, distributed as an inverse triangle. The spread is to the medial surface of the thighs | 14.9 12.7–17.1 |

**Table 14.2** Gonadotoxic chemotherapeutic agents and associated cumulative doses that impact male fertility

| Gonadotoxic agents | Cumulative doses |
|---|---|
| Cyclophosphamide | 7 g/m$^2$ |
| Ifosfamide | 42–60 g/m$^2$ |
| Nitrosoureas, e.g., BCNU and CCNU | 1 g/m$^2$ and 500 mg/m$^2$ |
| Chlorambucil | 1.4 g/m$^2$ |
| Melphalan | 140 mg/m$^2$ |
| Busulfan | 600 mg/m$^2$ |
| Procarbazine | 4 g/m$^2$ |
| Cisplatin | 500 mg/m$^2$ |

reported [30]. In summary, testicular damage is agent-specific and dose-related. The chance of recovery of spermatogenesis following cytotoxic chemotherapy and the extent and speed of recovery are related to the agent used and the dose received [48]. In contrast to the germinal epithelium, Leydig cells appear relatively resistant to the effects of chemotherapy [68]. However, a few studies have demonstrated a reduction in testosterone concentrations following treatment with gonadotoxic agents, and there is evidence to suggest that the Leydig cell impairment following chemotherapy may be relevant clinically.

### 14.2.2 Cytotoxic Effects of Testicular Irradiation

Soon after the discovery of X-rays by Roentgen, investigators noted that spermatogenesis is exquisitely sensitive to radiation [60]. The testes are directly irradiated in rare situations such as testicular involvement of acute lymphoblastic leukemia (ALL). Although the testes are usually not directly in the radiation field, they can still receive irradiation via body scatter. Scatter occurs when X-rays interact with tissues near the target of interest, resulting in secondary X-rays that then hit the target [37]. The amount of scattered radiation is a function of the proximity of the radiation field to the target, the field size and shape, the X-ray energy, and the depth of the target. Of these, distance from the field edge is the most important factor. Scatter dose to the testes becomes a real issue when treating a field that extends into the pelvis as in some cases of Hodgkin's disease or soft tissue sarcoma of the thigh. Small children, because of their short trunk length, can be at greater risk from scattered radiation than larger individuals.

The germinal epithelium is most sensitive to radiation effects and some effect on spermatogenesis will be seen at doses of 10 cGy (Table 14.3) [3]. Permanent sterilization may be seen with doses as low as 100 cGy [3]. Speiser et al. reviewed experimental data in mammals that indicated that the total radiation dose required to induce permanent azoospermia was lower if a

**Table 14.3** Impairment of spermatogenesis and Leydig cell function after fractionated radiotherapy [3]

| Testicular dose (cGy) | Effect on spermatogenesis | Effect on Leydig cell function |
|---|---|---|
| <10 | No effect | No effect |
| 10–30 | Temporary oligospermia | No effect |
| 30–50 | Temporary azoospermia at 4–12 months after radiation. 100 % recovery by 48 months | No effect |
| 50–100 | 100 % temporary azoospermia for 3–17 months after radiation Recovery begins at 8–26 months | |
| 100–200 | 100 % azoospermia from 2 months to at least 9 months. Recovery begins at 11–20 months | Transient rise in LH No change in testosterone |
| 200–300 | 100 % azoospermia beginning at 1–2 months. May lead to permanent azoospermia. If recovery takes place, it may take years | Transient rise in LH No change in testosterone |
| 1,200 | Permanent azoospermia | Elevated LH. Some patients may have decreased basal testosterone or in response to HCG stimulation. Replacement therapy not needed to ensure pubertal changes in most boys |
| 2,400 | Permanent azoospermia | Elevated LH. Many patients, but not all, will have decreased testosterone. Replacement therapy needed to ensure pubertal changes in most boys |

fractionated regimen was used than if a single dose was given [74]. The details of these experiments cannot be extrapolated to humans because there are significant differences in germ cell radiosensitivity between different species. However, the general conclusion that fractionated radiation is more effective than single doses in destroying germ cells appears to be true in humans as well. The explanation given for this is that at any given time, some percentage of the spermatogonia are relatively radioresistant because they are not proliferating. A single large dose of radiation may not kill these cells. However, when fractionated radiation is delivered, there is a chance that these cells will enter the proliferating compartment and be susceptible to radiation-induced killing. Therefore, the most efficient regimen for spermatogonial killing would be one in which each fraction is maximally efficient in causing death in proliferating spermatogonia but in which there are a sufficient number of fractions such that all the spermatogonia are eventually irradiated when they are in a proliferative, radiosensitive state.

More attention has been focused on the effects of radiation on spermatogenesis than on its effects on Leydig cell function [30]. The data available indicates that chemical changes in Leydig cell function are observable following direct testicular irradiation with the effect more pronounced with 2,400 cGy than with 1,200 cGy [71]. The severity of the effect is more marked the younger the patient at the time of radiotherapy [9]. In general, progression through puberty and testosterone production proceeds normally in males subjected to radiation therapy.

## 14.3  Clinical Manifestations

### 14.3.1  Effects of Chemotherapy

The extent and reversibility of cytotoxic damage generally depends on the agent and cumulative dose received, although significant individual variation has been observed consistently. The effects of alkylating agents on testicular function have been studied extensively.

Cyclophosphamide, either alone or in combination with other agents, is known to damage the germinal epithelium. Meta-analysis of 30 studies

that examined gonadal function following various chemotherapy regimens noted that gonadal
dysfunction correlated with total cumulative dose
of cyclophosphamide; more than 300 mg/kg was
associated with >80 % risk of gonadal dysfunction [61]. A study of men treated for pediatric
solid tumors reported permanent azoospermia in
90 % of men treated with cyclophosphamide
doses >7.5 g/m$^2$ [78]. Other studies have also
found that 7.5–9 g/m$^2$ of cyclophosphamide is
associated with a significant risk of testicular
injury [4, 36].

Although tumor cytotoxicity data indicates
that 1.1 g/m$^2$ cyclophosphamide is approximately
equivalent to 3.8 g/m$^2$ ifosfamide [13], the relative gonadotoxic effect is not well known. In a
recent series of male childhood survivors of
osteosarcoma with a median age of 9 years (range
4–17 years) from completion of therapy, the incidence of azoospermia related to ifosfamide therapy (median 42 g/m$^2$) versus no ifosfamide was
statistically significant ($P=0.005$). Six patients
were normospermic: five received no ifosfamide
and one received low-dose ifosfamide (24 g/m$^2$).
Fifteen of the 19 azoospermic patients received
ifosfamide. Infertility in the others may have
been related to cisplatin (560–630 mg/m$^2$). One
patient had oligospermia [45]. Recent studies
support that doses of ifosfamide in excess of
60 mg/m$^2$ are associated with a significant risk of
infertility in male patients [34, 84].

Hodgkin's disease (HD) patients treated with
six or more courses of mechlorethamine, vincristine, procarbazine, and prednisone (MOPP) have
also demonstrated permanent azoospermia attributable to both of the alkylating agents: mechlorethamine and procarbazine. Procarbazine appears
to play a major role in this process. Hassel et al.
studied testicular function after OPA/COMP
(vincristine, prednisone, adriamycin/cyclophos-
phamide, vincristine, methotrexate, prednisone)
chemotherapy without procarbazine in boys with
HD. These patients showed no major testicular
damage compared to boys who had received
OPPA/COPP (includes procarbazine), again
pointing out that procarbazine is a potent gonadotoxic agent [25]. Treatment of Hodgkin's disease
with combination chemotherapy regimens such

as ChlVPP (chlorambucil, vinblastine, procarbazine, and prednisolone) or COPP (cyclophosphamide, vincristine, procarbazine, and prednisolone)
have also been reported in a number of studies to
result in permanent azoospermia in 99–100 % of
patients treated with six to eight courses of these
regimens [12, 28, 46]. After ChlVPP, FSH and
LH were elevated in 89 % and 24 % respectively,
with azoospermia in all seven patients tested.
Charak and coworkers found azoospermia in all
92 patients following treatment with six or more
cycles of COPP; 17 % of patients had been
treated more than 10 years previously, suggesting
that germinal epithelial failure is likely to be permanent [12]. CHOP (cyclophosphamide, doxorubicin, vincristine, prednisolone) or CHOP-like
regimens such as those which are used for non-
Hodgkin's lymphoma (NHL) are generally less
gonadotoxic than those used for HD, presumably
due to the absence of procarbazine in the treatment for NHL (e.g., VAPEC-B, VACOP-B,
MACOP) [51, 59]. Azoospermia occurring on
therapy for NHL is likely to recover within the
following year [58]. Efforts to reduce the risk of
sterility after Hodgkin disease include the use of
ABVD (adriamycin, bleomycin, vinblastine,
dacarbazine – an effective combination that does
not contain the alkylating agents chlorambucil or
procarbazine) [40, 82] and other related regimens. Viviani and coworkers showed that while
recovery of spermatogenesis after MOPP was
rare, all who experienced oligospermia after
ABVD recovered completely by 18 months [82].
Hybrid regimens (i.e., alternating cycles of
ABVD with ChlVPP or MOPP) are also less
gonadotoxic than MOPP, ChlVPP, or COPP
given alone.

Nitrosoureas, used in the treatment of brain
tumors in childhood, may also cause gonadal
damage in boys [1, 44, 66]. In nine children
treated for medulloblastoma with craniospinal
radiation and a nitrosourea (carmustine or lomustine plus vincristine in four and procarbazine in
three), there was clinical and biochemical evidence of gonadal damage. Specifically, these
children presented with elevated serum FSH and
small testes for the stage of pubertal development
(compared with eight children similarly treated

but without chemotherapy). The authors concluded that nitrosoureas were responsible for the gonadal damage, with procarbazine also contributing in the three children who received this drug.

PVB (cisplatin, vinblastine, and bleomycin) is standard chemotherapy with minimal effects on long-term testicular function that is used in patients with germ cell tumors. Such patients, however, can be affected by ejaculatory failure caused by damage to the thoracolumbar sympathetic plexus during retroperitoneal lymph node dissection and by preexisting germ cell defects. Hansen et al. found that for patients treated with orchiectomy or orchiectomy plus PVB, sperm production was similar 1.5 years after treatment. Approximately half in each group had sperm counts below the normal control reference level [24]. Lampe et al. analyzed data on 170 patients with testicular germ cell cancers who underwent treatment with either cisplatin- or carboplatin-based chemotherapy [41]. A median of 30 months after completion of chemotherapy, 54 (32 %) were azoospermic and 43 (25 %) were oligospermic. The probability of recovery to a normal sperm count was higher in men: (a) with a normal pretreatment sperm count, (b) men who received carboplatin rather than cisplatin-based therapy, and (c) men treated with less than five cycles of chemotherapy. Recovery continued for more than 2 years, with the calculated chance of spermatogenesis at 2 years being 48 %, and a calculated chance of spermatogenesis at 5 years being 80 % [31, 41].

Heyn and colleagues described the late effects of therapy on testicular function in patients aged 10 months to 19 years with paratesticular rhabdomyosarcoma as a result of cyclophosphamide, radiation, and retroperitoneal lymph node dissection. Tanner staging was normal in 45 patients for whom it was recorded. However, eight had loss of normal ejaculatory function. Elevated FSH values and/or azoospermia occurred in greater than half the patients where data was available. Testicular size was decreased in those who received cyclophosphamide or testicular irradiation [27].

The importance of alkylating agents in the induction of gonadal toxicity is noted by contrasting the above outcomes to those of children with acute lymphoblastic leukemia (ALL). In general, testicular function is normal in boys after chemotherapy for ALL. All 37 survivors of childhood ALL evaluated at two time points after the completion of treatment (median age 9.7 years and again 18.6 years later) completed pubertal development normally and had a testosterone concentration within the normal adult range [83]. Six men showed evidence of severe damage to the germ epithelium with azoospermia or elevated FSH; all of these patients had received cyclophosphamide as part of their chemotherapy regimen [83]. In contrast to alkylating agents, the classic antimetabolites used in the treatment of childhood ALL are not associated with long-term gonadal toxicity [30]. Both vincristine and corticosteroids can cause immediate inhibition of spermatogenesis; however, following the cessation of these agents, spermatogenesis recovery occurs [39].

### 14.3.1.1 Treatment-Induced Leydig Cell Failure from Chemotherapy

Leydig cells are much less vulnerable to damage from cancer therapy than germ cells, likely due to their slow rate of turnover [68]. For example, chemotherapy-induced Leydig cell failure resulting in androgen insufficiency and requiring testosterone-replacement therapy is rare. However, studies suggest that Leydig cell dysfunction may be observed following treatment with alkylator-based regiments. Specifically, raised plasma concentrations of LH combined with low levels of testosterone are the hallmarks of Leydig cell dysfunction. When Leydig cell dysfunction occurs prior to or during puberty, affected individuals will experience delayed and/or arrested pubertal maturation and lack of secondary sexual characteristics [70]. If the insult follows completion of normal pubertal development, observed symptoms include loss of libido, erectile dysfunction, decreased bone density, and decreased muscle mass [70]. Measurements of testosterone and gonadotropin concentrations are therefore warranted following chemotherapy treatment. Males with a raised LH concentration in the presence of a low testosterone levels should be considered for androgen replacement therapy.

## 14.3.2 Effects of Radiation

The data for gonadal function following fractionated radiotherapy in humans comes from patients with cancers who have been treated with either fields near the testes in which there is scatter dose or diseases such as testicular cancers or ALL in which the testes are thought to be at risk of harboring disease and irradiated directly. One of the potentially confounding issues is that some of these cancers may themselves be associated with decreased gonadal function independent of irradiation. For example, Hodgkin's disease is well documented to cause oligospermia in some patients [29]. Patients with testicular tumors may have preexisting gonadal dysfunction [29]. In ALL, the leukemic cells may infiltrate into the interstitium of the testis and conceivably affect Leydig cell function.

Ash summarized data from several older studies [21, 62, 74] that examined testicular function following radiation for patients who were treated for a range of cancers including Hodgkin's disease, prostate cancer, and testicular cancer [3] (see Table 14.3). They found that oligospermia occurred at doses as low as 10 cGy and azoospermia at 35 cGy, which was generally reversible. However, 200–300 cGy could result in azoospermia that did not reverse even years after irradiation.

These results have been supported by other reports. In a study of 17 males treated for Hodgkin's disease who received 6–70 cGy of scatter dose to the testes, in those patients who received <20 cGy, FSH levels stayed within the normal range [38]. Those receiving ≥20 cGy had a dose-dependent increase in serum FSH levels with a maximum difference seen at 6 months following radiation. In all patients the FSH normalized within 12–24 months. Eight patients had normal pretreatment sperm counts. Most of these patients continued to have high sperm counts following irradiation although two developed transient oligospermia with complete recovery of sperm count by 18 months. Four patients, all of whom had received 23 cGy or less, went on to father children. Ortin et al. reported on children treated for Hodgkin's disease [53]. Seven boys

received pelvic radiation as part of their treatment without any chemotherapy. Three of them fathered children. Three had azoospermia 10–15 years after irradiation, and one had testicular atrophy diagnosed by biopsy a year after irradiation. However, these results are difficult to interpret because there was no measurement or estimate of dose received to the testes in these children.

Similar data exist for patients treated for soft tissue sarcomas (median age at diagnosis 49 years; range 14–67) [69]. These patients were estimated to have received between 1 and 2,500 cGy (median dose 80 cGy) of scatter dose to the testes. Patients who received 50 cGy or more to the testes had a greater elevation in FSH than did those who received less than 50 cGy. Only the latter group showed normalization of FSH levels by 12 months, whereas in the former, FSH levels remained above baseline as long as 30 months out.

There are also data on germ cell function after treatment for testicular cancer. Hahn et al. examined gonadal function in 14 patients who were irradiated to the paraaortic and ipsilateral pelvic/inguinal lymphatics with a "hockey stick" field following orchiectomy for seminoma [22]. The scatter dose to the remaining testicle in these 14 patients ranged from 32 to 114 cGy (median 82 cGy). Ten patients, all of whom received ≥70 cGy to the testes, developed azoospermia between 10 and 30 weeks following radiation. All patients except for two had recovery of spermatogenesis, and the recovery time from azoospermia was dose-dependent. Centola et al. studying males with seminoma also showed that the recovery time from oligospermia/azoospermia was dose-dependent [10].

The previous data includes only patients who received incidental irradiation to the testes; however, there are situations in which children receive direct irradiation to the testes. Sklar et al. examined testicular function in 60 long-term survivors of childhood ALL [71]. All the patients had received identical chemotherapy; however, the RT fields varied significantly: (1) craniospinal radiation and 1,200 cGy to the abdomen and testes ($n=11$), (2) craniospinal RT with 1,800 or

2,400 cGy (estimated gonadal dose 36–360 cGy; $n = 23$), or (3) cranial RT with 1,800 or 2,400 cGy (negligible testicular dose; $n = 26$). Based on measurements of serum FSH and testicular volume, which commenced at either 12 years of age or 7 years after diagnosis of ALL, gonadal function abnormalities occurred in 55 %, 17 %, and 0 % of patients in groups 1, 2, and 3, respectively. Because many of the patients were adolescents at the time of testing, when evaluation of germ cell function can be difficult, this study probably underestimated the incidence of this problem. Castillo et al. (1992) examined 15 boys with ALL given 1,200–2,400 cGy to the testes prior to puberty (median age 6.8 years; range 5–12 years), either as prophylaxis or for testicular relapse [9]. Semen analyses, performed at least 9 years following testicular irradiation, showed azoospermia in seven out of seven cases. Six of these patients had received 1,200 cGy and one had received 1,500 cGy.

### 14.3.2.1 Leydig Cell Function Following RT

Leydig cells in the testes are more resistant to radiation than germ cells. In the study cited previously of patients with Hodgkin's disease who received 6–70 cGy of scatter dose to the testes, no patient showed any elevation in LH levels or decrease in testosterone levels [38]. In the study of men treated for sarcomas by Shapiro et al. discussed above [69], maximal increases in LH levels relative to baseline were seen at 6 months following radiation, but these elevations were statistically significant only in the group that received >200 cGy of scatter irradiation to the testes, not for the groups that received 50–200 cGy or <50 cGy. For those receiving >200 cGy, the elevation in LH levels persisted until the last follow-up, 30 months out. No statistically significant changes in testosterone levels were seen for any of these three dose levels.

Higher doses to the testes result in more marked Leydig cell damage. In one study, 18 men who had undergone orchiectomy for a unilateral testicular cancer were subsequently found to have carcinoma in situ for which they received 2,000 cGy in ten fractions to the remaining testis

[20]. Eight of the men already had evidence of Leydig cell dysfunction even before they received radiation, a finding previously described in patients with testicular cancers [29, 65]. There was a statistically significant increase in LH levels and decrease in HCG-stimulated testosterone levels over the course of the study.

Petersen et al. followed 48 patients who received 1,400–2,000 cGy of radiation for carcinoma in situ in a remaining testis following orchiectomy for testicular carcinoma [57]. Out of 42 men for whom data was available, 18 received hormonal supplementation therapy because of symptoms of androgen insufficiency. All patients had serial hormone analyses and at least one testicular biopsy more than a year after irradiation. 2,000 cGy led to a complete eradication of germ cells; however, Sertoli and Leydig cells were still present in the seminiferous tubules and in the intertubular space, respectively.

Data regarding Leydig cell function in boys following radiation comes primarily from studies following boys who received direct testicular irradiation for ALL. In the analysis by Sklar et al. (1990) mentioned previously, only 1 out of 53 boys tested for gonadotropins had an increased LH levels, and only 2 out of 50 patients tested had a reduced testosterone level [71]. None of the boys in this study had received greater than 1,200 cGy to the testes. In the study by Castillo et al., out of 15 boys who received testicular radiation, only 2 showed evidence of Leydig cell failure, both of which had received 2,400 cGy [9]. The remaining 13 boys who had received 1,200–1,500 cGy to the testes, all had normal pubertal development and normal testosterone levels basally and in response on to HCG stimulation. Another study examined 12 boys with ALL who received 2,400 cGy of testicular irradiation for either overt disease or prophylaxis [8]. Ten of the 12 patients had evidence of impaired Leydig cell function by either low serum testosterone in response to HCG stimulation or elevated LH levels basally and/or after LHRH stimulation. Similarly, Blatt et al. followed seven boys who received 2,400 cGy testicular irradiation for relapsed ALL [7]. All seven had elevated FSH levels. Four of these boys had documented bilateral testicular disease, and three of these showed delayed sexual maturation with low testosterone levels.

There are data that suggest that the prepubertal testis is more susceptible to Leydig cell injury than the adult testis. Shalet et al. (1989) examined Leydig cell function in three groups of patients: (1) 16 adults who underwent unilateral orchiectomy for testicular teratoma and did not receive postoperative RT, (2) 49 adults who underwent orchiectomy for testicular seminoma and then received radiation during adulthood to the remaining testis (3,000 cGy in 20 fractions), and (3) 5 adults who had received scrotal irradiation (2,750–3,000 cGy) between the ages of 1 and 4 years for various pediatric malignancies [68]. The median LH level was lower in group 1 than in group 2 (6 IU vs. 16 IU; $p < 0.0001$), an expected result since the former group had not received radiation. However, group 3 patients had far higher LH levels than either group 2 or group 1, 20 IU/l in one patient and greater than 32 IU/l in four patients. Similarly, the median testosterone level was lower in group 2 than in group 1 (12.5 vs. 16 nmol/l; $p < 0.02$). However, the median testosterone level in group 3 was 0.7 nmol/l. Four subjects had prepubertal levels (<2.5 nmol/l) and the fifth had a level of 4.5 nmol/l. Likewise, Brauner et al. also found that younger children were more vulnerable than older ones to Leydig cell dysfunction following testicular radiation for ALL. Other studies have confirmed that a significant proportion of boys with ALL who are prepubertal at the time when they receive 2,400 cGy to the testes will develop overt Leydig cells failure and require androgen replacement therapy [42, 67].

Based on statistical analysis of the raw data in the studies mentioned above as well as several others, Izard estimated that approximately 20 % of males who receive 100 cGy in fractionated doses to the testes will have an abnormally high LH level, while approximately 1,200 cGy is required to see an abnormal testosterone in the same percentage of men (see Fig. 14.1) [33]. The estimated doses needed to see these effects in 50 % of men were correspondingly higher, 1,400 cGy for LH and 3,300 cGy for testosterone.

Consistent with the high tolerance of the Leydig cells to radiation injury, Sklar reported that two men who received more than 4,000 cGy to the testes in late adolescence still maintained normal testosterone levels as adults [70].

### 14.3.2.2 Testicular Function Following Total Body Irradiation (TBI)

There are data on germ cell function following TBI as part of transplant conditioning. Sarafoglou et al. followed 17 boys who had received cyclophosphamide and TBI (either 1,375 cGy or 1,500 cGy in 125 cGy three per day fractionation) prior to puberty as part of a transplantation regimen for leukemia [64]. Fourteen of 17 patients (82 %) entered puberty spontaneously, with 13 having normal testosterone levels. Of the three that did not enter puberty spontaneously, one had received a 1,200 cGy testicular boost in addition to the TBI, and in the remaining two, the levels of FH and LH were very low, consistent with a prepubertal state.

Couto-Silva (2001) followed 29 boys who received TBI for different malignancies in association with a variety of chemotherapy regimens [15]. The TBI was given as a single 1,000 cGy fraction in 12 patients and in 200 cGy×6 fractions (1,200 cGy) in 17 patients. At the last follow-up, 19/29 (66 %) had tubular failure associated with elevated FSH. Eight (28 %) also had Leydig cell failure. There was no relationship

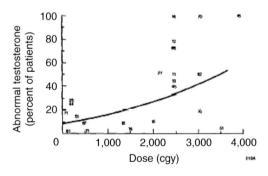

**Fig. 14.1** This graph shows the percentage of patients with an abnormal testosterone value compared against the stated dose of radiation to the testes based on a review of the literature. A curve showing best fit was extrapolated from the values by log-rank regression (Taken from Izard [33])

between the age at BMT and serum FSH, LH, or testosterone levels.

Bakker et al. followed 25 boys who were prepubertal at the time of bone marrow transplantation for hematological malignancy [5]. Transplantation included cyclophosphamide and TBI (single doses of 500 cGy, 750 cGy or 800 cGy or 1,200 cGy in six fractions). Nineteen boys who had not received additional testicular boost as part of their treatment all underwent puberty normally and achieved normal adult testosterone levels at some point following the onset of puberty. However, episodic elevations of LH were seen in ten of the patients, and in five patients, these elevations were accompanied by decreased testosterone. Elevation of FSH was seen in all patients.

These reports and others [43, 52] indicate that most boys who receive TBI, either single dose or fractionated as part of a transplantation regimen, will proceed through puberty and have normal testosterone levels. In contrast to this, Sanders [63], reporting the Seattle Marrow Transplant Team's experience, found a higher incidence of pubertal developmental delay in boys undergoing transplantation for leukemia using cyclophosphamide and TBI (900–1,000 cGy in a single fraction or 1,200–1,575 cGy in 200–225 cGy daily fractions over 6–7 days). There were 31 boys who were prepubertal at the time of transplantation and between the ages of 13 and 22 at the time of the study. Twenty-one out of 31 of these patients had delayed development of secondary sexual characteristics. Serum gonadotropins were obtained in 25 of the 31 boys and showed elevated LH levels in 10, normal levels in 12, and prepubertal levels in 3. It is not clear why this particular report showed such a high incidence of pubertal developmental delay compared to other studies, but it is possible that some of these boys had received prior testicular irradiation. Alternatively, the differences could be due to variations in exposure to alkylating agents or in total dose/fractionation schedule.

### 14.3.2.3 Summary

The spermatogenic capacity of the testes can be suppressed by extraordinarily low doses of radiation. As little as 10–20 cGy of scattered radiation in a fractionated regimen can lead to transient oligospermia and elevated FSH levels. Complete loss of sperm production appears to require somewhat higher doses and has been observed following 35 cGy. However, this effect may be transient. Permanent (or at least very long term) azoospermia has been seen after 140–260 cGy of fractionated scatter radiation. Doses used for testicular ALL which are an order of magnitude larger than these doses (1,200–2,400 cGy) are expected to lead to permanent azoospermia in virtually all patients.

In marked contrast to spermatogenic cells, doses of 70 cGy or less do not result in any increases in LH levels that might be suggestive of subclinical Leydig cell damage. LH elevation can be seen following fractionated regimens delivering 200 cGy to the testes. However, clinically relevant damage (failure of normal pubertal maturation; decreases in testosterone requiring replacement therapy) requires much higher doses, perhaps an order of magnitude greater. 1,200 cGy does not appear to cause loss of pubertal development in most boys who were prepubertal at the time of irradiation. However, this problem will occur in most prepubertal boys given 2,400 cGy. The data between 1,200 and 2,000 cGy are less clear cut with some studies showing normal sexual maturation in prepubertal boys who received these doses [9, 64] but others showing decreases in testosterone levels and subsequent requirement for androgen supplementation in a significant percentage of boys and men treated to these doses [57, 63]. The reason for the conflicting data regarding Leydig cell function at these intermediate doses probably has to do with the heterogeneity of patients in the various studies with differences in the underlying diseases, which might themselves affect Leydig cell function (i.e., testicular carcinoma, testicular ALL), the age of the patients at the time of irradiation, the use of alkylating agents, especially in transplantation studies, and the frequency and timing of the subsequent laboratory investigations to identify Leydig cell dysfunction.

## 14.4 Detection and Screening

### 14.4.1 Assessment of Testicular Function

The male reproductive tract is very susceptible to the toxic effects of chemotherapy and radiation, which may disrupt the endocrine axis or damage the testes directly. Assessment of testicular maturation and function involves pubertal staging, plasma hormone analysis, and semen analysis. Pubertal staging provides clinical information about both of the testicular functions. The development of normal secondary sexual characteristics would suggest intact Leydig cell function with normal steroidogenesis, while testicular volumes are an important indicator of spermatogenesis. Testicular volume of <12 ml, determined using the Prader orchidometer, is strongly suggestive of impaired spermatogenesis.

Hormone analysis involves measurement of plasma FSH, LH, and sex steroids. However, in prepubertal children, this is an unreliable predictor of gonadal damage since the prepubertal hypothalamic-pituitary-testicular axis is quiescent. In postpubertal boys, elevated LH and diminished testosterone levels would indicate Leydig cell dysfunction, while elevated FSH and diminished inhibin B would support germ cell failure. HCG may be given to confirm the diagnosis of end-organ failure as a cause of hypogonadism. An abnormal response to HCG is suggestive of disturbed Leydig cell function. Patients with hypogonadotrophic hypogonadism should have a brisk response, while those with decreased Leydig cell function will have little or none. GnRH may be administered to determine whether the primary defect is in the hypothalamus, in which case the pituitary and testicles themselves should respond normally to exogenous GnRH, or in the pituitary itself, in which case there will be an inadequate response. An exaggerated response of FSH and LH to GnRH suggests a "failing" testis, so this test may be useful in detecting early testicular failure. Depressed gonadotropins may also be found in patients after the administration of exogenous androgen. Determination of elevated FSH along with small

testicular size may offer the most practical approach for predicting subsequent testicular damage in boys with malignancies.

Recently, there has been an interest in estimating the gonadal function of male cancer survivors directly by measuring the serum levels of the bioactive gonadal peptide hormone inhibin B using a newly developed enzyme-linked immunosorbent assay [2, 81]. It is postulated that inhibin B is produced by the Sertoli cells and the germ cells of the testes and reflects the degree of seminiferous tubular damage [35, 56, 66]. Furthermore, inhibin B exerts negative feedback regulation of pituitary production and FSH release [17]. In a study examining gonadal status of childhood brain tumor survivors, researchers found a significant inverse correlation between basal FSH and inhibin B, and a significant correlation between inhibin B and total testicular volume [66].

Following pubertal staging and hormone analysis, semen analysis is necessary to confirm spermatogenesis (Table 14.4). The sample should be fresh and properly collected. This usually involves abstaining from sexual intercourse for and collecting the specimen by masturbation. Sperm count and quality can provide useful information about the likelihood of natural fertility or whether assisted reproduction may be required. Since recovery from damage to germinal epithelium may occur 5–10 years (or even later) after therapy, these counts should be repeated from time to time as indicated.

## 14.5 Management of Established Problems

### 14.5.1 Method to Minimize Testicular Radiation Dose

As discussed above, in most cases, the testicular dose from a radiation treatment is mostly due to internal scatter, not direct irradiation. Internal scatter is difficult to prevent, but methods have been developed to decrease this dose. Frass et al. reported on a gonadal shield that formed a cup around the testes to reduce the testicular dose

**Table 14.4** Assessment of fertility status

| Test | Interpretation |
| --- | --- |
| Inhibin B | Low levels indicate impaired spermatogenesis |
| FSH | Elevated levels indicate impaired spermatogenesis |
| Semen analysis | Sperm count best indicator of fertility status |

[19, 69]. They found that this led to a three- to tenfold reduction in the dose to the testes, depending on the distance from the proximal edge of the field. In almost all cases, the measured dose to the testes was less than 1 % of the prescription dose. Therefore, for a patient receiving 5,000 cGy to a pelvic field, the dose to the testes would be less than 50 cGy, which would most likely prevent permanent azoospermia and almost certainly prevent a decline in testosterone levels.

## 14.5.2 Prevention of Testicular Damage

The cytotoxic effect of chemotherapy on germinal epithelia function launched a search for possible fertility preservation strategies in men undergoing therapy. Cryopreservation of sperm has become a standard practice and should be offered to all newly diagnosed postpubertal males at risk for potential infertility. Many improvements have been made in the techniques used to store sperm, and advances in assisted reproductive technology using intracytoplasmic sperm injection (ICSI) have increased the chance of successful pregnancies using banked sperm [18, 54].

Ejaculatory azoospermia is not the same as testicular azoospermia [11]. Therefore, studies on the gonadotoxicity of chemotherapy have to be interpreted in the era of assisted reproductive technology in which it is possible to use testis sperm to conceive. The level of sperm necessary for sperm to exist in the testis is far less than that required for sperm in the ejaculate [11]. Therefore, with testis sperm extraction (TESE), followed by ICSI, it is now possible for patients who did not sperm bank, and have azoospermia

on semen analysis, to be evaluated for TESE/ICSI. A retrospective study by Damani et al. evaluated 23 men with ejaculatory azoospermia and a history of chemotherapy. They underwent TESE in search of usable sperm. Spermatozoa were found on TESE in 15 (65 %) of 23 men. The subsequent fertility rate was 65 % and pregnancy occurred in 31 % of cycles [16]. Men with post-chemotherapy azoospermia must be fully evaluated before they are considered sterile [32].

Unfortunately, at this time, there are no feasible options for prepubertal male patients. There has been no demonstrated protective effect of using GnRH analogues with and without testosterone to suppress testicular function during chemotherapy [53]. As pediatric oncologists, we must continue to attempt to reduce the gonadotoxicity of our treatment regimens while maintaining superior cure rates.

## References

1. Ahmed SR, Shalet SM, Campbell RH, Deakin DP (1983) Primary gonadal damage following treatment of brain tumors in childhood. J Pediatr 103:562–565
2. Andersson AM, Muller J, Skakkeaek NE (1998) Different roles of prepubertal and postpubertal germ cells and sertoli cells in the regulation of serum inhibin b levels. J Clin Endocrinol Metab 83:4451–4458
3. Ash P (1980) The influence of radiation on fertility in man. Br J Radiol 53:271–278
4. Aubier F, Flamamant F, Brauner R, Caillaud JM, Chaussain JM, Lemerle J (1989) Male gonadal function after chemotherapy for solid tumors in childhood. J Clin Oncol 7:304–309
5. Bakker B, Massa GG, Oostdijk W, Van Weel-Sipman MH, Vossen JM, Wit JM (2000) Pubertal development and growth after total-body irradiation and bone marrow transplantation for haematological malignancies. Eur J Pediatr 159(1–2):31–37
6. Ben Arush MW, Solt I, Lightman A, Linn S, Kuten A (2000) Male gonadal function in survivors of childhood Hodgkin and non-Hodgkin lymphoma. Pediatr Hematol Oncol 17(3):239–245
7. Blatt J, Sherins RJ, Niebrugge D, Bleyer WA, Poplack DG (1985) Leydig cell function in boys following treatment for testicular relapse of acute lymphoblastic leukemia. J Clin Oncol 3(9):1227–1231
8. Brauner R, Czernichow P, Cramer P, Schaison G, Rappaport R (1983) Leydig-cell function in children after direct testicular irradiation for acute lymphoblastic leukemia. N Engl J Med 309:25–28

9. Castillo LA, Craft AW, Kernahan J, Evans RG, Aynsley-Green A (1990) Gonadal function after 12-Gy testicular irradiation in childhood acute lymphoblastic leukaemia. Med Pediatr Oncol 18:185–189

10. Centola GM, Keller JW, Henzler M, Rubin P (1994) Effect of low-dose testicular irradiation on sperm count and fertility in patients with testicular seminoma. J Androl 15:608–613

11. Chan PTK, Palermo GD, Veeck LL, Rosenwaks Z, Schlegel PN (2001) Testicular sperm extraction combined with intracytoplasmic sperm injection in the treatment of men with persistent azoospermis post-chemotherapy. Cancer 92:1632–1637

12. Charak BS, Gupta R, Mandrekar P, Sheth NA, Banavali SD, Saikia TK, Gopal R, Dinshaw KA, Advani SH (1990) Testicular dysfunction after cyclophosphamide-vincristine-procarbazine-prednisolone chemotherapy for advanced Hodgkin's disease. A long-term follow-up study. Cancer 65:1903–1906

13. Colvin M (1982) The comparative pharmacology of cyclophosphamide and ifosfamide. Semin Oncol 9:2–7

14. Conte FA, Grumbach MM (1990) Pathogenesis, classification, diagnosis and treatment of anomalies of sex. In: Degroot LJ (ed) Endocrinology. WB Saunders, Philadelphia

15. Couto-Silva AC, Trivin C, Thibaud E, Esperou H, Michon J, Brauner R (2001) Factors affecting gonadal function after bone marrow transplantation during childhood. Bone Marrow Transplant 28:67–75

16. Damani MN, Masters V, Meng MV, Burgess C, Turek P, Oates RD (2002) Postchemotherapy ejaculatory azoospermia: fatherhood with sperm from testis tissue with intracytoplasmic sperm injection. J Clin Oncol 20:930–936

17. de Kretser DM, McFarlane JR (1996) Inhibin in the male. J Androl 17:179–182

18. Feldschuh J, Brassel J, Durso N, Levine A (2005) Successful sperm storage for 28 years. Fertil Steril 84:1017

19. Fraass BA, Kinsella TJ, Harrington FS, Glatstein E (1985) Peripheral dose to the testes: the design and clinical use of a practical and effective gonadal shield. Int J Radiat Oncol Biol Phys 11:609–615

20. Giwercman A, von der Maase H, Berthelsen JG, Rorth M, Bertelsen A, Skakkebaek NE (1991) Localized irradiation of testes with carcinoma in situ: effects on leydig cell function and eradication of malignant germ cells in 20 patients. J Clin Endocrinol Metab 73:596–603

21. Hahn EW, Feingold SM, Nisce L (1976) Aspermia and recovery of spermatogenesis in cancer patients following incidental gonadal irradiation during treatment: a progress report. Radiology 119:223–225

22. Hahn EW, Feingold SM, Simpson L, Batata M (1982) Recovery from aspermia induced by low-dose radiation in seminoma patients. Cancer 50:337–340

23. Hansen PV, Hansen SW (1993) Gonadal function in men with testicular germ cell cancer: the influence of cisplatin-based chemotherapy. Eur Urol 23:153–156

24. Hansen PV, Trykker H, Helkjoer PE, Andersen J (1989) Testicular function in patients with testicular cancer treated with orchiectomy alone or orchiectomy plus cisplatin-based chemotherapy. J Natl Cancer Inst 81:1246–1250

25. Hassel JU, Bramswig JH, Schlegel W, Schellong G (1991) Testicular function after OPA/COMP chemotherapy without procarbazine in boys with Hodgkin's disease. Results in 25 patients of the DAL-HD-85 study. Klin Padiatr 203:268–272

26. Heikens J, Behrendt H, Adriaanse R, Berghout A (1996) Irreversible gonadal damage in male survivors of pediatric Hodgkin's disease. Cancer 78:2020–2024

27. Heyn R, Raney RB Jr, Hays DM, Tefft M, Gehan E, Webber B, Maurer HM (1992) Late effects of therapy in patients with paratesticular rhabdomyosarcoma. Intergroup Rhabdomyosarcoma Study Committee. J Clin Oncol 10:614–623

28. Hobbie WL, Ginsberg JP, Ogle SK, Carlson CA, Meadows AT (2005) Fertility in males treated for Hodgkins disease with COPP/ABV hybrid. Pediatr Blood Cancer 44:193–196

29. Howell SJ, Shalet SM (2002) Effect of cancer therapy on pituitary-testicular axis. Int J Androl 25:269–276

30. Howell SJ, Shalet SM (2005) Spermatogenesis after cancer treatment: damage and recovery. J Natl Cancer Inst Monogr 34:12–17

31. Howell SJ, Shalet SM (2001) Testicular function following chemotherapy. Hum Reprod Update 7:363–369

32. Hsiao W, Stahl PJ, Osterberg EC, Nejat E, Palermo GD, Rosenwaks Z, Schlegel PN (2011) Successful treatment of postchemotherapy azoospermia with microsurgical testicular sperm extraction: the Weill Cornell experience. J Clin Oncol 29:1607–1611

33. Izard MA (1995) Leydig cell function and radiation: a review of the literature. Radiother Oncol 34:1–8

34. Janeway KA, Grier HE (2010) Sequelae of osteosarcoma medical therapy: a review of rare acute toxicities and late effects. Lancet Oncol 11:670–678

35. Jensen TK, Andersson AM, Hjollund NH (1997) Inhibin b as a serum marker of spermatogenesis: correlation to differences in sperm concentration and follicle-stimulating hormone levels. A study of 349 danish men. J Clin Endocrinol Metab 82:4059–4063

36. Kenney LB, Laufer MR, Grant FD, Grier H, Diller L (2001) High risk of infertility and long term gonadal damage in males treated with high dose cyclophosphamide for sarcoma during childhood. Cancer 91:613–621

37. Khan F (2003) The physics of radiation therapy, 3rd edn. Lippincott, Williams and Wilkins, Philadelphia

38. Kinsella TJ, Trivette G, Rowland J, Sorace R, Miller R, Fraass B, Steinberg SM, Glatstein E, Sherins RJ (1989) Long-term follow-up of testicular function

following radiation therapy for early-stage Hodgkin's disease. J Clin Oncol 7:718–724

39. Kreuser ED, Hetzel WD, Heit W, Hoelzer D, Kurrle E, Xiros N, Heimpel H (1988) Reproductive and endocrine gonadal functions in adults following multidrug chemotherapy for acute lymphoblastic or undifferentiated leukemia. J Clin Oncol 6:588–595

40. Kulkarni SS, Sastry PS, Saikia TK, Parikh PM, Gopal R, Advani SH (1997) Gonadal function following abvd therapy for Hodgkin's disease. Am J Clin Oncol 20:354–357

41. Lampe H, Horwich A, Norman A, Nicholls J, Dearnaley DP (1997) Fertility after chemotherapy for testicular germ cell cancers. J Clin Oncol 15:239–245

42. Leiper AD, Grant DB, Chessells JM (1986) Gonadal function after testicular radiation for acute lymphoblastic leukaemia. Arch Dis Child 61:53–56

43. Leiper AD, Stanhope R, Lau T, Grant DB, Blacklock H, Chessells JM, Plowman PN (1987) The effect of total body irradiation and bone marrow transplantation during childhood and adolescence on growth and endocrine function. Br J Haematol 67:419–426

44. Livesey EA, Brook CG (1988) Gonadal dysfunction after treatment of intracranial tumours. Arch Dis Child 63:495–500

45. Longhi A, Macchiagodena M, Vitali G, Bacci G (2003) Fertility in male patients treated with neoadjuvant chemotherapy for osteosarcoma. J Pediatr Hematol Oncol 25:292–296

46. Mackie EJ, Radford M, Shalet SM (1996) Gonadal function following chemotherapy for childhood Hodgkin's disease. Med Pediatr Oncol 27:74–78

47. Marshall WA, Tanner JM (1970) Variation in pattern of pubertal changes in boys. Arch Dis Child 45:13–23

48. Meistrich ML (2009) Male gonadal toxicity. Pediatr Blood Cancer 53:261–266

49. Moore KL (1988) The urogenital system. In: The developing human, 4th edn. W.B. Saunders, Toronto

50. Morris ID (1996) The testis: endocrine function. In: Hiller SG, Kitchener HC, Neilson JP (eds) Scientific essentials of reproductive medicine. W.B. Saunders, London, pp 160–171

51. Muller U, Stahel RA (1993) Gonadal function after MACOP-B or VACOP-B with or without dose intensification and ABMT in young patients with aggressive non-Hodgkin's lymphoma. Ann Oncol 4:399–402

52. Ogilvy-Stuart AL, Clark DJ, Wallace WH, Gibson BE, Stevens RF, Shalet SM, Donaldson MD (1992) Endocrine deficit after fractionated total body irradiation. Arch Dis Child 67:1107–1110

53. Ortin TT, Shostak CA, Donaldson SS (1990) Gonadal status and reproductive function following treatment for Hodgkin's disease in childhood: the Stanford experience. Int J Radiat Oncol Biol Phys 19:873–880

54. Palermo GD, Cohen J, Alikani M, Adler A, Rosenwaks Z (1995) Intracytoplasmic sperm injection: a novel treatment for all forms of male factor infertility. Fertil Steril 63:1231–1240

55. Papadakis V, Vlachopapadopoulou E, Van Syckle K, Ganshaw L, Kalmanti M, Tan C, Sklar C (1999) Gonadal function in young patients successfully treated for Hodgkin disease. Med Pediatr Oncol 32:366–372

56. Petersen PM, Andersson AM, Rorth M, Daugaard G, Skakkeaek NE (1999) Undetectable inhibin B serum levels in men after testicular irradiation. J Clin Endocrinol Metab 84:213–215

57. Petersen PM, Giwercman A, Daugaard G, Rorth M, Petersen JH, Skakkeaek NE, Hansen SW, von der Maase H (2002) Effect of graded testicular doses of radiotherapy in patients treated for carcinoma-in-situ in the testis. J Clin Oncol 20(6):1537–1543

58. Pryzant RM, Meistrich ML, Wilson G (1993) Long-term reduction in sperm count after chemotherapy with and without radiation therapy for non-Hodgkin's lymphomas. J Clin Oncol 11:239–247

59. Radford JA, Clark S, Crowther D, Shalet SM (1994) Male fertility after VAPEC-B chemotherapy for Hodgkin's disease and non-Hodgkin's lymphoma. Br J Cancer 69:379–381

60. Regaud C, Blanc J (1906) Extreme sensibilite des spermatogonies a ces rayons. C R Soc Biol Paris 61:163–165

61. Rivkees SA, Crawford JD (1988) The relationship of gonadal activity and chemotherapy-induced gonadal damage. JAMA 259:2123–2125

62. Sandeman TF (1966) The effects of x irradiation on male human fertility. Br J Radiol 39:901–907

63. Sanders JE, Pritchard S, Mahoney P, Amos D, Buckner CD, Witherspoon RP, Deeg HJ, Doney KC, Sullivan KM, Appelbaum FR et al (1986) Growth and development following marrow transplantation for leukemia. Blood 68:1129–1135

64. Sarafoglou K, Boulad F, Gillio A, Sklar C (1997) Gonadal function after bone marrow transplantation for acute leukemia during childhood. J Pediatr 130:210–216

65. Schilsky RL (1989) Infertility in patients with testicular cancer: testis, tumor, or treatment? J Natl Cancer Inst 81:1204–1205

66. Schmiegelow M, Lassen S, Poulsen HS, Schmiegelow K, Hertz H, Andersson AM, Skakkebaek NE, Muller J (2001) Gonadal status in male survivors following childhood brain tumors. J Clin Endocrinol Metab 86:2446–2452

67. Shalet SM, Horner A, Ahmed SR, Morris-Jones PH (1985) Leydig cell damage after testicular irradiation for lymphoblastic leukaemia. Med Pediatr Oncol 13:65–68

68. Shalet SM, Tsatsoulis A, Whitehead E, Read G (1989) Vulnerability of the human leydig cell to radiation damage is dependent upon age. J Endocrinol 120:161–165

69. Shapiro E, Kinsella TJ, Makuch RW, Fraass BA, Glatstein E, Rosenberg SA, Sherins RJ (1985) Effects

of fractionated irradiation of endocrine aspects of testicular function. J Clin Oncol 3:1232–1239

70. Sklar C (1999) Reproductive physiology and treatment-related loss of sex hormone production. Med Pediatr Oncol 33:2–8

71. Sklar CA, Robison LL, Nesbit ME, Sather HN, Meadows AT, Ortega JA, Kim TH, Hammond GD (1990) Effects of radiation on testicular function in long-term survivors of childhood acute lymphoblastic leukemia: a report from the Children Cancer Study Group. J Clin Oncol 8:1981–1987

72. Smith EP, Boyd J, Frank GR (1994) Estrogen resistance caused by a mutation in the estrogen-receptor gene in a man. N Engl J Med 331:1056–1061

73. Smith KD, Rodgriguez-Rigau LJ (1989) Laboratory evaluation of testicular function. In: Degroot LJ (ed) Endocrinology. W.B. Saunders, Philadelphia

74. Speiser B, Rubin P, Casarett G (1973) Aspermia following lower truncal irradiation in Hodgkin's disease. Cancer 32:692–698

75. Spitz S (1948) The histological effects of nitrogen mustards on human tumors and tissues. Cancer 1:383–398

76. Steinberger E (1989) Structural consideration of the male reproductive system. In: DeGroot LJ (ed) Endocrinology. W.B. Saunders, Philadelphia

77. Styne DM (1982) The testes: disorders of sexual differentiation and puberty. In: Kaplan SA (ed) Clinical pediatric endocrinology. WB Saunders, Philadelphia

78. Thomson AB, Campbell AJ, Irvine DC, Anderson RA, Kelnar CJ, Wallace WH (2002) Semen quality and spermatozoal DNA integrity in survivors of childhood cancer: a case-control study. Lancet 360: 361–367

79. Tsatsoulis A, Shalet SM, Morris ID, de Kretser DM (1990) Immunoactive inhibin as a marker of sertoli cell function following cytotoxic damage to the human testis. Horm Res 34:254–259

80. van Beek RD, Smit M, van den Heuvel-Eibrink MM, de Jong FH, Hakvoort-Cammel FG, van den Bos C, van den Berg H, Weber RF, Pieters R, de Muinck Keizer-Schrama SM (2007) Inhibin B is superior to FSH as a serum marker for spermatogenesis in men treated for Hodgkin's lymphoma with chemotherapy during childhood. Hum Reprod 22:3215–3222

81. van Casteren NJ, van der Linden GH, Hakvoort-Cammel FG, Hahlen K, Dohle GR, van den Heuvel-Eibrink MM (2009) Effect of childhood cancer treatment on fertility markers in adult male long-term survivors. Pediatr Blood Cancer 52:108–112

82. Viviani S, Santoro A, Ragni G, Bonfante V, Bestetti O, Bonadonna G (1985) Gonadal toxicity after combination chemotherapy for Hodgkin's disease. Comparative results of MOPP vs ABVD. Eur J Cancer Clin Oncol 21:601–605

83. Wallace WH, Shalet SM, Lendon M, Morris-Jones PH (1991) Male fertility in long-term survivors of childhood acute lymphoblastic leukaemia. Int J Androl 14:312–319

84. Williams D, Crofton PM, Levitt G (2008) Does ifosfamide affect gonadal function? Pediatr Blood Cancer 50:347–351

# Genitourinary

# 15

Nicole Larrier

## Contents

N. Larrier, MD, MSc
Department of Radiation Oncology, Duke University Medical Center, Durham, NC 27710, USA
e-mail: nicole.larrier@duke.edu

## 15.1 Introduction

This chapter addresses the long-term effects of the treatment of childhood cancer on the genitourinary (GU) tract, primarily focusing on the kidneys, ureters, bladder, urethra, prostate, vagina, and uterus. The effects on ovaries and testes are reviewed in Chaps. 13 and 14. The most common pediatric cancers that occur in the GU tract include Wilms' tumor, neuroblastoma, and rhabdomyosarcoma. The median age of children affected with these tumors ranges from 3 years (Wilms' tumor, neuroblastoma) to 6 years (rhabdomyosarcoma). Growth and development of the GU tract in the following years may be compromised by the cancer treatment, including surgery, radiation therapy (RT), or chemotherapy; see Table 15.1. Recent changes in cancer therapy, including bone marrow transplantation, intraoperative radiation therapy, and high-dose rate brachytherapy, pose new risks that have not been clearly defined. Furthermore, GU organs may be incidentally damaged by therapies used to treat tumors in non-GU organs. For example, many of the chemotherapeutic agents used to treat both GU and non-GU tumors are potentially toxic to the kidney and/or bladder. In addition, radiation fields designed to treat the liver or pelvic bones usually include portions of the kidney or bladder.

## 15.2 Pathophysiology

### 15.2.1 Normal Organ Development

Normal fetal development of the GU structures begins with successive development of pronephric, mesonephric, and metanephric tubules around the third, sixth, and twelfth weeks of gestation in the embryo, respectively. After 12 weeks, the urinary bladder has developed and separated from the rectum. The prostate and testes in boys, and the ovaries and uterus in girls, are also formed at approximately 12 weeks gestation. The vagina develops somewhat later. After birth, prostatic and vaginal-uterine growth proceeds very slowly until adolescence, when the organs enlarge during pubertal growth.

### 15.2.2 Organ Damage and Developmental Problems

The multimodal treatment of cancers with surgery, RT, and chemotherapy may cause structural or functional impairment of the GU organs and tissues. Table 15.1 summarizes late organ damage to the GU system.

### 15.2.3 Surgery

Removal of a paired structure, such as a kidney, is not usually associated with subsequent functional impairment, unless the remaining organ has been damaged from either therapy or the tumor. (In fact, the remaining kidney may undergo compensatory hypertrophy [1].) Conversely, the removal of a nonpaired structure such as the bladder, prostate, or uterus can produce severe and life-long impairment, such as urinary incontinence or infertility. Urinary diversion after total cystectomy for bladder sarcoma in childhood can be associated with infection and eventual renal impairment from pyelonephritis, ureteral, or stomal obstruction or both [2, 3]. In addition, ureterocolic diversion and bladder augmentation have occasionally been associated with early development of colon cancer [4]. It is also seen with reconstruction of the neurogenic bladder. The hypothesis is that the irritation of urine on bowel mucosa can be carcinogenic. An interesting canine study showed hyperplasia at the anastomoses [5]. Continent diversion techniques, using repeated catheterization of an indwelling ileal or colonic bladder, may provide better results [6]. Continent diversion is accomplished by creating a reservoir usually of bowel

**Table 15.1** Summary of late organ damage

| Organ | Surgery | Radiation therapy | Chemotherapy |
|---|---|---|---|
| Kidney | Late proteinuria possible with single kidney<br>Renal failure if bilateral | A single normal kidney usually provides good function<br>Bilateral injury can lead to renal dysfunction | Glomerular and tubular injury (cisplatin, ifosfamide) |
| Ureter | Urinary diversion may be necessary | Fibrosis rare: may occur after high-dose or intraoperative irradiation | |
| Bladder | Dysfunction due to partial or total organ loss may occur | Fibrosis, focal ulceration possible<br>Loss of capacity if large fraction of kidney irradiated | Contracture and functional loss possible after hemorrhagic cystitis (cyclophosphamide, ifosfamide)<br>Secondary bladder cancer (cyclophosphamide, ifosfamide) |
| Urethra | Stricture requiring dilation possible | | |
| Vagina | Dysfunction with partial or total organ loss | Fibrosis, ulceration, fistula, and maldevelopment possible | |
| Uterus | Dysfunction due to partial or total organ loss may occur | Maldevelopment and fibrosis possible | |
| Prostate | Dysfunction due to partial or total organ loss may occur | Loss of glandular function is possible | |

that the patient empties periodically via catheterization throughout the day.

## 15.2.4 Radiation Therapy

Organ injury following RT is generally classified as acute (occurring during or soon after therapy) and late (occurring months to years following therapy). Whereas the acute effects are usually transient, late effects are usually progressive. Acutely, RT frequently causes irritation of the mucosa of the bladder and urethra (causing cystitis and urethritis) or of the vagina and vulva (causing pruritus, discomfort, and candidal overgrowth). These symptoms usually occur after approximately 20 Gy of radiation. Since almost all children receiving GU tract irradiation are also receiving chemotherapy, normal acute tissue toxicities are seen earlier than they would be seen without concurrent chemotherapy. Typically, cystitis occurs after 3–4 weeks of radiation, but it can occur after 2 weeks with concurrent therapy. Occasionally, some morbidity is seen after doses as low as 8–10 Gy. Acute injury of the kidney, prostate, and uterus is generally not clinically apparent. The later effects of RT are dose dependent and due to progressive vascular and parenchymal cell damage, generally leading to scarring, fibrosis, and sometimes necrosis. Malignant tumors can be seen following irradiation, generally occurring a minimum of 4–5 years following completion of radiation [7]. A discussion of the late effects for each organ follows.

### 15.2.4.1 Kidney

Irradiation appears to cause renal dysfunction secondary to tubular damage. Nephropathy generally occurs when doses in excess of 20–25 Gy are delivered to both kidneys [8]. When chemotherapeutic agents are used as well, lower doses (10–15 Gy) can cause significant injury. In general, if only a portion (less than one-half to one-third) of the kidney is irradiated, then higher doses may be tolerated without demonstrable functional deficits. The sequelae may be more prominent and occur at lower doses in infants. Hyper-renin hypertension can also occur secondary to radiation-induced renal artery narrowing. This phenomenon has been noted most often in children (especially infants) and should be distinguished from other types of renal radiation-induced hypertension. Irradiation to the remaining kidney following nephrectomy may hinder the normal hypertrophic response.

### 15.2.4.2 Bladder, Ureter, and Urethra

Radiation can induce inflammation and fibrosis and cause dysfunction due to a reduction in bladder capacity and contractility. Although it is not certain, the underlying etiology seems to be radiation-induced vascular ischemia of the muscular wall [9–11]. The risk of developing bladder dysfunction is related to both the radiation dose and the percentage of the bladder wall irradiated [9, 12]. In data compiled in adults, it is clear that a small volume of the bladder can tolerate fairly high doses of radiation [9, 12]. (Radiation for prostate or bladder cancer in adults routinely results in irradiation of portions of the bladder with 60–70 Gy.) However, high doses may cause focal injury to part of the bladder wall, resulting in bleeding and stone formation [13–17]. It is believed that stone formation is associated with bacteriuria, which can occur after damage to the bladder. When the entire bladder is irradiated, doses of >50 Gy may result in severe contraction and secondary whole organ dysfunction. Consequently, both the radiation dose and volume of organ irradiated must be considered when assessing the risk of injury. Similarly, scarring and fibrosis can occur in the urethra and ureter, causing dysfunction of these structures [17–19]. Doses less than 50 Gy may slow or hamper the full development of the bladder, due to lesser degrees of fibrosis (Fig. 15.1).

### 15.2.4.3 Prostate, Uterus, and Vagina

The exact pathophysiology of radiation-induced late effects is less well defined than for the kidneys and bladder. When irradiated to high doses in an adult, the vagina undergoes loss of the epithelium and slow reepithelialization over a 2-year period. It is likely that the prominent late effects in the uterus and vagina are related to progressive fibrosis, leading to loss of function [20]. The

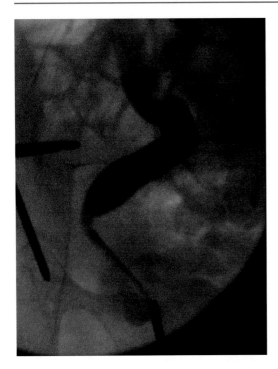

**Fig. 15.1** Stenosis (*arrow*) in ureter in a 13-year-old who received 41.4 Gy pelvic radiotherapy at age 2 for rhabdomyosarcoma

prostate may lose its secretory capacity, resulting in ejaculatory dysfunction.

## 15.2.5 Chemotherapy

The major chemotherapeutic agents that cause damage to the GU tract are the platinum compounds (cisplatin and carboplatin) and alkylating agents (cyclophosphamide and ifosfamide). The toxicity of the antimetabolite, methotrexate, is largely preventable and reversible [21].

### 15.2.5.1 Kidney

Cisplatin causes both glomerular and renal tubular damage, with wasting of divalent and monovalent cations (magnesium, calcium, and potassium). Cumulative doses as low as 450 mg/$m^2$ are associated with some renal toxicity. Proximal tubular damage predominates, especially in a low chloride environment [22]. Elevated serum concentration of creatinine and decreased glomerular filtration rate (GFR) with azotemia also occur and are dose and age related.

These effects vary both in severity and chronicity [22, 23]. Prior cisplatin administration may delay the renal clearance of methotrexate [24]. Carboplatin has a better renal toxicity profile than cisplatin. The replacement of cisplatin with carboplatin in standard regimens is being tested in adult studies, but in some instances, the tumor efficacy is not equivalent. Carboplatin at doses used in stem cell transplantation has been associated with renal dysfunction [25]. At present, the routine use of amifostine to protect renal integrity and function is not indicated [26, 27]. Its routine use as a renal protector is being investigated in clinical trials; a COG study did not show this approach to be effective in germ cell tumors [28].

The acute effects of ifosfamide, seen most commonly in young (<3-year-old) children or those with prior renal dysfunction or nephrectomy, include renal tubular damage with hyperphosphaturia, glycosuria, and aminoaciduria, followed by the inability to acidify the urine – the so-called Fanconi syndrome [29–31]. Hypophosphatemia and acidosis can lead to inhibition of statural growth, as well as to bone deformity (renal rickets) in prepubertal and pubertal children. Glomerular damage may accompany the tubular damage, leading to diminished GFR, with increased serum creatinine and azotemia. Median doses of 54 g/$m^2$ have been reported to cause progressive glomerular toxicity [32], and chronic glomerular and tubular toxicity has been reported [32, 33]. Risk factors include total ifosfamide dose [33], prior cisplatin administration [30, 31], and age. Recovery of renal function is possible over time [34].

Methotrexate toxicity is usually acute and reversible. The drug and its metabolites precipitate in the renal tubules. Adequate hydration and leucovorin administration will prevent most renal damage. (Doses up to 12 g/$m^2$ can be given safely if the appropriate precautions are taken [35].)

### 15.2.5.2 Bladder

Bladder damage, including hemorrhagic cystitis, fibrosis, and occasional bladder shrinkage, can occur following chronic administration of alkylating agents such as cyclophosphamide [36] and ifosfamide [37]. The metabolic by-products of these drugs include acrolein (of the same chemical class as the aniline dyes), which is excreted in the urine and irritates the bladder mucosa. This leads to exposure of submucosal blood vessels and subsequent bleeding [38]. Fortunately, drug-induced hemorrhagic cystitis and related fibrosis can nearly always be prevented by increased hydration during drug administration and the concomitant administration of intravenous or oral mercaptoethane sulfonate (MESNA). MESNA serves as a chemical sponge that binds the metabolites, thereby inactivating them and preventing their toxic action on the urothelium. Cyclophosphamide has also been associated with the induction of bladder tumors [39]. The interaction between RT and chemotherapy and their effects on hemorrhagic cystitis are discussed in Sect. 15.3.

Radiation may interact with a number of chemotherapeutic agents in an additive or synergistic fashion. The most notable example for the organs of the GU tract, particularly the kidneys, is the interaction between radiation and the antibiotics, actinomycin-D and doxorubicin [40]. There is a significant enhancement of the radiation effects when the agents are given concurrently, but this may also occur when the modalities are used sequentially. Radiation may also interact with cyclophosphamide, increasing the severity and chronicity of hemorrhagic cystitis. Therefore, great care is necessary when evaluating patients who have received or will receive RT to fields that include the kidney or bladder, if those patients also have received or will receive chemotherapy. This is of particular importance in patients who have nephrectomy or a fused or ectopic kidney, where the functional renal tissue may have been purposefully or inadvertently irradiated. It is critical in these cases to have precise information on the definition of the radiation portals.

Conditioning regimens for bone marrow transplantation (BMT) often include chemotherapy and total body irradiation. Data is emerging on late renal toxicity, such as hematuria and renal insufficiency [41, 42]. Renal biopsy reveals both parenchymal and vascular glomerular changes [43]. This data is from two published sources of the effects on ALL ($n=44$) and neuroblastoma ($n=15$) patients. Most patients received twice daily radiation (interfraction time of 4–6 h) to total doses equaling 12–14 Gy. Another group

has shown that many patients with hematologic malignancies already come into the BMT process with a decreased (but normal) GFR when compared to those undergoing the transplant for nonmalignant diseases [43]. This is likely related to the intensive systemic therapy that they have already received. Approximately 1 year after transplant, there is a significant decrease in GFR which stabilizes or slightly improves at over the ensuing 5 years. TBI-containing regimens show a greater decrease in the GFR. Hemorrhagic cystitis after bone marrow transplantation may also be associated with BK polyomavirus [44].

## 15.3 Clinical Manifestations

Table 15.2 summarizes the available data for the late genitourinary effects in childhood survivors of cancer. Each organ system is discussed below.

### 15.3.1 Kidney

#### 15.3.1.1 Surgery
Unilateral nephrectomy in childhood results in contralateral hyperplasia [45, 46]. Normal kidney function is usually seen following resection of one of the two kidneys [47, 48]. Normal function can continue with as little as one-third of one kidney remaining. Radiation in moderate doses (14–15 Gy) to the remaining kidney may decrease the amount of hyperplasia that otherwise would have taken place [49, 50].

#### 15.3.1.2 Radiation
Acute radiation nephropathy is an extremely uncommon occurrence, requiring greater than 30–40 Gy to the kidney. Subacute radiation nephropathy, characterized by hypertension and a decreased GFR, may occur 6–8 weeks to several months after doses equal to or greater than 15 Gy of radiation to both kidneys.

Significant late renal dysfunction occurs following radiation doses >20 Gy [51]. In children, even lower doses (5–20 Gy) can cause renal dysfunction. If a significant volume of the renal tissue is left unirradiated, the damage may not be clinically significant, although regional dysfunction within the irradiated portions of the kidney

**Table 15.2** Incidence of late genitourinary effects following treatment for childhood cancer

| Author | Tumor | Therapy | N | Follow-up (yrs) | Endpoint studied | Result |
|---|---|---|---|---|---|---|
| Barrera | Wilms' | Nephrectomy | 16 | >13 | Mild proteinuria tubular function DBP >90 | 2/16 25 % |
| Ritchey | Wilms': unilateral | Nephrectomy | 5,368 | >10 | Renal failure | 0.28 % |
| Makipernaa | Wilms' | Nephrectomy + ipsilateral RT (20–40 Gy) | 30 | 19 | HTN BUN/creatinine | 17 % normal |
| Paulino | Wilms' | Nephrectomy + RT (12–40 Gy) + CT | 42 | 15 | Serum BUN and creatinine HTN | Elevated in 1 patient 7 % |
| Thomas | Wilms' | Nephrectomy + RT (15–44 Gy) | 24 | 13 | Low-grade renal failure and UTIs | 4 % |
| Wikstad | Wilms | Nephrectomy + ipsilateral RT + contralateral kidney RT (5–15 Gy) | 22 | 13 | GFR | 82 % compared to normal controls; stable over time |
| | | | | | BP | Normal |
| Raney | Bladder or prostate sarcoma | Surgery + CT+/– RT (25–55 Gy) | 109 | 8 | Bladder dysfunction | 25 % |
| | | | | | Urinary diversion | 50 % |
| | | | | | HTN | 1 % |
| | | | | | Elevated BUN/Cr | 6 % |
| | | | | | Hematuria (intact bladder vs. diversion) | 20 % vs. 39 % |
| | | | | | Bacteriuria (intact bladder vs. diversion) | 8 % vs. 35 % |
| | | | | | Abnormal renal imaging (intact bladder vs. diversion) | 20 % vs. 37 % |
| Heyn | Paratesticular rhabdomyosarcoma | Surgery + RT (16–58 Gy) + CT | 86 | >4 | Ejaculatory dysfunction | 7 % |
| | | | | | Normal blood pressure | 96 % |
| | | | | | Normal BUN and creatinine | 100 % |
| | | | | | Ureteral obstruction | 3 % |
| | | | | | Hemorrhagic cystitis | 34 % |
| | | | | | Normal bladder function | 100 % |

| | | | Neurogenic bladder | 15 % |
|---|---|---|---|---|
| Hale | Germ cell tumors | 73 | 11 | Hemorrhagic cystitis | 13 % |
| | Surgery +/– RT (20–40 Gy) +/– CT | | | Recurrent UTI | 9 % |
| | | | | Ureteral/urethral stenosis | 3 % |
| | | | | Bladder atrophy | 75 % |
| | | | | Hydronephrosis | 100 % |
| Ritchey | Retroperitoneal tumors | 4 | 2 | Bilateral hydronephrosis | 50 % |
| | Surgery + EBRT (18–50 Gy) + IORT (10–25 Gy) | | | Renal artery stenosis | 4 % |
| | | | | Renal atrophy | 25 % |
| Stea | Pelvic sarcomas | 23 | 2 | Vaginal stenosis | 4 % |
| | CT + RT (55–60 Gy) +/–IORT +/– BMT (with TBI) | | | Cystitis | 4 % |
| | | | | Fistulas (IORT) | 100 % |
| Tarbell | ALL | 28 | 2 | Renal dysfunction | 32 % |
| Guinan | Leukemia | 115 | 3 | GFR | 41 % |
| Esiashvili | Leukemia | 60 | | Elevated Cr | Acute: 45 % |
| | BMT (with TBI) | | | | Delayed:25 % |
| Guinan | Neuroblastoma | 11 | | Renal dysfunction | 64 % |

Refs. [2, 43, 46, 51, 66, 75–85]

can be demonstrated. However, if all or the majority of the patient's renal tissue is irradiated, clinical renal dysfunction will result.

The more frequent use of three-dimensional and four-dimensional RT planning is prompting investigations into the volume-based analysis of clinical damage. The first of these studies suggests that over 2 years low-grade nephrotoxicity may be associated with the volume of kidney receiving 20 Gy or more [52]. The volume of kidney within the high-dose RT envelope may also be reduced by a better understanding of the individual motion of the organ using sophisticated computed tomography during the treatment planning and frequent (sometimes daily) verification of the set up during the treatment course [53, 54].

### 15.3.1.3 Chemotherapy

A variety of metabolic effects of chemotherapy on renal function have been noted. Long-term glomerular injury secondary to cisplatin may improve slowly over time [23]. However, tubular injury manifested by hypomagnesemia appears to persist. Chronic glomerular and tubular toxicity from ifosfamide has been observed [30]. However, whether these are long-lasting is unclear [55]. There is controversy regarding whether the age of the child affects the impact or severity of toxicity.

### 15.3.1.4 Aging Effects

The influence of aging on the expression of damage is primarily related to growth of the patient. Renal functional impairment may not become prominent until the growing child reaches a size that exceeds the ability of the remaining renal tissue to accommodate the need for metabolic adjustments and excretion. The child may therefore outgrow the kidney and require management of renal failure.

## 15.3.2 Bladder

### 15.3.2.1 Surgery

Bacteriuria is more prevalent in patients with urinary diversion than those with an intact bladder [2]. However, the clinical significance of this is unclear. Neurogenic bladder has been reported in 14 % of patients undergoing surgery and RT for pelvic germ cell tumors [51].

### 15.3.2.2 Radiation

Bladder dysfunction after irradiation for bladder and prostate sarcomas (median dose of 40 Gy) is reported to be 27 % [2]. This includes incontinence, urinary frequency, and nocturia. It should be noted that most of these patients also received cyclophosphamide.

### 15.3.2.3 Chemotherapy

The onset and timing of hemorrhagic cystitis secondary to the administration of chemotherapeutic agents varies, with some patients experiencing this complication during therapy and others developing it several months following cessation of therapy [2]. The hematuria may be microscopic or macroscopic, including clot passage, and can even result in significant anemia. Urgency, increased frequency of urination, and difficulty voiding can also occur. Cyclophosphamide appears to be associated with the development of transitional cell carcinoma of the bladder [39].

The impact of aging on the bladder is similar to the effects of aging on the kidney.

## 15.3.3 Prostate

The effects of surgical and radiation injury are not seen until puberty, because the gland is nonfunctional during the prepubescent years. Atrophy of the normal glandular tissue in the prostate can be seen following moderate or high doses of radiation [56]. Impaired growth of the seminal vesicles, with consequent decreased production of and storage capacity for seminal fluid, may result in a diminished ejaculum volume. Since the normal ejaculate is a combination of fluids derived from the gonads, seminal vesicles, and prostate, dysfunction of any of these structures theoretically can lead to abnormalities in ejaculation or the ejaculate volume.

## 15.3.4 Vagina

Fibrosis and diminished growth secondary to surgical procedures or RT have been described [57–59]. Vaginal mucositis can occur acutely during RT or following chemotherapy, notably with methotrexate, actinomycin-D, and doxorubicin. In patients who have received prior RT, the administration of actinomycin-D or doxorubicin can result in a "radiation recall" reaction with vaginal mucositis. Significant fibrosis of the vagina can occur after high-dose RT, or after more modest doses of radiation, when combined with chemotherapy. These therapies interfere with normal development of the vagina and therefore have a negative impact on sexual function. Both the size and flexibility of the vagina may be adversely affected. At extremely high doses of RT, soft tissue necrosis of the vaginal wall can occur. In adults, this appears to be more common in the posterior and inferior portions of the vagina [60]. Fistula formation (rectovaginal, vesicovaginal, and urethrovaginal) is the end stage of this event [61].

## 15.3.5 Uterus

Decreased uterine growth can be seen following exposure to 20 Gy of radiation [57, 62–64]. Scarring may be produced at higher doses. The resultant decreased uterine size may prevent the successful completion of pregnancy or result in low-birth-weight babies [62]. Decreased uterine blood flow has been seen in women who received pelvic irradiation as children. This may be related to smooth muscle proliferation surrounding small- and medium-sized arterioles [61].

## 15.3.6 Ureter

Limited data exist for ureteral damage in children [52, 65]. The data in adults suggest that the ureter is fairly resistant to irradiation [9, 18]. Injury appears to be related to the dose and length of the ureter in the radiation field. A higher incidence of ureteral injury is seen when the ureter is included in the field during intraoperative RT [66].

## 15.3.7 Urethra

There is no good data related to urethral injury and long-term sequelae of cancer therapy in children. The limited information in adults suggests that ureteral stricture occurs very infrequently (0–4 %) following RT alone. However, stricture is more commonly seen (5–16 %) in patients who undergo surgical manipulation of the urethra in addition to RT [9].

## 15.4  Detection and Screening

### 15.4.1 Evaluation of Overt Sequelae

The structure and function of the GU tract can be assessed by a variety of techniques. Simple screening methodologies include the history, with particular attention to urinary incontinence, urine volumes, and urine character (bloody or foamy), as well as the urinalysis. Creatinine clearance is a simple, cost-effective screen of kidney function. Structural abnormalities can be investigated by several tests, including ultrasound, IVP, CT scan, and MRI. Retrograde studies may be useful for structural and functional evaluation of the bladder and ureters. Cystoscopy may be necessary to evaluate hematuria in the long-term survivor. In patients with late-onset hemorrhagic cystitis, cystoscopy may be useful to assess the degree of mucosal damage and to evaluate the etiology of the hematuria. Patients with late-onset hemorrhagic cystitis are at risk for transitional cell carcinomas of the bladder that may be accompanied by hematuria. An IVP or retrograde study of the upper tracts may be necessary to identify other abnormalities that can cause bleeding.

For young girls who have had pelvic tumors, gynecologic examinations may be necessary at a young age. The vagina, cervix, and uterus are best examined under direct visualization using a speculum. General anesthesia may be required to produce adequate relaxation and to decrease motion. The uterus may be examined by ultrasound, CT and MRI; injection of contrast-enhancing dye is not generally necessary. Young women who have difficulty becoming pregnant need to be evaluated for hormonal dysregulation versus late structural (uterine) injury.

Young boys with pelvic tumors may also need imaging studies to evaluate the growth of their pelvic organs. The bladder and prostate are readily visualized with ultrasound.

Consultation with an experienced radiologist, nephrologist, urologist, and gynecologist may assist in planning individualized investigations.

## 15.4.2 Screening for Preclinical Injury

Because the kidneys have a large functional reserve, clinical renal function usually remains normal until there is serious derangement of glomerular or tubular function. Urinalysis is not very quantitative, but it is the cheapest, simplest, and most useful test along with the assessment of blood pressure for periodically reevaluating patients for the development of nephropathy. Elevated serum concentrations of blood urea nitrogen (BUN) and creatinine suggest a need for a more accurate assessment of glomerular function. Creatinine clearance and radionuclide scanning both provide quantitative measures of glomerular function. Tubular dysfunction may be identified by quantitative tests of phosphate,

bicarbonate, magnesium, potassium, glucose, amino acids, and beta-2 microglobulin. Injury to the bladder wall may be screened by urinalysis, looking for microscopic hematuria.

## 15.4.3 Guidelines for Follow-Up of Asymptomatic Patients

A detailed annual history and physical examination are recommended (Table 15.3) for all patients. Patients who have received therapies with known renal toxicities may benefit from simple screening tests (including hemoglobin or hematocrit, urinalysis, BUN, and creatinine), as well as from blood pressure monitoring [65–69]. A determination of the serum electrolyte concentrations and more definitive tests, such as creatinine clearance, may be indicated in selected cases.

After nephrectomy, preservation of the residual kidney function is essential. Participation in contact sports, especially football, is not advised. Kidney guards are often recommended, although there is no data regarding their efficacy in injury prevention. More likely, the appliance serves to remind the individual of vulnerability. Although urinary tract infection should be treated aggressively in all patients, this is especially important in those with a single kidney or with renal

**Table 15.3** Methods of evaluating organ function

| Organ | History | Physical | Laboratory | Radiologic | Surgical |
|---|---|---|---|---|---|
| Kidney | Hematuria fatigue | Blood pressure | Blood pressure growth parameters | BUN, creatinine, creatinine clearance, urinalysis, serum and urine electrolytes, beta-2 microglobin, hemoglobin/hematocrit | |
| Ureter | | | | IVP, retrograde ureterograms | |
| Bladder | Urinary frequency hematuria | | Urinalysis | IVP, retrograde studies, ultrasound | Cystoscopy volumetrics |
| Urethra | Urinary stream Urinary frequency hematuria | | | Voiding cystogram | |
| Prostate | Ejaculatory function | | | Ultrasound | |
| Vagina | Painful intercourse dryness | Pelvic examination | | | |
| Uterus | Abnormal menses difficult pregnancies | Pelvic examination | | | |

dysfunction. To rule out obstruction, patients with anatomic alteration of the GU tract may need periodic imaging studies; they may also need periodic urine cultures to assess urine sterility. The role of chronic antimicrobial prophylaxis in patients with urinary diversion is controversial [68, 70]. Urinalysis is a good screening tool following therapy for assessing possible damage to the bladder wall [71].

## 15.4.4 Management of Established Problems

### 15.4.4.1 Therapy

#### Kidney

If preclinical abnormalities are found, serial follow-ups at 3–6 month intervals are recommended. A pediatric nephrologist may need to follow such patients. Although little evidence is available that improvement in renal plasma flow or GFR occurs with time, tubular function does appear to undergo some recovery; therefore, efforts to support and treat the patient until such recovery occurs are appropriate. In the event of severe renal failure, the choice between dialysis and renal transplantation should rest with the patient, the family, the oncologist, and the nephrologist. Due to improved renal graft survival, using organs from living donors, this should be considered in the decision-making process. For children who have undergone irradiation to one kidney and who develop renal-vascular hypertension, unilateral nephrectomy is potentially curative if no contralateral renal changes have occurred. The medications for controlling hypertension and electrolyte imbalances should also be prescribed.

#### Bladder

Hemorrhagic cystitis may require cystoscopy and cauterization of bleeding sites. Persistent or refractory late-onset hemorrhagic cystitis may be treated with formalin instillation into the bladder. However, this procedure is not without risk. A complication rate as high as 14 % has been reported using higher concentrations of formalin [72]. Hyperbaric oxygen has become widely used

in the adult population and may be considered [73]. Severe bleeding may necessitate partial or total cystectomy, with reconstruction.

#### Ureter and Urethra

Stricture of the urethra is usually relieved by dilatation. Obstruction of the ureter can usually be treated with a stent. Urinary diversion is, at times, necessary [3].

#### Prostate, Vagina, and Uterus

Late structural defects may be treated using reconstruction with plastic surgery. Topical estrogen and vaginal dilators are described in the adult population, but their role has not been established in the pediatric group.

#### Rehabilitation

As the patient matures, rehabilitation efforts may well be needed both for physical and psychological problems. For example, children undergoing urinary diversion will need education and psychosocial support in dealing with their stoma and its proper hygiene. As the child grows older and learns that he or she is physically different from other children, careful discussion of this problem with the pediatric oncologist, the surgeon and a psychologist is of paramount importance in defining the rehabilitative treatments and allaying the patient's anxiety about the future. Adult cancer survivors report significant sexual dysfunction and decreased sexual activity [59]. Adult survivors of childhood cancer will likely experience similar problems. This information may not be volunteered, and careful questioning at follow-up is needed to ensure appropriate referral for psychological counseling. In addition, some survivors are not knowledgeable about the treatment that they received as a child [74]. Therefore, they may not recognize certain symptoms as late effects of cancer therapy.

---

#### Conclusion

This chapter described the risk, evaluation, and treatment of the late genitourinary effects of cancer therapy in children. Unfortunately, some studies do not provide systematic reporting of such effects. Effects on the kidney and bladder have been described the most. The effects on the ureters, urethra, prostate, vagina and uterus are less well documented. Additionally, the data on psychological effects, especially related to sexual matters, in the pediatric population are difficult to find. Newer reporting systems will hopefully provide a clearer sense of the problem. In the field of radiation oncology, volume-based predictors of injury are in their infancy with regard to pediatric patients. Biologic and genetic predictors for chemotherapy and radiation injury are also under investigation.

We have learned through following childhood cancer survivors over several decades that there is no substitute for a caring, knowledgeable primary physician as captain of the team. Internists should also be involved in the care of patients who reach adulthood. Ideally, these physicians should be knowledgeable about pediatric cancer patients; however, if this is not the case, the pediatric oncologist will need to provide information about the late effects of treatment to the patient's other physicians. Good communication between the initial treatment team and follow-up clinic and consultants should lead to optimum care of the long-term survivor of childhood cancer.

**Acknowledgements** The author wishes to acknowledge L. Marks, B. Raney, R. Heyn, and R. Cassaday.

# References

1. Schmidt A (1992) Long term results after partial and unilateral nephrectomy in childhood. Eur J Pediatr Surg 2:269–273
2. Raney B et al (1993) Sequelae of treatment of 109 patients followed for five to fifteen years after diagnosis of sarcoma of the bladder and prostate: a report from the Intergroup Rhabdomyosarcoma Study (IRS Committee). Cancer 71:2387–2394
3. Wespes E, Stone AF, King LR (1986) Ileocaecocystoplasty in urinary tract reconstruction in children. Br J Urol 58:266–272
4. Filmer RB, Spencer JR (1990) Malignancies in bladder augmentations and intestinal conduits. J Urol 122:163–164
5. Gitlin J et al (1999) New concepts of histological changes in experimental augmentation cystoplasty. Urology 162:1096–1100
6. Golomb J, Klutke CG, Raz S (1989) Complications of bladder substitution and continent urinary diversion. Urology 34:329–338
7. Meadows AT et al (1985) Second malignant neoplasms in children: an update from the late effects study group. J Clin Oncol 3:532–538
8. Cassady JR (1995) Clinical radiation nephropathy. Int J Radiat Oncol Biol Phys 31:1249–1256
9. Marks LB et al (1995) The response of the urinary bladder, urethra, and ureter to radiation and chemotherapy. Int J Radiat Oncol Biol Phys 31:1257–1280
10. Stewart FA (1986) Mechanism of bladder damage and repair after treatment with radiation and cytostatic drugs. Br J Cancer 53:280–291
11. Suresh UR et al (1993) Radiation disease of the urinary tract: histological features of 18 cases. J Clin Pathol 46:228–231
12. Dewit L, Ang KK, Vanderschueren E (1983) Acute side effects and late complications after radiotherapy of localized carcinoma of the prostate. Cancer Treat Rep 10:79–89
13. Montana GS, Fowler WC (1989) Carcinoma of the cervix: analysis of bladder and rectal radiation dose and complications. Int J Radiat Oncol Biol Phys 16:95–100
14. Perez CA et al (1984) Radiation therapy alone in the treatment of carcinoma of the uterine cervix II. Analysis of complications. Cancer 54:235–246
15. Perez CA et al (1986) Radiation therapy alone in the treatment of carcinoma of the uterine cervix: a 20-year experience. Gynecol Oncol 23:127–140
16. Pourquier H et al (1987) A quantified approach to the analysis and prevention of urinary complications in radiotherapeutic treatment of cancer of the cervix. Int J Radiat Oncol Biol Phys 12:1025–1033
17. Ryu JK et al (2002) Interim report of toxicity from 3D conformal radiation therapy (3D-CRT) for prostate cancer 3dOG/RTOG 9406, level III (79.2 Gy). Int J Radiat Oncol Biol Phys 54:1036–1046
18. Buglione M et al (2002) Post-radiation pelvic disease and ureteral stenosis: pathophysiology and evolution in the patient treated for cervical carcinoma. Review of the literature and experience of the Radium Institute. Arch Ital Urol Androl 71:6–11
19. Kontturi M, Kauppila A (1982) Ureteric complications following treatment of gynaecological cancer. Ann Chir Gynaecol 71:232–238
20. Abitol MM, Davenport JH (1974) The irradiated vagina. Obstet Gynecol 44:249–256
21. Kapoor M, Chan G (2001) Malignancy and renal disease. Crit Care Chirurgy 17(3):571–598
22. Stewart DJ et al (1985) Renal and hepatic concentrations of platinum: relationship to cisplatin time, dose and nephrotoxicity. J Clin Oncol 3:1251–1256
23. Brock PR et al (1991) Partial reversibility of cisplatin nephrotoxicity in children. J Pediatr 118:531
24. Crom WR et al (1984) The effect of prior cisplatin therapy on the pharmacokinetics of high-dose methotrexate. J Clin Oncol 2:655–661

25. Grigg A et al (1996) Multi-organ dysfunction associated with high-dose carboplatin therapy prior to autologous transplantation. Bone Marrow Transplant 17(1):67–74

26. Petrilli AS et al (2002) Use of amifostine in the therapy of osteosarcoma in children and adolescents. J Pediatr Hematol Oncol 24:188–191

27. Renner S et al (2000) Effect of amifostine on neuroblastoma during high dose chemotherapy: in vivo and in vitro investigations. Anticancer Res 20:4531–4538

28. Marina N et al (2005) Amifostine does not protect against the ototoxicity of high-dose cisplatin combined with etoposide and bleomycin in pediatric germ-cell tumors: a Children's Oncology Group study. Cancer 104(4):841–847

29. Skinner R et al (1996) Risk factors for ifosfamide nephrotoxicity in children with cancer. Lancet 348(80):578

30. Skinner R et al (1990) Nephrotoxicity after ifosfamide. Arch Dis Child 65:732–738

31. Vogelzang NJ (1991) Nephrotoxicity from chemotherapy: prevention and management. Oncology 5:97–112

32. Prasad et al (1996) Progressive glomerular toxicity of ifosfamide in children. Med Pediatr Oncol 27:149

33. Skinner R, Cotterill SK, Stevens MC (2000) Risk factors for nephrotoxicity after ifosfamide treatment in children: a UKCCSG late effects group study. Br J Cancer 82:1636–1645

34. Raney B et al (1992) Renal toxicity in patients treated with ifosfamide in intergroup rhabdomyosarcoma study (IRS)IV pilot regimens. Med Pediatr Oncol 20:429

35. Hempel L (2003) Influence of high-dose methotrexate therapy (HD-MTX) on glomerular and tubular kidney function. Med Pediatr Oncol 40:348–354

36. Levine LA, Richie JP (1989) Urological complications of cyclophosphamide. J Urol 141:1063–1069

37. Sarosy G (1989) Ifosfamide pharmacologic overview. Semin Oncol 16:2–8

38. Sklar CA, LaQuaglia MP (2000) The long term complications of chemotherapy in childhood genitourinary tumors. Urol Clin North Am 27:563–568

39. Samra Y, Hertz M, Lindner A (1985) Urinary bladder tumors following cyclophosphamide therapy: a report of two cases with a review of the literature. Med Pediatr Oncol 12:86–91

40. Tefft M et al (1976) Acute and later effects on normal tissues following combined chemo-and radiotherapy for childhood rhabdomyosarcoma and Ewing's sarcoma. Cancer 37:1201–1213

41. Tarbell NJ et al (1990) Renal insufficiency after total body irradiation for pediatric bone marrow transplantation. Radiother Oncol 18(Supp i):i39–i4239

42. Guinan EC et al (1988) Intravascular hemolysis and renal insufficiency after bone marrow transplantation. J Clin Oncol 72:451–455

43. Gronroos MH et al (2007) Long-term renal function following bone marrow transplantation. Bone Marrow Transplant 39(11):717–723

44. Vogeli TA (1999) Urological treatment and clinical course of BK polyomavirus-associated hemorrhagic cystitis in children after bone marrow transplantation. Eur Urol 36:252–257

45. Walker RD et al (1982) Compensatory renal growth and function in post-nephrectomized patients with Wilms' tumor. Urology 19:127

46. Wikstad I et al (1986) A comparative study of size and function of the remnant kidney in patients nephrectomized in childhood for Wilms' tumor and hydronephrosis. Acta Paediatr Scand 5:408

47. Luttenegger TJ et al (1975) Compensatory renal hypertrophy after treatment for Wilms' tumor. Am J Roentgenol 125:348

48. Cassidy MJD, Beck RM (1988) Renal functional reserve in live related kidney donors. Am J Kidney Dis 11:468–472

49. Cassidy JR et al (1981) Effect of low dose irradiation on renal enlargement in children following nephrectomy for Wilms' tumor. Acta Radiol Oncol 20:5–8

50. Vaeth JM (1964) The remaining kidney in irradiated survivors of Wilms' tumor. Am J Roentgenol 92:148

51. Hale GA et al (1999) Late effects of treatment for germ cell tumors during childhood and adolescence. J Pediatr Hematol Oncol 21:115–122

52. Bolling T et al (2011) Dose-volume analysis of radiation nephropathy in children: preliminary report of the risk consortium. Int J Radiat Oncol Biol Phys 80(3):840–844

53. Pai Panandiker AS et al (2012) Novel assessment of renal motion in children as measured via four-dimensional computed tomography. Int J Radiat Oncol Biol Phys 82(5):1771–1776

54. Nazmy MS et al (2012) Cone beam CT for organs motion evaluation in pediatric abdominal neuroblastoma. Radiother Oncol 102(3):388–392

55. Oberlin O et al (2009) Long-term evaluation of Ifosfamide-related nephrotoxicity in children. J Clin Oncol 27(32):5350–5355

56. Gill WB et al (1980) Sandwich radiotherapy (3000 and 4500 rads) around radical retropubic prostatectomy for stage C prostatic carcinoma. Urology 16:470–475

57. El-Mahdi AM et al (1974) Sequelae of pelvic irradiation in infancy. Radiology 110:665–666

58. Flamant F et al (1979) Embryonal rhabdomyosarcoma of the vagina in children. Conservative treatment with curietherapy and chemotherapy. Eur J Cancer 15:527–532

59. Flamant F et al (1990) Long-term sequelae of conservative treatment for vulvar and vaginal rhabdomyosarcoma in children. J Clin 8:1847–1853

60. Rotman M, Aziz H, Choi KN (1989) Radiation damage of normal tissues in the treatment of gynecologic cancers. In: Vaeth JM, Meyer JL (eds) Frontiers of radiation therapy and oncology, vol 23, Radiation tolerance of normal tissues. Karger, Basel

61. Grigsby PW et al (1995) Late injury of cancer therapy on the female reproductive tract. Int J Radiat Oncol Biol Phys 31:1281–1299

62. Li FP et al (1987) Outcome of pregnancies in survivors of Wilms' tumor. JAMA 257:216–219

63. Piver MS, Rose PG (1988) Long-term follow-up and complications of infants with vulvovaginal embryonal rhabdomyosarcoma treated with surgery, radiation therapy and chemotherapy. Obstet Gynecol 71:435–437

64. Kalapurakal JA et al (2004) Pregnancy outcomes after abdominal irradiation that included or excluded the pelvis in childhood Wilms tumor survivors: a report from the National Wilms Tumor Study. Int J Radiat Oncol Biol Phys 58(5):1364–1368

65. Gronroos ML et al (1996) Renal failure in Wilms' tumor patients: a report from the National Wilms' Tumor Study Group. Med Pediatr Oncol 26:75–80

66. Ritchey ML et al (1990) Pediatric urological complications with intraoperative radiation therapy. J Urol 143(1):89–91

67. Langer T et al (2000) Basic method and the developing structure of a late effects surveillance system (LESS) in the long-term follow up of pediatric cancer patients in Germany. Med Pediatr Oncol 34:348–351

68. Oeffinger KC et al (2000) Grading of late effects in young adult survivors of childhood cancer followed in an ambulatory adult setting. Cancer 88:1687–1695

69. Schwartz CL (1999) Long-term survivors of childhood cancer: the late effects of therapy. Oncologist 4:45–54

70. Cronan JJ et al (1989) Antibiotics and nephrostomy tube care: preliminary observations, part II. Bacteremia. Radiology 172:1043–1045

71. Wood DP et al (2003) Incidence and significance of positive urine culture in patients with an orthotopic neobladder. J Urol 169:2196–2199

72. Dewan AK, Mohan GM, Ravi R (1996) Intravesical formalin for hemorrhagic cystitis following irradiation of cancer of the cervix. Int J Gynaecol Obstet 42:131

73. Corman JM et al (2003) Treatment of radiation induced hemorrhagic cystitis with hyperbaric oxygen. J Urol 169:2200–2202

74. Kadan-Lottick NS et al (2002) Childhood survivors' knowledge about their past diagnosis and treatment: childhood cancer survivor study. JAMA 287:1832–1839

75. Barrera RLP, Stevens M (1989) Long-term follow-up after unilateral nephrectomy and radiotherapy for Wilms' tumor. Pediatr Nephrol 3:430–432

76. Heyn R et al (1992) Late effects of therapy in patients with paratesticular rhabdomyosarcoma. J Clin Oncol 10:614–623

77. Jaffe N (1987) Renal toxicity with cumulative doses of cis-diamminedichloroplatinum-II in pediatric patients with osteosarcoma. Effect on creatinine clearance and methotrexate excretion. Cancer 59:1577–1581

78. Makipernaa A et al (1991) Renal growth and function 11–28 years after treatment for Wilms' tumors. Eur J Pediatr 150:444–447

79. Ritchey ML et al (1996) Renal failure in Wilms' tumor patients: a report from the National Wilms' Tumor Study Group. Med Pediatr Oncol 26(2):75–80

80. Paulino AC et al (2000) Late effects in children treated with radiation therapy for Wilms' tumor. Int J Radiat Oncol Biol Phys 46:1239–1246

81. Stea B et al (1987) Treatment of pelvic sarcomas in adolescents and young adults with intensive combined modality therapy. Int J Radiat Oncol Biol Phys 13:1797–1805

82. Thomas PRM et al (1983) Late effects of treatment for Wilms' tumor. Int J Radiat Oncol Biol Phys 9:651–657

83. Tarbell NJ et al (1990) Renal insufficiency after total body irradiation for pediatric bone marrow transplantation. Radiother Oncol 18(Suppl 1):139–142

84. Esiashvili N et al (2009) Renal toxicity in children undergoing total body irradiation for bone marrow transplant. Radiother Oncol 90(2):242–246

85. Guinan EC et al (1988) Intravascular hemolysis and renal insufficiency after bone marrow transplantation. Blood 72(2):451–455

# Musculoskeletal, Integument

# 16

Robert B. Marcus Jr. and Natia Esiashvili

## Contents

## 16.1    Introduction

Multimodal therapy for childhood cancer resulted in improved survival [1]; however, many survivor do experience late effects affecting the musculoskeletal system. While the growth deficits of radiation are well known, it is important to realize that surgery and sometimes chemotherapy also affect the developing musculoskeletal system. In general, the treatment of sarcomas leads to the most severe late effects because the underlying malignancy originates in a muscle or bone and often an extremity. Despite the advances in modern surgery, the removal of a muscle or bone has permanent consequences that completely alter a child's life. Likewise, irradiation of developing bone and muscle yields permanent effects. Usually, the younger the child, the more severe are the late effects of therapy. It is important to understand the causes of and the rehabilitation for limb length discrepancies, amputation, scoliosis, and other complications of therapy. Therapy is often more successful if the consequences are properly anticipated and prevented, rather than waiting for deficits to develop.

In addition to musculoskeletal late effects, therapy can cause permanent deficits in the developing skin. At first, these may not appear as devastating as musculoskeletal issues, but they may be much more severe than appreciated by the treating physicians and other members of the treatment team.

R.B. Marcus Jr. (✉)
Radiation Oncology, Nemours Childrens
Hospital/Sacred Heart Cancer Center,
Pensacola, USA
e-mail: stargazer6@live.com

N. Esiashvili
Radiation Oncology, Winship Cancer Institute
of Emory University, Atlanta, USA

© Springer International Publishing 2015
C.L. Schwartz et al. (eds.), *Survivors of Childhood and Adolescent Cancer:*
*A Multidisciplinary Approach*, Pediatric Oncology, DOI 10.1007/978-3-319-16435-9_16

Along with physical consequences, it is necessary to anticipate the psychological and social consequences of treatment so that the child can understand the changes in his or her life. Treating the child and curing the cancer is not enough; understanding and dealing with the long-term consequences of treatment are critical as well.

## 16.2 Musculoskeletal

### 16.2.1 Pathophysiology

#### 16.2.1.1 Normal Organ Development

The musculoskeletal system develops from the mesoderm, which forms series of tissue blocks called somites on each side of the neural tube during the third week of embryogenesis. Different regions of the somite differentiate into the dermomyotome (dermal and muscle component) and sclerotome (forms the vertebral column) [64]. By the end of the fourth week of gestation, the sclerotome cells form a loose tissue called the mesenchyme, which then migrates and differentiates into fibroblasts, chondroblasts, and osteoblasts [92]. These cells initially form cartilage that eventually evolves into a bone through a lengthy process of ossification. Two main types of ossification occur in different bones: intramembranous (e.g., skull) and endochondral (e.g., limb long bones) ossification. Ossification continues postnatally, through puberty until the middle of the third decade of life.

In the flat bones of the skull and face, the mesenchyme develops directly into bone (membranous ossification); however, most of the remainder of the skeleton first forms hyaline cartilage, which in turn ossifies (endochondral ossification). Most of the ossification in the long bones occurs during fetal life.

In the adult skeleton, there are about 200 distinct bones, which are divided into the axial and appendicular groups. The long bones of the limbs (e.g., femurs, tibias, humeri) are found in the appendicular skeleton and create a system of levers to confer the power of locomotion. The axial skeleton consists of the skull, the vertebrae, the sternum, and the ribs. The bones of the axial skeleton

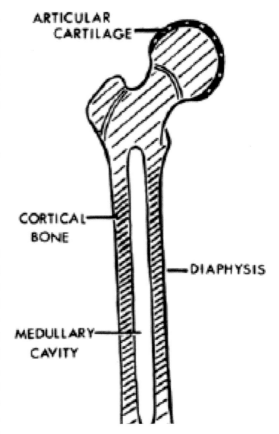

**Fig. 16.1** Schematic of a growing long bone. The shaft of the bone is called the diaphysis and contains the medullary cavity, which is filled with bone marrow. The two expanded ends are the epiphyses. The epiphysis at each end extends from the articular cartilage to the epiphyseal growth plate. The metaphysis is the region between the epiphyseal plate and the diaphysis (From [64], Fig. 2.3, p. 8)

are flat or irregularly shaped [93]. Each long bone has the following regions: shaft (diaphysis) with its medullary cavity and thickened ends called epiphysis, which extends from the growth plate to articular cartilage. The region between epiphysis and diaphysis is called the metaphysis (see Fig. 16.1). After initial ossification in utero, longitudinal growth of the bone occurs only at the epiphyseal plate (physis). The mechanism of growth at the physis is the proliferation of a layer of chondroblasts, which in turn form a layer of cartilage (Fig. 16.2). Small blood vessels invade the cartilage, increasing oxygen tension and stimulating the formation of osteoblasts. The osteoblasts create osteoid that calcifies into bone [89, 90].

**Fig. 16.2** A close-up of the region of the metaphysis and epiphysis. The proliferating cells (chondroblasts) are shown in the region of the physis (From [61])

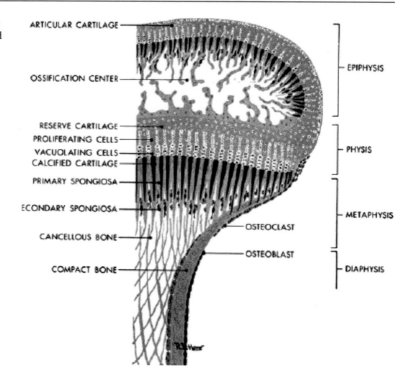

Most skeletal muscles also develop before birth, although some muscle formation continues until the end of the first year of life. Cells from the myotome region of the dermomyotomes become elongated spindle-shaped cells called myoblasts. These embryonic muscle cells fuse to form multinucleated muscle cells called muscle fibers. The dermatome regions of the dermomyotomes give rise to the dermis of the skin [64]. No new muscle cells are created after that time; muscle tissue enlarges due to increases in the number of myofilaments within each fiber, which result in an increase in the diameter of the individual muscle cells.

### 16.2.1.2 Organ Damage Induced by Cytotoxic Therapy

The surgical removal of parts of muscles or bone can lead to severe functional deficits; however, direct damage to the developing musculoskeletal system from cytotoxic therapy is most often caused by irradiation. The cells most sensitive to irradiation appear to be the growth plate chondrocytes [28, 79, 90]. Low total radiation doses reduce cell mitosis, promote premature terminal differentiation and apoptosis, and completely disrupt the cytoarchitecture. Surviving chondroblast clones repopulate the physis (although not always completely) if the total dose is below 20 Gy. Above this level, little repopulation occurs. Bones show a high capacity for repair after damage and fracture. After the initial damage takes place, inflammatory cells infuse from blood, secreting transforming growth factor β (TGF-β) to activate mesenchymal stem cells in the bone marrow, which can differentiate into chondrocytes, adipocytes, and stromal cells. Initially, a soft tissue callus (*procallus*) forms around the ends of the fractured bone, and osteoblasts begin to deposit immature woven bone. Although osteoblasts are damaged only by high doses of RT, radiation quickly increases vascularity of the bone, particularly in the metaphysis. This response in turn increases the resorption of bone, thereby increasing its porosity and the demineralization of the immature metaphysis [67]. Mesenchymal cells in the procallus start to form hyaline cartilage, which will undergo endochondral ossification and develop into a bony callus. Bone remodeling will eventually change woven bone into mature lamellar bone.

Recent evidence shows that the effect of radiation is very specific and leads to a decrease in the messenger ribonucleic acid (mRNA) expression of parathyroid hormone-related peptide (PTHrP), which is an important stimulus for mitosis of chondrocytes. The mechanism that triggers the decrease of the mRNA appears to be an increase in cytosolic calcium. The introduction of ethylene-glycotetraacetic acid (EGTA), a calcium chelator, inhibits the rise of cytosolic calcium and prevents most of the radiation damage [72]. Several hormones have a clear influence on bone formation and remodeling, including growth hormone (GH), parathyroid hormone (PTH), calcitonin, thyroid hormones, androgens and estrogens, and cortisol. Vitamin D acts directly on osteoblasts to secrete interleukin 1 (IL-1), which stimulates osteoclasts to increase bone resorption. In animal experiments, pentoxifylline can also decrease the effect of radiation on growth plate chondrocytes by mediating a decrease in cytosolic calcium [73].

The major risk factors for producing musculoskeletal late effects secondary to irradiation are as follows: (1) age at the time of treatment, (2) quality of radiation (dose per fraction and total dose), (3) volume irradiated, (4) growth potential of the treated site, (5) individual genetic and familial factors, and (6) coexisting therapy – surgery or chemotherapy [24].

There are too many variables to determine the effect of each variable individually. The current literature would imply that there is no threshold dose and that any dose of radiotherapy will affect the growth plate. Doses greater than 20 Gy will usually result in complete arrest. Nevertheless, the response to radiation is not an all-or-nothing phenomena; the higher the total dose and the younger the age at treatment, the greater the ultimate deficit [94]. This dose effect is probably because the epiphyseal plate appears to close more quickly with increasing levels of dose (Fig. 16.3a–c).

Some authors report that permanent bone growth arrest can be observed after total doses as low as 12 Gy delivered to the growth plate [19]. Various degrees of deformities are also reported at lower dose levels (range, 20–35 Gy), without a definite dose threshold [60, 74]. Silber et al. created a model to predict growth deficits from spinal irradiation based on the vertebral bodies treated, the total dose at normal fractionation, and the age of the child [97]. From these data, significant deficits would not be expected below 20 Gy. Investigators at St. Jude Children's Research Hospital (Memphis, TN) have attempted to use a random coefficient model for estimation of potential differences in volumetric bone growth in children with sarcoma treated with intensity-modulated radiation therapy (IMRT) and conformal radiation therapy (CRT) [45]. The model incorporated patient age, pretreatment bone volume, integral dose >35 Gy, and time since completion of radiation therapy and predicted that patients older than 10 years would maintain 98 % of normal growth, regardless of treatment method. Growth abnormalities are detected in almost all children treated with conventional fractionation to doses ranging from 40 to 55 Gy for extremity sarcomas [36, 74].

One of the goals of hyperfractionated radiotherapy (the use of small doses two or more times a day) is to decrease the extent of late effects. Studies are only now beginning to accumulate data, but Marcus and associates found that in the treatment of Ewing's sarcoma, fractions of 1.2 Gy twice daily to 50.4–63.2 Gy produce fewer musculoskeletal late effects than would be expected from similar doses using fractions of 1.8–2.0 Gy once a day (Fig. 16.4) [11, 57].

Other factors influence late sequelae. Orthovoltage irradiation, dose for dose, causes more growth deficits in the bone than megavoltage irradiation because of the increased bone absorption. Field size is also important: the larger the field of irradiation, the more significant the late effects [12].

Similar dose levels apply to muscle development as well. Doses <10 Gy cause virtually no detectable defect, and doses from 10 to 20 Gy produce some hypoplasia. Higher doses produce more significant problems.

Although high single doses of radiation can cause necrosis of muscle cells, in clinical practice, such an event is extremely rare. More commonly, even with fractionated treatment, radiation

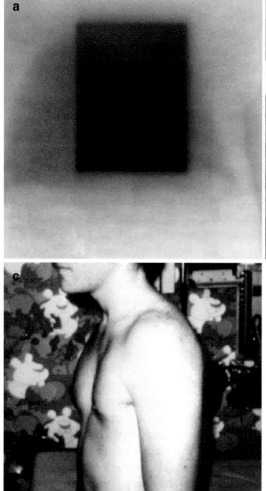
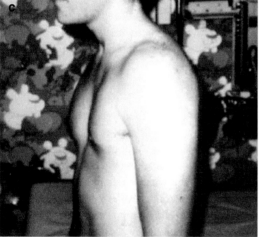

Fig. 16.3 (a–c) A 3-month-old boy who was treated in 1962 for a thoracic neuroblastoma using approximately 20 Gy in 10 fractions to the mediastinum and much of the left chest. (a) An AP-PA technique with 2-MEV photons was used. (b, c) The patient 20 years later. Mild hypoplasia of the left chest is present

damages the small vessels in muscles, preventing the full development of the muscle due to relative ischemia. Higher doses can give rise to atypical fibroblasts, which lay down excessive fibrin in the tissues, causing fibrosis [114].

There are sparse data on the pathophysiology of damage to growing muscle and bone by cytotoxic drugs, although in animal models the use of chemotherapy has caused a reduction in the shear strength of the physis [7, 104].

Chemotherapeutics have been shown to retard the proliferation of growth plate chondrocytes in both in vitro and in vivo experiments [85]. Chemotherapy retards growth during the course of treatment, but after the end of active therapy, most reports indicate that patients return to their normal growth rate or even exhibit catch-up growth [78]. Histologic examination of human growth plates after neoadjuvant chemotherapy and surgical excision has shown maintenance of the overall epiphyseal architecture, with growth arrest and then resumption of growth [7]. Most evidence would indicate that the deficit is temporary or primarily caused by endocrine dysfunction [6, 14].

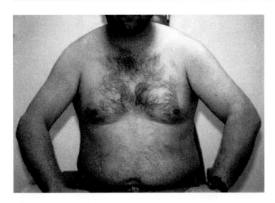

**Fig. 16.4** This man was treated for Ewing's sarcoma of the right humerus using 50.4 Gy in a fractionation scheme of 1.2 Gy twice daily when he was 14 years old. There was little noticeable difference in the muscle development in his upper arms until he started weight lifting. The left (untreated) arm responded, but the muscles in the radiation field did not increase as much in size or strength. In this picture, taken 11 years after treatment, the area of hypoplasia from the field of irradiation can be clearly seen

Methotrexate is a chemotherapeutic agent known to be associated with growth stunting, osteoporosis, and fracture [63, 66, 70]. The underlying pathophysiology for osteopathy in pediatric cancer patients receiving methotrexate chemotherapy remains unclear; however, animal experiments support the evidence that methotrexate interrupts bone resorption, inhibits bone turnover, and reduces recruitment of osteoblastic cells from proliferative precursor [29].

High or prolonged courses of steroids can cause the development of avascular necrosis of the femoral head. The exact mechanism is poorly understood, but there is evidence in animals to support a temporary decrease in blood flow through bones during treatment with steroids. Because the vasculature of the femoral and humeral heads is fragile, these structures are the most easily damaged by the decrease in blood flow, resulting in necrosis [25]. A class of drugs called bisphosphonates is used to treat patients with osteolytic metastasis, reducing skeletal complications by disruption of osteoclast-mediated bone resorption leading to decreased bone turnover. Some patients exposed to bisphosphonate therapy develop osteonecrosis [58, 113]. While the exact mechanism of osteonecrosis is still not known, the pathogenesis of localized

vascular insufficiency may be attributable to release of cytokines; interactions with growth hormone and insulin-like growth factor are known to play a role in regulation of blood circulation in bones, possibly from direct inhibition of endothelial cells. Metaphyseal sclerotic banding is another documented effect of periodic bisphosphonate treatment in growing children [110].

There is emergence of evidence about risk of osteonecrosis in patients treated with antiangiogenic drugs (bevacizumab), increasingly used in pediatric patients with newly diagnosed and recurrent malignancies. Rates of mandibular osteonecrosis have been increasingly observed in a combination of bevacizumab and bisphosphonates [13]. Recent evidence suggests that children treated with bevacizumab can be at risk for the development of lytic lesions and frank osteonecrosis in long bones [30, 98].

Retinoid acid derivative 13-cis-retinoic acid is used to treat minimal residual disease in patients with high-risk neuroblastoma. This agent is known to be associated with premature epiphyseal closure, and children were noticed to develop advanced bone age [40].

A more serious complication is rhabdomyolysis, a rare complication of cytarabine and other drugs, including cyclophosphamide, 5-azacytidine, interferon-α, and interleukin-2 [103]. It is thought that the ability of cytarabine to trigger the release of cytochrome-c from the mitochondria could lead to uncoupling of the oxidative phosphorylation with subsequent depletion of adenosine triphosphate (ATP) reserves at the skeletal muscle, resulting in rhabdomyolysis. Whatever the cause, the syndrome is complicated by acute renal failure often requiring hemodialysis.

## 16.2.2 Clinical Manifestations

Surgery, radiation therapy, and chemotherapy can all produce long-term sequelae in the developing musculoskeletal system; the effects of surgery and radiation have been more thoroughly studied than those of chemotherapy.

Most of the following text will focus on the late effects of irradiation; however, it is important to remember that the surgical removal of a portion of the musculoskeletal system can result in the same physical and psychological late effects as damage to the same tissue from radiation therapy or chemotherapy. The loss of a muscle group in the proximal lower extremity will cause weakness and gait disturbances; the amputation of an entire extremity will require the abrupt need for extensive rehabilitation. Limb length discrepancies often result from the unilateral surgical removal of one or more growth plates. The fact that the deficit is planned does not imply that the late effects should be discounted.

### 16.2.2.1 Bone

Some of the adverse effects of cancer therapy on growing bone are (1) bone density changes, (2) physical injuries, (3) pathologic fractures, and (4) avascular necrosis/osteonecrosis.

### Bone Density Changes

Radiation therapy can produce osteopenia in children. More information is needed to elucidate all the parameters involved, but the risk is probably between 8 % and 23 % at doses above 20 Gy, primarily seen in patients with cranial irradiation and could be attributed to growth hormone deficit. However, bone mineral loss up to 7–8 % can be detectable after 30 weeks following 20–25 Gy irradiation in rat femurs. The relationship between osteopenia and pathologic fracture remains unclear [43].

### Physeal Injury

The physical effects of radiation therapy are secondary to damage to the chondroblasts. This damage results in a slowing of, or arrested, physical growth, producing abnormal development of the involved bone, giving rise to (1) spinal abnormalities, (2) leg or arm length discrepancies, (3) angular deformities at joints, (4) slipped capitofemoral epiphyses, and (5) osteocartilaginous exostoses.

### Spinal Abnormalities

Spinal abnormalities most commonly include decreased stature or scoliosis, although lordosis or kyphosis can also occur [12, 67]. Except for decreased growth, severe spinal complications are less common after megavoltage RT, compared with the orthovoltage era, if the entire vertebral body is within the treatment field [83]. Although curvature can occur, it is usually a result of tethering that occurs with decreased muscle development as a result of irradiating just one side of the abdomen, as is often done in Wilms' tumor.

On standard radiographs, vertebral bodies show subcortical lucent zones within 9–12 months after completing RT. The subcortical lucent zones progress over the next 1–2 years to form growth arrest lines, which parallel the epiphysis of the vertebral body [91]. Following the development of these arrest lines, little or no further growth occurs. The higher the dose, the quicker the growth arrest occurs. Other changes may also be seen on radiographic examination. During the first few months after irradiation, vertebral bodies may have a more bulbous contour [49]. Scalloping of the physical cartilage plates may also be observed, and not infrequently, the final appearance is that of rounded vertebral bodies with central beaking [91].

Clinically, the deleterious effect of radiation on growing bone has been known for a long time. Neuhauser and associates reported on 24 children who received orthovoltage irradiation to the spine during their treatment for Wilms' tumor or neuroblastoma [67]. Doses below 10 Gy (using orthovoltage irradiation) caused no detectable vertebral abnormality regardless of the age at treatment. Higher doses caused severe late effects in the spine. Mayfield and coworkers reported on 28 children with neuroblastoma who received irradiation to their spine [60]. Scoliosis was the most common sequela and occurred most severely at doses above 30 Gy with orthovoltage irradiation. Megavoltage irradiation appears to cause fewer severe orthopedic complications. Rate et al. reported on a series of 31 Wilms' tumor patients irradiated between 1970 and 1984. Three out of ten patients treated with orthovoltage irradiation developed late orthopedic abnormalities requiring intervention [82]. None of the 21 patients receiving megavoltage treatment developed such complications, even at doses of 4,000 cGy. Scoliosis was related to

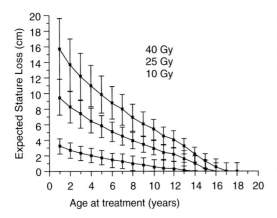

**Fig. 16.5** An example of the model for expected stature loss after radiation therapy to the spine during childhood, as proposed by Silber and coworkers. A hypothetical male patient was treated from T10–11 to L4–5, and his ideal adult stature was 176.8 cm. Each point corresponds to the age when irradiated, the dose in Gray, and stature loss, plus or minus one standard deviation (From [97], p. 309)

a higher median dose (2,890 cGy) and a larger field size (150 cm²); this sequela did not result for patients receiving smaller doses to a smaller field size (2,580 cGy–120 cm²). Paulino et al. report a lower incidence of scoliosis with doses <2,400 cGy than with higher doses [77]. Both orthovoltage and megavoltage irradiation were used. Probert and Parker were the first investigators to attempt to evaluate bone growth alterations secondary to megavoltage irradiation. They noted deficits sitting height for patients who received radiation to the spine for medulloblastoma, leukemia, and Hodgkin's disease [79]. Doses greater than 35 Gy were found to produce a significantly greater deficit in sitting height, compared with doses less than 25 Gy.

Silber and coworkers, using data from 36 children whose spine or pelvis was irradiated, have developed a mathematical model for predicting stature loss [97]. The model is based on the radiation dose in Gy, the location of the therapy (including whether or not the capitofemoral epiphysis was treated), gender, and the ideal adult height. Figure 16.5 shows an example of the model, based on four different irradiation doses. The model agrees closely with a report by Hogeboom et al. who calculated the height deficit after flank RT for Wilms' tumor patients at different ages and doses of radiation therapy [41]. In both reports, even a dose of 10 Gy at age 2 produced a height deficit of 2.3–2.4 cm by age 18 years. For infants less than 12 months of age receiving 10 Gy or more, the estimated height deficit was 7.0 cm. Although chemotherapy did not appear to increase the effect of radiation therapy in Hogeboom's study, there was a deficit associated with doxorubicin that – although it could be explained, at least partially, by other factors – does not completely rule out a permanent doxorubicin effect on bone growth.

Laminectomy is required in selected cases of children presenting with intraspinal or paraspinal tumors. Children undergoing laminectomy at a younger age are prone to development of kyphoscoliosis [20, 42]. Deformity risk increases significantly when postoperative radiotherapy is added [21, 48].

## Limb Length Discrepancy/Angular Deformity

Irradiation of the extremities or hip usually produces more long-term symptomatic sequelae than irradiation of the spine, particularly when an epiphysis is treated. Radiographic changes first reveal metaphyseal irregularities and epiphyseal widening. Later changes include sclerosis around the physis and eventually sclerosis and closure of the epiphyseal plate. Such premature closure can cause a discrepancy in ultimate length between the irradiated and unirradiated extremity. The degree of growth disturbance in long bones is dose and volume dependent; moreover, patient age plays a very important role [35]. In addition, if the entire physis is not included in the radiation port, then juxta-articular angular deformities can result [84]. It is possible to predict the effects of radiation on growth based on age and growth pattern. Altogether, about 65 % of leg growth occurs at the knee, 37 % from the distal femoral physis, and 28 % from the proximal tibial physis. Only 15 % occurs at the proximal femoral growth plate and 20 % from the distal tibial plate [5, 36]. This estimate may not be completely accurate because it assumes that no growth occurs after irradiation of the growth plate, but in reality, growth continues for at least a short period of time. Additionally, untreated physis in the same extremity can partially compensate for the affected one. Asymmetric dose delivery to the metaphysis can cause valgus and varus deformities [31].

Surgery may also have a significant effect on limb function. Limb preservation with expandable prosthesis has become a widely adopted method in the local management of bone malignancies in children [2, 10]. Repeat procedures for prosthesis, either lengthening or replacement, is often required [26], which potentially adversely affects the physical and emotional well-being of children [39, 102]. Rotationplasty is another durable reconstructive procedure which is associated with significant limb length discrepancy requiring prosthetics. Despite its complexity, children receiving this treatment appear to have reasonable physical and emotional resilience [32, 34]. Amputation is the most radical surgical procedure associated with the loss of a significant portion of the limb and can only be compensated with prosthetics. Despite significant differences between limb sparing, rotationplasty, and amputation, data suggests that survivors have fairly comparable physical and emotional outcomes with either approach [44].

## Craniofacial Deformities

Microcephaly, micrognathia, and other growth abnormalities are reported in children with retinoblastomas and rhabdomyosarcomas receiving external beam radiation to the craniofacial region [24, 62, 81].

Surgical management of tumors in the head and neck of young children may be associated with even more substantial cosmetic and functional disturbances. Given the anatomical challenges of these tumors, there is often concern about leaving microscopic or gross disease behind; thus, adjuvant radiotherapy is given [18]. This combined approach can result in more significant dysfunctions due to worse fibrosis developing over time. Reconstructive surgeries can correct these problems to an extent, but long-term outcomes are still far from satisfactory [16]. Anthropometric and descriptive methods are commonly used for documenting the extent of

deformities, but they are hard to quantify. Severe hypoplasia or asymmetry of tissues causing cosmetic and functional problems may require reconstructive surgery.

## Slipped Capitofemoral Epiphysis

Radiation therapy has been shown to increase the risk for slipped capital femoral epiphysis due to epiphyseal plate injury [9, 108, 112]. Patients with slipped capitofemoral epiphyses present with pain in the hip or knee (referred from the hip). The pain presents through either acute or chronic onset, since slippage of the capitofemoral epiphysis often proceeds slowly. Wolf and associates first reported cases of slipped capitofemoral epiphysis as a result of childhood irradiation [112]. These occurred 1–6 years after therapy with doses of 28.5–54 Gy and usually after the onset of puberty when there is a change in the angle of the femoral shaft in relation to the femoral neck and head (a change that increases the susceptibility to stress from excess weight and other factors). Children developing a slipped epiphysis after irradiation were generally 2–3 years younger than the average patient with idiopathic-slipped capitofemoral epiphysis, had twice the risk of bilateral involvement (20–50 %) if both proximal femurs were exposed to radiation, and, furthermore, did not usually fit the generally obese body habitus of the average patient presenting with the idiopathic variety. Paulino et al. reported on four infants (<6 months old) irradiated to the hip to doses of 20 Gy or higher for a neuroblastoma [75]. Two patients developed slipped capitofemoral epiphysis, at 25.5 Gy and 36 Gy. The other two patients received doses of 20 Gy and did not develop the problem. Slippage of the physis is thought to occur as a result of excess stress, either from obesity or from a weakening of the bone and physis secondary to radiation therapy. The threshold dose is thought to be around 25 Gy.

The use of chemotherapy has caused a reduction in the shear strength of the physis in an animal model [104]. Theoretically, chemotherapy would also appear to predispose patients to developing slipped capital femoral epiphysis, but this has not been studied in humans.

## Exostosis

Osteocartilaginous exostoses are benign outgrowths of the physis. They have been reported to occur in up to 18 % of children treated with radiation therapy [3], although the incidence in the megavoltage era is much lower. The etiology is unknown, but is thought to be due to an injury to the periphery of the growth plate. The lesion is a combination of a radiolucent cartilaginous cap with areas of ossification and calcification. It has a typical cauliflower appearance and the base may be narrow or broad. On physical examination, a hard mass is palpable adjacent to a joint [94]. Lesions may continue to grow slowly throughout childhood, although by the third decade growth should cease.

There is a small incidence of malignant degeneration that presents with pain and occurs after skeletal maturation.

## Pathologic Fractures

Irradiation of the metaphyseal portion of the bone may temporarily cause increased porosity and demineralization; radiographic examination will show cortical thinning and irregularities during this time. The irradiated segment of bone therefore acts as a stress concentrator and predisposes the bone to fracture [38]. This effect is particularly true in patients in whom the irradiated bone has been weakened by tumor involvement, such as in Ewing's sarcoma of the humerus and femur. This effect also occurs if the cortex of the bone has been biopsied, particularly in the area of the femoral neck [107]. Pathologic fractures usually occur within 3 years after treatment [38]. The most common site is the upper third of the femur, and since fractures can be caused by tumor recurrence, a full reevaluation of the patient should be performed to ensure that it is not related to relapse [107].

## Avascular Necrosis/Osteoradionecrosis

Avascular necrosis (AVN) of the femoral head has been reported as a complication of hip irradiation in children who have received doses exceeding 30 Gy [53]. Older age (usually >10 years old) appears to increase the risk, indicating that the rapidly growing and maturing bones of adolescents are more susceptible to the development of AVN [59]. High cumulative corticosteroid doses administered during the therapy strongly predispose patients to AVN, and dexamethasone seems to be more toxic than prednisone. AVN may be asymptomatic or result in joint swelling, pain, limited range of motion, and even joint damage and articular collapse. MRI is the best technique to detect early stages of AVN. The typical radiographic picture is shown in Fig. 16.6a–d.

Osteoradionecrosis (ORN) of the mandible is a rare complication of head-and-neck cancer therapy, and its incidence is quite variable in the literature, ranging from 0.9 % to 35 % [100, 105].

### 16.2.2.2 Muscle

The most common late effect of developing muscle tissues secondary to irradiation is diminished development of the muscle tissues (hypoplasia). The muscles treated are smaller and functionally not as strong as the patient's unirradiated muscle tissues. Still, the differences in strength are not pronounced, and, for the majority of patients, it is more of a cosmetic problem than a functional one. Nevertheless, it is a common problem. Macklis et al. reported that 13 of 14 long-term survivors of Wilms' tumor treated with low-dose pulmonary irradiation had musculoskeletal hypoplasia [55]. Long-term survivors treated with head-and-neck radiation therapy are reported to have a 77–100 % incidence of mild to severe radiation damage of soft tissues and bones [76, 80]. Radiotherapy for soft tissue sarcoma of the limb conventionally involves irradiation of the entire transverse cross section of the affected anatomical compartment [8]. Studies have shown that the functional outcome after radiotherapy to the limb is related to the radiotherapy volume and the size of the unirradiated corridor [4]. The total dose and dose per fraction of radiotherapy used are also a significant factor in determining range of movement, muscle power, and limb function [50]. Posttreatment function is paramount in the management of soft tissue sarcoma.

With higher doses, these tissues can develop marked fibrosis, which can produce stiffness, a decrease in range of motion of a joint, and even pain [88]. In mild cases, stiffness or pain occurs

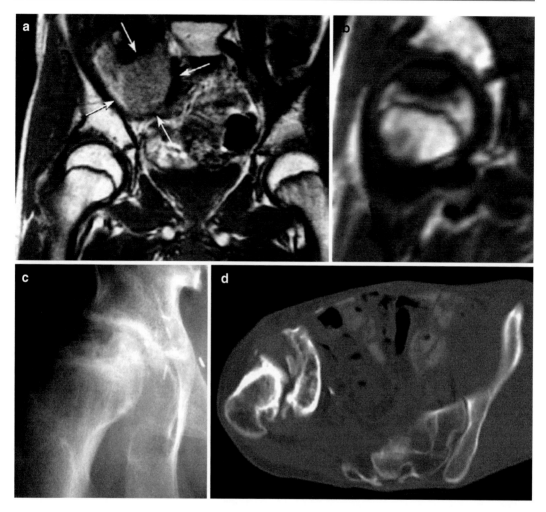

**Fig. 16.6** (**a–d**) A 14-year-old boy treated with preoperative irradiation (61 Gy) and chemotherapy for a synovial cell sarcoma of the right iliopsoas muscle. (**a**) Tumor (*arrows*) and normal femoral heads. (**b**) An MR scan 6 months later showing a close-up of the right femoral head. The scalloped, non-enhancing lesion in the femoral head is typical for an osteonecrosis. (**c**) A plain radiograph 1 year later, showing healing of the femoral head (**b–d**, see next page). (**d**) The early healing was not permanent, however, and a computed tomography scan 13 years after treatment demonstrates collapse of the femoral head, chronic dislocation of the femoral head, and extensive degenerative changes. Severe scoliosis resulted as well

primarily in the early morning and is improved by use of the involved muscles. Occasionally, the patient may have pain that is more persistent, lasts all day, and, even with use, does not improve.

A specific type of fibrosis is trismus, which is an inability to fully open the mouth. When the masticator muscles and the temporomandibular joint are included in the irradiated field, musculoskeletal fibrosis can cause trismus and mandibular dysfunction. It has been reported in about 5–10 % of children treated for head-and-neck malignancies [71, 105]. Since doses are lower in RMS of the head and neck, trismus is less common in RMS than in nasopharyngeal carcinoma [76].

## 16.2.3 Impact of Aging

In general, growth deficits of the musculoskeletal system from irradiation are amplified with increasing years after treatment. Obviously, when all epiphyses are closed, further bone growth deficits do not occur. However, other late effects of bone will continue to occur, and muscular hypoplasia (and fibrosis) may become more significant.

## 16.2.4 Detection/Screening

A thorough history and physical examination is critical in the evaluation of musculoskeletal treatment sequelae. It is necessary to know exactly when a deformity becomes symptomatic, the symptom complex, and the details of the previous cytotoxic treatment related to the deformity. Attention should be given to the types of surgical procedures, location of the radiation fields, radiation doses used, and details (including doses) of the chemotherapy regimen.

The physical examiner should look for skin changes from the cytotoxic treatment as well as any obvious deformity. The musculoskeletal assessment should include serial measures of weight, height, and sitting height (crown to rump). These measurements should be plotted on growth velocity charts to assess whether growth rate is within normal limits. Most normal children will grow a minimum of 5 cm per year between age 3 years and puberty. A patient in that age group who grows <5 cm per year, or whose serial heights on growth charts begin to fall into the lower percentiles, may be experiencing growth failure [65].

Any joints involved in the radiation fields, or affected by surgery, should be put through passive and active ranges of motion, and comparisons should be made with the contralateral side. Joint measurements should be taken if indicated by abnormalities in "performance" range of motion – for example, if the active motion of a particular joint is less than the passive range of motion. In the event that there are performance range-of-motion abnormalities, further assessments are indicated. Other joint problems that can occur include pain, crepitation, swelling, loss of mobility, and weakness [56].

Observation of gait and posture must be included in the musculoskeletal assessment. As indicated by treatment received, the muscles to be examined can be assessed by functional groups, and comparisons can be made bilaterally for symmetry, tone, size, and strength. Any areas of deformity, swelling, atrophy, or weakness should be noted [65].

The patient should be assessed for level of functioning and participation in normal daily activities, such as school and after-school activities. Normal growth and development parameters should be incorporated into this assessment, as developmental stages may influence the patient's participation in some activities. Another influence on the level of functioning or decreased participation in activities could be the lack of adjustment to body image changes.

There is no current method of completely preventing the development of late musculoskeletal effects from surgery or radiotherapy. The patient who has experienced an amputation or a significant growth deficit due to radiotherapy may or may not have incorporated this long-term effect into a new, positive body image. Many other factors contribute to general growth and development, such as nutritional deficits, other tissue damage, and hormonal influences. The examiner should not rush to attribute the entire problem to the cytotoxic treatment [65]. If the right assessment is made, intervention can sometimes prevent an asymptomatic or mildly symptomatic problem from becoming more clinically significant. At the very least, the appropriate intervention may be able to assist the patient in adapting to body image changes.

### 16.2.4.1 Spinal Sequelae

The evaluation of spinal sequelae should include the region of curvature, the magnitude of the curve, the deviation from vertical, the degree of shoulder asymmetry, the position of any rib humps or rib flare, and the type and degree of any gait abnormality. Usually, the best way to examine the back is with the patient bending over with the arms touching the toes and the knees straight. At each visit, measurements should be taken of the standing and sitting heights. The spinal shortening that occurs as a direct effect of irradiation is not correctable, but, except for an ultimate decrease in height, does not usually cause major problems, unless spinal curvature develops. Anteroposterior and lateral films of the entire spine should be used to screen for this. It is also important to be able to inform the patients of the height deficit to be expected. Figure 16.5 shows a model of expected stature loss by age at treatment for three dose levels for a hypothetical male patient receiving radiation from T10–T11 to L4–5 [97].

If the spine has been irradiated, standard radiographic images should be taken every 1–2 years until skeletal maturity to detect early scoliosis or kyphoscoliosis (Fig. 16.7). After that, films should still be taken every 1–2 years if some curvature is already present. It is rare to develop curvature after skeletal maturity if none was present before.

The most common method for measuring spinal curvature is the Cobb technique. The two end vertebrae of the curvature, the ones most tilted from the horizontal on the upright film, are selected. A line is drawn along the upper end plate of the upper end vertebra and along the lower end plate of the lower end vertebra. The angle of intersection of the perpendiculars from these lines is the angle of the curvature (see Fig. 16.8). It is extremely important to perform these measurements carefully. Since progression of any defect may be more important than the occurrence of the defect, the amount of curvature, both sites should be measured.

### 16.2.4.2 Limb Length Discrepancy

Limb length discrepancies are usually more significant. Differences in length between upper extremities are not often a problem, but leg length discrepancies can cause significant functional deficits. It is therefore important to be able to predict the ultimate outcome when radiotherapy is chosen. To do so, knowledge of the future growth of all epiphyses is necessary. In the lower extremity, 65 % of future growth comes from the knee, 37 % from the distal femoral physis, and 28 % from the proximal tibial physis. Only 15 % occurs at the proximal femoral plate and 20 % from the distal tibial plate [65]. Table 16.1 provides rough estimates, by age of the patient, of the growth remaining for the four major lower extremity

epiphyses. Information such as this can be used to calculate the probable discrepancy that may develop assuming that there is no growth of the irradiated physis after treatment. This is not completely accurate, since some growth may occur for a short time, and other untreated growth plates in the same extremity may partially compensate for the closed physis.

The evaluation of a limb length discrepancy on physical examination is also primarily based on accurate measurements. The patient should be undressed completely for the measurements to avoid tenting of the tape around folds in the patient's clothes. The *real* length of each leg is measured from the anterior superior iliac spine to the tip of the medial malleolus (Fig. 16.9a). The *apparent* length is measured from the umbilicus to the tip of the medial malleolus. The *real* length is the more important measurement because pelvic obliquity does not influence this measurement. The apparent length informs the evaluating physician of the compensation by the patient for the limb length discrepancy. To detect developing leg length discrepancies, measurements should also be taken at least once a year to follow the extent of the evolving discrepancy. If there is a high chance of a significant discrepancy developing, then film measurements should be taken as well. There are several accepted radiographic methods for evaluating limb length differences, and mistakes are easy to make in such measurements. Because of this, it is ideal if the same physician is able to evaluate the patient repetitively, but, as this is not always possible, it is important for any evaluating physician to carefully review the previous films (not just the reports) before using surgery to correct the defect. To evaluate the radiographic difference, a single exposure is taken of both legs on a long film, usually with the patient standing, and a radiographic ruler is placed on the cassette. The *real* length can then be measured from the anterior iliac spine to the medial malleolus [65] (Fig. 16.9b).

### 16.2.4.3 Other Bony Sequelae

Other bony sequelae are usually acutely symptomatic. A slipped capitofemoral epiphysis causes pain and can be diagnosed using a

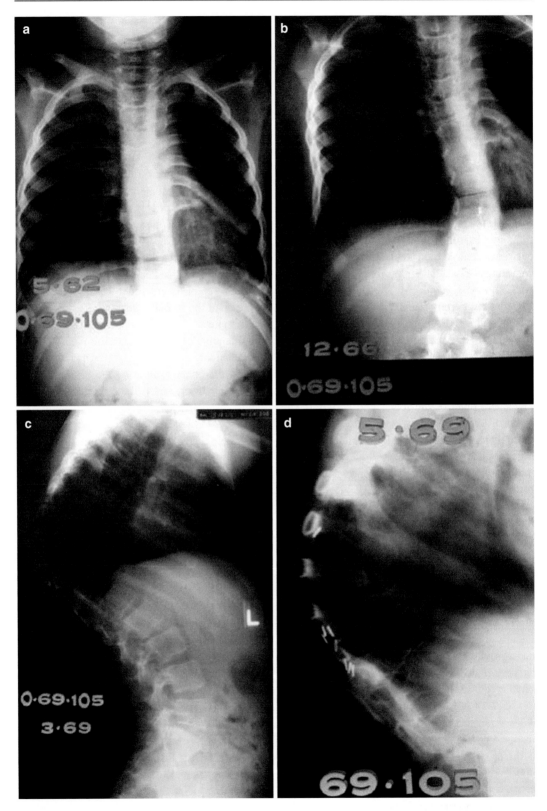

**Fig. 16.7** (**a–d**) A 2-year-old girl treated with orthovoltage irradiation to the abdomen and spine (dose unknown) for a neuroblastoma in 1960. (**a**) Two years after treatment, mild scoliosis developed. (**b–c**) Progression of kyphoscoliosis occurred over the next 7 years. (**d**) A close-up of the spine 9 years after therapy shows osteoporosis of vertebral bodies and wedge-shaped compression fractures

radiograph of the involved hip (Fig. 16.10a, b). A pathologic fracture also will be symptomatic and readily apparent on radiography.

### 16.2.4.4 Muscle

To evaluate a deficit in muscle development, measurements of the circumferences of the involved extremity should be performed, and a determination of the range of motion of all joints in the involved limb should be made. Measurements of the opposite normal extremity should be taken as well for comparison.

### 16.2.5 Management of Established Problems

#### 16.2.5.1 Management

It is not possible to prevent many of the late effects of irradiation. Of the common deficits that develop, scoliosis and leg length discrepancies need intervention most often.

Scoliotic curve progression beyond 30° (or curves over 20° with rapid progression) generally requires bracing. Curves greater than 40°, particularly in skeletally immature patients, should be instrumented and fused [51].

Table 16.2 shows the recommended treatment for categories of leg length discrepancies [65]. Small differences (0–2 cm) usually require no intervention. Greater differences require an orthopedic evaluation. Differences of 2–6 cm can be corrected with a shoe lift or a contralateral epiphysiodesis, an operation creating a premature fusion of an epiphysis in the contralateral limb to arrest growth. This prevents further exaggeration of the deficit. Greater inequality (6–15 cm) requires more aggressive management. Contralateral limb shortening or ipsilateral lengthening procedures are usually necessary to restore a functional gait. Differences of greater than 15–20 cm are difficult to manage.

Other less common late effects may also need intervention. Partial epiphyseal plate injury results in juxta-articular angular deformities of long bones. These uncommon growth aberrations are difficult to treat and often require complete physical arrest and osteotomies for correction. Their

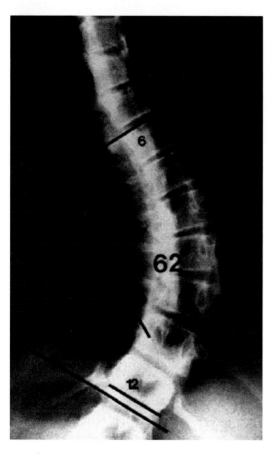

**Fig. 16.8** The Cobb technique for measuring the angle of spinal curvature. See text for a description (From Winter [111])

**Table 16.1** Average growth (in cm) remaining for each lower extremity epiphysis by age and sex

| Epiphysis | Boys (age in years) | | | | | Girls (age in years) | | | | |
|---|---|---|---|---|---|---|---|---|---|---|
| | 8 | 10 | 12 | 14 | 16 | 8 | 10 | 12 | 14 | 16 |
| Proximal femur | 3.5 | 3.0 | 2.0 | 0.8 | <0.5 | 2.8 | 1.9 | 0.8 | <0.5 | 0 |
| Distal femur | 8.5 | 7.5 | 5.0 | 2.0 | 0.5 | 7.0 | 4.7 | 2.0 | 0.8 | 0 |
| Proximal tibia | 6.0 | 5.0 | 3.5 | 1.0 | <0.5 | 4.5 | 3.0 | 1.0 | <0.5 | 0 |
| Distal tibia | 4.2 | 3.7 | 2.5 | 1.0 | <0.5 | 3.4 | 2.3 | 1.0 | <0.5 | 0 |

Adapted from Anderson [5] Table V, p.11

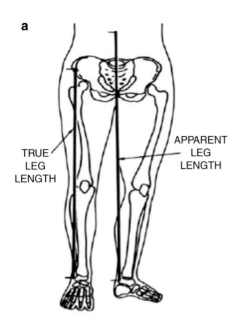

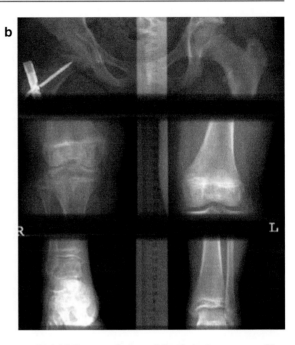

**Fig. 16.9** (**a**, **b**) Measurement of leg length discrepancy. See text for details. (**a**) Clinical measurement (From Mosely [65]). (**b**) Leg length scanogram of a 12-year-old girl initially treated at age 6 for Ewing's sarcoma of her right femur. The scanogram is more accurate than a clinical measurement

infrequent occurrence now is ascribed to more careful attention to irradiation technique so that the entire physis is incorporated within the portal.

The occurrence of a slipped capitofemoral epiphysis is a medical emergency requiring immediate referral to an orthopedic surgeon. Correcting the problem requires an in situ pin fixation to prevent a slipped capitofemoral epiphysis in the other leg if it also has been irradiated. Prophylactic pinning of the capitofemoral epiphysis in the other leg should be considered as well. Severe slips (greater than 60°) may require a proximal femoral osteotomy and osteoplasty [9]. Total hip replacement may be needed at times, although every attempt should be made to manage the condition more conservatively in children.

A few exostoses may require excision because of symptoms or malignant degeneration.

Pathologic fractures in the irradiated field, more common if the irradiated bone was biopsied or involved with tumor, rarely heal without internal fixation [38, 54]. Fractures through irradiated bone are a challenging problem and often require long periods of treatment and multiple procedures to obtain union. The concomitant radiation changes in the surrounding soft tissue that envelope the bone further complicate the management of these fractures. These compromised tissues greatly increase the risk of postoperative infection. Rigid internal fixation is mandatory, and bone grafts should be utilized liberally (Fig. 16.11a–c). Vascularized bone grafts are the gold standard for obtaining union in patients whose fractures have failed to unite after other procedures [99] (Fig. 16.12a, b). In the event of severe wound complication and nonunion, an amputation should be considered.

Muscular atrophy is usually a cosmetic problem for which there is no treatment. Even patients who strenuously pursue weight lifting or similar activities to build muscle strength find that the irradiated area rarely responds. However, appropriate exercise will prevent contractures and further decreases in muscle strength, as well as prevents the loss of the range of motion of joints.

Radiation-induced fibrosis (RIF) has been reported to respond to a combination of

**Fig. 16.10** (**a, b**) A 4-year-old boy treated for a lymphoma of the testicle. (**a**) At age 9, a routine follow-up radiograph shows hypoplasia of the left ischium and pubis, with a normal left femoral head and neck. (**b**) Two years later, at age 11, slippage of the left femoral capital epiphysis developed (From Wolf [112], p. 783)

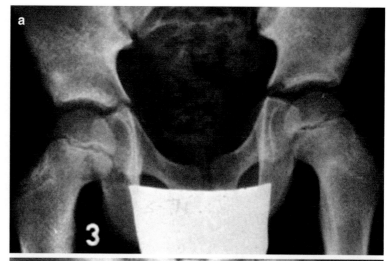

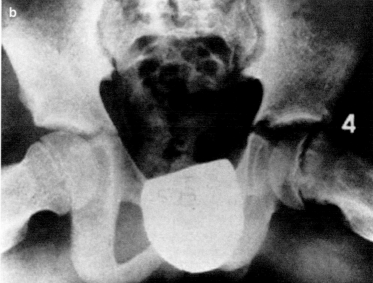

**Table 16.2** Recommended treatment for categories of leg length discrepancies

| Leg length discrepancy | Treatment |
| --- | --- |
| 0–2 cm | None required |
| 2–6 cm | Shoe lift, epiphysiodesis |
| 6–15 cm | Leg lengthening |
| >15 cm | Prosthetic fitting |

From Mosely [65], p. 784, list on p 795

pentoxifylline and tocopherol (vitamin E). In a series of 43 patients with 50 distinct zones of significant RIF who were given 400 mg of pentoxifylline and 500 IU of tocopherol twice a day, clinical improvement occurred in 83 % of lesions at 12 months. The average time from the end of treatment until the start of therapy in this group was 8.5 years. Treatment was given for 6 months or until clinical improvement had ceased. The mean SOMA score changed from 13.2 at the start of treatment to 6.9 at 12 months [22].

### 16.2.5.2 Rehabilitation

In most cases, late effects from cytotoxic therapy involve both the muscles and the bones of an anatomic region. While it is preferable to prevent major problems, this cannot always be done, and

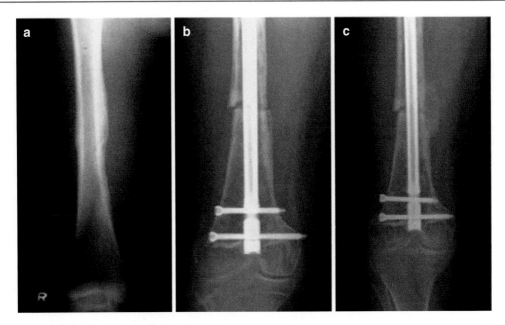

**Fig. 16.11** (**a**) AP radiograph of a 15-year-old girl treated with radiation therapy to her right femur at age 12 years. Shortly after this film was taken, she developed a fatigue fracture of the femur. (**b**) Internal fixation is required for pathologic fractures after radiation therapy, and she underwent intramedullary rodding of the fracture. Despite the rodding, a nonunion occurred, as shown in this radio- graph 2 years after the fracture. (**c**) The internal fixation was revised with the application of an autograph from her iliac crest to the nonunion site. As shown on this radio- graph, there is consolidation of the graph and bridging union across the old fracture site. She is currently pain- free. It is often necessary to bring unirradiated bone into the fracture zone to produce healing

moderate to severe sequelae do develop (Fig. 16.13). Whether or not surgery is required, one necessary portion of the management is a good exercise program. Range-of-motion exer- cises should progress slowly to weight bearing, then muscle-strengthening exercises. The battle with sequelae may be lifelong, and a proper exer- cise program will combat the progression of damage and may even help retrieve functionality previously lost. Nevertheless, caution should be used in recommending vigorous exercise regi- mens for patients who have received high doses of doxorubicin, since cardiac decompensation may result.

The psychological adaptations to the long- term sequelae of treatment also need attention. Novotny [69] observed that one's body image is composed of fluctuating physical, psychological, and social aspects. A positive adjustment to changes in body image requires discarding the previously held perception of one's body and incorporating the changes into a new perception. If the previous body image cannot be put aside so that the changes can be integrated and accepted, a negative body image may result.

Medical personnel can assist patients and their families in making a positive adaptation to changes in body image. Strategies for promot- ing acceptance of treatment-related body image changes must be individualized to each situa- tion [69]. The initial approach should begin with facilitating open, honest communication within the family about their previous experi- ences, current and anticipated concerns, and their educational needs. This information can then serve as the foundation on which to develop a plan of care.

Novotny provided general guidelines for building an individualized plan to assist the patient and family in positive coping with body image changes [69]. The guidelines included are as follows:

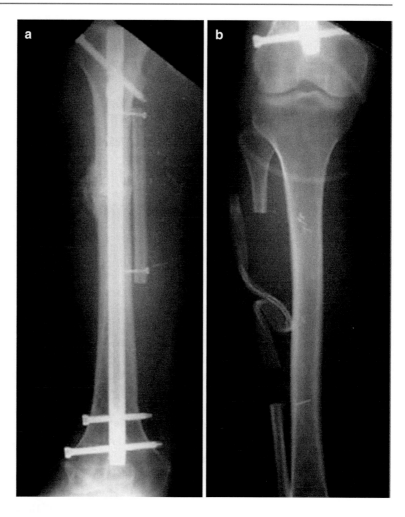

**Fig. 16.12** (**a**, **b**) Another method of repairing a pathologic fracture from radiation therapy is the application of a vascularized fibula graft. (**a**) Anterior-posterior view of the femur shows an intramedullary rod stabilizing the fracture and the fibula graft; the rod has been placed medially along the femur and is held in place with two screws. The graft is typically placed medially to allow close proximity to the femoral vessels for facilitating vessel anastomosis to the fibular vessels. (**b**) Radiograph of the donor site from the ipsilateral leg

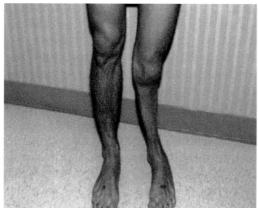

**Fig. 16.13** An 18-month-old boy was treated postoperatively with 50 Gy in 25 fractions for a primary rhabdomyosarcoma of the left calf. His leg is shown 16 years after treatment. The muscles are extremely hypoplastic, and the distal leg is shortened and alopecic. An epiphysiodesis was performed on the other leg to prevent the occurrence of too large a limb length discrepancy

1. Assessing the level of knowledge and adaptation:
   (a) Encouraging patient and family verbalization of fears, concerns, and questions
   (b) Providing anticipatory guidance for the expected physical changes
2. Promoting family unity and coping skills:
   (a) Assisting parents, siblings, significant friends, and school personnel in creating a supportive environment
   (b) Providing education and emotional support to the significant others in the patient's life
3. Reaffirming adaptive behaviors:
   (a) Promoting participation in the "normal" activities of the peer group to meet developmental and psychosocial needs
   (b) Advocating school attendance and participation

4. Changing maladaptive behaviors:
   (a) Supporting the initiative and independence of the patient
   (b) Encouraging the maintenance of usual family roles and discipline
   (c) Emphasizing abilities instead of disabilities

These strategies can be implemented on an ongoing basis. As the patient grows older, adjustments will need to be made continuously. Alteration in body image is a fluid process, and assisting the patient with coping during the various stages of life may be necessary.

Another ongoing process is meeting the educational needs of the patient and family. Patients who were diagnosed at a young age should be educated and reeducated at age-appropriate levels about their diseases, treatments, and actual, as well as potential, late effects [17]. The musculoskeletal physical examination is a good opportunity to explain what the examiner is looking for and why. Patients who have not evidenced musculoskeletal late effects within a short time after treatment may still be at risk for the remainder of their lives. Awareness of potential problem areas may assist in future detection of late effects.

In general, patient and family education about musculoskeletal late effects should include the following information and recommendations [61]:

1. Nutritional influences on musculoskeletal growth and nutritional counseling
2. The importance of avoiding excessive weight gain
3. Participation in noncontact sports/refraining from contact sports
4. Realistic expectations about functional abilities and growth patterns
5. General health education, especially cancer prevention
6. The importance of lifelong surveillance care by knowledgeable healthcare professionals

The patient who is biologically cured of cancer must still live with the aftereffects of the disease and its treatment. A thorough assessment of the many factors affecting each patient's growth and development, promoting positive coping with changes, and providing ongoing education can result in an overall improved quality of life for the patient and family.

## 16.3 Integument

### 16.3.1 Pathophysiology

#### 16.3.1.1 Brief Overview of Normal Organ Development

**Skin**

The skin develops from two sources: the superficial layer (*epidermis*) from the surface ectoderm and the deep layer (*dermis*) from the mesoderm. Early in development, the fetus is covered with a single layer of ectodermal cells. In the beginning of the second month through the fourth month, the following four layers of the epidermis form: (1) the basal layer, which is responsible for the production of new cells and is known as the *germinative layer*; (2) a thick, *spinous layer*, consisting of large polyhedral cells; (3) the *granular layer*, the cells of which contain small keratohyalin granules; and (4) the *horny layer*, forming the tough, scale-like surface of the epidermis and made up of closely packed dead cells loaded with keratin. Also during the first 3 months, cells of neural crest origin invade the epidermis. These cells (*melanocytes*) synthesize melanin pigment, which can be transferred to other cells of the epidermis through the dendritic processes.

The dermis develops during the third and fourth months. The dermis consists of a layer of connective tissue and fatty tissue and contains a number of structures, including hair. Hair starts as solid epidermal proliferations penetrating the underlying dermis. Nerve endings and blood vessels develop with the hair papillae, and cells from outbuddings of the follicle walls form the *sebaceous glands,* which degenerate, thereby forming a fatlike substance that is secreted into the hair follicle and then to the skin.

### 16.3.1.2 Organ Damage Induced by Cytotoxic Therapy

**Skin**

Both radiation therapy and chemotherapy can cause acute and late effects on the skin and subcutaneous tissues. Radiation damage to the skin is primarily owing to effects on the germinative layer of the epidermis. Even low doses quickly diminish mitotic activity, so that cell replacement is nearly zero. The cells of the basal layer become swollen and vacuolated, with nuclear pleomorphism and binucleation. The epidermis becomes thin, with flattening of the papillae. Epidermal cell maturation no longer occurs, causing incomplete keratinization of the superficial cells and, thus, producing desquamation. The desquamation is caused by intracellular edema with enhancement of the intercellular bridges. With high enough doses, the epidermis may slough, exposing the dermal surface, which becomes coated with a layer of fibrin. After treatment, reepithelialization occurs, although the effectiveness of this process will depend upon the extent of the damage. If all the basal cells are not killed, there is a radiation-induced increase in enzyme activity in the melanocytes, which is transmitted to the newly formed squamous cells, causing them to become very dark as they shed.

In the dermis, radiation first causes signs of acute inflammation: edema and a lymphocytic infiltrate. High doses produce nuclear swelling and unequal nuclear divisions of the fibroblasts. Because the papilla of the hair follicle is easily damaged, radiation quickly stops mitotic activity, and the hair root eventually separates from the papilla and is shed. Sweat glands are about 2–3 mm below the surface of the skin, have long lives, and only occasionally undergo mitosis. However, the cells that compose sweat glands can be destroyed by high doses of radiation. Sebaceous glands are more easily destroyed, partially because the normal life cycle includes cell death to produce sebum, and, thus, there is a need for continual replacement through cellular proliferation.

Late dermal reactions are caused by the development of subendothelial fibrous hyperplasia in the blood vessels, which causes telangiectasia and a decreased blood supply to the dermis resulting in increased fibroblastic activity. The skin then takes on a woody texture called fibrosis [4].

The skin changes resulting from radiation therapy are related to the total dose and fractionation of the radiation employed. There are differences between acute and late effects, however. Acute effects are dependent primarily upon the total dose and the overall time in which the radiation is delivered from the beginning to the end of the treatment course. The higher the total dose and the shorter the overall time, the more significant are the acute effects. Late effects are heavily dependent on the dose per fraction and the total dose. Doses greater than 2 Gy per fraction cause an increase in late effects to the skin and subcutaneous tissues. Most "curative" fractionation schemes include doses per fraction of less than 2 Gy. This is particularly true when treating children, in whom late effects are of even more concern.

Modern megavoltage irradiation is "skin sparing," which means that the full buildup of irradiation does not occur at the surface of the skin, but rather at some depth below. The higher the energy of the beam used, the deeper the maximum dose to the tissue. Thus, the severe skin changes seen in orthovoltage irradiation used before the 1960s or 1970s (depending upon the institution), in which the maximum dose was at the surface of the skin, do not occur as often now, unless for some clinical reason it is necessary to produce a high dose at the surface of the skin. With the skin-sparing capabilities of high-energy beams and the use of multiple fields to converge on the tumor, thus further limiting the dose to the skin in each treatment field, the true skin dose usually is not enough to cause severe skin injury. At times, during the treatment of skin lesions – or in the event of unusual situations – the skin receives a dose high enough to cause desquamation. Technical factors in the delivery of the radiation can also cause a higher dose to the skin; these factors include a tangential arrangement of the radiation beams employed, a bolus (tissue-equivalent material) on the skin, or lead blocks and a blocking tray used to shape the radiation fields that are too close to the patient.

A number of chemotherapy-induced skin changes occur, since antineoplastic drugs interfere with nucleic acid formation, ribosomal function, and other components of protein synthesis. Rapidly dividing tissues are the most sensitive; the skin damage is, therefore, primarily to the germinative layer, the hair follicles, and the melanocytes. Certain drugs, bleomycin, in particular, occasionally cause increased melanogenesis. Biopsies of the epidermis after bleomycin have shown larger melanocytes, with larger and more complex dendritic processes [15].

## 16.3.2 Clinical Manifestations

Damage to skin can be divided into acute effects and late effects. During a course of high-dose irradiation to the skin, the first sign of a skin reaction is faint erythema around the hair follicles. If the radiation is conventionally fractionated (less than 2 Gy per fraction), a dose of 20 Gy will usually produce erythema. Higher doses cause a progression to a generalized erythema, epilation, and a decrease in sweating, as well as diminished sebaceous gland secretion. The skin next becomes brightly erythematous, warm, and edematous as well as painful to touch, all of which are sharply limited to the irradiation field. Dry desquamation occurs (at 30 Gy), then moist desquamation follows (occurring at about 40 Gy), leaving the dermis bare with a layer of fibrin covering it. After treatment, these effects heal, usually within 1–2 weeks. Most children never develop such a severe reaction, since usually the dose to any region of skin is considerably less than the dose to the tumor, and a total dose of 40 Gy to the skin is rarely reached. However, any cream or other foreign substance present on the skin during treatment will enhance the skin reaction to radiation.

Doses of even a few Gy will cause temporary alopecia. Recovery takes 8–12 weeks after the end of treatment; the hair starts regrowing at that point and usually grows at a normal rate thereafter. The hair can return a different texture or color; the same phenomenon occurs after chemotherapy. Doses of 40 Gy and above to the hair follicles will cause permanent alopecia. High doses of radiation may cause a skin necrosis and destruction of tissue in the area treated, although these responses are extremely rare now with megavoltage therapy.

The first noticeable late effect consists of very slowly progressing atrophy, starting in the first few months after radiotherapy. The skin also loses its elasticity. If the injury is severe, telangiectasia (a spidery pattern of small blood vessels easily visible beneath the surface) will occur. In the dermis, fibrosis develops, with contraction and scarring in the field treated. Epilation can persist and nails will become brittle. Glands will no longer function normally; the involved skin will not sweat nor produce sebaceous secretions. The formation of comedones has been reported, although this is rare [109]. Related skin structures, such as the breast bud, will not develop normally nor secrete normally. This means that breast development may be hypoplastic or not occur at all.

Radiation effectively accelerates skin aging. Therefore, as the irradiated person grows older, the skin prematurely develops changes consistent with aging. It becomes drier, less flexible, and it may develop "aging" spots or other discolorations. The extent of all these changes is dose related. Doses below 10 Gy (to the skin) rarely cause noticeable problems, while the risk of such late effects increases above 30 Gy [33].

Another potential late sequela of treatment is the risk of the development of a secondary skin cancer, usually a basal cell carcinoma [33, 86]. Basal cell carcinomas are observed in patients with no evidence of chronic skin changes secondary to radiotherapy [33]. The exact risk of a secondary basal cell carcinoma is small; in one series, the calculated excess risk was 0.31/104 patient-years per Gy [86]. The latency period is usually at least 20 years. There may be no excess risk for a skin surface dose of less than 10 Gy for patients receiving standard fractionations, but this conclusion is controversial.

Radiation therapy in childhood has also been implicated in the development of malignant melanoma later in life. In a study utilizing data from Nordic National Cancer Registries, as well as eight centers in France and Great Britain, it was found that between 1960 and 1987, children receiving greater than 15 Gy had a risk of developing melanoma 13 times as great as the risk in nonirradiated children. The risk was in the radiation therapy field [37].

There are at least three skin reactions to chemotherapy: (1) changes related to cytotoxicity, (2) pigment alterations, and (3) rashes and eruptions. Cytotoxic changes related to nucleic acid synthesis, ribosomal function, etc., rarely appear after chemotherapy alone. However, "radiation recall" may be owing to cytotoxic changes in the skin. This phenomenon consists of erythema, blistering, and, sometimes, moist desquamation in an area previously irradiated. It usually occurs a few weeks to a few months after radiotherapy subsequent to a course of chemotherapy containing doxorubicin HCl or dactinomycin (or, occasionally, a number of other drugs, particularly if given in high doses). The same drugs cause increased radiation reactions if given concomitantly with radiation therapy. The etiology is probably renewed damage by chemotherapy to stem cells, which have residual injury from irradiation.

Alopecia occurs through damage to the hair follicles. It is the most predictable skin reaction to chemotherapy. Drugs that cause alopecia include cyclophosphamide, doxorubicin, dactinomycin, and others – the list of agents is very long. Alopecia of the scalp does not appear to require a large threshold dose and occurs after each cycle of the drug; however, it is almost always reversible. Alopecia involving the eyelids and eyelashes is less predictable. Usually, it requires higher and more prolonged courses of chemotherapy, but when it happens, it may sometimes be permanent [95]. In addition, permanent alopecia of the scalp and other hair-bearing regions has been noted after a busulfan-/cyclophosphamide-conditioning regimen for bone marrow transplantation. Over 30 % of patients receiving busulfan as part of a chemotherapy-alone conditioning regimen experience some degree of permanent alopecia [106]. The presence of chronic graft-versus-host disease increases the risk.

**Table 16.3** Pigment changes from chemotherapy

| Abnormality | Associated drugs |
|---|---|
| Generalized hyperpigmentation | 5-Fluorouracil, busulfan |
| Localized hyperpigmentation | Adriamycin, cyclophosphamide, and other alkylating agents, bleomycin, mithramycin, dactinomycin, various hormones |
| Hyperpigmentation of nails | Adriamycin, cyclophosphamide, nitrogen mustard, 5-fluorouracil, methotrexate, nitrosoureas, DTIC, others |
| Linear hyperpigmentation | Most cytotoxics (along veins), bleomycin (on trunk and extremities separate from venous channels) |

From Nixon et al. [68]

Drugs reported to cause pigment changes are shown in Table 16.3. While some, including doxorubicin, have been postulated to have a direct effect on melanocytes [23], the mechanism essentially remains undefined. Generalized hyperpigmentation from bleomycin therapy is probably the most common of these abnormalities, but other drugs such as busulfan, cyclophosphamide, dactinomycin, 5-fluorouracil, hydroxyurea, and methotrexate can also do this on occasion [23]. This generalized hyperpigmentation usually resolves slowly with time, but it can be permanent.

Antimitotic agents can also cause banding of the nails, either vertical or horizontal, as well as black pigmentation. The latter occurs first at the base of the nails and then moves distally [68, 96]. Although usually these changes reverse when the drug is withdrawn, nail hyperpigmentation can be permanent [96].

The drug 5-fluorouracil and high doses of methotrexate, dactinomycin, and doxorubicin can cause skin eruptions, including urticaria – a generalized erythematous rash. They can also cause hyperpigmented, brawny, indurated plaques, particularly of the hands and feet, as well as nodularity of the hands and feet [15, 27]. These effects are temporary.

Children receiving chemotherapy have been reported to develop increased numbers of benign melanocytic nevi after treatment [46].

## 16.3.3 Detection/Screening

It is usually not difficult to predict the extent of the acute changes during treatment based on the radiotherapy dose and fractionation schedule and based on the chemotherapy regimen. The patient (and parents) can therefore anticipate the severity of the reaction. This will usually diminish some of the anxiety that inevitably accompanies the reaction.

Late effects progress with time and may be subtle at first. Careful physical examinations are necessary to detect any cutaneous late effects. These examinations should be performed by a physician who is knowledgeable of the treatment received. Areas of pigmentation changes, dryness, atrophy, telangiectasia, contraction, and scarring should be noted and carefully recorded. If chemotherapy has been given, then skin coloration should be checked as well, along with the status of the nail beds.

While a reversal of skin changes secondary to irradiation and chemotherapy is not possible (although subcutaneous tissues will occasionally soften with time), education of the patient and family can be effective in decreasing the long-term effects. Since radiation damage and sun damage to the skin are similar, it is important for the patient to avoid severe sun exposure after treatment. Sun exposure will increase the aging process started by irradiation. If heavy sun exposure is anticipated, a strong sunscreen (SPF 15 or above) must be used on the treated region.

Most chemotherapy-related skin changes require no specific care, but it is important to carefully check the status of all benign nevi after treatment with chemotherapy. Increased numbers of benign melanocytic nevi appears to be one of the strongest risk factors in the development of malignant melanoma. Since it has been reported that children treated with chemotherapy have more nevi than normal, careful assessments are required [46, 101].

## 16.3.4 Management of Established Problems

### 16.3.4.1 Management and Rehabilitation

Although the acute effects of irradiation are less common now, they can be alarming when they occur. It is important to remember that healing will generally occur spontaneously within 2–4 weeks.

There is no clinically accepted way to reverse late radiation skin changes, though celecoxib has been reported to decrease skin damage after radiation in mice [52]. Because of the lack of sebaceous secretions after treatment, it may be helpful to use Vaseline or a moisturizing cream for patient comfort.

Temporary alopecia from radiotherapy or chemotherapy needs no particular treatment and will resolve in time. Permanent alopecia from radiation therapy cannot be reversed, but hair transplants have been reported to be effective. This can only be done if there remains a large portion of unaffected scalp from which to harvest plugs of normal hair and if the area of alopecia involves well-healed scalp [47]. Hair transplantation has also been reported to be effective following permanent busulfan-induced alopecia, as occurs during bone marrow transplantation. Although allotransplantation is usually unsatisfactory, it will work if the hair grafts are harvested from the same patient that provided the donor marrow [87].

## References

1. American Cancer Society. Cancer Facts and Figures (2007) American Cancer Society http://www.cancer.org/downloads/STT/CAFF2007PWSecured.pdf
2. Aboulafia AJ, Wilkerson J (2012) Lower-limb preservation with an expandable endoprosthesis after tumor resection in children: is the cup half full or half empty? Commentary on an article by Eric R. Henderson, MD, et al.: "Outcome of lower-limb preservation with an expandable endoprosthesis after bone tumor resection in children". J Bone Joint Surg Am 94(6):e39
3. Ackman JD, Rouse L, Johnston CE II (1988) Radiation induced physeal injury. Orthopaedics 11:343–349
4. Alektiar KM, Zelefsky MJ, Brennan MF (2000) Morbidity of adjuvant brachytherapy in soft tissue sarcoma of the extremity and superficial trunk. Int J Radiat Oncol Biol Phys 47(5):1273–1279

5. Anderson M, Green W, Messner MB (1963) Growth and predictions of growth in the lower extremities. J Bone Joint Surg 45:1–14

6. Bajorunas DR et al (1980) Endocrine sequelae of antineoplastic therapy in childhood head and neck malignancies. J Clin Endocrinol Metab 50:329–335

7. Bar-On E et al (1993) Effects of chemotherapy on human growth plate. J Pediatr Orthop 13:220–224

8. Barnett GC, Hoole AC, Twyman N, Jefferies SJ, Burnet NG (2005) Post-operative radiotherapy for soft tissue sarcoma of the anterior compartment of the thigh: should the sartorius muscle be included? Sarcoma 9(1–2):1–6

9. Barrett I (1985) Slipped capitol femoral epiphysis following radiotherapy. J Pediatr Orthop 5:268–273

10. Baumgart R, Lenze U (2009) Expandable endoprostheses in malignant bone tumors in children: indications and limitations. Recent Results Cancer Res 179:59–73

11. Bolek T et al (1996) Local control and functional results after twice-daily radiotherapy for Ewing's sarcoma of the extremities. Int J Radiat Oncol Biol Phys 35:687–692

12. Butler MS et al (1990) Skeletal sequelae of radiation therapy for malignant childhood tumors. Clin Orthop 251:235–240

13. Christodoulou C, Pervena A et al (2009) Combination of bisphosphonates and antiangiogenic factors induces osteonecrosis of the jaw more frequently than bisphosphonates alone. Oncology 76(3):209–211

14. Clayton P et al (1988) Growth in children treated for acute lymphoblastic leukaemia. Lancet 1:460–462

15. Cohen I et al (1973) Cutaneous toxicity of bleomycin therapy. Arch Dermatol 107:553–555

16. Cohen SR, Bartlett SP, Whitaker LA (1990) Reconstruction of late craniofacial deformities after irradiation of the head and face during childhood. Plast Reconstr Surg 86(2):229–237

17. D'Angio G (1988) Cure is not enough: late consequences associated with radiation treatment. J Assoc Pediatr Oncol Nurses 5:20–23

18. Daw NC, Mahmoud HH, Meyer WH, Jenkins JJ, Kaste SC, Poquette CA, Kun LE, Pratt CB, Rao BN (2000) Bone sarcomas of the head and neck in children: the St Jude children's research hospital experience. Cancer 88(9):2172–2180

19. Dawson WB (1968) Growth impairment following radiotherapy in childhood. Clin Radiol 19(3):241–256

20. De Bernardi B, Pianca C, Pistamiglio P, Veneselli E, Viscardi E, Pession A, Alvisi P, Carli M, Donfrancesco A, Casale F, Giuliano MG, di Montezemolo LC, Di Cataldo A, Lo Curto M, Bagnulo S, Schumacher RF, Tamburini A, Garaventa A, Clemente L, Bruzzi P (2001) Neuroblastoma with symptomatic spinal cord compression at diagnosis: treatment and results with 76 cases. J Clin Oncol 19(1):183–190

21. de Jonge T, Slullitel H, Dubousset J, Miladi L, Wicart P, Illes T (2005) Late-onset spinal deformities in children treated by laminectomy and radiation therapy for malignant tumours. Eur Spine J 14(8):765–771

22. Delanian S, Balla-Medias S, Lefaix JL (1999) Striking regression of chronic radiotherapy damage in a clinical trial of pentoxifylline and tocopherol. J Clin Oncol 17:3283–3290

23. DeSpain J (1992) Dermatologic toxicity of chemotherapy. Semin Oncol 19:501–507

24. Donaldson S (1992) Effects of irradiation on skeletal growth and development. Wiley-Liss, New York

25. Drescher W, Schneider T, Becker C, Hobolth J (2001) Selective reduction of bone blood flow by short-term treatment with high-dose methylprednisolone. An experimental study in pigs. J Bone Joint Surg Br 83:274–277

26. Eckardt JJ, Kabo JM, Kelley CM, Ward WG Sr, Asavamongkolkul A, Wirganowicz PZ, Yang RS, Eilber FR (2000) Expandable endoprosthesis reconstruction in skeletally immature patients with tumors. Clin Orthop Relat Res 373:51–61

27. Etcubanas E, Wilbur J (1974) Uncommon side effects of adriamycin (letter). Cancer Chemother Rep 58:757–758

28. Fajardo L (1982) Pathology of radiation injury. Masson, New York

29. Fan C, Cool JC et al (2009) Damaging effects of chronic low-dose methotrexate usage on primary bone formation in young rats and potential protective effects of folinic acid supplementary treatment. Bone 44(1):61–70

30. Fangusaro J, Gururangan S et al (2013) Bevacizumab-associated osteonecrosis of the wrist and knee in three pediatric patients with recurrent CNS tumors. J Clin Oncol 31(2):e24–e27

31. Fletcher DT, Warner WC, Neel MD, Merchant TE (2004) Valgus and varus deformity after wide-local excision, brachytherapy and external beam irradiation in two children with lower extremity synovial cell sarcoma: case report. BMC Cancer 4:57

32. Forni C, Gaudenzi N, Zoli M, Manfrini M, Benedetti MG, Pignotti E, Chiari P (2012) Living with rotationplasty – quality of life in rotationplasty patients from childhood to adulthood. J Surg Oncol 105(4):331–336

33. Fragu P et al (1991) Long-term effects in skin and thyroid after radiotherapy for skin angiomas: a French Retrospective Cohort study. Eur J Cancer 27:1215–1222

34. Fuchs B, Kotajarvi BR, Kaufman KR, Sim FH (2003) Functional outcome of patients with rotationplasty about the knee. Clin Orthop Relat Res 415:52–58

35. Goldwein JW, Meadows AT (1993) Influence of radiation on growth in pediatric patients. Clin Plast Surg 20(3):455–464

36. Gonzalez DG, Breur K (1983) Clinical data from irradiated growing long bones in children. Int J Radiat Oncol Biol Phys 9(6):841–846

37. Guerin S et al (2003) Radiation dose as a risk factor for malignant melanoma following childhood cancer. Eur J Cancer 39:2379–2386

38. Helmstedter C et al (2001) Pathologic fractures after surgery and radiation for soft tissue tumors. Clin Orthop 389:165–172

39. Henderson ER, Pepper AM, Marulanda G, Binitie OT, Cheong D, Letson GD (2012) Outcome of lower-limb preservation with an expandable endoprosthesis after bone tumor resection in children. J Bone Joint Surg Am 94(6):537–547

40. Hobbie WL, Mostoufi SM et al (2011) Prevalence of advanced bone age in a cohort of patients who received cis-retinoic acid for high-risk neuroblastoma. Pediatr Blood Cancer 56(3):474–476

41. Hogeboom C et al (2001) Stature loss following treatment for Wilms' tumor. Med Pediatr Oncol 36:295–304

42. Hoover M, Bowman LC, Crawford SE, Stack C, Donaldson JS, Grayhack JJ, Tomita T, Cohn SL (1999) Long-term outcome of patients with intraspinal neuroblastoma. Med Pediatr Oncol 32(5):353–359

43. Hopewell J (2003) Radiation therapy effects on bone density. Med Pediatr Oncol 41:208–211

44. Hopyan S, Tan JW, Graham HK, Torode IP (2006) Function and upright time following limb salvage, amputation, and rotationplasty for pediatric sarcoma of bone. J Pediatr Orthop 26(3):405–408

45. Hua C, Shukla HI, Merchant TE, Krasin MJ (2007) Estimating differences in volumetric flat bone growth in pediatric patients by radiation treatment method. Int J Radiat Oncol Biol Phys 67(2):552–558

46. Hughes BR, Cunliffe W, Bailey CC (1989) Excess benign melanocytic naevi after chemotherapy for malignancy in childhood. Br Med J 299:88–91

47. Jacobs J, Monell C (1979) Treatment of radiation-induced alopecia. Head Neck Surg 2:154–159

48. Katzenstein HM, Kent PM et al (2001) Treatment and outcome of 83 children with intraspinal neuroblastoma: the Pediatric Oncology Group experience. J Clin Oncol 19(4):1047–1055

49. Katzman H, Waugh T, Berdon W (1969) Skeletal changes following irradiation of childhood tumors. J Bone Joint Surg Am 51-A:825–842

50. Keus RB, Rutgers EJ, Ho GH, Gortzak E, Albus-Lutter CE, Hart AA (1994) Limb-sparing therapy of extremity soft tissue sarcomas: treatment outcome and long-term functional results. Eur J Cancer 30A(10):1459–1463

51. King J, Stowe S (1982) Results of spinal fusion for radiation scoliosis. Spine (Phila Pa 1976) 7(6):574–585

52. Liang L, Dongping H, Weimin L (2003) Celecoxib reduces skin damage after radiation: selective reduction of chemokine and receptor mRNA expression in irradiated skin but not in irradiated mammary tumor. Am J Clin Oncol 26:S114–S121

53. Libshitz HI, Edeiken BS (1981) Radiotherapy changes of the pediatric hip. AJR Am J Roentgenol 137(3):585–588

54. Lin PP, Boland P, Healey JH (1998) Treatment of femoral fractures after irradiation. Clin Orthop 352:168–178

55. Macklis RM, Oltikar A, Sallan SE (1991) Wilms' tumor patients with pulmonary metastases. Int J Radiat Oncol Biol Phys 21:1187–1193

56. Malasonos L et al (1981) Musculoskeletal assessment. Mosby, St Louis

57. Marcus RB Jr, Cantor A, Heare TC, Graham-Pole J, Mendenhall NP, Million RR (1991) Local control and function after twice-a-day radiotherapy for Ewing's sarcoma of bone. Int J Radiat Oncol Biol Phys 21(6):1509–1515

58. Marx RE (2003) Pamidronate (Aredia) and zoledronate (Zometa) induced avascular necrosis of the jaws: a growing epidemic. J Oral Maxillofac Surg 61(9):1115–1117

59. Mattano LA Jr, Sather HN et al (2000) Osteonecrosis as a complication of treating acute lymphoblastic leukemia in children: a report from the Children's Cancer Group. J Clin Oncol 18(18):3262–3272

60. Mayfield JK, Erkkila JC, Winter RB (1981) Spine deformity subsequent to acquired childhood spinal cord injury. J Bone Joint Surg Am 63(9):1401–1411

61. Meadows A (1988) The concept of care for life. J Assoc Pediatr Oncol Nurses 5:7–9

62. Meadows AT, Silber J (1985) Delayed consequences of therapy for childhood cancer. CA Cancer J Clin 35(5):271–286

63. Meister B, Gassner I et al (1994) Methotrexate osteopathy in infants with tumors of the central nervous system. Med Pediatr Oncol 23(6):493–496

64. Moore K (1988) Essentials of human embryology. Decker, Toronto

65. Mosely C (1990) Leg-length discrepancy. Lippincott, Philadelphia

66. Nesbit M, Krivit W et al (1976) Acute and chronic effects of methotrexate on hepatic, pulmonary, and skeletal systems. Cancer 37(2 Suppl):1048–1057

67. Neuhauser E et al (1952) Irradiation effects of roentgen therapy on the growing spine. Radiology 59:637–650

68. Nixon D et al (1981) Dermatologic changes after systemic cancer therapy. Cutis 27:181–194

69. Novotny M (1986) Body image changes in amputee children: how nursing theory can make the difference. J Assoc Pediatr Oncol Nurses 3:8–13

70. O'Regan S, Melhorn DK et al (1973) Methotrexate-induced bone pain in childhood leukemia. Am J Dis Child 126(4):489–490

71. Ozyar E, Cengiz M, Gurkaynak M, Atahan IL (2005) Trismus as a presenting symptom in nasopharyngeal carcinoma. Radiother Oncol 77(1):73–76

72. Pateder D et al (2001) The role of autocrine growth factors in radiation damage to the epiphyseal growth plate. Radiat Res 155:847–857

73. Pateder D et al (2002) Role of pentoxifylline in preventing radiation damage to epiphyseal growth plate chondrocytes. Radiat Res 157:62–68

74. Paulino AC (2004) Late effects of radiotherapy for pediatric extremity sarcomas. Int J Radiat Oncol Biol Phys 60(1):265–274

75. Paulino AC, Mayr NA, Simon JH, Buatti JM (2002) Locoregional control in infants with neuroblastoma:

role of radiation therapy and late toxicity. Int J Radiat Oncol Biol Phys 52(4):1025–1031

76. Paulino AC, Simon JH, Zhen W, Wen BC (2000) Long-term effects in children treated with radiotherapy for head and neck rhabdomyosarcoma. Int J Radiat Oncol Biol Phys 48(5):1489–1495

77. Paulino A et al (2000) Late effects in children treated with radiation therapy for Wilms' tumor. Int J Radiat Oncol Biol Phys 46:1239–1246

78. Pinkel D (1971) Five-year follow-up of "total therapy" of childhood lymphocytic leukemia. JAMA 216:648–652

79. Probert J, Parker BR (1975) The effects of radiation therapy on bone growth. Radiology 114:155–162

80. Raney RB, Anderson JR, Kollath J, Vassilopoulou-Sellin R, Klein MJ, Heyn R, Glicksman AS, Wharam M, Crist WM, Maurer HM (2000) Late effects of therapy in 94 patients with localized rhabdomyosarcoma of the orbit: report from the Intergroup Rhabdomyosarcoma Study (IRS)-III, 1984–1991. Med Pediatr Oncol 34(6):413–420

81. Raney RB, Asmar L, Vassilopoulou-Sellin R, Klein MJ, Donaldson SS, Green J, Heyn R, Wharam M, Glicksman AS, Gehan EA, Anderson J, Maurer HM (1999) Late complications of therapy in 213 children with localized, nonorbital soft-tissue sarcoma of the head and neck: a descriptive report from the Intergroup Rhabdomyosarcoma Studies (IRS)-II and – III. IRS Group of the Children's Cancer Group and the Pediatric Oncology Group. Med Pediatr Oncol 33(4):362–371

82. Rate WR, Butler MS, Robertson WW Jr, D'Angio GJ (1991) Late orthopedic effects in children with Wilms' tumor treated with abdominal irradiation. Med Pediatr Oncol 19(4):265–268

83. Riseborough E et al (1976) Skeletal alterations following irradiation for Wilms' tumor. J Bone Joint Surg Am 58A:526–536

84. Robertson W et al (1991) Leg length discrepancy following irradiation of childhood tumors. J Pediatr Orthop 11:284–287

85. Robson H, Anderson E, Eden OB, Isaksson O, Shalet S (1998) Chemotherapeutic agents used in the treatment of childhood malignancies have direct effects on growth plate chondrocyte proliferation. J Endocrinol 157:225–235

86. Ron E et al (1991) Radiation-induced skin carcinomas of the head and neck. Radiat Res 125:318–325

87. Rosati P, Bergarno A (1999) Allogenic hair transplant in a bone marrow transplant recipient. Dermatol Surg 25:664

88. Rowin J, Cheng G, Lewis SL, Meriggioli MN (2006) Late appearance of dropped head syndrome after radiotherapy for Hodgkin's disease. Muscle Nerve 34(5):666–669

89. Rubin P (1964) Dynamic classification of bone dysplasia. Year Book Medical Publishers, Chicago

90. Rubin P et al (1959) Radiation induced dysplasias of bone. Am J Roentgenol 82:206–216

91. Rutherford H, Dodd GD (1974) Complications of radiation therapy: growing bone. Semin Roentgenol 9:15–27

92. Sadler T (1990) Langman's medical embryology. Williams and Wilkins, Baltimore

93. Salter R (1983) Textbook of disorders and injuries of the musculoskeletal system. Williams and Wilkins, Baltimore

94. Schriock E et al (1991) Abnormal growth patterns and adult short stature in 115 long-term survivors of childhood leukemia. J Clin Oncol 9:400–405

95. Seipp C (2001) Adverse effects of treatment: hair loss. Lippincott Williams and Wilkins, Philadelphia

96. Shah P, Rao KRP, Patel AR (1978) Cyclophosphamide induced nail pigmentation. Br J Dermatol 98:675–680

97. Silber J, Littman PS, Meadows AT (1990) Stature loss following skeletal irradiation for childhood cancer. J Clin Oncol 8:304–312

98. Smith AR, Hennessy JM et al (2008) Reversible skeletal changes after treatment with bevacizumab in a child with cutaneovisceral angiomatosis with thrombocytopenia syndrome. Pediatr Blood Cancer 51(3):418–420

99. Springeld D, Pagliarulo PAC (1985) Fractures of long bones previously treated for Ewing's sarcoma. J Bone Joint Surg Am 67A:477–481

100. Sulaiman F, Huryn JM et al (2003) Dental extractions in the irradiated head and neck patient: a retrospective analysis of Memorial Sloan-Kettering Cancer Center protocols, criteria, and end results. J Oral Maxillofac Surg 61(10):1123–1131

101. Swerdlow A et al (1986) Benign melanocytic naevi as a risk factor for malignant melanoma. Br Med J 292:1555–1559

102. Tabone MD, Rodary C, Oberlin O, Gentet JC, Pacquement H, Kalifa C (2005) Quality of life of patients treated during childhood for a bone tumor: assessment by the child health questionnaire. Pediatr Blood Cancer 45(2):207–211

103. Truica C, Frankel SR (2002) Acute rhabdomyolysis as a complication of cytarabine chemotherapy for acute myeloid leukemia: a case report and review of the literature. Am J Hematol 70:320–323

104. Van Leeuwen B et al (2003) Chemotherapy decreases epiphyseal strength and increases bone fracture risk. Clin Orthop 413:243–254

105. Vissink A, Jansma J et al (2003) Oral sequelae of head and neck radiotherapy. Crit Rev Oral Biol Med 14(3):199–212

106. Vowels M et al (1993) Factors affecting hair regrowth after bone marrow transplantation. Bone Marrow Transplant 23:347–350

107. Wagner L et al (2001) Fractures in pediatric Ewing's sarcoma. J Pediatr Hematol Oncol 23:568–571

108. Walker S et al (1981) Slipped capital femoral epiphysis following radiation and chemotherapy. Clin Orthop Relat Res 159:186–193

109. Walter J (1980) Cobalt radiation-induced comedones. Arch Dermatol 116:1073–1074

110. Whyte MP, Wenkert D et al (2003) Bisphosphonate-induced osteopetrosis. N Engl J Med 349(5):457–463

111. Winter R (1990) Spinal problems in pediatric ortho-
     paedics. Lippincott, Philadelphia
112. Wolf E et al (1977) Slipped femoral capital epiphy-
     sis as a sequela to childhood irradiation for malig-
     nant tumors. Radiology 125:781–784
113. Woo SB, Hellstein JW et al (2006) Narrative [cor-
     rected] review: bisphosphonates and osteonecrosis
     of the jaws. Ann Intern Med 144(10):753–761
114. Zeman W, Solomon M (1971) Effects of radiation on
     striated muscle. Williams and Wilkins, Baltimore

# Breast Chapter

# 17

Tara O. Henderson and Lisa Diller

## Contents

Impairment of breast development, disruption of breast function, and breast cancers are all late consequences that have been observed in survivors of childhood cancer. Normal breast development can be impaired by exposure to radiation, prior surgery, and by decreased estrogen exposure associated with therapy-induced ovarian or hypothalamic disruption. Normal function of the breast as the lactation organ has not been well studied in survivors. Most studies have focused on breast cancer risks in survivors of childhood cancer, with a particular concern for breast cancers after radiation to the chest. Recent work has focused on surveillance strategies, prophylaxis, and changes in primary cancer therapy that might reduce the risk of secondary breast cancer. Finally, understanding of the underlying genetic risk factors for secondary breast cancers may determine future strategies for prevention of breast malignancy after childhood cancer. In this chapter, we review normal breast development, risk factors for secondary breast cancer, surveillance, and prevention strategies, as well as what is known about management of breast hypoplasia and lactation impairment in survivors.

T.O. Henderson, MD, MPH (✉)
Pediatric Hematology, Oncology and Stem Cell Transplantation, University of Chicago, Comer Children's Hospital, Chicago, IL, USA

L. Diller, MD
Pediatric Oncology, Dana-Farber Cancer Institute/ Harvard Medical School, Boston, MA, USA

## 17.1 Brief Overview of Normal Development

The mammary glands consist of a branching network of ducts ending in buds, which during puberty evolve into increasing numbers of alveolar lobules. During pregnancy and lactation, these lobules become secretory. In human embryonic development, the first sign of mammary glands are found in the form of a band-like thickening of epidermis, the *mammary line* or *ridge*. This extends on each side of the body from the base of the forelimb to the region of the hind limb by the seventh week of gestation. Most of the mammary line disappears quickly, but a small portion in the thoracic region persists and penetrates the underlying mesenchyme, forming the breast bud. The bud sprouts 16–24 cords, which ultimately form the lactiferous ducts surrounded by the alveoli of the gland. The ducts at first open into a small epithelial pit in the bud, but shortly after birth, this pit matures into the *nipple* by proliferation of the underlying mesenchyme [1]. At birth, the breast of both the male and female is identical. At puberty the female breast bud enlarges, followed by development of the mammary glands and, subsequently, deposition of fat. The nipple and areola enlarge as well [2]. These developmental changes are determined by circulating levels of female pituitary and gonadotropic hormones; specifically, estrogen generates ductal growth, progesterone stimulates alveolar lobules, prolactin stimulates the alveoli to produce milk products, and oxytocin then stimulates the letdown and release of milk [3].

## 17.2 Breast Hypoplasia After Childhood Cancer

### 17.2.1 Breast Hypoplasia Due to Radiation Exposure

In the growing breast, the most sensitive structure is the breast bud. As little as 10 Gy to the breast bud will cause breast hypoplasia (underdevelopment); doses above 20 Gy may ablate development altogether [4]. In patients treated with pulmonary irradiation for Wilms' tumor, four out of ten females had hypoplastic breast development, including two who received less than 20 Gy [5].

## 17.2.2 Breast Hypoplasia as a Consequence of Ovarian Failure

A consequence of premature ovarian failure prior to or in the midst of puberty due to exposure to alkylator chemotherapy, radiation involving the pelvis and/or surgery requiring removal of the ovaries, is the failure of breast development. Survivors with primary ovarian failure will not go through puberty without hormone replacement therapy (HRT). Decisions around timing and dosage of HRT need to be individualized for the patient, considering chronological age, stage of secondary sexual characteristics, as well as psychological issues, such as desire to match peers with respect to pubertal development [6]. It should also be recognized that there is a fine balance which needs to be achieved when prescribing estrogen replacement in girls with premature ovarian failure – while at low doses it stimulates longitudinal growth, at higher doses it can result in premature epiphyseal closure and ultimately reduction in adult height. Thus, initiation of HRT should take into account maximizing longitudinal growth. In the absence of any breast development, it has been recommended by age 12 years; girls with known ovarian failure should start low-dose estrogen to stimulate breast development [6]. After about 6–18 months of this initial therapy, based on the amount of breast development prior to initiating HRT and the desired rate of progressing through puberty, the estrogen dose should be increased. Once breast development is complete (usually after 12–24 months of the higher-dose estrogen treatment), cyclic dosed progestins [such as combined estrogen-progestin products, such as oral contraceptive pills (OCPs), or transvaginal or transdermal formulations] can be incorporated to the HRT in order to maintain the health of the endometrium. Progesterone does not play a significant role in breast development and early puberty. In order to mimic "typical" puberty, it is considered most appropriate to begin HRT with estrogen monotherapy.

### 17.2.3 Breast Hypoplasia Detection

In females who were exposed to over 10 Gy to the breast (including chest, whole-lung, mediastinal, axilla, mini-mantle, mantle, extended mantle, total-body irradiation), in particular those who were treated when they were prepubertal, yearly breast exams should be performed to identify failure of breast development [7].

### 17.2.4 Breast Hypoplasia Management

Breast hypoplasia may be corrected by breast augmentation. Upon completion of growth and puberty, females may be referred for surgical consultation for breast reconstruction. Optimally, surgeons should be familiar with hypoplasia in survivors as healing may be impaired in previously irradiated areas. Providers should consider the survivors' emotional and psychological status when determining this referral [7]. A downside of the procedure is that breast augmentation may make breast cancer surveillance more difficult, though studies to date suggest that breast cancer stage at diagnosis and subsequent outcomes are similar in women with and without previous breast augmentation [8].

## 17.3 Lactation After Childhood Cancer

The functioning of the mammary glands is dependent on an interplay of neuroendocrine factors, as well as health of breast tissue, skin, and glands. Prolactin, produced in the anterior pituitary, is necessary for milk production, and oxytocin, produced in the posterior pituitary, controls milk letdown and ejection. Disruption in the hypothalamic-pituitary axis known to result from cancer therapies, such as cranial radiation for central nervous system tumors or leukemia, may result in dysfunctional lactation [9]. Other therapies that can interfere with the normal anatomy of the breast can also interfere with the ability to successfully lactate. For example, chest radiation or surgeries resulting in hypoplasia or asymmetry can result in decreased ability to successfully lactate. McCullough and colleagues reported a cross-sectional survey study of 81 survivors of childhood and young adult Hodgkin lymphoma, who received chest radiotherapy at a median dose of 41 Gy (range: 27–46 Gy), and found 57 out of 94 (61 %) breast-feeding attempts were reported as successful as compared to 74 of 94 (79 %) attempts in sibling controls [10]. While these findings were encouraging, the researchers did note that lactation compromise was a previously unreported late effect of Hodgkin lymphoma therapy.

### 17.3.1 Lactation Issues Detection and Surveillance

In patients who were exposed to radiation of the hypothalamic-pituitary axis, patients should be counseled about potential lactation dysfunction. Yearly screening with LH, FSH, prolactin, GH, TSH, and T4 may indicate that lactation dysfunction may be an issue. In females who received radiation to the breast, particularly in those who received over 40 Gy radiation, providers should counsel them that there is an increased risk of lactation failure upon childbearing. However, providers should stress to survivors the health benefits of breast-feeding in order not to dissuade them from attempting breast-feeding.

### 17.3.2 Lactation Issues Management

For women with hypothalamic-pituitary axis damage, hormone replacement in the case of central hypothyroidism or central GNRH failure may correct inability to lactate. For women exposed to chest radiation, there is not a known treatment for women unable to lactate. Like the general population, these women should be counseled to follow up with their obstetrician, pediatrician, and/or a lactation consultant in the event there is a correctable latch issue or other correctable issue not related to the previous cancer therapy.

## 17.4 Breast Cancer After Childhood Cancer

Adult survivors of childhood cancer are at an increased risk of breast cancer due to a complex interplay of constitutional factors, exposures through treatment with chemotherapy and radiation, and genetic predisposition [11–14]. Given the significant morbidities and mortality associated with a breast cancer diagnosis, especially given survivors' previous disease and treatment exposures, it is imperative that health-care providers understand the risks, the biology and genetics, the recommended surveillance guidelines for early detection, and potential prevention strategies available for care of survivors at increased risk for breast cancer.

### 17.4.1 Risk of Breast Cancer in Childhood Cancer Survivors

Women who were treated with chest radiation therapy for a childhood, adolescent, or young adult malignancy are at significantly increased risk of developing breast cancer at a young age [11, 13, 14].

Hodgkin lymphoma survivors treated with high-dose mantle radiation (over 40 Gy) carry the highest risk of developing breast cancer, though risk is quite high in those who received 30–35 Gy [13, 14]. However, the risk is also significantly elevated in women who received moderate-dose radiation for other childhood and young adult malignancies, such as Wilms' tumor, non-Hodgkin lymphoma, neuroblastoma, and sarcomas [12, 13]. In light of the improved cure rates for pediatric and young adult cancers over the past several decades, it is estimated that there are currently 50,000–55,000 women in the United States at high risk for breast cancer due to earlier treatment with moderate- to high-dose chest radiation (≥20 Gy) [15–17].

A systematic review [18] of studies focused on breast cancer in women treated with chest radiation for a pediatric or young adult cancer showed significant increased risk of breast cancer, with standardized incidence ratios (SIR) ranging from 13.3 to 55.5 and the absolute excess risks ranging from 18.6 to 79.0 per 10,000 person-years [12, 19–23]. Risk increased as early as 8 years following chest radiation and did not plateau with increasing length of follow-up [12, 19, 24–26]. The cumulative incidence of breast cancer by 40–45 years of age was 13–20 % (12–26 % by 25–30 years of follow-up) [12, 19, 23, 26] (see Fig. 17.1). This incidence is similar to that in women with a BRCA gene mutation, where the cumulative incidence ranges from 10 % to 19 %

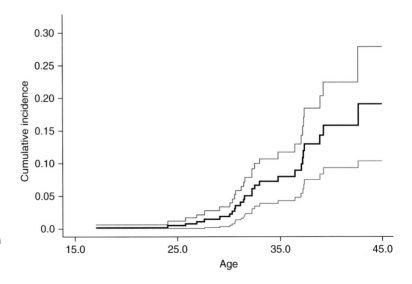

**Fig. 17.1** Cumulative incidence of breast cancer in HL survivors (From Bhatia et al. [19])

by age 40 [27–29]. In comparison, the cumulative incidence of invasive breast cancer is 1 % by age 45 in the general population [18].

Radiation dose modifies the risk of breast cancer in this population. Travis and colleagues estimated that among women diagnosed with Hodgkin lymphoma at age 15 years and counseled for screening at the age of 25, 9.2 % of those treated with 20–39 Gy and 11.1 % of those treated with ≥40 Gy would develop breast cancer

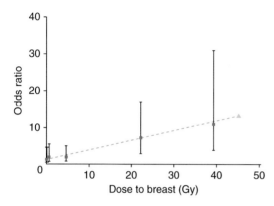

**Fig. 17.2** Breast cancer risk by radiation dose to the breast (Permission requested for use from ASCO/JCO, Inskip et al. [13])

by age 45 [30]. Inskip and colleagues examined the women with breast cancer in the North American cohort, the Childhood Cancer Survivor Study (CCSS), and found a linear radiation dose-response (see Fig. 17.2), reaching an odds ratio (OR) of 10.8 (95 % CI, 3.8–31) for 40 Gy compared to no radiation exposure [13]. De Bruin and colleagues found that a reduced volume of radiation was associated with decreased risk of breast cancer in Hodgkin survivors [31]; mantle field radiation (cervical, supraclavicular, axillary, mediastinal nodes) was associated with a 2.7-fold increased risk (95 % CI, 1.1–6.9) as compared with similarly dosed (36–44 Gy) mediastinal radiation alone (see Fig. 17.3).

In the 1980s, the field and dose of radiation used to treat Hodgkin lymphoma was reduced, and therapy was combined with chemotherapy in response to other late effects, such as growth deformities, infertility, and cardiovascular disease. In the most modern pediatric Hodgkin trials, physicians are continuing to examine how to further minimize chest radiation in this population. Ultimately, the breast cancer risk (along with other late effects risks) is not yet known in the more recent large cohorts of Hodgkin

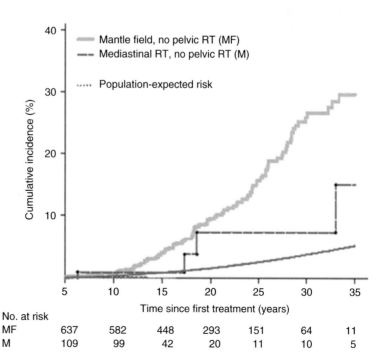

**Fig. 17.3** Breast cancer risk in Hodgkin lymphoma survivors exposed to mantle and mediastinal fields as compared to the general population (From De Bruin et al. [31])

| No. at risk | | | | | | |
|---|---|---|---|---|---|---|
| MF | 637 | 582 | 448 | 293 | 151 | 64 | 11 |
| M | 109 | 99 | 42 | 20 | 11 | 10 | 5 |

survivors treated with lower-dose radiation. However, one report of 112 childhood Hodgkin lymphoma survivors treated with chemotherapy and lower-dose 15–25.5 Gy involved-field radiation described an elevated excess risk of second malignant neoplasms (SMNs) similar to that observed in earlier cohorts [32]. However, the irradiated volume in that study appears to have been more extensive than used in more recent treatment cohorts.

While chest radiation appears to be the most influential factor in a childhood cancer survivor's risk of breast cancer, other factors have been identified which appear to modify that risk. A family history of breast cancer or sarcoma modestly increases the likelihood women exposed to chest radiation will develop breast cancer [12, 33]. In fact, in Kenney and colleagues' CCSS study, almost one quarter of the women with early-onset breast cancer in the cohort had not been exposed to chest radiation, suggesting a genetic predisposition to breast cancer [12]. Estrogen exposure may modulate risk, as male breast cancer after radiation is rare. Similarly, in women exposed to breast radiation *and* ovarian radiation, the risk of breast cancer is substantially reduced compared to women who received chest radiation without gonadal radiation [12, 13, 23, 31, 34]. Finally, high-dose alkylating agent chemotherapy reduces the risk of breast cancer by inducing premature ovarian failure and thereby lowering endogenous estrogens [12, 23, 30, 34].

Earlier studies have indicated that women exposed to chest radiation prior to puberty have lower risk of breast cancer than those treated adolescence [35]. However, Yasui and colleagues identified a methodological issue in the analysis of second malignant neoplasms which did not account for the natural age-associated increase of risk [36]. More recent studies in this population, which incorporate extended years of follow-up and thus account for this natural age-associated risk, have not shown a difference in breast cancer risk among females treated with chest radiation prior to puberty compared with those treated in adolescence [12, 13, 19].

## 17.4.2 Breast Cancer Biology and Clinical Characteristics

In women treated with chest radiation before the age of 20, the median age of initial breast cancer diagnosis is 32–35 years [12, 26]. Risk begins to increase as early as 8 years following chest radiation exposure. Of note, the median age of diagnosis for breast cancer in the general population is 61 years of age, with 1.9 % of cases occurring between ages 20–34 and 10.6 % between ages 35 and 44 [17].

The majority (77–85 %) of breast cancers in childhood, adolescent, and young adult cancer survivors are characterized by invasive ductal carcinoma, which is comparable to the proportion of invasive ductal carcinomas among breast cancer cases in the general population [37, 38]. In a case-control study of 253 women with breast cancer following Hodgkin lymphoma compared with 741 women with sporadic breast cancer who were matched for age, race, and age at breast cancer, there were no statistically significant differences between groups in histology (including DCIS, invasive ductal carcinoma, and invasive lobular carcinoma), estrogen receptor status, HER2 status, or proportion of patients with multifocal disease [38].

The risk of *bilateral* breast cancer is increased in women treated at young age with chest radiation. Henderson et al. found, reviewing three studies of Hodgkin lymphoma survivors, that of 219 women with breast cancer, 12.8 % had bilateral disease: 5.5 % synchronous and 7.3 % metachronous [18, 39–41]. This is contrasted to studies of breast cancer in the general population where 3–5 % of cases show bilateral disease, about half of which are synchronous and half metachronous [39–41]. Lastly, while Elkin and colleagues found in their case-control study of breast cancer in Hodgkin survivors as compared to sporadic breast cancer a significantly increased rate of bilateral breast cancer, the overall incidence was lower than in previous studies – 6 % of Hodgkin survivors presented with bilateral disease as compared with 2 % of controls [38]. It is important to note that the average age of childhood cancer survivors at risk for breast cancer following chest radiation is relatively young, so the percent of cases with metachronous disease will likely increase over time.

## 17.4.3 Breast Cancer Genetics

To date, there is no single gene that has been determined to account for most breast cancer after childhood cancer. Genetic predisposition to cancer can be classified into two categories: genes that are highly penetrant and result in a high risk to individual carriers and low-penetrant genes which may more broadly increase risk to a lesser degree across a population. The genetic predisposition to breast cancer after childhood cancer may involve both types of genes. Nonetheless, several defined cancer family syndromes with known cancer predisposition genes include both childhood cancers and breast cancer.

Li-Fraumeni syndrome (LFS) is a familial cancer syndrome associated with a germline mutation of the *TP53* gene [42–44]. A family with a child with a sarcoma whose mother has developed very early-onset breast cancer is perhaps pathognomonic for germline *TP53* mutation [45]. However, pedigrees of LFS families are characterized by children with a wide variety of tumor types including not only bone and soft tissue sarcomas, but also brain tumors, adrenocortical carcinomas, leukemias, and other rare tumors. Young women with a history of nearly any diagnosis of cancer as a child should be considered at risk for breast cancer, and care should include querying family history as well as consideration of genetic counseling. Genetic testing for germline TP53 mutations may result in a diagnosis of LFS in these survivors and may inform breast cancer prevention and screening strategies for these survivors and their female relatives [46]. LFS should be suspected in survivors of childhood cancers who subsequently develop breast cancer as young adults and in those rare patients who develop primary breast cancer during adolescence. Although a genetic mutation may be the major underlying factor in developing breast

cancer in survivors with LFS, radiation in the field of the first cancer may also further increase the risk of developing breast cancer [47].

Evaluation of the two major familial breast cancer genes, *BRCA1* and *BRCA2*, is now a routine for patients with early-onset breast cancer or strong family history of breast cancer. In a study of a large cohort of *BRCA1* and *BRCA2* breast cancer families, there did not appear to be an excess of childhood cancers associated with either gene [48]. However, Magnussen et al. demonstrated a substantial risk of childhood cancers in *BRCA2* but not *BRCA1* families [49]. Biallelic mutations of *BRCA2* are associated Fanconi anemia (FA), but have also been reported in Wilms' tumor patients as well as patients with CNS tumors, some of whom may not have the classic Fanconi features [50, 51]. While these patients are rare and data on FA survivors is lacking (as there are few long-term survivors of FA), the strong association of *BRCA2* in the heterozygous form with breast cancer would suggest that survivors of childhood cancers who carry germline biallelic *BRCA2* mutations would also carry a high risk of breast cancer.

Hereditary retinoblastoma associated with germline *RB1* has historically been a paradigm of how a germline mutation, coupled with cancer treatment effects, results in second cancers in adult life. While the majority of these *RB1* patients develop sarcomas after bilateral retinoblastoma, other tumors occur in excess, including breast cancer [52, 53].

The genetics of breast cancer after Hodgkin lymphoma remains an enigma. Although radiation to the mantle area has been considered a major underlying risk factor, the high risks of breast cancer specific to Hodgkin patients have suggested a host factor as well as a treatment factor. Several cancer-related genes have been excluded in the search for genetic etiologies of breast cancer after Hodgkin lymphoma, and these have included *BRCA1*, *BRCA2*, and *ATM* [33, 54–56]. A polymorphism in the *MLH1* gene has been suggested in a single study to increase the risk of breast cancer after chemotherapy for Hodgkin lymphoma [57]. Recently, Best and colleagues identified two variants at chromosome 6q21 associated with the risk of second malignant neoplasms in Hodgkin lymphoma survivors (mainly breast cancers and thyroid cancers). These variants regulate *PRDM1* (also known as *BLIMP1*) and suggest that common variants can have large effect sizes in the context of a specific exposure to radiation therapy (as *PRDM1* variants are not associated with non-radiation-associated breast cancer) [58]. Along with further examination of this promising finding, researchers continue to search for both major genes as well as low-penetrant modifier genes that increase the risk for breast and other SMN in Hodgkin lymphoma as well as other cancer survivors.

### 17.4.4 Breast Cancer Detection and Surveillance

Recognizing that women treated for a pediatric or young adult cancer with chest radiation ($\geq 20$ Gy) or those with familial or genetic risk (e.g., LFS) have a substantially elevated risk of breast cancer at a young age, many groups have recommended early breast cancer surveillance in those survivors at highest risk. A prospective trial examining early screening and its impact on mortality would be the gold standard for informing surveillance recommendations, but the population is too small to provide the power for such a study. Thus, available evidence regarding the clinical characteristics of this population, as well as evidence from other high-risk and general populations, has informed the current available guidelines. Similar to the general population, it appears that early stage at diagnosis is associated with improved breast cancer outcomes. Thus, there would appear to be a clinical benefit associated with early detection.

Studies have demonstrated that screening mammography can identify breast cancers in women with breasts previously exposed to chest radiation [59–63]. Dershaw et al. reported in a retrospective review that mammography demonstrated 90 % of the cancers in 27 women (55 % under the age of 45 years), with 38 % being detected only by mammography [62]. Wolden et al. retrospectively examined 71 cases of breast cancer in 65 women and noted 27 % of breast cancers were initially detected by screening mammograms [64]. Notably, 75 % of the women at time of breast cancer diagnosis were premenopausal (median age, 43 years). Prospective studies have also demonstrated that mammograms can detect breast cancers in this population, but the data is unclear as to the benefit of breast self-exam, especially in younger women whose tumors are not radiographically distinct from glandular breast tissue [59–61]. Diller et al. followed 90 women treated with chest radiation for Hodgkin lymphoma for a median of 3.1 years [59]. During this study, 12 breast cancers were detected at a median age of 43 years (range, 29–50 years); 2 were diagnosed upon entry to the study and 10 were diagnosed during the follow-up. Henderson and colleagues examined the rate of false-positive screens in this prospective study in combination with the prospective screening study by Kwong et al. and reported that over 12.3 % of 178 women had a false-positive mammogram, 8.4 % of whom were recalled and needed additional imaging and 3.9 % who required a biopsy [18, 59, 65].

Mammography appears to detect the majority of cancers in these women. However, more than half of mammograms in women who had previous chest radiation have moderate to very dense breast tissue, thus limiting the sensitivity of mammography in detecting early cancers in this population. Studies examining MRI for surveillance in this population are limited. The use of MRI has been in examined in women at high risk for breast cancer due to BRCA mutation or strong family history. A systematic review of 11 prospective studies reported that screening with both MRI and mammography among women with a hereditary risk of breast cancer appears to detect cancerous lesions better than mammography alone [66]. While all 11 studies reported a higher sensitivity for MRI than mammography for invasive cancer, mammography was more sensitive than MRI for ductal carcinoma in situ. It is not possible to estimate the impact of this early detection on lifetime breast cancer mortality.

Despite available data in other high-risk populations, it is not proven that the combination of mammography and MRI enhance the specificity and sensitivity of detecting breast cancer in women exposed to chest radiation. Expert panels developing surveillance recommendations have extrapolated this data to women treated to chest radiation, given similarities in incidence rates, age of the women at risk, and the superior cure rate in earlier-stage cancers. A prospective study of 148 women treated for Hodgkin lymphoma between the age of 12 and 35 and screened with both MRI and mammography reveals that utilization of MRI *and* mammography as a screening strategy improved sensitivity of screening above the rate observed with either modality alone [67]. In this study, 5/16 cancers were detected on MRI only; there are too few survivors of pediatric radiation to draw separate conclusions regarding this subgroup. Currently, for women treated for a pediatric or young adult cancer with chest radiation ≥20 Gy, the Children's Oncology Group recommends annual surveillance mammography and MRI, starting at age 25 or 8 years after completion of radiation therapy, whichever occurs last [18]. Meanwhile, the American Cancer Society recommends that physicians discuss with at-risk women starting mammography and MRI at age 30 [68]. These recommendations as well as those recommended internationally are summarized in Table 17.1. Of note, recently there was an international harmonization effort for childhood cancer survivor surveillance guidelines, including breast cancer. In this effort, it was concluded that there is strong evidence for the following recommendations: mammography or breast MRI or a combination is recommended for female CAYA cancer survivors treated with ≥20 Gy chest radiation; initiation of breast cancer surveillance is recommended at age 25 years or ≥8 years from radiation (whichever occurs last); and annual breast cancer surveillance is recommended until at least 50 years of age [69].

## 17.4.5 Prevention Strategies

In addition to early surveillance, risk reduction strategies utilized in other populations with elevated breast cancer risk (i.e., familial risk, BRCA carriers) should be considered in pediatric cancer survivors. Prophylactic bilateral mastectomy is associated with a 90–95 % reduction in risk in women with familial breast cancer [70]. This risk reduction strategy has been the intervention of choice in women at highest risk for breast cancer, including those with known TP53 germline mutations. Of note, not all women feel comfortable with this surgical option [71]. As observed in the CCSS report, many women exposed to chest radiation (including bilateral breasts) with unilateral radiogenic breast cancer choose to have bilateral mastectomies, thus reducing the risk of contralateral cancer. In the Kenney study, for example, 12/95 women with unilateral breast cancer after childhood cancer elected to have prophylactic mastectomies [12].

Tamoxifen, a synthetic selective estrogen receptor modifier (SERM), was demonstrated to decrease the risk for breast cancer by 50 % in women at moderately increased risk for developing breast cancer [72, 73]. This outcome is consistent with the finding that reduction of endogenous estrogen exposure (often by chemotherapy induced ovarian failure) reduces risk of breast cancer in the radiation-exposed breast. Of note, the Consortium of Pediatric Interventional Research has an ongoing multiinstitutional, NCI-supported trial of low-dose tamoxifen in this population. Other breast cancer chemoprevention strategies have not been explored in childhood cancer survivors, although women who have experienced a unilateral breast cancer after chest radiation may choose chemoprophylaxis for prevention of a contralateral cancer.

## 17.4.6 Treatment Management and Survival

Treatment and reconstruction options are more limited in women who have been previously treated with chest radiation compared to women with breast cancer in the general population [21, 62, 64, 74]. Mastectomy is recommended as the standard treatment [63, 74]. Breast-conserving surgery with radiation is controversial because of the potential for tissue necrosis given previous radiation exposure [64, 74] and the fact that the

**Table 17.1** Summary of consensus-based recommendations for breast imaging surveillance from different national and international organizations

| Organization | Breast imaging surveillance recommendation | Source/public link |
|---|---|---|
| Children's Oncology Group | For women treated with ≥20 Gy radiation to the chest for a childhood, adolescent, or young adult cancer, initiate annual screening mammography with adjunct breast MRI at 25 years of age or 8 years after completion of radiation therapy, whichever occurs last | Long-Term Follow-Up Guidelines for Survivors of Childhood, Adolescent, and Young Adult Cancers (Version 3) www.survivorshipguidelines.org |
| American Cancer Society | For women treated with radiation to the chest between the ages of 10 and 30 years, recommend annual screening mammography with adjunct breast MRI, beginning at 30 years of age or as determined by the patient and her physician based upon her personal circumstances and preferences | Can Breast Cancer Be Found Early? (guide for patients) http://www.cancer.org/docroot/CRI/content/CRI_2_4_3X_Can_breast_cancer_be_found_early_5.asp |
| United Kingdom Department of Health; United Kingdom Children's Cancer Study Group | For women treated with mediastinal radiation prior to age 17, recommend annual breast MRI from 25 to 29 years of age, followed by a baseline 2-view mammogram at 30 years of age. Thereafter, annual 2-view mammography is recommended from 30 to 50 years of age. For women with dense breast tissue at the baseline mammogram, an annual breast MRI is combined with mammography. If the breast tissue becomes predominantly fatty prior to age 50, surveillance continues with annual mammography alone. Over the age of 50, recommendations do not differ from the standard NHS Breast Cancer Screening Programme | Therapy Based Long Term Follow Up: Practice Statement (2nd Edition) http://ukccsg.org/public/followup/PracticeStatement/16.pdf |
| The Netherlands Cancer Institute | Screening based upon the dose and type of radiation. For women treated with chest RT ≥20 Gy or with total-body irradiation of any dose, an annual breast MRI is recommended, starting at age 25. Then, starting at age 30, a mammogram is recommended with the MRI. For women treated with 7–19 Gy chest RT, an annual mammogram without an MRI is recommended, starting at age 30 | Website not currently available |

entire breast is at risk for malignancy. Options for chemotherapy and radiation are limited by prior therapies.

Similar to the general population, where the 5-year survival rate for localized disease is 98 % and 24 % for distant disease, survival rates in this population are strongly associated with stage/advanced disease at diagnosis, similar to the general population [64, 74–76].

# References

1. Sadler T (1990) Langman's medical embryology, 6th edn. Williams and Wilkins, Baltimore
2. Moore K (1988) Essentials of human embryology. Decker, Toronto
3. Biochemical society S, Rudland PS (1998) Mammary development and cancer. Portland, London
4. Furst CJ, Lundell M, Ahlback SO et al (1989) Breast hypoplasia following irradiation of the female breast in infancy and early childhood. Acta Oncol 28:519–523
5. Macklis RM, Oltikar A, Sallan SE (1991) Wilms' tumor patients with pulmonary metastases. Int J Radiat Oncol Biol Phys 21:1187–1193
6. Divasta AD, Gordon CM (2010) Hormone replacement therapy and the adolescent. Curr Opin Obstet Gynecol 22:363–368
7. Long term follow-up guidelines for survivors of childhood, adolescent and young adult Cancer, Version 4.0 (2013) Group CsO, Arcadia
8. Holmich LR, Mellemkjaer L, Gunnarsdottir KA et al (2003) Stage of breast cancer at diagnosis among women with cosmetic breast implants. Br J Cancer 88:832–838
9. Ogg SW, Hudson MM, Randolph ME et al (2011) Protective effects of breastfeeding for mothers surviving childhood cancer. J Cancer Surviv Res Pract 5:175–181
10. McCullough L, Ng A, Najita J et al (2010) Breastfeeding in survivors of Hodgkin lymphoma treated with chest radiotherapy. Cancer 116:4866–4871
11. Henderson TO, Amsterdam A, Bhatia S et al (2010) Systematic review: surveillance for breast cancer in women treated with chest radiation for childhood, adolescent, or young adult cancer. Ann Intern Med 152:444–455, W144–54
12. Kenney LB, Yasui Y, Inskip PD et al (2004) Breast cancer after childhood cancer: a report from the Childhood Cancer Survivor Study. Ann Intern Med 141:590–597
13. Inskip PD, Robison LL, Stovall M et al (2009) Radiation dose and breast cancer risk in the childhood cancer survivor study. J Clin Oncol 27:3901–3907
14. Moskowitz CS, Chou JF, Wolden SL et al (2014) Breast cancer after chest radiation therapy for a childhood cancer. J Clin Oncol 32:2217–2223
15. Hewitt M, Weinder S, Simone JV (eds) Childhood cancer survivorship: improving care and quality of life (2003) National Academies Press, Washington, DC
16. Bleyer AOLM, Barr R, Ries LAG (2006) Cancer epidemiology in older adolescents and young adults 15 to 29 years of age, including SEER incidence and survival, 1975–2000. National Cancer Institute, Bethesda
17. Ries LAG, Krapcho M, Stinchcomb DG, Howlader N, Horner MJ et al (eds) SEER Cancer Statistics Review, 1975–2007 (2013). National Cancer Institute, Bethesda
18. Henderson TO, Amsterdam A, Bhatia S et al (2009) Surveillance for breast cancer in women treated with chest radiation for a childhood, adolescent or young adult cancer: a report from the Children's Oncology Group. Ann Intern Med 152:444–455, W144–54
19. Bhatia S, Yasui Y, Robison LL et al (2003) High risk of subsequent neoplasms continues with extended follow-up of childhood Hodgkin's disease: report from the Late Effects Study Group. J Clin Oncol 21:4386–4394
20. Ng AK, Bernardo MV, Weller E et al (2002) Second malignancy after Hodgkin disease treated with radiation therapy with or without chemotherapy: long term risks and risk factors. Blood 100:1989–1996
21. Wolden SL, Lamborn KR, Cleary SF et al (1998) Second cancers following pediatric Hodgkin's disease. J Clin Oncol 16:536–544
22. Constine LS, Tarbell N, Hudson MM et al (2008) Subsequent malignancies in children treated for Hodgkin's disease: associations with gender and radiation dose. Int J Radiat Oncol Biol Phys 72:24–33
23. De Bruin ML, Sparidans J, Van't Veer MB et al (2009) Breast cancer risk in female survivors of Hodgkin's lymphoma: lower risk after smaller radiation volumes. J Clin Oncol 27:4239–4246
24. Alm El-Din MA, Hughes KS, Finkelstein DM et al (2009) Breast cancer after treatment of Hodgkin's lymphoma: risk factors that really matter. Int J Radiat Oncol Biol Phys 73:69–74
25. Metayer C, Lynch CF, Clarke EA et al (2000) Second cancers among long-term survivors of Hodgkin's disease diagnosed in childhood and adolescence. J Clin Oncol 18:2435–2443
26. Taylor AJ, Winter DL, Stiller CA et al (2007) Risk of breast cancer in female survivors of childhood Hodgkin's disease in Britain: a population-based study. Int J Cancer 120:384–391
27. Begg CB, Haile RW, Borg A et al (2008) Variation of breast cancer risk among BRCA1/2 carriers. JAMA 299:194–201
28. Easton DF, Ford D, Bishop DT (1995) Breast and ovarian cancer incidence in BRCA1-mutation carriers. Breast Cancer Linkage Consortium. Am J Hum Genet 56:265–271
29. Easton DF, Steele L, Fields P et al (1997) Cancer risks in two large breast cancer families linked to BRCA2 on chromosome 13q12-13. Am J Hum Genet 61:120–128
30. Travis LB, Hill D, Dores GM et al (2005) Cumulative absolute breast cancer risk for young women treated for Hodgkin lymphoma. J Natl Cancer Inst 97:1428–1437

31. De Bruin ML, Sparidans J, van't Veer MB et al (2009) Breast cancer risk in female survivors of Hodgkin's lymphoma: lower risk after smaller radiation volumes. J Clin Oncol 27:4239–4246

32. O'Brien MM, Donaldson SS, Balise RR et al (2010) Second malignant neoplasms in survivors of pediatric Hodgkin's lymphoma treated with low-dose radiation and chemotherapy. J Clin Oncol 28:1232–1239

33. Hill DA, Gilbert E, Dores GM et al (2005) Breast cancer risk following radiotherapy for Hodgkin lymphoma: modification by other risk factors. Blood 106:3358–3365

34. Travis LB, Hill DA, Dores GM et al (2003) Breast cancer following radiotherapy and chemotherapy among young women with Hodgkin disease. JAMA 290:465–475

35. Bhatia S, Robison LL, Oberlin O et al (1996) Breast cancer and other second neoplasms after childhood Hodgkin's disease. N Engl J Med 334:745–751

36. Yasui Y, Liu Y, Neglia JP et al (2003) A methodological issue in the analysis of second-primary cancer incidence in long-term survivors of childhood cancers. Am J Epidemiol 158:1108–1113

37. DeVita VH, Hellman S, Rosenberg SA (2005) Cancer of the breast. In: Vea D (ed) Cancer: principles & practice of oncology, 7th edn. Lippincott, Philadelphia

38. Elkin EB, Klem ML, Gonzales AM et al (2011) Characteristics and outcomes of breast cancer in women with and without a history of radiation for Hodgkin lymphoma: a multi-institutional, matched cohort study. J Clin Oncol Off J Am Soc Clin Oncol 29:2466–2473

39. Hartman M, Czene K, Reilly M et al (2007) Incidence and prognosis of synchronous and metachronous bilateral breast cancer. J Clin Oncol 25:4210–4216

40. Quan G, Pommier SJ, Pommier RF (2008) Incidence and outcomes of contralateral breast cancers. Am J Surg 195:645–650; discussion 650

41. Verkooijen HM, Chatelain V, Fioretta G et al (2007) Survival after bilateral breast cancer: results from a population-based study. Breast Cancer Res Treat 105:347–357

42. Relling MV, Hancock ML, Boyett JM et al (1999) Prognostic importance of 6-mercaptopurine dose intensity in acute lymphoblastic leukemia. Blood 93:2817–2823

43. Friedman DL, Meadows AT (2002) Late effects of childhood cancer therapy. Pediatr Clin N Am 49:1083–1106

44. Malkin D, Li FP, Strong LC et al (1990) Germ line p53 mutations in a familial syndrome of breast cancer, sarcomas, and other neoplasms. Science 250:1233–1238

45. Levine AB, Aaron EZ, Criniti SM (2008) Screening for depression in pregnant women with HIV infection. J Reprod Med 53:352–356

46. Clarke AJ, Gaff C (2008) Challenges in the genetic testing of children for familial cancers. Arch Dis Child 93:911–914

47. Menu-Branthomme A, Rubino C, Shamsaldin A et al (2004) Radiation dose, chemotherapy and risk of soft tissue sarcoma after solid tumours during childhood. Int J Cancer 110:87–93

48. Robison S, Rapmund A, Hemmings C et al (2009) False-positive diagnosis of metastasis on positron emission tomography-computed tomography imaging due to hibernoma. J Clin Oncol 27:994–995

49. Shih YC, Elting LS, Levin B (2008) Disparities in colorectal screening between US-born and foreign-born populations: evidence from the 2000 National Health Interview Survey. J Cancer Educ 23:18–25

50. Lynch BM, Cerin E, Newman B et al (2007) Physical activity, activity change, and their correlates in a population-based sample of colorectal cancer survivors. Ann Behav Med 34:135–143

51. Hirsch B, Shimamura A, Moreau L et al (2004) Association of biallelic BRCA2/FANCD1 mutations with spontaneous chromosomal instability and solid tumors of childhood. Blood 103:2554–2559

52. Fletcher O, Easton D, Anderson K et al (2004) Lifetime risks of common cancers among retinoblastoma survivors. J Natl Cancer Inst 96:357–363

53. Levin B, Lieberman DA, McFarland B et al (2008) Screening and surveillance for the early detection of colorectal cancer and adenomatous polyps, 2008: a joint guideline from the American Cancer Society, the US Multi-Society Task Force on Colorectal Cancer, and the American College of Radiology. Gastroenterology 134:1570–1595

54. Offit K, Gilad S, Paglin S et al (2002) Rare variants of ATM and risk for Hodgkin's disease and radiation-associated breast cancers. Clin Cancer Res Off J Am Assoc Cancer Res 8:3813–3819

55. Broeks A, Russell NS, Floore AN et al (2000) Increased risk of breast cancer following irradiation for Hodgkin's disease is not a result of ATM germline mutations. Int J Radiat Biol 76:693–698

56. Nichols KE, Levitz S, Shannon KE et al (1999) Heterozygous germline ATM mutations do not contribute to radiation-associated malignancies after Hodgkin's disease. J Clin Oncol Off J Am Soc Clin Oncol 17:1259

57. Worrillow LJ, Smith AG, Scott K et al (2008) Polymorphic MLH1 and risk of cancer after methylating chemotherapy for Hodgkin lymphoma. J Med Genet 45:142–146

58. Best T, Li D, Skol AD, Kirchhoff T, Jackson SA, Yasui Y, Bhatia S, Strong LC, Domchek SM, Nathanson KL, Olopade O, Mack TM, Conti DV, Offit K, Cozen W, Robison LL, Onel K (2011) Variants at 6q21 implicate PRDM1 in the etiology of therapy-induced second malignancies after Hodgkin lymphoma. Nat Med 17:941–943

59. Diller L, Medeiros Nancarrow C, Shaffer K et al (2002) Breast cancer screening in women previously treated for Hodgkin's disease: a prospective cohort study. J Clin Oncol 20:2085–2091

60. Lee L, Pintilie M, Hodgson DC et al (2008) Screening mammography for young women treated with supradiaphragmatic radiation for Hodgkin's lymphoma. Ann Oncol Off J Eur Soc Med Oncol/ESMO 19:62–67

61. Kwong A, Hancock SL, Bloom JR et al (2008) Mammographic screening in women at increased risk

of breast cancer after treatment of Hodgkin's disease. Breast J 14:39–48

62. Dershaw DD, Yahalom J, Petrek JA (1992) Breast carcinoma in women previously treated for Hodgkin disease: mammographic evaluation. Radiology 184: 421–423

63. Wolden SL, Hancock SL, Carlson RW et al (2000) Management of breast cancer after Hodgkin's disease. J Clin Oncol Off J Am Soc Clin Oncol 18:765–772

64. Wolden SL, Hancock SL, Carlson RW et al (2000) Management of breast cancer after Hodgkin's disease. J Clin Oncol 18:765–772

65. Kwong A, Cheung PS, Wong AY et al (2008) The acceptance and feasibility of breast cancer screening in the East. Breast 17:42–50

66. Warner E, Messersmith H, Causer P et al (2008) Systematic review: using magnetic resonance imaging to screen women at high risk for breast cancer. Ann Intern Med 148:671–679

67. Ng A, Garber J, Diller L et al (2013) A prospective study of the efficacy of breast magnetic resonance imaging and mammographic screening in Hodgkin lymphoma survivors. J Clin Oncol 31:2282–2288

68. Saslow D, Boetes C, Burke W et al (2007) American Cancer Society guidelines for breast screening with MRI as an adjunct to mammography. CA Cancer J Clin 57:75–89

69. Kremer LC, Mulder RL, Oeffinger KC et al (2012) A worldwide collaboration to harmonize guidelines for the long-term follow-up of childhood and young adult cancer survivors: a report from the international late effects of Childhood Cancer Guideline Harmonization Group. Pediatr Blood Cancer 60:543–549

70. Hartmann LC, Sellers TA, Schaid DJ et al (2001) Efficacy of bilateral prophylactic mastectomy in BRCA1 and BRCA2 gene mutation carriers. J Natl Cancer Inst 93:1633–1637

71. Schwartz MD, Lerman C, Brogan B et al (2004) Impact of BRCA1/BRCA2 counseling and testing on newly diagnosed breast cancer patients. J Clin Oncol 22:1823–1829

72. Fisher B, Costantino JP, Wickerham DL et al (1998) Tamoxifen for prevention of breast cancer: report of the national surgical adjuvant breast and bowel project P-1 study. J Natl Cancer Inst 90:1371–1388

73. Gail MH, Brinton LA, Byar DP et al (1989) Projecting individualized probabilities of developing breast cancer for white females who are being examined annually. J Natl Cancer Inst 81:1879–1886

74. Yahalom J, Petrek JA, Biddinger PW et al (1992) Breast cancer in patients irradiated for Hodgkin's disease: a clinical and pathologic analysis of 45 events in 37 patients. J Clin Oncol 10:1674–1681

75. Cutuli B, Borel C, Dhermain F et al (2001) Breast cancer occurred after treatment for Hodgkin's disease: analysis of 133 cases. Radiother Oncol 59: 247–255

76. Ries L, Eisner M, Kosary C (eds) (2005) SEER cancer statistics review, 1975–2002. National Cancer Institute, Bethesda

# Hematopoietic Stem Cell Transplantation

# 18

Anne Wohlschlaeger, Sogol Mostoufi-Moab, and Nancy Bunin

## Contents

Hematopoietic stem cell transplant (HSCT) is increasingly used for the treatment of both malignancies and nonmalignant diseases. This has been made possible by several factors, including expansion of the unrelated donor pool, advances in mobilization and collection of autologous cells, and reduced intensity conditioning regimens. Although transplant-related mortality and relapse remain obstacles, an increasing number of children are surviving following HSCT. Both the HSCT antecedent therapy and the posttransplant complications have multisystem effects, and understanding and anticipating these are important in caring for the children affected. This chapter will provide a brief overview, as many of these complications are discussed in more depth in other chapters of this book.

A. Wohlschlaeger (✉) • N. Bunin
Division of Oncology, The Children's Hospital of Philadelphia, PA, USA
e-mail: wohlschlaeger@email.chop.edu

S. Mostoufi-Moab
Division of Endocrinology and Oncology,
The Children's Hospital of Philadelphia, PA, USA

## 18.1    Conditioning

All children undergoing HSCT for malignancies receive conditioning prior to the infusion of the hematopoietic stem cells. The agents and doses used are determined by the underlying disease,

© Springer International Publishing 2015
C.L. Schwartz et al. (eds.), *Survivors of Childhood and Adolescent Cancer:
A Multidisciplinary Approach*, Pediatric Oncology, DOI 10.1007/978-3-319-16435-9_18

patient condition, and the type of graft. The goals of conditioning may include eradication of malignancy, creation of space for new cells, and immunosuppression to allow donor cell engraftment. Patients with hematologic malignancies generally received myeloablative conditioning with high-dose chemotherapy +/− total body irradiation. Total body irradiation is now generally delivered over several days in fractions of 150–200 cGy, with total doses ranging from 1,000 to 1,450 cGy. Fractionation allows for partial recovery of normal tissues between fractions. This may reduce the risk of long-term complications (e.g., cataracts and pulmonary restrictive disease) that are commonly noted with single-fraction total body irradiation (TBI). Complications such as graft versus host disease (GVHD) after allogeneic HSCT may play a significant role in the development of sequelae.

Reduced intensity or non-myeloablative conditioning regimens are increasingly used in patients undergoing allogeneic HSCT for nonmalignant diseases [29, 51]. The drugs commonly used are alemtuzumab, fludarabine, melphalan, and "mini" busulfan or low-dose (200–300 cGy) total body irradiation. These regimens are extremely immunosuppressive, as is necessary to permit engraftment, but may be less toxic in the immediate posttransplant period and in the long term. GVHD remains a significant potential complication with these regimens.

HSCT for solid tumors usually uses autologous hematopoietic cells that have been collected and cryopreserved prior to conditioning. Chemotherapy agents selected for solid tumor conditioning regimens are those that can be safely dose escalated and have differing methods of action and nonoverlapping extramedullary toxicities. Local irradiation may also be used for tumor control, either before or after the HSCT. To improve survival, tandem or sequential transplants over a period of several months are sometimes used for diseases, such as neuroblastoma and brain tumors.

## 18.2    Endocrine System

The endocrine system is affected in many patients who receive myeloablative conditioning. The extent of damage is dependent upon prior cytotoxic therapy and the particular agents selected for the conditioning regimen. Growth, reproduction, thyroid function, and glucose metabolism may be affected.

### 18.2.1    Growth

The growth of those who have undergone an HSCT is affected by many factors, including genetic, nutritional, hormonal, and therapeutic factors. Effects are most commonly attributed to radiation of the hypothalamic-pituitary axis, which can result in either radiation-induced growth hormone deficiency or abnormal secretion of growth hormone. Direct impairment of bone growth may also occur following radiation damage to the growth plates, commonly seen with the inadequate pubertal spine growth after craniospinal radiation therapy [10]. TBI and cranial irradiation as components of prior therapy increase the risk of growth failure. Higher risk is also associated with young age at the time of HSCT and male gender [10, 19, 27, 73]. Children with neuroblastoma who have received radiation are at particular risk, due to their young age at the time of transplant [26, 45]. The greatest effect on growth occurs in children with leukemia who received cranial irradiation prior to TBI [27].

Impaired growth manifests as a decrease in growth velocity or in height standard deviation score (SDS). In general, growth hormone deficiency increases with time from TBI [19]. Growth of peri-pubertal patients at HSCT may be further impacted by impairment of normal mechanisms leading to the pubertal growth spurt [38]. Although the production of growth hormone plays an important role in determining height, many other factors play a role such as thyroid function, nutritional status, corticosteroid therapy, and production of sex hormones during puberty [13]. Current leukemia treatment protocols use only low-dose cranial irradiation (1,200–1,800 cGy) for very-high-risk patients only. Patients who have CNS relapses generally receive higher radiation doses resulting in greater incidence of growth hormone deficiency that varies widely in different studies, ranging from 20 to 70 % [6, 19, 26, 27]. Some studies fail to show a correlation between growth rate and growth hormone secretion with stimulation testing [7, 11]. IGF-1 and IGFBP-3 studies are not useful predictors of GH deficiency, although lower IGF-1 and IGFBP-3 values are noted in those who receive TBI, compared with those not given TBI [7]. In one study with repeated evaluation of GH status, improvement was noted over time [25], although further confirmation of these results is needed.

The role of growth hormone replacement is controversial. Growth hormone replacement has been found to ameliorate poor growth rate as a result of radiation [7, 19, 27]. In a study by Brauner et al. no catch-up growth was observed [7]. Patients who received fractionated TBI were less affected at 2 years post HSCT than those who received single-fraction TBI, but at 5 years, both groups demonstrated similar height decrements [7]. Resistance of the bone to IGF-1 induced by radiation has been proposed as the explanation for the lack of catch-up growth observed. Skeletal abnormalities including slipped capital femoral epiphysis (SCFE) and osteochondromas have been more commonly noted in children younger than 8 years who were given TBI [16]. TBI and chemotherapy exposure at a young age, such as high-risk neuroblastoma therapy, significantly increase the risk of SCFE during GH therapy [40]. In addition, treatment with cis-retinoic acid can result in advanced bone age further contributing to reduced final height potential [22] (Table 18.1).

There have been some reports following chemotherapy-only conditioning of growth disturbances [1, 4]. However, most children who receive chemotherapy-only conditioning regimens have relatively normal growth, although both the long-term use of steroids for chronic GVHD and prior cranial irradiation negatively affect growth [38, 72, 73].

## 18.2.2 Thyroid

Thyroid dysfunction is a well-described complication after HSCT. Although it occurs most commonly after TBI, there are reports of thyroid dysfunction in patients who received chemotherapy alone. The developing thyroid gland may be more susceptible to damage as the incidence is increased in children below the age of 10 years and the highest risk group is patients undergoing mantle radiation for treatment of Hodgkin's lymphoma with an overall incidence of 73 % [13]. The incidence varies widely in studies, depending upon the technique of TBI. Patients who receive fractionated TBI have a 15–20 % incidence of hypothyroidism [6, 32, 68]. Compensated primary hypothyroidism has a median time of onset of 12 months post HSCT and may be transient [32]. Replacement therapy is indicated for persistent elevation of TSH. Patients who received TBI should have annual physical assessments of the thyroid gland as radiation increases the risk of thyroid cancer.

Compensated primary hypothyroidism has been noted in 10–15 % of patients who received chemotherapy without radiation therapy [2, 70]. The etiology of hypothyroidism in this group is unclear; but it is believed that the high doses of drugs associated with chemotherapy may be involved. Chemotherapy-only regimens have been

**Table 18.1** Endocrine: summary and suggested follow-up

| Evaluation | | |
|---|---|---|
| Growth | Height, bone age, somatomedin C, IGFBP-3 | TBI and/or cranial irradiation: refer to endocrinologist for GH provocative testing; growth hormone may be indicated |
| Thyroid | Physical assessment, free T4, T3, TSH | Elevated TSH: may repeat in 3–6 months if mild elevation; thyroxine replacement |
| Reproductive | Tanner assessment | Postpubertal females: estrogen replacement; prepubertal children: refer to endocrinologist if delayed puberty or low testosterone/estradiol |
| | Males: FSH, LH, testosterone (>13 years) Females: FSH, LH, estradiol (>12 years) | |
| Glucose metabolism | Height, weight, fasting cholesterol, triglycerides | |

associated with euthyroid sick syndrome, in which the T3 and T4 are low, while the TSH is either normal or low. This syndrome has been reported in 29 % of patients at 14 months post therapy [70]. The clinical significance of this is not clear.

### 18.2.3 Diabetes and Metabolic Syndrome

Survivors of HSCT may be at risk for insulin resistance, impaired glucose tolerance, and type 2 diabetes [66]. Risk factors relevant to the development of these problems include obesity, family history of diabetes, inactivity, inadequate diet, use of growth hormone, and race. In one study of 748 patients evaluated for type 2 diabetes, 34 had developed this condition at a median follow-up of 11 years. The prevalence of type 2 diabetes was 9 % among the survivors of leukemia, with CML patients at highest risk [23]. The prevalence was age-related, with 12 % occurring among leukemia survivors 20–39 years old and 43 % occurring among survivors 40–49 years. The prevalence of diabetes type 1, although less common, was three times higher than in the general population. Most patients evaluated were not obese and experienced a relatively early onset of type 2 diabetes. Racial minorities were more likely to develop diabetes; TBI was not a risk factor in this analysis (Table 18.2).

Hyperinsulinemia and hypertriglyceridemia [23] have been described post HSCT. Therefore, post-HSCT patients, particularly those who were treated for leukemia, merit close observation for the development of diabetes, as well as lipid abnormalities.

### 18.2.4 Reproductive

Gonadal dysfunction is common following HSCT, a finding attributable to the use of alkylating agents, such as cyclophosphamide, and radiation therapy. Busulfan, as a stem cell toxin, also causes a high incidence of gonadal failure [2, 67]. Gonadal dysfunction results in infertility in most affected patients, with some patients also having difficulties with pubertal development.

**Table 18.2** Organ systems: suggested follow-up

| Organ | Suggested evaluation |
|---|---|
| Heart | ECG, echocardiogram, exercise stress test: yearly to every 3–5 years |
| Pulmonary | PFTs: yearly to every 3–5 years |
| Renal | Blood pressure, urinalysis, BUN, creatinine, erythropoietin level if evidence of thrombotic microangiopathy |
| Dental | Semiannual dental evaluation |
| Hearing | Audiogram for patients at risk (prior cisplatin, carboplatin, cranial irradiation) |
| Eyes | Annual ophthalmologic evaluation, artificial tears if sicca syndrome |
| Bone | Physical assessment, bone density evaluation (DXA, pQCT) |
| Brain | Neuropsychologic assessment 1–3 years post BMT in patients at risk (<6 years with TBI, hearing loss) |

In males, the Sertoli and germ cells are more vulnerable to radiation and chemotherapy than the Leydig cells. FSH levels are usually elevated, with normal LH levels. Testosterone levels may be normal with reduced or absent spermatogenesis. Most boys will undergo spontaneous pubertal development without the addition of testosterone. Testicular irradiation used for treatment of leukemic testicular relapse is associated with damage to Leydig cells and low testosterone levels. Boys who have undergone testicular irradiation should be followed closely as most will need long-term testosterone replacement.

Estrogen is necessary for breast development and for the normal pubertal growth spurt. In prepubertal females who undergo HSCT, the recovery of ovarian function may be more likely than in postpubertal [55], but approximately 70 % will have hypergonadotropic hypogonadism and require estrogen replacement therapy [56]. Failure of progression through puberty is often an indication for the need for estrogen replacement. Patients without breast development who have increased FSH and LH levels should be treated with estrogen/progestin. The dose of hormonal replacement will require adjustment with age in order to ensure progression through puberty and cyclic menstruation. Estrogen replacement for postpubertal females should be initiated 3–6 months after HSCT. It has been suggested that replacement be stopped for 2 months at around

1 year post HSCT to evaluate for ovarian recovery [67]. The incidence of pregnancy is less than 3 % for females who received TBI or busulfan, although there are a few reports of successful pregnancies following TBI [54, 55]. Most males will also be sterile after TBI. However, recent studies show that male recipients younger than 25–30 years at time of transplant and without chronic GVHD have a reasonable likelihood of spermatogenesis recovery even those receiving myeloablative TBI based conditioning. Recovery can be incomplete, resulting in oligospermia [74]. Options for preservation of fertility should be discussed prior to HSCT. For pubertal males, sperm banking should be encouraged. Prior therapy may limit this option for some males. Cryopreservation of testicular tissue in prepubertal males is being done on research basis only as well as cryopreservation of ovarian tissue for prepubertal females. For postpubertal females, cryopreservation of ovarian tissue or oocytes is feasible. Gamete preservation is not yet available on a non-research basis. There have been reports of pregnancy from embryos with donated oocytes, with hormonal support [53]. Pregnancies that do occur following TBI are more likely to result in miscarriage, preterm labor, and low-birth-weight infants [55].

With non-myeloablative conditioning regimens, the endocrine effects, particularly gonadal function, are unknown. Effects may be dependent upon the dose and timing of the agents used.

## 18.3 Pulmonary

The assessment of the effects of HSCT conditioning on pulmonary function is usually limited by the age of the patient, as very young children cannot perform pulmonary function tests. The spectrum of long-term pulmonary complications differs among patients who received allogeneic vs. autologous HSCT. This is due to the effects of chronic GVHD, which may result in changes called bronchiolitis obliterans. Other factors that may impact pulmonary function post HSCT include prior chemotherapies such as bleomycin, TBI during conditioning, and thoracic irradiation.

There are three categories of PFT abnormalities: obstructive, restrictive, and those that result from a decrease in diffusion capacity. Obstructive abnormalities result in decreased FEV1 and in a decreased FEV1/FVC ratio. These occur as a result of small airway closure or obstruction of expiration. Bronchiolitis obliterans is the most common cause of obstructive abnormalities post HSCT. Radiation, pulmonary infection, and pneumonitis may all result in restrictive lung disease, with decreased total lung capacity (TLC) and preserved FEV1/FVC ratio. Decreased DLCO, or diffusion capacity for carbon monoxide, may be a result of an abnormal alveolar–capillary interface. Anemia will result in a low DLCO as well.

Up to 85 % of patients will have abnormal PFTs 3–6 months post HSCT, with a restrictive pattern being the most common abnormality [9]. Late abnormalities are often associated with chronic GVHD, although prior aggressive therapy for advanced-stage disease may also have a negative impact on pulmonary function [9]. The most common late abnormality is a decrease in DLCO, followed by restrictive defects [37]. GVHD is associated with the risk of chronic aspiration pneumonia, particularly in patients with esophageal involvement. GVHD is also associated with the risk of bronchiolitis obliterans (BO) in up to 37 % [59] of post-HSCT patients and with the risk of bronchiolitis obliterans organizing pneumonia (BOOP).

Patients with BO do not present with fever, but have complaints of exercise intolerance, cough, and wheezing. Chest radiograph may be normal, and PFTs will show obstructive defects. Immunosuppressant agents are usually not therapeutically helpful. Patients with bronchiolitis obliterans organizing pneumonia (BOOP) present with fever, cough, dyspnea, and rales. BOOP may be present as early as 1 month post HSCT, but is more common after 3 months. In patients suffering from this condition, there is a patchy distribution of granulation tissue plugs filling the lumens of airways and extending into the alveoli [17]. BOOP is strongly associated with prior acute or chronic GVHD, as well as prior leukemia [17]. Radiographic findings may include patchy alveolar opacities and asymmetric infiltrates.

In a small study of children who received autologous HSCT, restrictive impairment was found in 20 % of patients at 5–10 years [18], but there was stabilization after the first year. Obstructive impairment was rare, but diffusion impairment was found in over 50 % of patients at 10 years. TBI was associated with decreased lung volumes.

## 18.4    Cardiac

Cardiotoxic drugs, particularly the anthracyclines, used for disease treatment prior to HSCT conditioning may increase the risk of cardiotoxicity post HSCT, although most patients are asymptomatic despite changes on ECG and echocardiograms. Factors that may increase the risk of cardiotoxicity include young age at the time of treatment, high-dose cyclophosphamide, and chest irradiation. In addition, HSCT survivors are at an increased risk for developing cardiovascular risk factors such as hypertension and metabolic syndrome [4, 42]. Posttransplant echocardiograms have been reported as normal in most children [38], but some studies have reported decreased systolic function [32, 48]. However, pre-transplant anthracycline administration and TBI increase risk for reduced cardiac function [71]. Exercise testing may be a more sensitive tool for detecting changes in cardiovascular function over time; however, it is limited to patients who are old enough to perform such testing. A retrospective study of serial cardiopulmonary exercise tests noted that despite decreases in all parameters of exercise performance, both aerobic and physical working capacity increase over time [24]. This study suggests that oxygen extraction becomes more efficient with recovery and that it may compensate for impaired cardiac ability.

## 18.5    Renal

Renal toxicity post HSCT may occur as a result of TBI or as a result of nephrotoxic drugs commonly used such as cyclosporine or tacrolimus, a history of cisplatin administration, or conditioning with carboplatin. Thrombotic microangiopathy, a syndrome which includes endothelial injury resulting in microangiopathic hemolytic anemia and platelet consumption, may increase the risk of chronic renal injury [34]. This syndrome may be associated with GVHD and TBI, and patients requiring dialysis have a poor prognosis [21]. Nephrotic syndrome has also been associated with chronic GVHD [52].

## 18.6    Ocular

Cataract formation and keratoconjunctivitis sicca (dry eye) syndrome are the two most common ocular complications for patients post HSCT. Risk factors for cataracts include TBI schedule, type of transplant, development of GVHD, and prolonged use of steroids. Cataracts are usually posterior subcapsular, in contrast to those seen in older adults, which appear in the central part of the lens. Cataracts are seen in up to 80 % of patients who received unfractionated TBI, but are less common in patients receiving fractionated TBI, with incidences of approximately 20 % [38]. They may often occur after 4 years (median, 98 months after fractionated TBI); annual follow-up is, therefore, extremely important. Surgical repair may be necessary for some patients, but this is not commonly required. Clinically significant cataracts are noted only occasionally in patients who received non-TBI regimens, and more often than not, this may be related to corticosteroid exposure.

The incidence of keratoconjunctivitis sicca syndrome reaches 20 % 15 years after stem cell transplantation. The ocular manifestations include reduced tear flow, conjunctivitis, corneal defects, and corneal ulcerations. Chronic GVHD is the greatest risk factor, with late-onset keratoconjunctivitis occurring in 40 % of patients with chronic GVHD, versus 10 % of patients without GVHD. Other risk factors for late-onset keratoconjunctivitis include female gender, age greater than 20 years, single-dose TBI, and the use of methotrexate for GVHD prophylaxis [3].

## 18.7 Dental

Damage to dentition associated with HSCT is generally the result of irradiation. Side effects that have been reported include disruption in normal enamel development, hypoplasia, microdontia of the crowns of erupted permanent teeth, and thinning and tapering of the roots of erupted permanent molars. Cranial irradiation prior to TBI may further increase the risk of tooth agenesis [68] as can chemotherapy in young children.

Chronic GVHD may result in damage to the oral cavity and salivary glands. A significant reduction in the show of saliva, as measured by sialometry and salivary gland scintigraphy, has been noted in patients with acute and chronic GVHD. This reduction may persist in patients who received TBI [41]. Decreased salivation and poor oral hygiene post HSCT may increase the risk of dental caries.

## 18.8 Ototoxicity

Children who receive platinum-based agents prior to, or as part of, the conditioning are at the highest risk for developing hearing loss after transplantation, and more than 80 % may experience significant loss [46, 49]. Depending on the chemotherapy history, local or total body irradiation can accentuate hearing loss in children with solid tumors such as neuroblastoma and brain tumors. For patients with neuroblastoma, hearing loss prior to transplant portends significant hearing loss after a regimen containing high-dose carboplatin [46]. However, even those children who did not have a hearing loss prior to transplant developed hearing loss after receiving carboplatin as part of the conditioning.

## 18.9 Bone Mineral Density

There are increasing data on the effects of HSCT upon bone mineral density (BMD). Factors that may impact BMD include prior therapy for malignancies, conditioning regimens, lack of physical activity, poor nutrition, and post-HSCT therapy with calcineurin inhibitors and cortico-

steroids [44]. Post-HSCT hypogonadism may also negatively impact bone mineral density. One recent study showed nadir BMD at month 24 for total body and femoral neck [58] in patients who received allogeneic HSCT. BMD continuously declined at the femoral neck sites. Steroids and cyclosporine use, as well as loss of muscle mass, were associated with low BMD. Only very young patients were protected from bone loss. The relationship between BMD changes and fracture risk is not yet established post HSCT.

Osteochondromas are benign bone tumors that consist of projecting mature bone capped by cartilage. Radiation, including TBI, is generally believed to be the cause of osteochondromas. The pathogenesis of these bone tumors is not well understood. The mean latent time from HSCT to the development of osteochondromas was 4.6 years in one study [65] (NBL paper by Ginsberg et.al most recent), and younger patients (less than 5 years old) were at increased risk. Of patients less than 5 years old at the time of TBI, an osteochondroma occurred in 24 % [65]. There is a low malignant potential for these tumors, but they do cause a great deal of anxiety when found and can be painful depending on the location.

Osteonecrosis (ON) is a condition that presents as vague, diffuse bone pain, most likely because of increased intraosseous pressure, or joint-related pain because of an effusion. It was first reported as a posttransplant complication in 1980s. Once subchondral collapse occurs, arthritic-type joint pain predominates and is accompanied by decreased range of motion. The most common sites of destruction in children are knees, hips, and shoulders [8].

There are multiple risk factors for the development of ON which are TBI-based conditioning regimens and the use of corticosteroids both before and after HSCT [14]. Treatment involves minimizing exposure to corticosteroids, use of analgesics for pain, and physical therapy designed to focus on non-weight-bearing exercise [31]. If symptomatic, treatment is targeted to preserve the joint and control the pain. Some of these include core decompression, use of bisphosphonates, and joint replacement [50]. Guidelines and consensus on treatment are lacking.

## 18.10    Neuropsychologic

Conditioning regimens containing high drug doses and radiation that may be neurotoxic can result in neuropsychologic sequelae. Agents that are associated with neurotoxicity include busulfan, thiotepa, and melphalan. Although much is known about the neuropsychologic effects of cranial irradiation for leukemias and brain tumors, there is relatively little known about the outcomes of children post HSCT. Doses of radiation used for central nervous system leukemia are between 1,800 and 2,400 cGy and for brain tumors up to 6,000 cGy. Although the total doses used for TBI are may be lower (1,000–1,400 cGy) than used in other situations, the biologic effect enhanced by the shorter duration of radiation over 3–4 days compared to radiation therapy for leukaemia or solid tumors. Children of different ages may be impacted by TBI in different ways; children under 3 years old may be at higher risk than older children, and they may experience declines in cognition and school performance [33, 60]. Other small studies have suggested that no cognitive impairment occurs even with TBI [47, 61]. However, executive functioning has not been well studied, and it is suggested that this may be affected by conditioning. Chemotherapy-only regimens rarely show a detrimental effect of cognitive function, although hearing loss in children with neuroblastoma may have a significant effect on verbal IQ [43]. Prior cranial radiation increases the risks.

## 18.11    Other Issues Post HSCT

### 18.11.1  Chronic GVHD

The incidence of chronic GVHD is lower in children compared with adults, but is responsible for significant post-HSCT morbidity. Chronic GVHD occurs in approximately 20 % of children who receive matched sibling donor transplants and 40–60 % who receive unrelated donor hematopoietic stem cells. The use of mobilized peripheral stem cells increases the risk of chronic GVHD [36, 57]. The most significant risk factor for chronic GVHD is prior acute GVHD; other risk factors include older age, a female multiparous donor, or an unrelated or partially matched related donor [35]. Chronic GVHD may be classified as progressive, evolving from acute GVHD; quiescent, following a period of resolution from acute GVHD; or de novo, in patients who had no prior acute GVHD. Chronic GVHD is associated with a decrease in leukemic relapse risk, although it may come at a price with a significant impact upon quality of life and increase in transplant-related mortality. Classification of chronic GVHD is difficult and currently undergoing revision.

Current classification of chronic GVHD is "limited" or "extensive." Limited GVHD refers to localized skin involvement with or without hepatic test abnormalities, and extensive refers to generalized skin involvement or involvement of other organs. Poor prognostic factors include progressive onset, platelets $<100 \times 10^9$/ml, and poor performance status.

The etiology of chronic GVHD is not well understood. Many manifestations resemble autoimmune diseases, with loss of normal T-cell regulation considered to be a possible cause.

### 18.11.2  Clinical Features

The manifestations of chronic GVHD usually occur after day 100 post HSCT. Almost all patients are diagnosed within the first year post HSCT. The effects of chronic GVHD vary, depending upon location and severity of involvement (Table 18.3). The skin is the most commonly affected organ, with over 50 % of patients with chronic GVHD having some degree of skin involvement. Diagnosis may be confirmed with a biopsy if other diagnoses (particularly infection) are being considered.

### 18.11.3  Evaluation and Therapy

Most patients will be in the care of their primary oncologists when chronic GVHD is diagnosed. It is important that physicians be aware of the subtle manifestations and that particular care be

**Table 18.3** Chronic GVHD: clinical features

| Organ | Features | Symptoms |
|---|---|---|
| Skin | Dyspigmentation, lichen planus, atrophy, scleroderma, alopecia, onychodystrophy, sweat gland loss | Pruritus, erythema, inflexibility, alopecia, onychodystrophy, sweat gland loss, heat insensitivity |
| Liver | Elevated transaminases, alkaline phosphatase, bilirubin | |
| Oral cavity | Lichen planus, erythema, ulcers, xerostomia, fibrosis | Pain, dry mouth |
| Eyes | Sicca syndrome | Dry eyes, photophobia |
| GI | Esophageal strictures, abnormal motility, malabsorption | Dysphagia, cramping, diarrhea, anorexia, weight loss |
| Pulmonary | Obstructive pattern, bronchiolitis obliterans, bronchiectasis | Cough, dyspnea, exercise intolerance |
| Musculoskeletal | Arthritis, joint contractures | Myalgia, stiffness |
| Genitourinary | Phimosis, vaginal strictures | Pain |
| Hematologic | Thrombocytopenia, eosinophilia | |
| Immunologic | Hypogammaglobulinemia, decreased T lymphocytes | Increased infectious risks, particularly streptococcus and pneumococcus |

**Table 18.4** Infectious risks and prophylaxis

| | |
|---|---|
| *Pneumocystis carinii* | Sulfamethoxazole/ trimethoprim or dapsone |
| Varicella/herpes zoster | Acyclovir |
| Encapsulated organisms | Daily penicillin or erythromycin, Prevnar, Pneumovax |
| Hypogammaglobulinemia (IgG <500 g/L) | Monthly intravenous immunoglobulin |
| *Candida albicans* | Fluconazole |
| *Aspergillosis* | Voriconazole |

taken during the physical examination of the skin, oral mucosa, nails, range of motion, and lungs [15]. Infection is the greatest risk to these patients due to inadequate immune recovery and functional hyposplenism. Prophylactic antibiotics and IVIG may be necessary (Table 18.4). To control or improve the symptoms of chronic GVHD, at least two immunosuppressant drugs may be necessary in order to impede the immune recovery already compromised by chronic GVHD-induced immune dysregulation.

Therapy for chronic GVHD generally includes a regimen with prednisone and a calcineurin inhibitor, such as cyclosporine or tacrolimus. An alternate day regimen of prednisone and the calcineurin inhibitor may help decrease the side effects of both while retaining disease control. Therapy and weaning should be done

in conjunction with the transplant center, and close communication is required. For patients who do not respond to this regimen, other drugs may be added with the guidance of the transplant team.

## 18.12 Immune Reconstitution and Reimmunization

The duration and severity of immunodeficiency post HSCT depend upon several factors, including graft type and manipulation, graft vs. host disease, and the age of the recipient. There are significant differences in the kinetics of immune reconstitution between autologous and allogeneic HSCT. However, the pattern of immune reconstitution with various types of allogeneic grafts, including cord blood, appears similar [69]. NK cells generally recover within the first few months and may be elevated for up to 2 years, but recovery of B lymphocytes and in particular T lymphocytes takes much longer. Children may have more active thymic tissue than adults, which may be the reason why their immune reconstitution appears to be faster than that seen in adults [63]. In general, most patients will have complete immune reconstitution by 2 years, unless they have chronic

GVHD. Chronic GVHD has an adverse effect upon reconstitution, not only due to the effects of immune suppressive drugs required for its control, but also due to the aberrant T-cell function of the GVHD process itself. In the absence of GVHD, recipients of T-replete allogeneic or autologous grafts will have near normal CD3+ cells 3 months post HSCT. However, CD4+ is decreased during this period, with higher proportions of CD8+ cells. With chronic GVHD, this inverted CD4+/CD8+ ratio persists for up to a year or longer. However, even recipients of autologous HSCT may experience delayed T-cell reconstitution, and up to one-third may have subnormal CD4+ cells at 1 year [30]. In the absence of GVHD, the response to mitogens usually returns to normal within several months, as does the production of IgG and IgM. IgA may take longer to recover. The delay in immune recovery may be responsible for infections, including *Pneumocystis carinii* pneumonia, varicella, CMV, and EBV

### 18.12.1 Reimmunization After HSCT

Most recipients of HSCT will lose their immunity to the vaccinations they have received prior to HSCT. In addition, patients with chronic GVHD are at risk for infections with *Streptococcus pneumoniae* and *H. influenza*. Therefore, reimmunization of HSCT recipients is essential. There are guidelines detailing vaccination schedules [62], but longitudinal analysis of antibody response has revealed low antibody titers following reimmunization for pertussis, measles, mumps, and hepatitis B [28]. In general, at 12 months post HSCT in patients without chronic GVHD, vaccinations can be given on a schedule similar to that used with normal infants; however, the 23-valent pneumococcal polysaccharide vaccine may not result in adequate antibody response, even when administration is delayed to 12 months [20]. The 7-valent pneumococcal conjugate vaccine is linked to a protein carrier and may enhance immune response. A recent study showed early immunization with this 7-valent vaccine resulted in protection in most patients. The authors of the

**Table 18.5** Recommended vaccinations for allogeneic and autologous hematopoietic stem cell transplant recipients

| Time after HSCT | |
|---|---|
| Inactivated vaccine or toxoid | |
| Diphtheria, tetanus, pertussis | |
|   Children aged <7 years | DTP or DT at 12, 14, and 24 months |
|   Children aged ≥7 years | Td at 12, 14, and 24 months |
| Inactivated polio | 12, 14, and 24 months |
| Hepatitis B | 12, 14, and 24 months |
| 13-valent pneumococcal | |
| 23-valent pneumococcal polysaccharide (PPV23) | 12 and 24 months |
| Influenza | Seasonal administration ≥6 months after HSCT |
| Meningococcal | Patients at risk |
| Live attenuated vaccine | |
| Measles–mumps–rubella | 24 months |
| Varicella vaccine | 24 months |

study suggest an administration schedule of 3, 6, and 12 months [39]. Vaccines that are contraindicated include BCG, oral polio, and varicella (see Table 18.5).

## 18.13 Secondary Malignancies

Patients are at increased risk for secondary malignancies following HSCT. This is the consequence of many factors, including chemotherapy used before HSCT and for conditioning and radiation therapy.

In one large study, the solid cancer risk increased to an estimated 11 % at 15 years post HSCT; patients who were under 5–10 years of age at HSCT had the highest risk [12, 64]. These patients received total body irradiation. Both chronic GVHD and irradiation may play a role in the development of secondary cancers [5]. The most common types of cancers include liver, oral cavity, thyroid, and cervical. Squamous cell cancer of the skin and oral cavity are increased in patients with chronic GVHD [12]. There are a few studies that support an increased risk of secondary cancers in children who received non-TBI regimens, but no large studies have been done.

# References

1. Adan L, Laversin M et al (1997) Growth after bone marrow transplantation in young children conditioned with chemotherapy alone. Bone Marrow Transplant 19(3):253–256
2. Afify Z, Shaw P et al (2000) Growth and endocrine function in children with acute myeloid leukaemia after bone marrow transplantation using busulfan/ cyclophosphamide. Bone Marrow Transplant 25(10):1087–1092
3. Anderson N, Regillo C (2004) Ocular manifestations of graft versus host disease. Curr Opin Ophthalmol 15:503–507
4. Baker K, Ness K et al (2007) Diabetes, hypertension, and cardiovascular events in survivors of hematopoietic cell transplantation: a report from the bone marrow transplantation survivor study. Blood 109:1765–1772
5. Bhatia S, Louie AD et al (2001) Solid cancers after bone marrow transplantation. J Clin Oncol 19(2):464–471
6. Boulad F, Bromley M et al (1995) Thyroid dysfunction following bone marrow transplantation using hyperfractionated radiation. Bone Marrow Transplant 15(1):71–76
7. Brauner R, Adan L et al (1997) Contribution of growth hormone deficiency to the growth failure that follows bone marrow transplantation. J Pediatr 130(5):785–792
8. Burger B, Beier R et al (2005) Osteonecrosis: a treatment related toxicity in childhood acute lymphoblastic luekemia (ALL)- experiences from trial ALL-BFM-95. Pediatr Blood Cancer 44:220–225
9. Cerveri I, Fulgoni P et al (2001) Lung function abnormalities after bone marrow transplantation in children: has the trend recently changed? Chest 120(6):1900–1906
10. Chow EJ, Friedman DL, Yasui Y et al (2007) Decreased adult height in survivors of childhood acute lymphoblastic leukemia: a report from the Childhood Cancer Survivor Study. J Pediatr 150:370–375
11. Cohen A, Rovelli A et al (1999) Final height of patients who underwent bone marrow transplantation for hematological disorders during childhood: a study by the Working Party for Late Effects-EBMT. Blood 93(12):4109–4115
12. Curtis RE, Rowlings et al (1997) Solid cancers after bone marrow transplantation. N Engl J Med 336(13):897–904
13. Dvorak CC, Gracia CR et al (2011) NCI, NHLBI/ PBMTC first international conference on late effects after pediatric hematopoietic cell transplantation: endocrine challenges-thyroid dysfunction, growth impairment, bone health, & reproductive risks. Biol Blood Marrow Transplant 17(12):1725–1738
14. Faraci M, Calevo M et al (2006) Osteonecrosis after allogeneic stem cell transplantation in childhood. A case-control study in Italy. Haematologica 91:1096–1099
15. Filipovich A, Weisdorf D et al (2005) National Institutes of Health consensus development project on criteria for clinical trials in chronic graft-versus-host disease: I. Diagnosis and staging working group report. Biol Blood Marrow Transplant 11:945–955
16. Fletcher BD, Crom DB et al (1994) Radiation-induced bone abnormalities after bone marrow transplantation for childhood leukemia. Radiology 191(1):231–235
17. Freudenberger TD, Madtes DK et al (2003) Association between acute and chronic graft-versus-host disease and bronchiolitis obliterans organizing pneumonia in recipients of hematopoietic stem cell transplants. Blood 102(10):3822–3828
18. Frisk P, Arvidson J et al (2004) Pulmonary function after autologous bone marrow transplantation in children: a long-term prospective study. Bone Marrow Transplant 33:645–650
19. Giorgiani G, Bozzola M et al (1995) Role of busulfan and total body irradiation on growth of prepubertal children receiving bone marrow transplantation and results of treatment with recombinant human growth hormone. Blood 86(2):825–831
20. Guinan EC, Molrine DC et al (1994) Polysaccharide conjugate vaccine responses in bone marrow transplant patients. Transplantation 57(5):677–684
21. Hingoarani S, Guthrie K et al (2007) Chronic kidney disease in long-term survivors of hematopoietic cell transplant. Bone Marrow Transplant 39:223–229
22. Hobbie WL, Mostoufi-Moab S, Carlson CA, Gruccio D, Ginsberg JP (2011) Prevalence of advanced bone age in a cohort of patients who received cis-retinoic acid for high-risk neuroblastoma. Pediatr Blood Cancer 56:474–476
23. Hoffmeister PA, Storer BE et al (2004) Diabetes mellitus in long-term survivors of pediatric hematopoietic cell transplantation. J Pediatr Hematol Oncol 26(2):81–90
24. Hogarty AN, Leahey A et al (2000) Longitudinal evaluation of cardiopulmonary performance during exercise after bone marrow transplantation in children. J Pediatr 136(3):311–317
25. Holm K, Nysom K et al (1996) Growth, growth hormone and final height after BMT. Possible recovery of irradiation-induced growth hormone insufficiency. Bone Marrow Transplant 8(1):163–170
26. Hovi L, Saarinen-Pihkala UM et al (1999) Growth in children with poor-risk neuroblastoma after regimens with or without total body irradiation in preparation for autologous bone marrow transplantation. Bone Marrow Transplant 24(10):1131–1136
27. Huma Z, Boulad F et al (1995) Growth in children after bone marrow transplantation for acute leukemia. Blood 86(2):819–824
28. Inaba H, Hartford CM et al (2012) Longitudinal analysis of antibody response to immunization in paediatric survivors after allogeneic haematopoietic stem cell transplantation. Br J Haematol 156(1):109–117
29. Jacobsohn D, Duerst R et al (2004) Reduced intensity haematopoietic stem-cell transplantation for treatment of non-malignant diseases in children. Lancet 364:156–162

30. Kamani N, Kattamis A et al (2000) Immune reconstitution after autologous purged bone marrow transplantation in children. J Pediatr Hematol Oncol 22(1):13–19

31. Kaste S, Shidler T et al (2004) Bone mineral density and osteonecrosis in survivors of childhood allogeneic bone marrow transplantation. Bone Marrow Transplant 33:435–441

32. Katsanis E, Shapiro RS et al (1990) Thyroid dysfunction following bone marrow transplantation: long-term follow-up of 80 pediatric patients. Bone Marrow Transplant 5(5):335–340

33. Kramer J, Crittenden M et al (1997) Cognitive and adaptive behavior 1 and 3 years following bone marrow transplantation. Bone Marrow Transplant 19:607–613

34. Laskin B, Goebel J et al (2011) Small vessels, big trouble in the kidneys and beyond: hematopoietic stem cell transplantation-associated thrombotic microangiopathy. Blood 118:1452–1462

35. Lee S, Vogelsang G et al (2003) Chronic graft-versus-host disease. Biol Blood Marrow Transplant 9:215–233

36. Levine J, Wiley J et al (2000) Cytokine-mobilized allogeneic peripheral blood stem cell transplants in children result in rapid engraftment and a high incidence of chronic GVHD. Bone Marrow Transplant 25:13–18

37. Marras TK, Szalai JP et al (2002) Pulmonary function abnormalities after allogeneic marrow transplantation: a systematic review and assessment of an existing predictive instrument. Bone Marrow Transplant 30(9):599–607

38. Michel G, Socie G et al (1997) Late effects of allogeneic bone marrow transplantation for children with acute myeloblastic leukemia in first complete remission: the impact of conditioning regimen without total-body irradiation–a report from the Societe Francaise de Greffe de Moelle. J Clin Oncol 15(6):2238–2246

39. Molrine DC, Antin JH et al (2003) Donor immunization with pneumococcal conjugate vaccine and early protective antibody responses following allogeneic hematopoietic cell transplantation. Blood 101(3):831–836

40. Mostoufi-Moab S, Isacoff EJ, Spiegel D et al (2013) Childhood cancer survivors exposed to total body irradiation are at significant risk for slipped capital femoral epiphysis during recombinant growth hormone therapy. Pediatr Blood Cancer 6D(11):1766–1771

41. Nagler R, Marmary Y et al (1996) Major salivary gland dysfunction in human acute and chronic graft-versus-host disease (GVHD). Bone Marrow Transplant 17(2):219–224

42. Nieder ML, McDonald GB et al (2011) National Cancer Institute-National Heart, Lung and Blood Institute/pediatric Blood and Marrow Transplant Consortium First International Consensus Conference on late effects after pediatric hematopoietic cell transplantation: long-term organ damage and dysfunction. Biol Blood Marrow Transplant 17(11):1573–1584

43. Notteghem P, Soler et al (2003) Neuropsychological outcome in long-term survivors of a childhood extracranial solid tumor who have undergone autologous bone marrow transplantation. Bone Marrow Transplant 31(7):599–606

44. Nysom K, Holm et al (2000) Bone mass after allogeneic BMT for childhood leukaemia or lymphoma. Bone Marrow Transplant 25:191–196

45. Olshan JS, Willi SM et al (1993) Growth hormone function and treatment following bone marrow transplant for neuroblastoma. Bone Marrow Transplant 12(4):381–385

46. Parsons SK, Neault MW et al (1998) Severe ototoxicity following carboplatin-containing conditioning regimen for autologous marrow transplantation for neuroblastoma. Bone Marrow Transplant 22(7):669–674

47. Phipps S, Dunavant M et al (2000) Cognitive and academic functioning in survivors of pediatric bone marrow transplantation. J Clin Oncol 18(5):1004–1011

48. Pihkala J, Saarinen UM et al (1994) Effects of bone marrow transplantation on myocardial function in children. Bone Marrow Transplant 13(2):149–155

49. Punnett A, Bliss B et al (2004) Ototoxicity following pediatric hematopoietic stem cell transplantation: a prospective cohort study. Pediatr Blood Cancer 42:598–603

50. Ramachandran M, Ward K et al (2007) Intravenous bisphosphonate therapy for traumatic osteonecrosis of the femoral head in adolescents. J Bone Joint Surg Am 89:1727–1734

51. Rao K, Amrolia P et al (2005) Improved survival after unrelated donor bone marrow transplantation in children with primary immunodeficiency using a reduced-intensity conditioning regimen. Blood 105:879–885

52. Reddy P, Johnson K et al (2006) Nephrotic syndrome associated with chronic graft-versus-host disease after allogeneic hematopoietic stem cell transplantation. Bone Marrow Transplant 38:351–357

53. Rio B, Letur-Konirsch H et al (1994) Full-term pregnancy with embryos from donated oocytes in a 36-year-old woman allografted for chronic myeloid leukemia. Bone Marrow Transplant 13(4):487–488

54. Sanders JE, Buckner CD et al (1988) Ovarian function following marrow transplantation for aplastic anemia or leukemia. J Clin Oncol 6(5):813–818

55. Sanders JE, Hawley J et al (1996) Pregnancies following high-dose cyclophosphamide with or without high-dose busulfan or total-body irradiation and bone marrow transplantation. Blood 87(7):3045–3052

56. Sanders JE, Pritchard S et al (1986) Growth and development following marrow transplantation for leukemia. Blood 68(5):1129–1135

57. Schmitz N, Beksac M et al (2002) Transplantation of mobilized peripheral blood cells to HLA-identical siblings with standard risk leukemia. Blood 100:761–767

58. Schulte CM, Beelen DW (2004) Bone loss following hematopoietic stem cell transplantation: a long-term follow-up. Blood 103(10):3635–3643

59. Schultz KR, Green GJ et al (1994) Obstructive lung disease in children after allogeneic bone marrow transplantation. Blood 84(9):3212–3220

60. Shah A, Epport K et al (2008) Progressive declines in neurocognitive function among survivors of hematopoietic stem cell transplantation for pediatric hematologic malignancies. J Pediatr Hematol-Oncol 30:411–418

61. Simms S, Kazak A et al (2002) Cognitive, behavioral and social outcome in survivors of childhood stem cell transplantation. J Pediatr Hematol-Oncol 24:115–119

62. Singhal S, Mehta J (1999) Reimmunization after blood or marrow stem cell transplantation. Bone Marrow Transplant 23(7):637–646

63. Small TN, Papadopoulos EB et al (1999) Comparison of immune reconstitution after unrelated and related T-cell-depleted bone marrow transplantation: effect of patient age and donor leukocyte infusions. Blood 93(2):467–480

64. Socie G, Curtis RE et al (2000) New malignant diseases after allogeneic marrow transplantation for childhood acute leukemia. J Clin Oncol 18(2):348–357

65. Taitaz J, Cohn R et al (2003) Osteochondroma after total body irradiation: an age-related complication. Pediatr Blood Cancer 42:225–229

66. Taskinen M, Saarinen-Pihkala UM et al (2000) Impaired glucose tolerance and dyslipidaemia as late effects after bone-marrow transplantation in childhood. Lancet 356(9234):993–997

67. Thibaud E, Rodriguez-Macias K et al (1998) Ovarian function after bone marrow transplantation during childhood. Bone Marrow Transplant 21(3):287–290

68. Thomas BC, Stanhope R et al (1993) Endocrine function following single fraction and fractionated total body irradiation for bone marrow transplantation in childhood. Acta Endocrinol 128(6):508–512

69. Thomson BG, Robertson KA et al (2000) Analysis of engraftment, graft-versus-host disease, and immune recovery following unrelated donor cord blood transplantation. Blood 96(8):2703–2711

70. Toubert ME, Socie G et al (1997) Short- and long-term follow-up of thyroid dysfunction after allogeneic bone marrow transplantation without the use of preparative total body irradiation. Br J Haematol 98(2):453–457

71. Uderzo C, Pillon M et al (2007) Impact of cumulative anthracycline dose, preparative regimen and chronic graft-versus-host disease on pulmonary and cardiac function in children 5 years after allogeneic hematopoietic stem cell transplantation: a prospective evaluation on behalf of the EBMT Pediatric Diseases and Late Effects Working Parties. Bone Marrow Transplant 39:667–675

72. Urban C, Schwingshandl J et al (1988) Endocrine function after bone marrow transplantation without the use of preparative total body irradiation. Bone Marrow Transplant 3(4):291–296

73. Wingard JR, Plotnick LP et al (1992) Growth in children after bone marrow transplantation: busulfan plus cyclophosphamide versus cyclophosphamide plus total body irradiation. Blood 79(4):1068–1073

74. Joshi S, Savani BN et al (2014) Clinical Guide to fertility preservation in hematopoietic cell transplant recipients. Blood Marrow Transplant (49): 477–484

# Second Malignancies Following Treatment for Childhood Cancer

# 19

Smita Bhatia

## Contents

## 19.1 Epidemiology of Subsequent Malignant Neoplasms

Second or subsequent malignant neoplasms (SMNs) are defined as histologically distinct cancers developing after the occurrence of a first cancer and are one of the most devastating consequences of cancer therapy in children with cancer. Studies following large cohorts of childhood cancer survivors have reported a three- to sixfold increased risk of SMNs compared with the background incidence of cancer in the general population; this risk continues to increase as the cohort ages. Follow-up of a Nordic cohort of 47,697 patients diagnosed with their first cancer at 19 years of age or younger between 1943 and 2005 resulted in the identification of 1,180 SMNs [1]. The cohort was at a 3.3-fold increased risk of developing an SMN when compared with an age- and gender-matched healthy population. The relative risk (RR) was statistically significantly increased in all age groups, even for cohort members approaching 70 years of age. Another population-based cohort of 17,981 5-year survivors of childhood cancer diagnosed before the age of 15 years in Great Britain between 1940 and 1991 was followed for a median of 24 years; 1,354 SMNs were observed, and the cohort was at a fourfold increased risk of developing a new cancer, when compared with the general population [2]. A retrospective cohort of 14,359 children

S. Bhatia, MD, MPH
Cancer Outcomes and Survivorship, University of Alabama, 1600 7th Ave South, Lowder 500, Birmingham, AL 35223, USA
e-mail: sbhatia@peds.uab.edu

© Springer International Publishing 2015
C.L. Schwartz et al. (eds.), *Survivors of Childhood and Adolescent Cancer: A Multidisciplinary Approach*, Pediatric Oncology, DOI 10.1007/978-3-319-16435-9_19

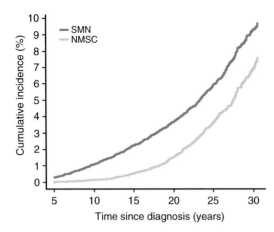

**Fig. 19.1** Cumulative incidence of second neoplasms after initial cancer diagnosis (Friedman et al. [3])

diagnosed between 1970 and 1986 in the USA before the age of 21 years, and surviving at least 5 years, was followed by the Childhood Cancer Survivor Study (CCSS) [3]. The estimated 30-year cumulative incidence was 7.9 % for SMNs (excluding nonmelanoma skin cancers, Fig. 19.1). Overall, the cohort was at a sixfold increased risk of developing a second cancer. Female sex, older age at diagnosis, earlier treatment era, and treatment with radiation were associated with an increase in risk of SMNs. Childhood cancer survivors are at risk for the development of multiple primaries; the cumulative incidence of a third primary approaches 47 % at 20 years after the second primary [4]. Radiation-exposed survivors, who developed a nonmelanoma skin cancer as an SMN, carry a higher risk of a subsequent invasive SMN when compared with those without a history of a non-melanoma skin cancer.

Unique associations with specific therapeutic exposures have resulted in the classification of SMNs into two distinct groups: chemotherapy-related myelodysplasia and acute myeloid leukemia (t-MDS/AML) and radiation-related solid SMNs. Characteristics of AML include a short latency (<5 years from primary cancer diagnosis) when associated with topoisomerase II inhibitors vs. AML/MDS that usually occur with a longer latency extending 10–15 years after therapeutic exposure when associated with alkylating agents. Solid SMNs have a well-defined association with

radiation and are characterized by a latency that typically exceeds 10 years [3, 5–7]. The most frequently observed solid SMNs include the breast, skin, thyroid, and central nervous system (CNS) tumors and bone/soft tissue sarcomas and carcinomas [8–10] (Table 19.1).

t-MDS/AML have been reported after successful treatment of Hodgkin lymphoma (HL), non-Hodgkin lymphoma (NHL), acute lymphoblastic leukemia (ALL), and bone/soft tissue sarcomas [5, 8, 11–15] (Table 19.1). The risk of t-MDS/AML is generally low, approaching 2 % at 15 years after conventional therapy [5]. Using the WHO classification, two types of t-MDS/AML are recognized, related closely to the therapeutic exposure (Table 19.2): alkylating agents/radiation and topoisomerase II inhibitors [16]. The alkylating agent-related t-MDS/AML typically develops ~5 years after exposure. Cytopenias are common. Two-thirds of the patients present with myelodysplasia; the remaining present with AML but carry myelodysplastic features. Abnormalities involving chromosomes 5 (−5/del[5q]) and 7 (−7/del[7q]) are frequently seen. AML secondary to topoisomerase II inhibitors presents as overt leukemia, without a preceding myelodysplastic phase. The latency is brief, ranging from 6 months to 5 years, and is associated with balanced translocations involving chromosome bands 11q23 or 21q22. Epipodophyllotoxin-associated t-AML depends more on the schedule of drug administration than total cumulative dose [17].

Solid SMNs are clearly related to radiation therapy used to treat the primary cancer and thus will usually arise within the radiation field [5, 6, 8, 18, 19]. However, solid SMNs can also occur outside of radiation fields and also in children treated with chemotherapy alone. The latency for radiation-related solid SMNs usually exceeds 10 years [5, 6, 8, 19]. The risk is highest when radiation exposure occurs at a younger age [5, 7, 19–26] and increases with increasing doses of radiation and with increasing time since radiation [6, 8]. Eighty percent of the entire burden of SMNs is accounted for by radiation-related solid SMNs. Some of the well-established radiation-related solid SMNs include breast cancer, thyroid cancer, CNS tumors, sarcomas, and basal cell carcinomas (BCCs) [3, 5–8, 24, 27].

**Breast Cancer** Breast cancer is the most commonly reported second malignancy among female survivors of childhood HL treated with mantle field irradiation (SIR = 24.7, 95 % CI, 19.3–31.0), and the risk remains markedly elevated for many decades after exposure [5, 19, 27–30]. The survivors have up to a 55-fold increased risk of breast cancer compared with the general population, and the cumulative incidence of developing a secondary breast cancer approaches 20 % at 45 years of age [8]. Moreover,

40 % of the patients with radiation-related breast cancer develop contralateral disease, usually within 1–3 years. The incidence is also increased among those exposed to TBI as the only source of radiation to the chest when compared with those who did not receive TBI (17 % vs. 3 %) [31]. The risk of breast cancer increases in a linear fashion with radiation dose, reaching 11-fold for local breast doses of ~40 Gy relative to no radiation [32]. Conversely, a reduction in irradiated breast volume, at least in patients irradiated for Hodgkin lymphoma, decreases the risk for breast cancer. The risk of radiation-related breast cancer declines with age at radiation, such that

**Table 19.1** Characteristics of second cancers among childhood cancer survivors – by primary cancer type

| Primary cancer | Secondary cancer | Median latency | Risk factors |
|---|---|---|---|
| Hodgkin lymphoma | Breast cancer | 15–20 | Radiation |
| | | | Female sex |
| | Myelodysplastic syndrome/acute myeloid leukemia | 3–5 years | Alkylating agents |
| | | | Topoisomerase II inhibitors |
| | Thyroid cancer | 13–15 years | Radiation |
| | | | Younger age |
| | | | Female sex |
| | Soft tissue sarcoma | 10–11 years | Radiation |
| | | | Younger age |
| | | | Anthracyclines |
| Bone tumor | Breast cancer | 15–20 years | Radiation |
| | | | Female sex |
| | Myelodysplastic syndrome/acute myeloid leukemia | 3–5 years | Alkylating agents |
| | | | Topoisomerase II inhibitors |
| | Thyroid cancer | 13–15 years | Radiation |
| | | | Younger age |
| | | | Female sex |
| | Other bone tumors | 9–10 years | Radiation |
| | | | Alkylating agents |
| | Soft tissue sarcomas | 10–11 years | Radiation |
| | | | Younger age |
| | | | Anthracyclines |
| Soft tissue sarcoma | Breast cancer | 15–20 years | Radiation |
| | | | Female sex |
| | Thyroid cancer | 13–15 years | Radiation |
| | | | Younger age |
| | | | Female sex |
| | Bone tumor | 9–10 years | Radiation |
| | | | Alkylating agents |
| | Other soft tissue sarcoma | 10–11 years | Radiation |
| | | | Younger age |
| | | | Anthracyclines |

(continued)

**Table 19.1** (continued)

| Primary cancer | Secondary cancer | Median latency | Risk factors |
|---|---|---|---|
| Acute lymphoblastic leukemia | Breast cancer | 15–20 years | Radiation |
| | | | Female sex |
| | Brain tumors | 9–10 years | Radiation |
| | | | Younger age |
| | Myelodysplastic syndrome/acute myeloid leukemia | 3–5 years | Alkylating agents |
| | | | Topoisomerase II inhibitors |
| | Thyroid cancer | 13–15 years | Radiation |
| | | | Younger age |
| | | | Female sex |
| | Bone tumors | 9–10 years | Radiation |
| | | | Alkylating agents |
| Brain tumor | Other brain tumors | 9–10 years | Radiation |
| | | | Younger age |
| | Breast cancer | 15–20 years | Radiation |
| | | | Female sex |
| | Thyroid cancer | 13–15 years | Radiation |
| | | | Younger age |
| | | | Female sex |
| Wilms tumor | Breast cancer | 15–20 years | Radiation |
| | | | Female sex |
| Non-Hodgkin lymphoma | Breast cancer | 15–20 years | Radiation |
| | | | Female sex |
| | Thyroid cancer | 13–15 years | Radiation |
| | | | Younger age |
| | | | Female sex |

**Table 19.2** Clinical characteristics of treatment-related myelodysplastic syndrome and acute myeloid leukemia

| Characteristics | Alkylating agents | Epipodophyllotoxins |
|---|---|---|
| Median latency | 4–6 years (range, 1–20) | 1–3 years (range, 0.5–4.5) |
| Presentation | Myelodysplasia | Abrupt-onset leukemia – no pre-leukemic phase |
| Cytogenetic abnormalities | Loss of genetic material, often from chromosomes 5 and/or 7 | Balanced translocations (often include 11q23) |
| Age at onset | Typically older patients | Typically younger patients |

the relative risks in cancer patients who had received radiation after age 40 years are comparable to those of the general population [33, 34]. There appears to be a protective effect of early menopause induced either by alkylating agents or radiation dose >5 Gy to the ovaries, suggesting that ovarian hormones play an important role in promoting tumorigenesis once an initiating event has been produced by radiation [27, 32, 35, 36].

**Thyroid Cancer** Secondary thyroid malignancies, typically papillary carcinoma, are generally associated with radiation exposure to the thyroid gland as part of CNS irradiation, for treatment of CNS leukemia, as part of therapeutic irradiation of cervical lymph nodes in HL patients, or as part of conditioning with TBI for hematopoietic cell transplantation [5, 7, 8, 12, 19]. Thyroid malignancy typically develops 10 or more years from treatment. Veiga et al. analyzed multiple cohorts including CCSS, noting that a linear exponential model best described the relative risk of thyroid cancer; RR increased through 10 Gy (to 13.7 95 % CI: 8.0–24.0) and then reached a plateau until 30 Gy when a downturn in the dose-response relationship was observed[37]. This pattern is influenced by effect modification attributable to chemotherapy (alkylating agents, bleomycin, anthracyclines), which increases the RR for patients receiving <20 Gy. Sex (higher radiation risk among females), age at exposure (higher radiation risk at a younger age at exposure), and time since exposure (higher radiation risk with longer time) are significant modifiers of the radiation-related risk of thyroid cancer [38]. HCT recipients are at a 3.3-fold increased risk of thyroid cancer, when compared with age- and sex-matched general population [39]. Younger age at HCT (<10 years), neck radiation, female sex, and chronic GvHD are associated with an increased risk of thyroid cancer. Thyroid cancer usually develops after a latency of ~10 years, and, as is true of de novo thyroid malignancy, the long-term outcome for survivors diagnosed with a secondary thyroid malignancy is excellent.

**Central Nervous System Tumors** Brain tumors develop after cranial radiation for histologically distinct brain tumors [6] or for prophylaxis or treatment of CNS leukemia [7, 12, 19]. The risk is 16.9-fold higher than that of the general population for ALL survivors and is 14.2-fold increased for brain tumor survivors. Histologically, radiation-related late-occurring CNS tumors include high-grade gliomas (glioblastomas and malignant astrocytomas), peripheral neuroectodermal tumors, ependymomas, and meningiomas [7, 13, 40, 41]. Gliomas are diagnosed a median of 9 years from radiation; for meningiomas, the latency is longer (median latency = 17 years) [6]. Radiation exposure is associated with increased risk of both subsequent glioma (OR = 6.8) and meningiomas (OR = 9.9). The dose-response for the excess relative risk is linear. For gliomas, the excess relative risk per Gy is highest among children exposed at less than 5 years of age.

**Sarcomas** The risk of sarcoma after an initial diagnosis of childhood cancer is reported to be ninefold that in the general population; the risk is

particularly elevated after a primary soft tissue sarcoma (24.7-fold), bone tumor (10.6-fold), HL (11.7-fold), or renal tumors (14.6-fold) [42]. Patients with heritable retinoblastoma are at a particularly increased risk of radiation-related sarcomas (13.7-fold increased risk) [43]. Sarcomas develop within the radiation field after a latency of ~10 years.

**Carcinomas** With extended follow-up of cohorts of young survivors, increased risks of common adult carcinomas, including colorectal, lung, and stomach, have emerged, and these cancers are being diagnosed at younger ages than observed in the general population [8, 27, 44–46]. In a large population-based study, breast, lung, and gastrointestinal cancers accounted for almost two-thirds of the estimated excess number of cases [47]. In another population-based cohort of 5-year survivors, the greatest excess risk associated with SMNs among survivors older than 40 years of age was for digestive and genitourinary neoplasms [2]. The risk of carcinomas (other than breast, thyroid, skin) is sixfold higher than that expected [48]. The most common sites are the head and neck (mostly parotid gland), gastrointestinal tract, female genitourinary tract, and kidney. The risk is highest among survivors of neuroblastoma and soft tissue sarcoma; the risk is also elevated for patients who have received radiation therapy.

**Skin Cancer** Ionizing radiation is a well-established cause of nonmelanoma skin cancers (primarily basal cell and squamous cell carcinoma) [23, 49]; radiation is associated with a 6.3-fold increased risk. Over 90 % of nonmelanoma skin cancers develop within the radiation field [5–7, 12, 13, 19].

## 19.2 Pathogenesis of Subsequent Malignant Neoplasms

Although the role of chemotherapy and radiation in the development of second primary cancers is well established, the observed interindividual variability in risk suggests a role for genetic variation in the susceptibility to genotoxic exposures. The risk of chemotherapy- or radiation-related SMNs could potentially be modified by mutations in high-penetrance genes that lead to serious genetic diseases, e.g., Li-Fraumeni syndrome [50] and Fanconi anemia [51–54]. However, the attributable risk is expected to be very small because of the extremely low prevalence of the high-prevalence genes. The interindividual variability in the risk of SMNs is more likely related to common polymorphisms in low-penetrance genes that regulate the availability of active drug metabolite or those responsible for DNA repair. Genetic variation contributes 20–95 % of the variability in cytotoxic drug disposition [55]. Polymorphisms in genes involved in drug metabolism and transport are relevant in determining disease-free survival and drug toxicity [56]. Variation in DNA repair plays a role in susceptibility to de novo cancer [57–61] and likely modifies SMN risk after exposure to DNA-damaging agents, such as radiation and chemotherapy. Genetic predisposition and its interaction with therapeutic exposures can potentially exacerbate the toxic effect of treatment on normal tissues.

In order to understand the pathogenesis of SMNs, it is imperative to understand individual variability in the internal dose of the therapeutic agent, the alterations induced by the therapeutic agent to the structure or function of the tissue, and the consequent development of preclinical disease. Understanding the underlying etiopathogenetic pathways that lead to SMNs is critical in developing targeted prevention and intervention strategies, optimizing risk-based health care of cancer survivors, and improving quality of life.

**Drug Metabolism** Metabolism of genotoxic agents occurs in two phases. Phase I involves activation of substrates into highly reactive electrophilic intermediates that can damage DNA – a reaction principally performed by the cytochrome p450 (CYP) family of enzymes. Phase II enzymes (conjugation) function to inactivate genotoxic substrates. The phase II proteins comprise the glutathione S-transferase (GST), NAD(P)H:quinone oxidoreductase-1 (NQO1),

and others. The balance between the two sets of enzymes is critical to the cellular response to xenobiotics; e.g., high activity of phase I enzyme and low activity of a phase II enzyme can result in DNA damage from the excess of harmful substrates. The xenobiotic substrates of CYP proteins include cyclophosphamide, ifosfamide, thiotepa, doxorubicin, and dacarbazine [62]. The CYPs transfer singlet oxygen onto their substrates creating highly reactive intermediates which, unless detoxified by phase II enzymes, have a strong ability to damage DNA [63]. The expression of these enzymes is highly variable among individuals because of several functionally relevant genetic polymorphisms. GSTs detoxify reactive electrophiles via conjugation to reduced glutathione, preventing damage to DNA. Polymorphisms exist in cytosolic subfamilies: μ [M], π [P], θ [T], and others. GSTs detoxify doxorubicin, lomustine, busulfan, chlorambucil, cisplatin, cyclophosphamide, melphalan, etc. [64]. Quinone oxidoreductase NQO1 uses the cofactors NADH and NADPH to catalyze the electron reduction of its substrates, produces less reactive hydroquinones, and therefore prevents generation of reactive oxygen species and free radicals which may subsequently lead to oxidative damage of cellular components. Using a candidate gene approach, investigators have examined the association between polymorphisms in the glutathione S-transferase genes (*GSTM1*, *GSTT1*, and *GSTP1*) and t-MDS/AML [65]. Individuals with at least one *GSTP1* codon 105 Val allele were significantly overrepresented in t-AML cases compared with de novo AML cases (OR = 1.81, 95 % CI, 1.11–2.94). Also, relative to de novo AML, the *GSTP1* codon 105 allele occurred more often among t-AML patients with prior exposure to chemotherapy (OR = 2.66, 95 % CI, 1.39–5.09), particularly among those with prior exposure to known *GSTP1* substrates (OR = 4.34, 95 % CI, 1.43–13.20) and not among t-AML patients with exposure to radiation alone. While the genes implicated carried biological plausibility, they were not replicated in this study. Furthermore, the comparison groups consisting of healthy controls and patients with de novo AML could compromise the observations.

**DNA Repair** DNA repair mechanisms protect somatic cells from mutations in tumor suppressor genes and oncogenes that can lead to cancer initiation and progression. An individual's DNA repair capacity appears to be genetically determined [66]. A number of DNA repair genes contain polymorphic variants, resulting in large interindividual variations in DNA repair capacity [66]. Even subtle differences in an individual's DNA repair capacity may be important in the presence of large external influences such as chemotherapy or radiotherapy. Individuals with altered DNA repair mechanisms are likely susceptible to the development of genetic instability that drives the process of carcinogenesis as it relates to both chemotherapy-related t-MDS/AML and radiation-related solid SMNs.

*Mismatch repair* (*MMR*) functions to correct mismatched DNA base pairs that arise as a result of misincorporation errors that have avoided polymerase proofreading during DNA replication [67]. Defects in the MMR pathway result in genetic instability or a mutator phenotype, manifested by an elevated rate of spontaneous mutations characterized as multiple replication errors in simple repetitive DNA sequences (microsatellites) – functionally identified as microsatellite instability (MSI). Approximately 50 % of t-MDS/AML patients have MSI, associated with methylation of the MMR family member MLH1 [68, 69], low expression of MSH2 [70], or polymorphisms in MSH2 [71–74]. The appearance of MMR-deficient, drug-resistant clones during genotoxic treatment for a primary cancer could be a vital factor in SMN susceptibility, particularly because the mutator phenotype (inherent of MMR-deficient cells) would be expected to accelerate the accumulation of further mutations and eventually SMN initiation. In addition, loss of MMR may result in deregulation of homologous recombination repair and consequent chromosomal instability [75].

*Double-strand breaks* (*DSBs*) in DNA may lead to loss of genetic material, resulting in chromosomal aberrations. High levels of DSBs arise following ionizing radiation and chemotherapy exposures. Cellular pathways available to repair DSBs include homologous recombination (HR),

non-homologous end-joining (NHEJ), and single-strand annealing [76]. HR uses the second, intact copy of the chromosome as a template to copy the information lost at the DSB site on the damaged chromosome – a high-fidelity process. RAD51 is one of the central proteins in the HR pathway, functioning to bind to DNA and promote ATP-dependent homologous pairing and strand transfer reactions [77, 78]. *RAD51-G-135C* polymorphism is significantly overrepresented in patients with t-MDS/AML compared with controls (C allele: OR = 2.7) [79]. *XRCC3* also functions in the HR DSB repair pathway by directly interacting with and stabilizing *RAD51* [80, 81]. *XRCC3* is a paralog of *RAD51*, also essential for genetic stability [82, 83]. A polymorphism at codon 241 in the *XRCC3* gene results in a Thr→Met amino acid substitution [84]. The variant *XRCC3-241Met al*lele has been associated with a higher level of DNA adducts compared with cells with the wild-type allele, implying aberrant repair [85], and has also been associated with increased levels of chromosome deletions in lymphocytes after exposure to radiation [86]. Although *XRCC3-Thr241Met* was not associated with t-MDS/AML (OR = 1.4, 95 % CI, 0.7–2.9), a synergistic effect resulting in an eightfold increased risk of t-MDS/AML (OR = 8.1, 95 % CI, 2.2–29.7) was observed in the presence of *XRCC3-241Met and RAD51-135C* allele in patients with t-MDS/AML compared with controls [79]. NHEJ pathway joins broken DNA ends containing very little homology. This process is not always precise and can result in small regions of non-template nucleotides around the site of the DNA break, potentially relevant in MLL-translocation associated with t-MDS/AML. Many of the translocation junctions have been sequenced and found to contain regions of microhomology consistent with the operation of the NHEJ pathway, and an impairment of this pathway may modulate t-MDS/AML risk [87].

*Base excision repair* (*BER*) pathway corrects individually damaged bases occurring as a result of ionizing radiation and exogenous xenobiotic exposure. The *XRCC1* protein plays a central role in the BER pathway and also in the repair of single-strand breaks, by acting as a scaffold and recruiting other DNA repair proteins [88, 89]. The protein also has a *BRCA1* C-terminus (BRCT) domain – a characteristic of proteins involved in DNA damage recognition and response. The presence of variant *XRCC1-399Gln* has been shown to be protective for t-MDS/AML [90] and BCC [91].

*Nucleotide excision repair (NER)* removes structurally unrelated bulky damage induced by radiation and chemotherapy. The NER pathway is linked to transcription, and components of the pathway comprise the basal transcription factor IIH complex (TFIIH), which is required for transcription initiation by RNA polymerase II. One of the genes involved in the NER pathway (*ERCC2*) is a member of the TFIIH complex. The polymorphic Gln variant (*ERCC2 Lys751Gln*) is associated with t-MDS/AML [92].

Results from studies examining genetic susceptibility in the development of SMNs are summarized in Table 19.3; some of these studies are highlighted below.

Ellis et al. utilized a case-control study design and examined the association between t-MDS/AML and two common functional p53-pathway variants – the *MDM2* SNP309 and the *TP53* codon 72 polymorphism [93]. Neither polymorphism demonstrated a significant association. However, an interactive effect was detected such that individuals carrying both an *MDM2* G allele and a *TP53* Pro allele were at increased risk of chemotherapy-related t-MDS/AML. The strengths of the study included the utilization of a discovery set ($n = 80$ cases) and replication set ($n = 91$ cases). However, the investigators utilized healthy controls as a comparison group – thus precluding the ability to assess whether the case-control differences reflected differences in susceptibility to primary disease or t-MDS/AML.

Knight et al. conducted a GWAS in patients who had developed t-MDS/AML (cases) and controls [94]. The discovery set included 80 cases and healthy 150 controls. The relevant findings were replicated in an independent set of 70 cases and healthy 95 controls. The investigators identified three SNPs (rs1394384 [OR = 0.29, 95 % CI, 0.15–0.56], rs1381392 [OR = 2.08, 95 % CI, 1.29–3.35], and rs1199098 [OR = 0.46, 95 % CI,

0.27–0.79]) to be associated with t-MDS/AML with chromosome 5/7 abnormalities. rs1394384 is intronic to *ACCN1*, a gene encoding an amiloride-sensitive cation channel that is a member of the degenerin/epithelial sodium channel; rs1199098 is in LD with *IPMK*, which encodes a multikinase that positively regulates the prosurvival AKT kinase and may modulate Wnt/beta-catenin signaling; and rs1381392 is not near any known genes, miRNAs, or regulatory elements, although it lies in a region recurrently deleted in lung cancer. Although the investigators were able to confirm findings in an independent replication cohort, utilization of a noncancer healthy control group raises concerns about the case-control differences being generated by the genetics of the primary cancer vs. t-MDS/AML.

Best et al. performed a GWAS to identify variants associated with radiation-related solid malignancies in HL survivors [95]. They identified two variants at chromosome 6q21 associated with SMNs. The variants comprise a risk locus associated with decreased basal expression of *PRDM1* and impaired induction of the *PRDM1* protein after radiation exposure. These data suggest new gene-exposure interaction that may implicate *PRDM1* in the etiology of radiation therapy-induced second malignancies.

Understanding the pathogenesis of SMN will facilitate focused medical follow-up care and surveillance of the ever-growing population of childhood cancer survivors.

## 19.3 Screening

Several groups have developed recommendations for cancer surveillance on the basis of exposures to treatment, recognizing that these cancers are a leading cause of non-relapse late mortality [96] and serious morbidity [97]. The underlying premise for these surveillance recommendations is that almost half of the SMNs can be detected at an early stage by periodic surveillance [1, 3, 98, 99]. For example, young women treated for a childhood cancer with a moderate-to-high dose of chest radiation have a greatly increased risk of breast cancer, similar in

**Table 19.3** Role of genetic susceptibility in the development of treatment-related adverse events

| Study | GWAS vs. candidate gene | Study design | Replication | Sample size | Results |
|---|---|---|---|---|---|
| *Therapy-related leukemia – associated with exposure to alkylating agents and topoisomerase II inhibitors* | | | | | |
| Knight et al. [94] | GWAS | Case-control (healthy controls) | Yes | Discovery set: 80 cases; 150 controls Replication set: 70 cases; 95 controls | Among patients with acquired abnormalities of chromosomes 5 or 7; 3 SNPs (rs1394384 [OR = 0.29, 95 % CI, 0.15–0.56], rs1381392 [OR = 2.08, 95 % CI, 1.29–3.35], and rs1199098 [OR = 0.46, 95 % CI, 0.27–0.79]) were associated with t-MDS/AML |
| Ellis et al. [93] | Candidate gene (2 common functional p53-pathway variants, the *MDM2* SNP309 and the *TP53* codon 72 | Case-control (healthy controls) | Yes | Discovery set: 80 cases Replication set: 91 cases | Neither polymorphism alone influenced the risk of t-MDS/AML; however, an interactive effect was detected such that *MDM2* TT *TP53* Arg/Arg double homozygotes, and individuals carrying both a *MDM2* G allele and a *TP53* Pro allele, were at increased risk of t-MDS/AML (OR = 2.04, 95 % CI, 1.20–3.48, $P_{interaction} = 0.009$) |
| Allan et al. [65] | Candidate gene approach Polymorphisms in *GSTM1, GSTT1, GSTP1* | Case-control | No | 89 cases; 420 patients with de novo AML; 1,022 healthy controls | Individuals with at least one *GSTP1* codon 105 Val allele were significantly overrepresented in t-AML cases compared with de novo AML cases (OR = 1.81, 95 % CI, 1.11–2.94). Also, compared with de novo AML, the *GSTP1* codon 105 allele occurred more often among t-AML patients with prior exposure to chemotherapy (OR = 2.66, 95 % CI, 1.39–5.09), particularly among those with prior exposure to known *GSTP1* substrates (OR = 4.34, 95 % CI, 1.43–13.20) and not among t-AML patients with exposure to radiation alone |
| Worrillow et al. [71] | Candidate gene hMSH2 –6exon 13 polymorphism Evaluation of MSI | Case-control | No Verification performed by direct sequencing | 91 cases; 420 patients with de novo AML, 837 healthy controls | The variant (C) hMSH2 allele was significantly overrepresented in t-AML cases that had previously been treated with O6-guanine alkylating agents, including cyclophosphamide and procarbazine, compared with controls (OR = 4.02, 95 % CI 1.40–11.37); 38 % of the patients were MSI positive |
| Worrillow et al. [102] | Candidate gene Polymorphism of *MLH1* (position –93, rs1800734) | Case-control | No | 133 cases 420 patients with de novo AML, 242 patients with primary HL, 1,177 healthy controls | Carrier frequency of MLH1 –93 variant was higher in patients who developed t-AML or secondary breast cancer after alkylating agents exposure for HL, compared to patients without alkylating agent exposure. The MLH1 –93 variant allele was also overrepresented in t-AML cases when compared to de novo AML cases and was associated with increased risk of t-AML (OR = 5.31, 95 % CI, 1.40–20.15) among patients exposed to alkylating agents |
| Seedhouse et al. [90] | Candidate gene Polymorphisms in *XRCC1, XRCC3, XPD, NQO1* | Case-control | No | 34 cases; 134 patients with de novo AML; 178 healthy controls | Presence of at least one *XRCC1* 399Gln allele indicated a protective effect for the allele in controls compared with patients with t-AML (OR = 0.44, 95 % CI, 0.20–0.93) |

(continued)

**Table 19.3** (continued)

| Study | GWAS vs. candidate gene | Study design | Replication | Sample size | Results |
|---|---|---|---|---|---|
| Jawad et al. [78] | Candidate gene C/T-3′ untranslated region (UTR) polymorphism in HLX; polymorphism in RAD51 (135G/C-5′ UTR) | Case-control | No | 42 cases; 166 patients with de novo AML; 189 healthy controls | Presence of the variant HLX1 allele significantly increased the risk of t-AML (OR = 3.36, 95 % CI, 1.65–6.84). Polymorphism in RAD51 (135G/C-5′ UTR) also increased the risk of t-AML. Combined analysis revealed a synergistic 9.5-fold increase (95 % CI, 2.22–40.64) in risk for t-AML |
| *Subsequent solid malignancies – associated with exposure to radiation therapy* | | | | | |
| Best et al. [95] | GWAS | Case-control (controls: cancer survivors with no SMNs) | Yes | Discovery set: 100 cases; 89 controls Replication set: 62 cases; 71 controls | Two variants at chromosome 6q21 (rs4946728 [OR = 11.4, 95 % CI, 3.23–40.25]; rs1040411 [OR = 6.57, 95 % CI, 3.19–13.52]) were associated with SMNs in childhood Hodgkin lymphoma (HL) survivors, but not in adult-onset HL survivors |
| Mertens et al. [103] | Candidate gene Polymorphisms in GSTM1, GSTT1, XRCC1 | Cohort study | No | 650 patients with HL (178 with subsequent malignancy) | Individuals lacking GSTM1 were at increased risk of any subsequent malignancy (OR = 1.5, 95 % CI, 1.0–2.3). A nonsignificant increased risk for thyroid cancer was observed in individuals lacking either GSTM1 (OR, 2.9, 95 % CI, 0.8–10.9) or GSTT1 (OR, 3.7, 95 % CI, 0.6–23.5). Individuals with the genotype of the arginine/glutamine polymorphism at codon 399 in the XRCC1 gene (R399)r showed a nonsignificant increased risk of breast cancer (OR, 1.4, 95 % CI, 0.7–2.7) |

magnitude to that of carriers of the *BRCA* mutation [100]. In general, because survival rates are strongly associated with the stage of disease at diagnosis, early initiation of SMN surveillance is recommended. This early surveillance is even more necessary because options become limited for the treatment of SMNs because of prior therapeutic exposures. The COG LTFU Guidelines [101] recommend monitoring for t-MDS/AML with annual complete blood count for 10 years after exposure to alkylating agents or topoisomerase II inhibitors. Most other SMNs are associated with radiation exposure. Screening recommendations include careful annual physical examination of the skin and underlying tissues in the radiation field. Mammography, the most widely accepted screening tool for breast cancer in the general population, may not be the ideal screening tool by itself for radiation-related breast cancers occurring in relatively young women with dense breasts. Hence, the American Cancer Society recommends including adjunct screening with MRI. Thus, the COG LTFU recommendations for females who received radiation with potential impact to the breast (i.e., radiation doses of 20 Gy or higher to the mantle, mediastinal, whole lung, and axillary fields) include monthly breast self-examination beginning at puberty; annual clinical breast examinations beginning at puberty until age 25 years; a clinical breast examination every 6 months, with annual mammograms and MRIs beginning 8 years after radiation or at age 25 (whichever occurs later). Screening of those at risk for early-onset colorectal cancer (i.e., radiation doses of 30 Gy or higher to the abdomen, pelvis, or spine) should include colonoscopy every 5 years beginning at age 35 years or 10 years following radiation (whichever occurs last).

## 19.4   Summary and Future Directions

Our knowledge is constrained by the limited follow-up period (~3 decades) of the existing survivor cohorts. Not until there are large enough numbers of survivors in their fourth and fifth decade of life will we learn how normal aging processes and the natural increase of cancer in the general population influences the development of SMNs in survivors of childhood cancer.

More research is needed to understand the pathogenesis of treatment-related cancers and to characterize those individuals at highest risk. This information needs to be used to develop cancer-risk prediction models to estimate individual risk and help discussions between the doctor and patient about surveillance for SMNs. There is a crucial need to promote and optimize screening for these cancers and develop behavioral and pharmacologic intervention trials to stop or reverse the process of progression of pre-malignant lesions into overt malignant diseases. Finally, there is a critical need to use this information to modify upfront therapy while balancing cure with long-term morbidity.

## References

1. Olsen JH, Moller T, Anderson H et al (2009) Lifelong cancer incidence in 47,697 patients treated for childhood cancer in the Nordic countries. J Natl Cancer Inst 101:806–813
2. Reulen RC, Frobisher C, Winter DL, Kelly J, Lancashire ER, Stiller CA et al (2011) Long-term risks of subsequent primary neoplasms among survivors of childhood cancer. JAMA 305(22):2311–2319
3. Friedman DL, Whitton J, Leisenring W, Mertens AC, Hammond S, Stovall M et al (2010) Subsequent neoplasms in 5-year survivors of childhood cancer: the Childhood Cancer Survivor Study. J Natl Cancer Inst 102(14):1083–1095
4. Armstrong GT, Liu W, Leisenring W et al (2011) Occurrence of subsequent neoplasms in long-term survivors of childhood cancer: a report from the Childhood Cancer Survivor Study. J Clin Oncol 29:3056–3064
5. Bhatia S, Robison LL, Oberlin O, Greenberg M, Bunin G, Fossati-Bellani F et al (1996) Breast cancer and other second neoplasms after childhood Hodgkin's disease. N Engl J Med 334(12):745–751
6. Neglia JP, Robison LL, Stovall M, Liu Y, Packer RJ, Hammond S et al (2006) New primary neoplasms of the central nervous system in survivors of childhood cancer: a report from the Childhood Cancer Survivor Study. J Natl Cancer Inst 98(21):1528–1537
7. Neglia JP, Meadows AT, Robison LL, Kim TH, Newton WA, Ruymann FB et al (1991) Second neoplasms after acute lymphoblastic leukemia in childhood. N Engl J Med 325(19):1330–1336

8. Bhatia S, Yasui Y, Robison LL, Birch JM, Bogue MK, Diller L et al (2003) High risk of subsequent neoplasms continues with extended follow-up of childhood Hodgkin's disease: report from the Late Effects Study Group. J Clin Oncol 21(23):4386–4394

9. Ng AK, Bernardo MV, Weller E (2002) Second malignancy after Hodgkin disease treated with radiation therapy with or without chemotherapy: long-term risks and risk factors. Blood 100:1989–1996

10. Swerdlow AJ, Barber JA, Hudson GV (2000) Risk of second malignancy after Hodgkin's disease in a collaborative British cohort: the relation to age at treatment. J Clin Oncol 18:498–500

11. Bhatia S, Krailo MD, Chen Z, Burden L, Askin FB, Dickman PS et al (2007) Therapy-related myelodysplasia and acute myeloid leukemia after Ewing sarcoma and primitive neuroectodermal tumor of bone: a report from the Children's Oncology Group. Blood 109(1):46–51

12. Bhatia S, Sklar C (2002) Second cancers in survivors of childhood cancer. Nat Rev Cancer 2(2):124–132

13. Bhatia S, Sather HN, Pabustan OB, Trigg ME, Gaynon PS, Robison LL (2002) Low incidence of second neoplasms among children diagnosed with acute lymphoblastic leukemia after 1983. Blood 99:4257–4264

14. Travis LB, Andersson M, Gospodarowicz M, van Leeuwen FE, Bergfeldt K, Lynch CF et al (2000) Treatment-associated leukemia following testicular cancer. J Natl Cancer Inst 92(14):1165–1171

15. Travis LB, Holowaty EJ, Bergfeldt K, Lynch CF, Kohler BA, Wiklund T et al (1999) Risk of leukemia after platinum-based chemotherapy for ovarian cancer. N Engl J Med 340(5):351–357

16. Vardiman JW, Thiele J, Arber DA, Brunning RD, Borowitz MJ, Porwit A et al (2009) The 2008 revision of the World Health Organization (WHO) classification of myeloid neoplasms and acute leukemia: rationale and important changes. Blood 114(5):937–951

17. Smith MA, Rubinstein L, Anderson JR, Arthur D, Catalano PJ, Freidlin B et al (1999) Secondary leukemia or myelodysplastic syndrome after treatment with epipodophyllotoxins. J Clin Oncol 17:569–577

18. Sigurdson AJ, Ronckers CM, Mertens AC, Stovall M, Smith SA, Liu Y et al (2005) Primary thyroid cancer after a first tumour in childhood (the Childhood Cancer Survivor Study): a nested case-control study. Lancet 365(9476):2014–2023

19. Neglia JP, Friedman DL, Yasui Y, Mertens AC, Hammond S, Stovall M et al (2001) Second malignant neoplasms in five-year survivors of childhood cancer: childhood cancer survivor study. J Natl Cancer Inst 93(8):618–629

20. Boice JD Jr, Land C, Preston DL (1996) Ionizing radiation. In: Schottenfield D, Fraumeni JF Jr (eds) Cancer epidemiology and prevention. Oxford University Press, New York, pp 319–354

21. Preston DL, Kusumi S, Tomonaga M, Izumi S, Ron E, Kuramoto A et al (1994) Cancer incidence in atomic bomb survivors. Part III. Leukemia, lymphoma and multiple myeloma, 1950–1987. Radiat Res 137(2 Suppl):S68–S97

22. Thompson DE, Mabuchi K, Ron E, Soda M, Tokunaga M, Ochikubo S et al (1994) Cancer incidence in atomic bomb survivors. Part II: solid tumors, 1958–1987. Radiat Res 137(2 Suppl):S17–S67

23. Ron E, Modan B, Preston D, Alfandary E, Stovall M, Boice JD Jr (1991) Radiation-induced skin carcinomas of the head and neck. Radiat Res 125(3): 318–325

24. Wong FL, Boice JD Jr, Abramson DH, Tarone RE, Kleinerman RA, Stovall M et al (1997) Cancer incidence after retinoblastoma. Radiation dose and sarcoma risk. JAMA 278(15):1262–1267

25. Strong LC, Stine M, Norsted TL (1987) Cancer in survivors of childhood soft tissue sarcoma and their relatives. J Natl Cancer Inst 79(6):1213–1220

26. Land CE, Saku T, Hayashi Y, Takahara O, Matsuura H, Tokuoka S et al (1996) Incidence of salivary gland tumors among atomic bomb survivors, 1950–1987. Evaluation of radiation-related risk. Radiat Res 146(1):28–36

27. Kenney LB, Yasui Y, Inskip PD, Hammond S, Neglia JP, Mertens AC et al (2004) Breast cancer after childhood cancer: a report from the Childhood Cancer Survivor Study. Ann Intern Med 141(8):590–597

28. Metayer C, Lynch CF, Clarke EA, Glimelius B, Storm H, Pukkala E et al (2000) Second cancers among long-term survivors of Hodgkin's disease diagnosed in childhood and adolescence. J Clin Oncol 18(12):2435–2443

29. Wolden SL, Lamborn KR, Cleary SF, Tate DJ, Donaldson SS (1998) Second cancers following pediatric Hodgkin's disease. J Clin Oncol 16(2):536–544

30. Sankila R, Garwicz S, Olsen JH, Dollner H, Hertz H, Kreuger A et al (1996) Risk of subsequent malignant neoplasms among 1,641 Hodgkin's disease patients diagnosed in childhood and adolescence: a population-based cohort study in the five Nordic countries. Association of the Nordic Cancer Registries and the Nordic Society of Pediatric Hematology and Oncology. J Clin Oncol 14(5):1442–1446

31. Friedman DL, Rovo A, Leisenring W et al (2008) Increased risk of breast cancer among survivors of allogeneic hematopoietic cell transplantation: a report from the FHCRC and the EBMT-Late Effect Working Party. Blood 111:939–944

32. Inskip PD, Robison LL, Stovall M et al (2009) Radiation dose and breast cancer risk in the childhood cancer survivor study. J Clin Oncol 27:3901–3907

33. Travis LB, Hill D, Dores GM, Gospodarowicz M, van Leeuwen FE, Holowaty E et al (2005) Cumulative absolute breast cancer risk for young women treated for Hodgkin lymphoma. J Natl Cancer Inst 97(19):1428–1437

34. de Bruin ML, Sparidans J, van't Veer MB et al (2009) Breast cancer risk in female survivors of Hodgkin's lymphoma: lower risk after smaller radiation volumes. J Clin Oncol 27:4239–4246

35. Travis LB, Hill DA, Dores GM (2003) Breast cancer following radiotherapy and chemotherapy among young women with Hodgkin disease. JAMA 290:465–475
36. van Leeuwen FE, Klokman WJ, Stovall M (2003) Roles of radiation dose, chemotherapy, and hormonal factors in breast cancer following Hodgkin's disease. J Natl Cancer Inst 95:971–980
37. Veiga LHS, Lubin J, Anderson H et al (2012) A pooled analysis of thyroid cancer incidence following radiotherapy for childhood cancer. Radiat Res 178:365–376
38. Bhatti P, Veiga LHS, Ronckers CM et al (2010) Risk of second primary thyroid cancer after radiotherapy for a childhood cancer in a large cohort study: an update from the Childhood Cancer Survivor Study. Radiat Res 174:741–752
39. Cohen A, Rovelli A, Merlo DF et al (2007) Risk for secondary thyroid carcinoma after hematopoietic stem-cell transplantation: an EBMT Late Effects Working Party Study. J Clin Oncol 25: 2449–2454
40. Hijiya N, Hudson MM, Lensing S, Zacher M, Onciu M, Behm FG et al (2007) Cumulative incidence of secondary neoplasms as a first event after childhood acute lymphoblastic leukemia. JAMA 297(11):1207–1215
41. Pui CH, Cheng C, Leung W, Rai SN, Rivera GK, Sandlund JT et al (2003) Extended follow-up of long-term survivors of childhood acute lymphoblastic leukemia. N Engl J Med 349(7):640–649
42. Henderson TO, Whitton J, Stovall M, Mertens AC, Mitby P, Friedman D et al (2007) Secondary sarcomas in childhood cancer survivors: a report from the Childhood Cancer Survivor Study. J Natl Cancer Inst 99(4):300–308
43. MacCarthy A, Bayne AM, Brownhill PA et al (2013) Second and subsequent tumours among 1927 retinoblastoma patients diagnosed in Britain 1951–2004. Br J Cancer 108:2455–2463
44. Van Leeuwen FE, Klokman WJ, Stovall M, Hagenbeek A, van den Belt-Dusebout AW, Noyon R et al (1995) Roles of radiotherapy and smoking in lung cancer following Hodgkin's disease. J Natl Cancer Inst 87:1530–1537
45. Deutsch M, Wollman MR, Ramanathan R, Rubin J (2002) Rectal cancer twenty-one years after treatment of childhood Hodgkin disease. Med Pediatr Oncol 38(4):280–281
46. Dores GM, Metayer C, Curtis RE, Lynch CF, Clarke EA, Glimelius B et al (2002) Second malignant neoplasms among long-term survivors of Hodgkin's disease: a population-based evaluation over 25 years. J Clin Oncol 20(16):3484–3494
47. Hodgson DC, Glibert ES, Dores GM (2007) Long-term solid cancer risk among 5-year survivors of Hodgkin's lymphoma. J Clin Oncol 25:1489–1497
48. Bassal M, Mertens AC, Taylor L et al (2006) The risk of selected subsequent carcinomas in survivors of childhood cancer: a report from the Childhood Cancer Survivor Study. J Clin Oncol 24:476–483
49. Shore RE, Moseson M, Xue X et al (2002) Skin cancer after X-ray treatment for scalp ringworm. Radiat Res 157:410–418
50. Limacher JM, Frebourg T, Natarajan-Ame S, Bergerat JP (2001) Two metachronous tumors in the radiotherapy fields of a patient with Li-Fraumeni syndrome. Int J Cancer 96(4):238–242
51. Alter BP (2003) Cancer in Fanconi anemia, 1927–2001. Cancer 97(2):425–440
52. Tischkowitz M, Dokal I (2004) Fanconi anaemia and leukaemia – clinical and molecular aspects. Br J Haematol 126(2):176–191
53. Rosenberg PS, Alter BP, Ebell W (2008) Cancer risks in Fanconi anemia: findings from the German Fanconi Anemia Registry. Haematologica 93(4):511–517
54. Kennedy RD, D'Andrea AD (2005) The Fanconi Anemia/BRCA pathway: new faces in the crowd. Genes Dev 19(24):2925–2940
55. Kalow W, Ozdemir V, Tang BK, Tothfalusi L, Endrenyi L (1999) The science of pharmacological variability: an essay. Clin Pharmacol Ther 66(5):445–447
56. Evans WE, McLeod HL (2003) Pharmacogenomics–drug disposition, drug targets, and side effects. N Engl J Med 348(6):538–549
57. Berwick M, Vineis P (2000) Markers of DNA repair and susceptibility to cancer in humans: an epidemiologic review. J Natl Cancer Inst 92(11):874–897
58. Goode EL, Ulrich CM, Potter JD (2002) Polymorphisms in DNA repair genes and associations with cancer risk. Cancer Epidemiol Biomarkers Prev 11(12):1513–1530
59. Bhatti P, Doody MM, Alexander BH, Yuenger J, Simon SL, Weinstock RM et al (2008) Breast cancer risk polymorphisms and interaction with ionizing radiation among U.S. radiologic technologists. Cancer Epidemiol Biomarkers Prev 17(8):2007–2011
60. Bhatti P, Struewing JP, Alexander BH, Hauptmann M, Bowen L, Mateus-Pereira LH et al (2008) Polymorphisms in DNA repair genes, ionizing radiation exposure and risk of breast cancer in U.S. Radiologic technologists. Int J Cancer 122(1):177–182
61. Rajaraman P, Bhatti P, Doody MM, Simon SL, Weinstock RM, Linet MS et al (2008) Nucleotide excision repair polymorphisms may modify ionizing radiation-related breast cancer risk in US radiologic technologists. Int J Cancer 123(11):2713–2716
62. McFadyen MC, Melvin WT, Murray GI (2004) Cytochrome P450 enzymes: novel options for cancer therapeutics. Mol Cancer Ther 3(3):363–371
63. Park JY, Shigenaga MK, Ames BN (1996) Induction of cytochrome P4501A1 by 2,3,7,8-tetrachlorodibenzo-p-dioxin or indolo(3,2-b) carbazole is associated with oxidative DNA damage. Proc Natl Acad Sci U S A 93(6):2322–2327
64. Hayes JD, Flanagan JU, Jowsey IR (2005) Glutathione transferases. Annu Rev Pharmacol Toxicol 45:51–88

65. Allan JM, Wild CP, Rollinson S, Willett EV, Moorman AV, Dovey GJ et al (2001) Polymorphism in glutathione S-transferase P1 is associated with susceptibility to chemotherapy-induced leukemia. Proc Natl Acad Sci U S A 98(20):11592–11597

66. Collins A, Harrington V (2002) Repair of oxidative DNA damage: assessing its contribution to cancer prevention. Mutagenesis 17(6):489–493

67. Karran P, Offman J, Bignami M (2003) Human mismatch repair, drug-induced DNA damage, and secondary cancer. Biochimie 85(11):1149–1160

68. Casorelli I, Offman J, Mele L, Pagano L, Sica S, D'Errico M et al (2003) Drug treatment in the development of mismatch repair defective acute leukemia and myelodysplastic syndrome. DNA Repair (Amst) 2(5):547–559

69. Seedhouse CH, Das-Gupta EP, Russell NH (2003) Methylation of the hMLH1 promoter and its association with microsatellite instability in acute myeloid leukemia. Leukemia 17(1):83–88

70. Zhu YM, Das-Gupta EP, Russell NH (1999) Microsatellite instability and p53 mutations are associated with abnormal expression of the MSH2 gene in adult acute leukemia. Blood 94(2):733–740

71. Worrillow LJ, Travis LB, Smith AG, Rollinson S, Smith AJ, Wild CP et al (2003) An intron splice acceptor polymorphism in hMSH2 and risk of leukemia after treatment with chemotherapeutic alkylating agents. Clin Cancer Res 9(8):3012–3020

72. Horiike S, Misawa S, Kaneko H, Sasai Y, Kobayashi M, Fujii H et al (1999) Distinct genetic involvement of the TP53 gene in therapy-related leukemia and myelodysplasia with chromosomal losses of Nos 5 and/or 7 and its possible relationship to replication error phenotype. Leukemia 13(8):1235–1242

73. Fishel R, Lescoe MK, Rao MR, Copeland NG, Jenkins NA, Garber J et al (1993) The human mutator gene homolog MSH2 and its association with hereditary nonpolyposis colon cancer. Cell 75(5):1027–1038

74. Brentnall TA, Rubin CE, Crispin DA, Stevens A, Batchelor RH, Haggitt RC et al (1995) A germline substitution in the human MSH2 gene is associated with high-grade dysplasia and cancer in ulcerative colitis. Gastroenterology 109(1):151–155

75. Worrillow LJ, Allan JM (2006) Deregulation of homologous recombination DNA repair in alkylating agent-treated stem cell clones: a possible role in the aetiology of chemotherapy-induced leukaemia. Oncogene 25(12):1709–1720

76. O'Driscoll M, Jeggo PA (2006) The role of double-strand break repair – insights from human genetics. Nat Rev Genet 7(1):45–54

77. Baumann P, West SC (1998) Role of the human RAD51 protein in homologous recombination and double-stranded-break repair. Trends Biochem Sci 23(7):247–251

78. Jawad M, Seedhouse CH, Russell N, Plumb M (2006) Polymorphisms in human homeobox HLX1 and DNA repair RAD51 genes increase the risk of therapy-related acute myeloid leukemia. Blood 108(12):3916–3918

79. Seedhouse C, Faulkner R, Ashraf N, Das-Gupta E, Russell N (2004) Polymorphisms in genes involved in homologous recombination repair interact to increase the risk of developing acute myeloid leukemia. Clin Cancer Res 10(8):2675–2680

80. Bishop DK, Ear U, Bhattacharyya A, Calderone C, Beckett M, Weichselbaum RR et al (1998) Xrcc3 is required for assembly of Rad51 complexes in vivo. J Biol Chem 273(34):21482–21488

81. Liu N, Lamerdin JE, Tebbs RS, Schild D, Tucker JD, Shen MR et al (1998) XRCC2 and XRCC3, new human Rad51-family members, promote chromosome stability and protect against DNA cross-links and other damages. Mol Cell 1(6):783–793

82. Tebbs RS, Zhao Y, Tucker JD, Scheerer JB, Siciliano MJ, Hwang M et al (1995) Correction of chromosomal instability and sensitivity to diverse mutagens by a cloned cDNA of the XRCC3 DNA repair gene. Proc Natl Acad Sci U S A 92(14):6354–6358

83. Pierce AJ, Johnson RD, Thompson LH, Jasin M (1999) XRCC3 promotes homology-directed repair of DNA damage in mammalian cells. Genes Dev 13(20):2633–2638

84. Shen MR, Jones IM, Mohrenweiser H (1998) Nonconservative amino acid substitution variants exist at polymorphic frequency in DNA repair genes in healthy humans. Cancer Res 58(4):604–608

85. Matullo G, Palli D, Peluso M, Guarrera S, Carturan S, Celentano E et al (2001) XRCC1, XRCC3, XPD gene polymorphisms, smoking and (32) P-DNA adducts in a sample of healthy subjects. Carcinogenesis 22(9):1437–1445

86. Au WW, Salama SA, Sierra-Torres CH (2003) Functional characterization of polymorphisms in DNA repair genes using cytogenetic challenge assays. Environ Health Perspect 111(15): 1843–1850

87. Coiteux V, Onclercq-Delic R, Fenaux P, Amor-Gueret M (2007) Predisposition to therapy-related acute leukemia with balanced chromosomal translocations does not result from a major constitutive defect in DNA double-strand break end joining. Leuk Res 31(3):353–358

88. Caldecott KW, McKeown CK, Tucker JD, Ljungquist S, Thompson LH (1994) An interaction between the mammalian DNA repair protein XRCC1 and DNA ligase III. Mol Cell Biol 14(1):68–76

89. Kubota Y, Nash RA, Klungland A, Schar P, Barnes DE, Lindahl T (1996) Reconstitution of DNA base excision-repair with purified human proteins: interaction between DNA polymerase beta and the XRCC1 protein. EMBO J 15(23):6662–6670

90. Seedhouse C, Bainton R, Lewis M, Harding A, Russell N, Das-Gupta E (2002) The genotype distribution of the XRCC1 gene indicates a role for base excision repair in the development of therapy-related acute myeloblastic leukemia. Blood 100(10):3761–3766

91. Nelson HH, Kelsey KT, Mott LA, Karagas MR (2002) The XRCC1 Arg399Gln polymorphism, sunburn, and non-melanoma skin cancer: evidence of gene-environment interaction. Cancer Res 62(1):152–155

92. Allan JM, Smith AG, Wheatley K, Hills RK, Travis LB, Hill DA et al (2004) Genetic variation in XPD predicts treatment outcome and risk of acute myeloid leukemia following chemotherapy. Blood 104(13):3872–3877

93. Ellis NA, Huo D, Yildiz O, Worrillow LJ, Banerjee M, Le Beau MM et al (2008) MDM2 SNP309 and TP53 Arg72Pro interact to alter therapy-related acute myeloid leukemia susceptibility. Blood 112(3):741–749

94. Knight JA, Skol AD, Shinde A, Hastings D, Walgren RA, Shao J et al (2009) Genome-wide association study to identify novel loci associated with therapy-related myeloid leukemia susceptibility. Blood 113(22):5575–5582

95. Best T, Li D, Skol AD, Kirchhoff T, Jackson SA, Yasui Y et al (2011) Variants at 6q21 implicate PRDM1 in the etiology of therapy-induced second malignancies after Hodgkin's lymphoma. Nat Med 17(8):941–943

96. Mertens AC, Liu Q, Neglia JP, Wasilewski K, Leisenring W, Armstrong GT et al (2008) Cause-specific late mortality among 5-year survivors of childhood cancer: the Childhood Cancer Survivor Study. J Natl Cancer Inst 100(19):1368–1379

97. Oeffinger KC, Mertens AC, Sklar CA et al (2006) Chronic health conditions in adult survivors of childhood cancer. N Engl J Med 355:1572–1582

98. Jenkinson HC, Hawkins MM, Stiller CA, Winter DL, Marsden HB, Stevens MC (2004) Long-term population-based risks of second malignant neoplasm after childhood cancer in Britain. Br J Cancer 91:1905–1910

99. Meadows AT, Friedman DL, Neglia JP et al (2009) Second neoplasms in survivors of childhood cancer: findings from the Childhood Cancer Survivor Study cohort. J Clin Oncol 27:2356–2362

100. Begg CB, Haile RW, Borg A et al (2008) Variation of breast cancer risk among BRCA1/2 carriers. JAMA 299:194–201

101. Landier W, Bhatia S, Eshelman DA et al (2004) Development of risk-based guidelines for pediatric cancer survivors: the Children's Oncology Group long-term follow-up guidelines from the Children's Oncology Group Late Effects Committee and Nursing Discipline. J Clin Oncol 22:4979–4990

102. Worrillow LJ, Smith AG, Scott K, Andersson M, Ashcroft AJ, Dores GM et al (2008) Polymorphic MLH1 and risk of cancer after methylating chemotherapy for Hodgkin lymphoma. J Med Genet 45(3):142–146

103. Mertens AC, Mitby PA, Radloff G, Jones IM, Perentesis J, Kiffmeyer WR et al (2004) XRCC1 and glutathione-S-transferase gene polymorphisms and susceptibility to radiotherapy-related malignancies in survivors of Hodgkin disease. Cancer 101(6):1463–1472

# Psychological Aspects of Long-Term Survivorship

# 20

Mary T. Rourke, Kate K. Samson,
and Anne E. Kazak

## Contents

M.T. Rourke, PhD (✉) • K.K. Samson, MA
Institute for Graduate Clinical Psychology,
Widener University, One University Avenue,
Chester, PA 19013, USA
e-mail: mrourke@widener.edu

A.E. Kazak, PhD, ABPP
Pediatric Behavioral Health, Department of
Pediatrics, Nemours Children's Health System and
Thomas Jefferson University, Wilmington, DE, USA

Childhood cancer survivors and their families can be surprised by the realization that cancer does not end when treatment ends and that life does not automatically return to normal. As families manage the many transitions that accompany the end of treatment, they find that cancer survivorship has its own set of medical and psychological issues. Medical visits and monitoring continue – initially for disease recurrence and then for the emergence of medical late effects – and longer-term psychological reactions emerge. For these reasons, it is more accurate to conceive of cancer survivorship as a stage in a life-long chronic illness, rather than as an acute illness that ends with "cure" or the attainment of "survivorship" status [74]. The goal of this chapter is to provide an overview of psychological late effects of childhood cancer and present guidance for managing these effects.

The term "psychological late effects" refers to the influence of cancer, treatment, and survivorship on survivors' and family members' feelings, thoughts, behaviors, relationships, and development. Like medical late effects, psychological late effects can occur early (in the year or two after treatment ends) or may emerge later, including many years after treatment ends. The breadth of this definition reflects the impact that psychological late effects can have in many domains of a survivor's life. The development of psychological symptoms (e.g., depression, behavior disorders, posttraumatic stress), the functional impact

© Springer International Publishing 2015
C.L. Schwartz et al. (eds.), *Survivors of Childhood and Adolescent Cancer:
A Multidisciplinary Approach*, Pediatric Oncology, DOI 10.1007/978-3-319-16435-9_20

of cancer/quality of life, and peer relationships/ social skills are addressed in this chapter. Because childhood cancer is a powerful experience not only for the diagnosed child but also for those closely involved with him or her, we will examine psychological late effects that survivors' family members may experience.

## 20.1 Psychological Symptoms in Childhood Cancer Survivors

### 20.1.1 Depression and Behavior Disorders

Although health-care providers may assume that high rates of depression or behavioral disorders are common in childhood cancer survivors, there is actually little evidence for this. In fact, findings consistently report resilience and relatively good psychological health among pediatric cancer survivors [45]. Although early research focusing on young survivors of childhood cancer indicated that parents reported higher than average levels of somatic symptoms in children (e.g., headaches, stomachaches, toileting issues) [63, 69], most research has shown no unusual levels of psychological symptoms in survivors during childhood and adolescence. Across a number of studies, overall rates of depression [68], behavioral disorders [67, 69] and other general psychological symptoms [20, 52, 91] reported by children and their parents have been comparable to rates reported by children who never had cancer.

A more recent study of adolescent survivors (ages 12–17) found slight increases in psychological symptoms in survivors, relative to their siblings. Specifically, survivors were more likely to report depression/anxiety and antisocial/ behavior problems, as well as attentional difficulties [93]. Survivors of CNS tumors, leukemia, and neuroblastoma, and particularly those who received cranial radiation therapy and intrathecal methotrexate during treatment, were most at risk for developing psychological symptoms during survivorship [93].

Most recent research has aimed at examining longer-term psychological late effects in older survivors of childhood cancer. In general, adolescent and young adult (AYA) survivors' rates of depressive symptoms and general psychological distress are comparable to those of peers [43, 55] or to normative data [87]. A report from the Childhood Cancer Survivor Study (CCSS) identified higher levels of depressive and somatic symptoms in survivors than in their siblings, but survivors' overall rates of depressive and somatic symptoms were within the normal range [106, 109, 110]. A large-scale population-based study in the UK concluded that survivors of childhood cancer rate their mental health similarly to those in the general population [84], while a large Danish study found that overall rates of depression and other psychiatric disorders in survivors of childhood cancers other than brain tumor were consistent with national norms. In the latter study, however, survivors of brain tumors experienced higher levels of depression and other presumably organic disorders (e.g., psychoses, schizophrenia), as well as a higher rate of psychiatric hospitalization compared to survivors of other childhood cancers [87]. Aggression and antisocial behavior in young adult survivors occur at rates comparable to those in never-ill peers, while survivors' use of alcohol and illegal drugs may be less frequent than that of peers [102] or siblings [112].

Although most survivors are not depressed and report that they are doing well overall, a subset of patients does experience some form of significant psychological distress [112]. Compared to their siblings, childhood cancer survivors are twice as likely to report clinical levels of emotional distress [112]. One quarter to one third of AYA survivors report higher than average levels of global psychological distress [26, 52, 80], with a higher than expected percentage reporting that they have experienced suicidal symptoms [79, 80]. Certain risk factors predict higher levels of psychological distress. As is true in the general population, increased psychological distress in survivors is associated with being female, having lower levels of educational attainment, being unmarried, having a low household income, being unemployed, or having a major medical condition [112]. Some treatment-related variables are also associated with distress. There is some evidence that increased parental distress at diagnosis is related to young adult distress later in survivorship [86], and survivors with more intense treatment report more distress, particularly in the form of anxiety or somatic symptoms [43, 112]. In addition, poor current health, or severity of medical late effects, is associated with higher levels of distress; poor current health also predicts suicidality, even after adjusting for mood- and treatment-related variables [34, 79, 106, 111]. This finding suggests that cancer-related distress may be related to compromised physical health [106].

## 20.1.2  Posttraumatic Stress

Ratings of global distress, coupled with the lack of evidence for any one clear psychological diagnosis, have led researchers to speculate that more traditional or general measures of psychopathology and well-being may not capture the specific experiences of childhood cancer survivors [38]. One alternative is to view cancer (and, potentially, aspects of the cancer survivorship period) as traumatic events, which may in turn lead to the experience of posttraumatic stress in the survivorship years [38, 89, 97].

It is easy to see the ways in which childhood cancer can be traumatic. At diagnosis, parents are told explicitly that their child may die. Patients may hear this or may interpret life threat from their parents' urgency and intense emotional reactions, their own physical reactions to treatment, and the abrupt changes in their family routine. Cancer treatment can be experienced as a horrifying, scary, painful series of events for everyone involved, ranging from events like losing hair to feeling nauseous to experiencing repeated, painful, invasive procedures. Patients and their families may watch other children, with whom they have developed relationships, die of the same disease they are fighting. Likewise, survivorship can offer its own set of traumatic events. Just when survivors are reaching a stage of development at which they are becoming more independent, they may be faced with significant late effects – such as cardiovascular disease, infertility, or cognitive limitation – that limit or otherwise affect the life choices available to

them. Further, it is not uncommon for survivors to know fellow survivors who have died of a recurrence or medical late effect.

Posttraumatic stress reactions to these traumatic events can emerge soon after the initial traumatic event or many years later and can continue or recur for many years. Three kinds of posttraumatic stress symptoms may emerge: persistent reexperiencing of the traumatic parts of the cancer/survivorship experience (including intrusive thoughts, nightmares, or strong negative feelings triggered by reminders), actual or considered avoidance of cancer- or survivorship-related situations, and strong physiological responses when reminded about cancer or survivorship [3, 44]. Survivors may experience some of these posttraumatic stress symptoms (PTSS), resulting in varying levels of distress, or they can develop several symptoms in all three of the categories described above. If this happens, and if the symptoms significantly interfere with their normal activities, they may meet the criteria for diagnosis of posttraumatic stress disorder (PTSD).

Research has documented higher levels of both PTSS and PTSD in cancer survivors and in their family members. Rates of PTSD for adolescent survivors are generally low and roughly comparable to rates in non-ill adolescents (ranging from 5 to 10 %; [11, 22, 41]). Most adolescent survivors, however, do report at least some symptoms of PTSD; approximately 10–20 % scored in the clinical range on psychological measures, and more than 75 % meet at least one cluster criterion (i.e., reexperiencing, arousal) used to diagnose PTSD [10, 22, 43]. In one study, 50 % of adolescent survivors reported reexperiencing symptoms, and 29 % reported increased physiological responses when reminded of their cancer/survivorship experience [41].

Developmentally, PTSD and PTSS appear to be even more prominent for childhood cancer survivors during young adulthood, where 15–21 % of young adult survivors report experiencing PTSD. In addition, more than 75 % of young adult survivors report reexperiencing difficult moments of treatment/survivorship, nearly half reported increased physiological reactions when reminded of cancer/survivorship, and one quarter attempt to or want to avoid cancer-related situations [88]. Higher levels of posttraumatic stress were found among survivors diagnosed and treated during adolescence than those diagnosed at younger ages, and among those who experienced more intense treatment [43]. Data indicate that for child and adolescent survivors, traumatic reactions are associated with concrete events like losing hair or experiencing painful procedures. For young adult survivors, these reactions to concrete events persist but are accompanied by two kinds of additional distress: distress over the retrospective realization of the life threat that they experienced and worry over medical late effects that exist or may occur [41]. The presence of long-term medical complications may act as a trigger for posttraumatic stress, consistent with the finding that the experience of a significant medical condition is associated with higher levels of distress and anxiety [112].

Although PTS symptoms are often subclinical, they can significantly impede survivors' development and/or their ability to manage their health care. For example, an adolescent who is very upset when reminded of her treatment experience may avoid talking or thinking about her cancer. She may not feel comfortable socializing with friends or dating, even though she would like to do these things. A child or adolescent might become so distracted by a high level of worry or vigilance about his health that his ability to focus at school suffers, resulting in lower or inconsistent grades. For young adult survivors, concerns related to cognitive or physical limitations may prevent the establishment of independence, and worries about infertility and other medical late effects can interfere with intimate relationships and family planning. Young adults, who are assuming more responsibility for their health care, may avoid thinking about their medical needs and/or participating in recommended screenings. Data from the CCSS indicate that only 35 % of survivors recognize their cancer-related medical risks and more than half do not participate in regular follow-up care [66]. Because survivors may report no other significant areas of difficulty and their distress may be limited to cancer- or survivorship-related triggers that are not readily observable to others, it may

be difficult to discern that they are experiencing posttraumatic stress.

Family members also may experience PTSS and PTSD. Although rates of PTSD in mothers and fathers range from 5 to 20 % across studies [39, 41, 56, 57], at least one third of families of adolescent survivors have one or more members with cancer-related PTSD. In addition, subclinical rates of PTSS in family members are common. Mothers and fathers of survivors report significantly more PTSS than do parents of never-ill children [39, 42]. Nearly all families (99 %) have at least one family member with reexperiencing symptoms; over 80 % have one member with increased physiological reactions when reminded of cancer; and nearly half have a member who avoids reminders of cancer [40]. Adolescent siblings, too, appear to have mild to moderate levels of PTSS in response to a brother's or sister's cancer [1, 2]. Common sibling reactions include persistent worries about the survivor's health and distress when reminded of the cancer experience. Like the adolescent survivors, adolescent siblings may be functioning well overall, and the posttraumatic stress may not be readily apparent.

There is some evidence that certain treatment-related factors may predispose survivors and family members to develop PTSD or PTSS. For survivors, having more intense treatment and being diagnosed during adolescence (vs. school-age) appear to be related to PTSS. In addition, for young adult survivors, the presence of severe medical late effects is related to higher levels of posttraumatic stress [88, 112]. For both survivors and family members, what they *believe* about their treatment intensity, current and past life threat, and impact of cancer in their lives is related to posttraumatic stress [31, 47, 107].

## 20.2 Positive Psychological Outcomes After Childhood Cancer

Increasingly, researchers are challenging the assumption that the trauma and distress of the childhood cancer experience will result only in psychological difficulties and are exploring the possibility that childhood cancer survivorship may also be associated with positive psychological outcomes. Terms such as posttraumatic growth and benefit finding refer to the degree to which survivors construct a positive meaning or benefit to their experience and translate that benefit into psychological growth [4, 61, 108].

Research has supported the experience of benefit finding in childhood cancer. In a study of 150 adolescent survivors, nearly 85 % reported at least one positive consequence of their cancer experience, and almost one third of the sample reported four or more positive consequence [5]. Benefit finding has been documented, as well, in adolescents still on treatment [76] and in a British sample of adolescent survivors and parents [61]. The large Childhood Cancer Survivor Study, surveying more than 6,000 adult survivors of childhood cancer, documented higher levels of perceived positive impact of cancer in survivors, relative to their siblings [108]. Qualitative explorations of the positive psychological outcomes associated with childhood cancer survivorship have found that survivors report increased psychological maturity, greater levels of compassion and empathy, a reordered set of values and priorities that emphasize the importance of close relationships, and an appreciation of new strengths gained from dealing with the challenges of cancer and survivorship [73].

Across several studies, positive growth is associated with older age at diagnosis, less time since end of treatment, and with certain diagnoses (bone tumor and leukemia survivors report more growth; [5, 61, 108]). Much like negative psychological outcomes after cancer, positive outcomes may also be related to subjective appraisals. Individuals who perceive greater life threat and treatment severity [5] and who believe that the illness continues to affect them [61] reported more benefit finding. While few studies have explored the relationship between benefit finding in survivors and their family members, early literature does suggest that while parents, too, report benefit finding, there is not an association between child and parent benefit finding in the same family [61]. This emerging area of

research will continue to elaborate our knowledge of the complex interplay of both positive and negative outcomes associated with the childhood cancer experience.

## 20.3   Quality of Life and Functional Impact of Cancer

A number of studies have looked at the more global construct of quality of life to assess psychological late effects and overall functioning in the years after childhood cancer. These studies agree that, overall, AYA survivors of childhood cancer report good functioning in physical and general psychosocial domains [13, 19, 43, 53, 107, 109]. Despite good overall quality of life among survivors, a notable minority of survivors reports lower than average physical quality of life, with specific concerns over medical late effects, health issues in general, or the possibility that a second cancer may emerge [13, 53, 105, 112]. This lower physical quality of life is likely related to the increased number of health problems reported by survivors relative to siblings and age-matched peers [35, 95]. As in the general population, several factors predict lower quality of life in survivors, including female sex, lower educational attainment, unemployment, and being unmarried [112]. Cancer-related predictors of lower quality of life include having received cranial radiation, having had a CNS or bone tumor, and having a major medical late effect [43, 83, 107, 112]. Mothers report more negative quality of life for their adolescent survivors than survivors report themselves [19], suggesting the importance of asking both children and their mothers, independently, about quality of life issues.

Studies documenting the impact of childhood cancer on educational, employment, and achievement of developmental milestones are largely consistent with survivors' generally positive perceived quality of life. Overall, survivors finish high school and earn bachelor's degrees at rates comparable to those of their siblings [29, 54, 55]. Some survivors are at greater risk for difficulties. Those who were treated before the age of 6, who survived a brain tumor, or who received intrathecal methotrexate and/or cranial radiation (especially at doses higher than 24 Gy) are at risk for learning disabilities and special education placements and are less likely to finish high school and complete a bachelor's degree [29, 54, 62, 64]. Educational challenges for survivors of CNS tumors are likely related to well-documented cognitive effects of these tumors and their associated treatments. Multiple studies have documented significant and progressive declines in intellectual function and academic achievement in the years after brain tumor treatment [16], as well as deficits in executive functions, including attention, working memory, and processing speed [104].

While some studies suggest that survivors of non-CNS cancers have employment rates similar to those of the general population [7, 25], other research indicates that survivors report more unemployment than do their siblings [49, 64]. Cancer-related differences may exist even for those survivors who are employed. Survivors earn less and are less likely to hold managerial or professional positions than are their siblings [49]. As in other areas of function, survivors of CNS tumors have increased vulnerability in the employment domain and demonstrate higher rates of unemployment, lower income, and a decreased likelihood of working in a managerial/professional position than other survivors [7, 49]. Consistent with these findings, survivors with neurocognitive changes are also less likely to live independently as adults [51]. Differences in employment may lead to insurance challenges for childhood cancer survivors.

## 20.4  Survivors' Health Beliefs

Beliefs, or cognitive appraisals of oneself, the world, and future, provide important ways to understand survivors and to inform psychosocial treatment approaches. As noted above, survivors who believe that their treatment was more intense, that they did or do have a more significant life threat related to their cancer treatment, and/or those who have negative perceptions of cancer's impact report more distress and poorer quality of life [31, 107]. More focused exploration of survi-

vors' health beliefs can help clarify this link. Beliefs specific to health, termed "health competence beliefs," have been conceptualized to describe how AYAs (both with and without a cancer history) think about their health and well-being [15]. A study utilizing the Health Competence Beliefs Inventory (HCBI; [15]), a 21-item patient report scale that captures clinically relevant beliefs associated with four domains (Health Perceptions [e.g., I have a reason to worry about my health], Satisfaction with Healthcare [e.g., My doctor understands my concerns], Cognitive Competence [e.g., My memory is not as good as others], and Autonomy [e.g., I feel comfortable going to the doctor by myself]), AYA cancer survivors reported less positive health competence beliefs compared to AYAs without a significant medical history on all HCBI subscales except Satisfaction with Healthcare [43]. Health competence beliefs influenced the relationship between the number of health problems survivors reported and PTSS, such that having less positive health competence beliefs increased the likelihood that health problems would be associated with PTSS [94]. There is also some indication that more adaptive beliefs about cognitive competence are associated with positive health behaviors, specifically physical activity [32].

## 20.5  Effects on Social Development

Developing social relationships is a primary task of childhood and adolescence and provides children with the contextual experience necessary to build an understanding of who they are, as well as a sense of competence. Because cancer and treatment at least partially remove children from the normal everyday activities in which most children build these relationships, social development is an area of risk for survivors.

Several reports indicate that childhood cancer survivors show some social developmental differences. Overall, survivors are rated by teachers and peers to be more socially isolated and have fewer best friends than do other children [6, 101]. They participate in fewer than half as many normative peer activities (e.g., going to a friend's house, going out with friends, playing sports) as do their never-ill peers [75]. Children whose physical appearance and athletic ability were affected by their treatment may be at higher risk for some of these social challenges [82, 101].

For survivors of non-CNS malignancies, however, there seem to be few immediate consequences of these social differences. Despite being identified as more socially isolated and having fewer best friends, childhood cancer survivors are as well liked as their classmates [100]. Teachers rate survivors as less aggressive than other children and, in some studies, as more sociable [24]. Further, as mentioned above, survivors themselves do not report feeling lonely or depressed.

The evidence on social development is not as positive for children treated for a CNS malignancy [82]. Several studies identify difficulties in social competence and communication skills with peers, as well as social isolation [23, 33, 77, 92, 100]. Classmates recognize the changed social status of children treated for brain tumors and continue to view them as being "sick," even many years after treatment has ended [100].

It is likely that compromises in social competence are related to the cognitive changes that many brain tumor survivors experience as a result of their disease and treatment [92]. Specifically, cognitive impairments may impede children's ability to interpret and express nonverbal social information and respond appropriately to social cues. In one study of social skills, brain tumor survivors made significantly more errors interpreting adult facial expressions than children with juvenile rheumatoid arthritis [8]. In a different study of brain tumor survivors, verbal memory and learning problems accounted for much of the social withdrawal seen in the children, while difficulties in verbal fluency and decreased IQ were significantly related to difficulties with attention, inhibition, and social functioning [33].

Over time, brain tumor survivors may experience increasing challenges associated with social competence. In a large Danish study of long-term childhood cancer survivors, brain tumor survivors (but not survivors of non-CNS malignancies) were significantly more likely to experience psychiatric hospitalization and to demonstrate a higher risk of organically caused psychotic ill-

ness [87]. In a review of literature published between 2000 and 2009, time since diagnosis was consistently related to social adjustment, with social outcomes becoming increasingly negative as time since diagnosis increased [92].

For both survivors of CNS and non-CNS malignancies, the potential for longer-term problems associated with social competence differences exists, but has not been well researched. Being less involved with peers – a result of school absences and increased rates of social isolation – may deprive survivors of the social practice they will need as young adults. For survivors with less immediate social difficulties, challenges may emerge over time and might not be evident until several years after treatment ends. Although some research indicates that social functioning among young adult survivors is similar to that of comparison peers [25], other research suggests that adult survivors of childhood cancer have more difficulty with close friendships and romantic relationships, reporting shorter intimate relationships characterized by a lack of confiding or personal involvement [55]. Young adult survivors have fewer intimate relationships and romantic partners, which may relate to social factors as well as physical and cognitive changes [36, 81, 98]. For survivors of CNS tumors, these relational difficulties may be more pronounced [98]. Consistent with these findings, several studies have shown that survivors have lower marriage rates than siblings or population norms, with survivors of CNS tumors demonstrating the lowest marriage rates [54, 78]. More thorough work in this area is necessary to better understand different developmental pathways leading to long-term social outcomes for survivors.

### 20.5.1 Social Consequences for Survivors' Family Members

There has been very little research on the social consequences of childhood cancer for members of a survivor's family. Some research suggests that parents may feel lonely or isolated after treatment ends [99]. A qualitative study of parents' experiences at the end of treatment indicated that the transition off treatment is a confusing and complicated one for parents and requires significant adjustment in terms of personal coping skills and social support resources [60]. A review of literature from the past three decades documented the vulnerability experienced by many parents at the end of active treatment. While parents routinely celebrate as treatment ends, they also report significant fear of recurrence, fatigue, and loneliness [103].

Even many years into survivorship, parents may have continued concerns about their child's health, while the number of people available to hear and respond to those concerns decreases substantially. Medical teams are seen less frequently, while friends and family members – relieved by the victory of survival – may not understand a parent's medical concerns. In one study comparing survivor parents to parents of children currently on treatment, the two groups demonstrated comparable levels of distress, indicating that parents of survivors continue to feel vulnerable for many years after treatment ends [28]. Being aware that these feelings can emerge, and finding new ways to talk to supportive people in their lives about the stage of cancer survivorship, can help parents feel more connected and less isolated. Increasingly, parents are also turning to books, on-line support groups, websites, listservs, and other media to reduce feelings of isolation (see [48], for a particularly good resource for parents and others close to long-term survivors). Understanding parental concerns may be particularly relevant for CNS tumor survivors; given that their higher frequency of unemployment and lower rates of involvement in intimate relationships may keep families of origin more closely involved to meet survivors' needs.

## 20.6    Implications for the Transition to Follow-Up Care

Participation in regular follow-up care is strongly recommended for long-term survivors in order to provide prevention and/or early detection of medical late effects [17, 27, 30, 70, 85]. Despite clear guidelines for ongoing follow-up care,

fewer than half of adult survivors of childhood cancers successfully transition to adult medical care that is tailored to their cancer-related medical risks [65, 71].

Research has begun to explore the complex network of variables that support or undermine successful transition to adult follow-up care (see chapter on transitions in this volume). Psychosocial issues – including distress, beliefs, quality of life, and relationships with family and medical team members – represent an important set of factors that can contribute to the success of care transitions [27, 50, 96]. A model of psychosocial readiness for transition proposed by Schwartz, Tuchman, Hobbie, and Ginsberg [96] suggests that successful transition will be facilitated by a consideration of a nested set of individual and relational variables. On an individual level, the model suggests that demographics (older age at time of treatment, higher SES), cognitive status (average or higher levels of intelligence), and psychological health will facilitate survivors' readiness for transition. Further, they suggest that successful transition is more likely when survivors have access to care (they have insurance and providers are available), have a degree of developmental maturity and autonomy that matches the demands of the adult health-care system, have knowledge of their health-care needs, and have the ability to interact with family and medical providers about health-related issues with little distress [96]. The authors provide some evidence that pediatric survivorship providers use these criteria when making readiness decisions [96].

Evidence does suggest that individual and ecological variables relate to transition success. Patients who are non-White, who do not have medical insurance, and who have not had the urgency of a second cancer are less likely to attend follow-up visits and successfully transition to survivorship care [50]. It also makes good clinical sense that psychological distress would relate to participation in follow-up care. Even low to moderate symptoms of posttraumatic stress, common in survivors, can result in avoidance of care, which may be exacerbated when there is a transition in medical providers.

Participating in follow-up care itself may elicit distress. Survivors might become more upset and even be re-traumatized by follow-up visits, as they hear about medical complications possibly associated with their treatment. While there are few studies of the direct link between emotional responses and successful transition, a qualitative study of young adult survivors demonstrates how emotional responses can affect participation in follow-up care. All survivors interviewed for the study reported survivorship-related fear and anxiety; for some, the fear motivated them to seek care, and for others the fear prompted avoidance [27]. The same survivors also reported the power of positive emotions in facilitating transition. Those survivors who felt gratitude and significant personal change associated with cancer were more likely to transition successfully [27].

Survivors' beliefs may also be related in important ways to successful transition. As outlined above, there is some variability in survivors' beliefs about health competence (e.g., beliefs that one has autonomy, is satisfied with health care, and perceives oneself to be both cognitively competent and not in fragile health; [15]). These kinds of beliefs may also facilitate or hinder transition to care. For example, when interviewed, adult survivors of childhood cancers indicated that beliefs about their identity, the role of cancer in their current lives, and the impact of talking about cancer on their families affected whether or not they transitioned to follow-up care. Those survivors who integrated cancer into their identity in a positive way and who identified themselves as survivors were more likely to transition successfully [27]. Survivors who did not identify as a cancer survivor, who believed that cancer's impact was isolated to and belonged in the past, and who believed that talking about cancer was traumatic to family and should be avoided were less likely to transition successfully [12, 27].

Given the importance of follow-up care, successful transition may depend on medical teams, families, and patients themselves attending to indicators of transition readiness well before the transition occurs. Working with survivors to identify transition risk factors and to prepare them for transitions to follow-up care can minimize the percentage of patients who "fail" transition. Attention to psychosocial variables should begin during active treatment, at a time when trusted health-care providers can provide anticipatory guidance regarding the potential for normative medical and psychological late effects, as well as the availability of and need for long-term medical care [27].

On an individual level, identifying and addressing psychological needs both before and after transition is a critical element of providing survivorship care. An important component of psychosocially informed care is to institute comprehensive but brief psychosocial screening into every follow-up visit for every patient [80]. There is some evidence that survivors are receptive to psychosocial screening and interventions in the context of their follow-up care (e.g., [21, 43, 80]), although there is a lack of clarity regarding exactly what form of specific screening should take. Screenings will best inform subsequent referrals if they include assessments of issues specific to the cancer experience (rather than assessments of global distress). Although health-care providers may be able to use standardized symptom questionnaires, survivors may share more information directly relevant to their health-related experiences and concerns in direct face-to-face conversation about cancer-specific symptoms [88]. During annual clinic visits, for example, it is important for providers to ask specific questions about survivors' achievement of appropriate developmental milestones (e.g., education, employment, relationships), emotional distress, and about specific symptoms of posttraumatic stress (i.e., reexperiencing, avoidance, and arousal). Systematic assessment of symptoms of pain and fatigue should also be part of each assessment, given the relationship between these somatic symptoms and psychosocial distress. Treatment and demographic variables can be used during screening to identify patients at high risk for distress and, potential, transition risk. Specifically, patients who survived CNS tumors or leukemia, as well as those who report significant current health problems, should merit a more careful exploration of distress and quality of life concerns, as should those who are unemployed or report a low household income.

In addition, gathering an assessment of survivors' health-care beliefs can provide important information on ability to navigate important health-care activities [43]. Understanding the degree to which survivors see themselves as changed by cancer, as well as the degree to which they feel cancer should be kept in the past can direct pre-transition interventions; aligning survivors with group activities, for example, to build a positive cancer-related identity may ease transition [27]. Similar interventions aimed at building beliefs that will support transition, based on Health Competence Beliefs, are listed in Table 20.1. Knowing a survivor's strengths, as well as the specific symptoms he or she experiences, will round out a full picture of strengths and vulnerabilities of each patient.

Attending to developmental issues associated with survivorship can also facilitate good transition planning. Childhood cancer survivors may not have had full access to information during their treatments and often learn of their long-term medical risks for the first time during a follow-up visit [37]. Further, as childhood cancer survivors reach new developmental stages and new levels of cognitive understanding, it may be necessary to reteach health-related information. As survivors reach adulthood and take on the direct responsibility of managing their own health care,

this complex task that was formerly handled by parents and can be overwhelming and frightening – and might require more support and direction for the survivor. Being aware of each survivor's developmental trajectory and tailoring psychoeducation and support to that level can facilitate survivors' engagement in care.

In order to accommodate these concerns, it is critical to develop ways of responsibly educating survivors on their medical risk while minimizing the anxiety that such education may provoke [35]. Providers should be attuned to the potential psychological impact of the information they are delivering and should be sensitive to the fact that many survivors may be hearing the information directly for the first time or may feel independently responsible for managing this health-related issue for the first time. Being careful to ask about and listen to survivors' perceptions and health beliefs, and then carefully correcting misperceptions, can minimize anxiety-provoking misunderstandings that can impede participation in future medical care. Providing anticipatory guidance about psychosocial symptoms that are normative for many survivors (e.g., anxiety and worry about medical late effects, distress when reminded of cancer and late effects) can also minimize worry. Helping survivors recognize aspects of the situation that they control (e.g., participating in regular preventive care) and identifying their areas of strength in managing their own health may also decrease the chances that posttraumatic reactions could undermine their involvement in future medical care.

**Table 20.1** Adolescent and Young Adult (AYA) health belief subtypes, based on responses to the Health Competence Beliefs Inventory (HCBI; [14])

| Group | Health belief pattern | Appropriate intervention |
|---|---|---|
| Adaptive beliefs group | AYAs demonstrate high scores on all HCBI factors | Support that reinforces positive beliefs and reinforces adherence to recommendations and achieving personal goals |
| Low autonomy group | AYAs have primarily positive beliefs, but have low scores on independence/autonomy scale | Support should include a consideration of reasons for lower autonomy; work should include survivors and parents, with a focus on pursuing developmentally appropriate health-care management and personal goals |
| Vulnerable group | AYAs have low scores across all HCBI domains | Support may need to focus more intensively on negative beliefs and on setting goals to enhance disease management and quality of life |

Adapted from Brier et al. (2012)

Finally, while it is recommended that all patients receive this standard level of psychosocial care integrated into each follow-up visit, some survivors will demonstrate specific, and possibly intensive, psychological needs. It is therefore important to maintain a referral list of care providers who can deliver more intensive care, including psychotherapists and neuropsychologists.

## 20.7 Research and Practice: Developing Interventions Targeting Psychological Late Effects

A critical piece of providing comprehensive follow-up care is interdisciplinary research to develop and demonstrate the effectiveness of psychosocial interventions consistent with or integrated into follow-up care. There are relatively few evidence-based interventions for survivors, although the largest set of interventions available are helpful in targeting health behaviors (e.g., [14, 58, 59, 72]). As an example of an intervention targeting PTSS across members of the family, the Surviving Cancer Competently Intervention Program (SCCIP; [46]) integrates cognitive behavioral approaches to distressing symptoms of posttraumatic stress within a family systems intervention model. SCCIP has been shown to reduce PTSS in survivors and in their fathers [40]. Other more general pilot programs suggest the feasibility of interventions that aim to educate survivors during a follow-up visit on their medical vulnerability and on the need for continued participation in follow-up care (e.g., [18]) and that aim to provide sustained psychosocial via telephone contact after a follow-up visit [90]. The longer-term effectiveness of such programs is not yet known.

### Conclusion

Overall, survivors of childhood cancer report good psychological adjustment and have low rates of psychopathology. However, a significant minority may experience psychosocial challenges that threaten their ongoing development, including PTSD, impaired physical quality of life, and maladaptive beliefs about their health. Particularly for survivors of a central nervous system malignancy, these challenges may be associated with educational and employment challenges. Social and relationship differences, particularly in brain tumor survivors, are also vulnerabilities in many survivors. It is essential that comprehensive follow-up care includes sensitive assessment of these issues and referral to appropriate community resources, as well as health-care interventions that account for and are informed by any specific psychosocial concerns that a survivor demonstrates. Involvement of psychosocial professionals, including social workers, psychologists, and psychiatrists, on comprehensive follow-up care teams should therefore be seen as essential.

Finally, it is important to emphasize that the psychological experience after childhood cancer is not unidimensional and negative. Emerging theoretical models and early research explorations indicate many survivors and their parents experience positive psychological outcomes that they ascribe to the childhood cancer experience (e.g., [73, 108]). Many psychologists working with survivors have qualitative or anecdotal reports that parents and survivors grow to appreciate at least some parts of the cancer experience. Parents and survivors frequently explain that childhood cancer taught them to put things in perspective in ways that other people do not do and that they are not as materialistic and are more empathic. Survivors frequently feel that they are more mature than others their age and that they value their family relationships more. Family members and survivors may feel grateful to the medical professionals who worked with them and proud of their ability to manage – and survive – a challenge like childhood cancer [41]. Drawing on these strengths and the positive contributions of the cancer experience can help survivors and their family members weather any challenges they might face. Understanding the complicated interplay of these strengths with the more challenging psychological late effects experienced by some survivors can help providers work more effectively to promote positive adaptation and growth in the decades after childhood cancer survivorship.

# References

1. Alderfer MA, Hodges JA (2010) Supporting siblings of children with cancer: a need for family-school partnerships. Sch Ment Health 2:72–81
2. Alderfer M, Labay L, Kazak A (2003) Brief report: does posttraumatic stress apply to siblings of childhood cancer survivors? J Pediatr Psychol 28:281–286
3. American Psychiatric Association (1994) Diagnostic and statistical manual of the American Psychiatric Association, 4th edn. American Psychiatric Press, Washington, DC
4. Arpawong TE, Oland A, Milam JE, Ruccione K, Meeske KA (2013) Post-traumatic growth among an ethnically diverse sample of adolescent and young adult cancer survivors. Psychooncology 22(10):2235–2244
5. Barakat LP, Alderfer MA, Kazak AE (2006) Posttraumatic growth in adolescent survivors of cancer and their mothers and fathers. J Pediatr Psychol 31(6):413–419
6. Barrera M, Shaw AK, Speechley KN, Maunsell E, Pogany L (2005) Educational and social late effects of childhood cancer and related clinical, personal, and familial characteristics. Cancer 104(8):1751–1760
7. Boman KK, Lindblad F, Hjern A (2010) Long-term outcomes of childhood cancer survivors in Sweden. Cancer 116:1385–1391. doi:10.1002/cncr.24840
8. Bonner MJ, Hardy KH, Willard VW, Anthony KK, Hood M, Gururangan S (2008) Social functioning and facial expression recognition in survivors of pediatric brain tumors. J Pediatr Psychol 33(10):1142–1152
9. Brier MJ, Schwartz LA, Kazak AE (2015) Psychosocial, health-promotion, and neurocognitive interventions for survivors of childhood cancer. Syst Rev 34(2):130–148
10. Brown R, Madan-Swain A, Lambert R (2003) Posttraumatic stress symptoms in adolescent survivors of childhood cancer and their mothers. J Trauma Stress 16:309–318
11. Butler R, Rizzi L, Handwerger B (1996) Brief report: the assessment of posttraumatic stress disorder in pediatric cancer patients and survivors. J Pediatr Psychol 21:499–504
12. Casillias J, Kahn KL, Doose M et al (2010) Transitioning childhood cancer survivors to adult-centered healthcare: insights from parents, adoles-

cent and young adult survivors. Psychooncology 19:982–991
13. Crom DB, Chathaway DK, Tolley EA, Mulhern RA, Hudson MM (1999) Health status and health-related quality of life in long-term adult survivors of pediatric solid tumors. Int J Cancer 12:25–31
14. deMoor JS, Puleo E, Ford JS, Greenberg M, Hodgson DC, Tyc VL, Ostroff J, Diller LR, Levy AG, Sprunck-Harrild K, Emmons KM (2011) Disseminating a smoking cessation intervention to childhood and young adult cancer survivors: baseline characteristics and study design of the partnership for health-2 study. BMC Cancer 11:165
15. DeRosa BW, Kazak AE, Doshi K, Schwartz LA, Ginsberg J, Mao JJ, Straton J, Hobbie W, Rourke MT, Carlson C, Ittenbach RF (2011) Development and validation of the health competence beliefs inventory in young adults with and without a history of childhood cancer. Ann Behav Med 41(1):48–58
16. DeRuiter MA, Van Mourik R, Schouten-VanMeeteren AY, Grootenhuis MA, Oosterlaan J (2013) Neurocognitive consequences of a paediatric brain tumour and its treatment: a meta-analysis. Dev Med Child Neurol 55:408–417
17. Eiser C (2007) Beyond survival: quality of life and follow-up after childhood cancer. J Pediatr Psychol 32(9):1140–1150. doi:10.1093/jpepsy/jsm052
18. Eiser C, Hill JJ, Blacklay A (2000) Surviving cancer: what does it mean for you? An evaluation of a clinic based intervention for survivors of childhood cancer. Psychooncology 9:214–220
19. Eiser C, Vance YH, Glaser A, Galvin H (2003) The value of the PedsQTLM in assessing quality of life in survivors of childhood cancer. Child Care Health Dev 29(2):95–102
20. Elkin TD, Phipps S, Mulhern RK, Fairclough D (1997) Psychological functioning of adolescent and young adult survivors of pediatric malignancy. Med Pediatr Oncol 29:582–588
21. Emmons KM, Butterfield RM, Puleo E, Park ER, Mertens A, Gritz ER, Lahti M, Li FP (2003) Smoking among participants in the childhood cancer survivors cohort: the partnership for health study. J Clin Oncol 21(2):189–196
22. Erickson S, Steiner H (2001) Trauma and personality correlates in long term pediatric cancer survivors. Child Psychiatry Hum Dev 31:195–213
23. Fuemmeler BF, Elkin TD, Mullins LL (2001) Survivors of childhood brain tumors: behavioral, emotional, and social adjustment. Clin Psychol Rev 22:547–585
24. Gartstein MA, Noll RB, Vannatta K (2000) Childhood aggression and chronic illness: possible protective mechanisms. J Appl Dev Psychol 21(3):315–333
25. Gerhardt CA, Dixon M, Miller K, Vannatta K, Valerius KS, Correll J, Noll RB (2007) Educational and occupational outcomes among survivors of childhood cancer during the transition to emerging adulthood. J Dev Behav Pediatr 28:448–455

26. Glover DA, Byrne J, Mills JL, Robison LL, Nicholson HS, Meadows A, Zeltzer LK (2003) Impact of CNS treatment on mood in adult survivors of childhood leukemia: a report from the Children's Cancer Group. J Clin Oncol 21(23):4395–4401

27. Granek L, Nathan PC, Rosenberg-Yunger ZR, D'Agostino N, Amin L, Barr RD, Greenberg ML, Hodgson D, Boydell K, Klassen AF (2012) Psychological factors impacting transition from paediatric to adult care by childhood cancer survivors. J Cancer Survivorship Res Pract 6(3):260–269

28. Hardy KK, Bonner MJ, Masi R, Hutchinson KC, Willard VW, Rosoff PM (2008) Psychosocial functioning in parents of adult survivors of childhood cancer. J Pediatr Hematol Oncol 30(2):153–159

29. Haupt R, Fears TR, Robison LL, Mills JL, Nicholson S, Zeltzer LK, Meadows AT, Byrne J (1994) Educational attainment in long-term survivors of childhood acute lymphoblastic leukemia. JAMA 272(18):1427–1432

30. Hobbie W, Ogle S (2001) Transitional care for young adult survivors of childhood cancer. Semin Oncol Nurs 17(4):268–273

31. Hobbie W, Stuber M, Meeske K, Wissler K, Rourke M, Ruccione K, Hinkle A, Kazak A (2000) Symptoms of posttraumatic stress in young adult survivors of childhood cancer. J Clin Oncol 18:4060–4066

32. Hocking MC, Schwartz LA, Hobbie WL, DeRosa BW, Ittenback RF, Mao JJ, Ginsberg JP, Kazak AE (2012) Prospectively examining physical activity in young adult survivors of childhood cancer and healthy controls. Pediatr Blood Cancer, published online: 20 Mar 2012. doi:10.1002/pbc.24144

33. Holmquist LA, Scott J (2002) Treatment, age, and time-related predictors of behavioral outcome in pediatric brain tumor survivors. J Clin Psychol Med Settings 9(4):315–321

34. Howard RA, Inskip PD, Travis LB (2007) Suicide after childhood cancer. J Clin Oncol 25(6):731. doi:10.1200/jcoo.2006.09.2056

35. Hudson MM, Mertens AC, Yasui Y, Hobbie W, Chen H, Gurney JG, Yeazel M, Recklitis CJ, Marina N, Robison LR, Oeffinger KC (2003) Health status of adult long-term survivors of childhood cancer: a report from the Childhood Cancer Survivor Study. JAMA 290(12):1583–1592

36. Janson C, Leisenring W, Cox C, Termuhlen AM, Mertens AC, Whitton JA, Goodman P, Zeltzer L, Robison LL, Krull KR, Kadan-Lottick NS (2009) Predictors of marriage and divorce in adult survivors of childhood cancers: a report from the Childhood Cancer Survivor Study. Cancer Epidemiol Biomarkers Prev 18(10):2626–2635

37. Kadan-Lottick NS, Robison L, Gurney JG, Neglia JP, Yasui Y, Hayashi R, Hudson M, Greenberg M, Mertens A (2002) Childhood cancer survivors' knowledge about their past diagnosis and treatment: Childhood Cancer Survivor Study. JAMA 287(14):1832–1839

38. Kazak A (2005) Evidence-based interventions for survivors of childhood cancer and their families. J Pediatr Psychol 30(1):29–39

39. Kazak A, Alderfer M, Rourke M, Simms S, Streisand R, Grossman J (2004) Posttraumatic stress symptoms (PTSS) and Posttraumatic stress disorder (PTSD) in families of adolescent cancer survivors. J Pediatr Psychol 29(3):211–219

40. Kazak A, Alderfer M, Streisand R, Simms S, Rourke M, Barakat L, Gallagher P, Cnaan A (2004) Treatment of posttraumatic stress symptoms in adolescent survivors of childhood cancer and their families: a randomized clinical trial. J Fam Psychol 18(3):493–504

41. Kazak A, Barakat L, Alderfer M, Rourke M, Meeske K, Gallagher P, Cnaan A, Stuber M (2001) Posttraumatic stress in survivors of childhood cancer and their mothers: development and validation of the Impact of Traumatic Stressors Interview Schedule (ITSS). J Clin Psychol Med Settings 8:307–323

42. Kazak A, Barakat L, Meeske K, Christakis D, Meadows A, Casey R, Penati B, Stuber M (1997) Posttraumatic stress, family functioning, and social support in survivors of childhood leukemia and their mothers and fathers. J Consult Clin Psychol 65:120–129

43. Kazak AE, DeRosa BW, Schwartz LA, Hobbie W, Carlson C, Ittenback RF, Mao JJ, Ginsberg JP (2010) Psychological outcomes and health beliefs in adolescent and young adult survivors of childhood cancer and controls. J Clin Oncol 28(12):2002–2007. doi:10.1200/JCO.2009.25.9584

44. Kazak AE, Kassam-Adams N, Alderfer M, Rourke MT, Schneider S, Zelikovsky N (2006) A model for understanding pediatric medical traumatic stress. J Pediatr Psychol 31(4):343–355

45. Kazak AE, Noll RB (2015) The integration of psychology in pediatric oncology research and practice: A a family-centered model of collaboration to improve outcomes. Am Psychol 70(2):146–158, http://dx.doi.org/10.1037/a0035695

46. Kazak A, Simms S, Barakat L, Hobbie W, Foley B, Golomb V, Best M (1999) Surviving Cancer Competently Intervention Program (SCCIP): a cognitive-behavioral and family therapy intervention for adolescent survivors of childhood cancer and their families. Fam Process 38:175–191

47. Kazak A, Stuber M, Barakat L, Meeske K, Guthrie D, Meadows A (1998) Predicting posttraumatic stress symptoms in mothers and fathers of survivors of childhood cancer. J Am Acad Child Adolesc Psychiatry 37:823–831

48. Keene N, Hobbie W, Ruccione K (2012) Childhood cancer survivors: a practical guide to your future, 3rd edn. O'Reilly, Cambridge

49. Kirchhoff AC, Krull KR, Ness KK, Park ER, Oeffinger KC, Hudson MM, Stovall M, Robison LL, Wickizer T, Leisenring W (2011) Occupational outcomes of childhood cancer survivors. Cancer 117(13):3033–3044. doi:10.1002/cncr.25867

50. Klosky JL, Cash DK, Buscemi J, Lensing S, Zhao W, Ward S, Hudson M (2008) Factors influencing long-term follow-up clinic attendance among survivors of childhood cancer. J Cancer Surviv 2(4):225–232

51. Kunin-Batson A, Kadan-Lottick N, Zhu L, Cox C, Bordes-Edgar V, Srivastava DK, Zeltzer L, Robison LL, Krull KR (2011) Predictors of independent living status in adult survivors of childhood cancer. A report from the Childhood Cancer Survivor Study. Pediatr Blood Cancer 15:1197–1203

52. Kupst MJ, Natta M, Richardson C, Schulman J, Lavigne J, Das L (1995) Family coping with pediatric leukemia: ten years after treatment. J Pediatr Psychol 20:601–617

53. Langeveld NE, Stam H, Grootenhuis MA, Last BF (2002) Quality of life in young adult survivors of childhood cancer. Support Care Cancer 10:579–600

54. Langeveld NE, Ubbink MC, Last BF, Grootenhuis MA, Voute PA, DeHaan RJ (2003) Educational achievement, employment and living situation in long-term young adult survivors of childhood cancer in the Netherlands. Psychooncology 12:213–225

55. Mackie E, Hill J, Kondryn H, McNally R (2000) Adult psychosocial outcomes in long-term survivors of acute lymphoblastic leukaemia and Wilms' tumour: a controlled study. Lancet 355:1310–1314

56. Manne S, DuHamel K, Gallelli K, Sorgen K, Redd W (1998) Posttraumatic stress disorder among mothers of pediatric cancer survivors: diagnosis, comorbidity, and utility of the PTSD Checklists as a screening instrument. J Pediatr Psychol 23:357–366

57. Manne S, DuHamel K, Nereo N, Ostroff J, Parsons S, Martini R, Williams S, Mee L, Sexson S, Wu L, Difede J, Redd W (2002) Predictors of PTSD in mothers of children undergoing bone marrow transplantation: the role of cognitive and social processes. J Pediatr Psychol 27:607–617

58. Mays D, Black JD, Mosher RB, Heinly A, Shad AT, Tercyak KP (2011) Efficacy of the Survivor Health and Resilience Education (SHARE) program to improve bone health behaviors among adolescent survivors of childhood cancer. Ann Behav Med 42:91–98

59. Mays D, Black JD, Mosher RB, Shad AT, Tercyak KP (2011) Improving short-term sun safety practices among adolescent survivors of childhood cancer: a randomized controlled efficacy trial. J Cancer Surviv 5(3):247–254

60. Mckenzie S, Curle C (2012) 'The end of treatment is not the end': parents' experiences of their child's transition from treatment for childhood cancer. Psychooncology 21(6):647–654

61. Michel G, Taylor N, Absolom K, Eiser C (2009) Benefit finding in survivors of childhood cancer and their parents: further empirical support for the benefit finding scale for children. Child Health Care Dev 36(1):123–129

62. Mitby PA, Robison LL, Whitton JA et al (2003) Utilization of special education services and educational attainment among long-term survivors of childhood cancer: a report from the Childhood Cancer Survivor Study. Cancer 97(4):1115–26

63. Mulhern R, Wasserman AL, Friedman AG, Fairclough D (1989) Social, competence and behavioral adjustment of children who are long-term survivors of cancer. Pediatrics 83(1):18–25

64. Nagarajan R, Neglia JP, Clohisy DR, Yasui Y, Greenberg M, Hudson M, Zevon MA, Tersak JM, Ablin A, Robison LL (2003) Education, employment, insurance, and marital status among 694 survivors of pediatric lower extremity bone tumors: a report of the Childhood Cancer Survivor Study. Cancer 97(10):2554–2564

65. Nathan PC, Greenberg ML, Ness KK, Hudson MM, Mertens AC, Mahoney MC, Gurney JG, Donaldson SS, Leisenring WM, Robison LL, Oeffinger KC (2008) Medical care in long-term survivors of childhood cancer: a report from the Childhood Cancer Survivor Study. J Clin Oncol 26:4401–4409

66. Nathan PC, Ness KK, Greenberg ML, Hudson M, Wolden S, Davidoff A, Laverdiere C, Mertens A, Whitton J, Robison LL, Zeltzer L, Gurney JG (2007) Health-related quality of life in adult survivors of childhood Wilms tumor or neuroblastoma: a report from the Childhood Cancer Survivor Study. Pediatr Blood Cancer 49:704–715

67. Newby WL, Brown RT, Pawletko TM, Gold SH, Whitt JK (2000) Social skills and psychological adjustment of child and adolescent cancer survivors. Psychooncology 9:113–126

68. Noll R, Bukowski W, Davies W, Koontz K, Kularkrni R (1993) Adjustment in the peer system of children with cancer: a two-year follow-up study. J Pediatr Psychol 18:351–364

69. Noll RB, MacLean WE, Whitt JK, Kaleita TA, Stehbens JA, Waskerwitz MJ, Ruymann FB, Hammond GD (1997) Behavioral adjustment and social functioning of long-term survivors of childhood leukemia: parent and teacher reports. J Pediatr Psychol 22(6):827–841

70. Oeffinger KC (2003) Longitudinal risk-based health care for adult survivors of childhood cancer. Curr Probl Cancer 27:143–167

71. Oeffinger KC, Mertens AC, Hudson MM, Gurney JG, Casillas JC, Hegang W, Yeazel M, Yasui Y, Robison LL (2004) Health care of young adult survivors of childhood cancer: a report from the Childhood Cancer Survivor Study. Ann Fam Med 2(1):61–70

72. Park ER, Puleo E, Butterfield RM, Zorn M, Mertens AC, Gritz E, Li F, Emmons KM (2010) A process evaluation of a telephone-based peer-delivered smoking cessation intervention for adult survivors of childhood cancer: the partnership for health study. Prev Med Int J Devoted Pract Theory 42(6):435–442

73. Parry C, Chesler MA (2005) Thematic evidence of psychosocial thriving in childhood cancer survivors. Qual Health Res 15(8):1055–1073

74. Patenaude AF, Last B (2001) Editorial: cancer and children: where are we coming from? Where are we going? Psychooncology 10:281–283

75. Pendley JS, Dahlquist LM, Dreyer Z (1997) Body image and psychosocial adjustment in adolescent cancer survivors. J Pediatr Psychol 22(1):29–43

76. Phipps S, Long AM, Ogden J (2007) Benefit finding scale for children: preliminary findings from a childhood cancer population. J Pediatr Psychol 32(10):1264–1271

77. Radcliffe J, Bennett D, Kazak AE, Foley B, Phillips PC (1996) Adjustment in childhood brain tumor survival: child, mother, and teacher report. J Pediatr Psychol 21(4):529–539

78. Rauck AM, Green DM, Yasui Y, Mertens A, Robison LL (1999) Marriage in the survivors of childhood cancer: a preliminary description from the Childhood Cancer Survivor Study. Med Pediatr Oncol 33:60–63

79. Recklitis CJ, Lockwood RA, Rothwell MA, Diller LR (2006) Suicidal ideation and attempts in adult survivors of childhood cancer. J Clin Oncol 24(24):3852–3857

80. Recklitis C, O'Leary T, Diller L (2003) Utility of routine psychological screening in the childhood cancer survivor clinic. J Clin Oncol 21(5):787–792

81. Reimers TS, Mortensen EL, Nysom K, Schmiegelow K (2009) Health-related quality of life in long-term survivors of childhood brain tumors. Pediatr Blood Cancer 53(6):1086–1091

82. Reiter-Purtill J, Noll R (2003) Peer relationships of children with chronic illness. In: Roberts M (ed) Handbook of pediatric psychology, 3rd edn. Guilford, New York

83. Reulen RC, Winter DL, Lancashire ER, Zeegers MP, Jenney ME, Walters SJ, Jenkinson C, Hawkins MM (2007) Health-status of adult survivors of childhood cancer: a large-scale population-based study from the British Childhood Cancer Study. Int J Cancer 121:633–640. doi:10.1002/ijc.22658

84. Reulen RC, Winter DL, Lancashire ER, Zeegers MP, Jenney ME, Walters SJ, Jenkinson C, Hawkins MM (2009) Health-status of adult survivors of childhood cancer: a large-scale population-based study from the British Childhood Cancer Survivor Study. Int J Cancer 121(3):633–40

85. Richardson RC, Nelson MB, Meeske K (1999) Young adult survivors of childhood cancer: attending to emerging medical and psychosocial needs. J Pediatr Oncol Nurs 16(3):136–144

86. Robinson KE, Gerhardt CA, Vannatta K, Noll RB (2009) Survivors of childhood cancer and comparison peers: the influence of early family factors on distress in emerging adulthood. J Fam Psychol 23(1):23–31

87. Ross L, Johansen C, Dalton SO, Mellemkjaer L, Thornassen LH, Mortensen PB, Olsen JH (2003) Psychiatric hospitalizations among survivors of cancer in childhood or adolescence. N Engl J Med 349(7):650–657

88. Rourke M, Hobbie W, Kazak A (2002) Posttraumatic stress in young adult survivors of childhood cancer. 7th International conference on long-term complications of treatment of children and adolescents for cancer, Niagara on the Lake, Ontario, Canada

89. Rourke M, Stuber M, Hobbie W, Kazak A (1999) Posttraumatic stress disorder: understanding the psychosocial impact of surviving childhood cancer into young adulthood. J Pediatr Oncol Nurs 16:126–135

90. Santacroce SJ, Asmus K, Kadan-Lottick N, Grey M (2010) Feasibility and preliminary outcomes from a pilot study of coping skills training for adolescent-young adult survivors of childhood cancer and their parents. J Pediatr Oncol Nurs 27(1):10–20

91. Sawyer M, Antoniou G, Toogood I, Rice M, Baghurst P (2000) Childhood cancer: a 4-year prospective study of the psychological adjustment of children and parents. J Pediatr Hematol Oncol 22(3):214–220

92. Schulte F, Barrera M (2010) Social competence in childhood brain tumor survivors: a comprehensive review. Support Care Cancer 18(12):1499–1513. doi:10.1007/s00520-010-0963-1

93. Schultz KA, Ness KK, Whitton J, Recklitis C, Zebrack B, Robison LL, Zeltzer L, Mertens AC (2007) Behavioral and social outcomes in adolescent survivors of childhood cancer: a report from the Childhood Cancer Survivor Study. J Clin Oncol 25(24):3649–3656

94. Schwartz LA, Kazak AE, Derosa BW, Hocking MC, Hobbie WL, Ginsberg JP (2012) The role of beliefs in the relationship between health problems and posttraumatic stress in adolescent and young adult cancer survivors. J Clin Psychol Med Settings 19(2):138–146

95. Schwartz LA, Mao JJ, DeRosa BW, Ginsberg JP, Hobbie WL, Carlson CA, Mougianis ID, Ogle SK, Kazak AE (2010) Self-reported health problems of young adults in clinical settings: survivors of childhood cancer and healthy controls. J Am Board Fam Med 23(3):306–314. doi:10.3122/jabfm.2010.03.090215

96. Schwartz LA, Tuchman LK, Hobbie WL, Ginsberg JP (2011) A social-ecological model of readiness for transition for adult-oriented care for adolescents with chronic health conditions. Child Care Health Dev 37(6):883–885

97. Stuber M, Kazak A, Meeske K, Barakat L (1998) Is posttraumatic stress a viable model for understanding responses to childhood cancer? Psychiatr Clin N Am 7:169–182

98. Sundberg KK, Lampic C, Arvidson J, Helstrom L, Wettergren L (2011) Sexual function and experience among long-term survivors of childhood cancer. Eur J Cancer 47:397–403. doi:10.1016/j.ejca.2010.09.040

99. Van Dongen-Melman JEWM, Pruyn JFA, DeGroot A, Koot HM, Hahlen K, Verhulst FC (1995) Late psychosocial consequences for parents of children who survived cancer. J Pediatr Psychol 20(5):567–586

100. Vannatta K, Gartstein MA, Short A, Noll RB (1998) A controlled study of peer relations of children surviving brain tumors: teacher, peer, and self ratings. J Pediatr Psychol 23(5):279–287

101. Vannatta K, Zeller M, Noll RB, Koontz K (1998) Social functioning of children surviving bone marrow transplantation. J Pediatr Psychol 23(3):169–178

102. Verrill JR, Schafer J, Vannatta K, Noll RB (2000) Aggression, antisocial behavior, and substance abuse in survivors of pediatric cancer: possible protective effects of cancer and its treatment. J Pediatr Psychol 25(7):493–502

103. Wakefield CE, McLoone JK, Butow P, Lenthen K, Cohn RJ (2011) Parental adjustment to the completion of their child's cancer treatment. Pediatr Blood Cancer 56(4):524–531

104. Wolf K, Madan-Swain A, Kana RK (2012) Executive dysfunction in pediatric posterior fossa tumor survivors: a systematic literature review of neurocognitive deficits and interventions. Dev Neuropsychol 37(2):153–175

105. Zebrack BJ, Chesler M (2001) Health-related worries, self-image, and life outlooks of long-term survivors of childhood cancer. Health Soc Work 26(4):245–256

106. Zebrack BJ, Gurney JG, Oeffinger K, Whitton J, Packer RJ, Mertens A, Turk N, Castleberry R, Dreyer Z, Robison LL, Zeltzer LK (2004) Psychological outcomes in long-term survivors of childhood brain cancer: a report from the Childhood Cancer Survivor Study. J Clin Oncol 22(6):999–1006

107. Zebrack BJ, Landier W (2011) The perceived impact of cancer in quality of life for post-treatment survivors of childhood cancer. Qual Life Res 20:1595–1608. doi:10.1007/s11136-011-9893-8

108. Zebrack BJ, Stuber ML, Meeske KA, Phipps S, Krull KR, Liu Q, Yasui Y, Parry C, Hamilton R, Robison LL, Zeltzer LK (2012) Perceived positive impact of cancer among long-term survivors of childhood cancer: a report from the Childhood Cancer Survivor Study. Psychooncology 21(6):630–639

109. Zebrack BJ, Zeltzer LK, Whitton J, Mertens AC, Odom L, Berkow R, Robison LL (2002) Psychological outcomes in long-term survivors of childhood leukemia, Hodgkin's disease, and non-Hodgkin's lymphoma: a report from the Childhood Cancer Survivor Study. Pediatrics 110(1):42–52

110. Zebrack BJ, Zevon MA, Turk N, Nagarajan R, Whitton J, Robison LL, Zeltzer LK (2007) Psychological distress in long-term survivors of solid tumors diagnosed in childhood: a report from the Childhood Cancer Survivor Study. Pediatr Blood Cancer 49:47–51

111. Zeltzer LK, Lu Q, Leisenring W, Tsao JC, Recklitis C, Armstrong G, Mertens AC, Robison LL, Ness KK (2008) Psychosocial outcomes and health-related quality of life in adult childhood cancer survivors: a report from the Childhood Cancer Survivor Study. Cancer Epidemiol Biomark Prev 17(2):435–46

112. Zeltzer LK, Recklitis C, Buchbinder D, Zebrack B, Casillas J, Tsao JCI, Lu Q, Krull K (2009) Psychological status in childhood cancer survivors: a report from the Childhood Cancer Survivorship Study. J Clin Oncol 27(14):2396–2404. doi:10.1200/JCO.2008.21.1433

# Legal Issues

# 21

## Barbara Hoffman

## Contents

B. Hoffman
Rutgers School of Law, 123 Washington Street,
Newark, NJ USA
e-mail: bhoffman@kinoy.rutgers.edu

## 21.1 Introduction

A growing number of children in the United States are being diagnosed with and successfully treated for cancer. Approximately 83 % of all children diagnosed with cancer can expect to become long-term survivors [1]. Unlike adult survivors, whose average age of diagnosis is near retirement age, most childhood survivors offer decades of productive employment after cancer [2]. Young adult survivors entering the job market for the first time are a rapidly growing population. By 2010, approximately one of every 450 young adults was a childhood cancer survivor [3]. Although survivors once commonly experienced cancer-related barriers to employment, improvements in medical treatment and legal rights have reduced these barriers considerably.

This chapter reviews current studies of employment problems reported by cancer survivors, lists legal resources available for those whose rights have been violated, and provides suggestions for how to avoid and address these problems. This chapter also discusses childhood cancer survivors' rights to health insurance and education, referring to American law in effect in 2013.

© Springer International Publishing 2015
C.L. Schwartz et al. (eds.), *Survivors of Childhood and Adolescent Cancer:*
*A Multidisciplinary Approach*, Pediatric Oncology, DOI 10.1007/978-3-319-16435-9_21

## 21.2 The Scope of Cancer-Based Employment Problems

Of the more than 13.7 million cancer survivors in the United States, roughly one-half are of working age [4]. The majority of these individuals are willing and able to work [5]. Because of significant improvements in cancer care, most working-aged adults can work during and after cancer treatment [6]. For example, one survey of 10 studies that assessed return-to-work rates of 1,904 survivors from 1986 to 1999 found that a mean of 62 % returned to work [7].

The work issues of childhood cancer survivors differ somewhat from those of adult cancer survivors. Because childhood survivors first enter the workplace after diagnosis, they are often more concerned with how to obtain a job than with how to keep a job. Although many childhood survivors do not enter the job market for years or even decades after their diagnoses, some may find that their cancer histories affect their employability at any stage of their careers.

Most employers treat cancer survivors fairly and legally. Some employers, however, erect unnecessary and sometimes illegal barriers to job opportunities. Most personnel decisions are driven by economic factors, not by charitable or personal consideration. Employers may fear that an employee with a cancer history may affect insurance costs or be a less productive employee. Additionally, some employers fail to revise their personnel policies to comply with current antidiscrimination law. Even those who have updated personnel policies may not properly train their personnel managers to comply with these laws.

### 21.2.1 The Types of Employment Problems Encountered by Cancer Survivors

The employment problems of cancer survivors take many forms. A cancer diagnosis may affect any type of job action, including dismissal, failure to hire, demotion, denial of promotion, undesirable transfer, denial of benefits, and hostility in the workplace. Disparate treatments, such as blanket hiring bans against all individuals with a cancer history, are irrational and blatant. Other employment decisions, especially actions by legally sophisticated employers, are far more subtle.

Some survivors experience significant physical or mental limitations that affect their ability to work [8, 9]. One estimate is that 16.8 % of working-age survivors (compared with 5 % of matched controls) are unable to work because of physical, mental, or emotional problems; of those who could work, 7.4 % (compared with 3.2 % of matched controls) were limited in the kind or amount of work they could do [9].

Whether a cancer survivor continues to work during treatment or returns to work after treatment—and if so, whether that survivor's diagnosis or treatment will result in working limitations—depends on medical and socioeconomic factors:

Factors that affect a cancer survivor's ability to work [5].

| Medical factors | Socioeconomic factors | Job attributes |
|---|---|---|
| Age | Financial status | Essential job functions |
| Type of cancer | Education | Working hours |
| Stage of cancer | Access to health insurance | Commuting factors |
| Side effects of treatment | Access to transportation | Medical leave benefits |
| Other chronic health conditions | Access to quality cancer care | |

### 21.2.2 The Numbers of Cancer Survivors Who Encounter Employment Problems

Prior to the passage of state and federal employment rights laws, employment discrimination against cancer survivors was common. Such discrimination can have devastating physical, emotional, and financial consequences [10].

Survivors of childhood cancer once experienced significant employment problems similar to those encountered by adult cancer patients. For example, a 1986 Stanford study found that 43 % of 403 Hodgkin's disease survivors experienced difficulties at work that they attributed to their cancer history [11]. A 1982 study by Koocher and O'Malley of 60 childhood cancer survivors found that 25 % reported job discrimination (10 persons were refused a job at least once, 3 were denied benefits, 3 experienced illness-related conflict with a supervisor, 4 reported job task problems, and 11 were rejected by the military) [12]. A 1986 study by Teta found a large disparity in the civilian and military employment rates of childhood cancer survivors compared with their siblings [13]. Eighty percent of the male survivors were rejected from the military compared with 18 % of their siblings, and 32 % were rejected from job opportunities compared with 19 % of their siblings. Although female survivors faced disproportionate rejection from the military (75 % compared with 13 % for siblings), the percentage of women rejected from employment was the same for survivors as for their siblings (19 %).

Hays and colleagues surveyed 219 childhood survivors and matched controls who were treated between 1945 and 1975 and were at least 30 years old at the time of the survey [14]. They found that childhood survivors, with the exception of survivors of central nervous system tumors, experienced relatively the same employment history as the controls [14]. The controls, however, reported somewhat more annual income than did the survivors [14]. Hays' results suggest that as the length of time between diagnosis and initial employment increases, the incidence of employment problems may decrease.

Only those survivors who sought entry into the military faced increased rates of discrimination (15.2 % of survivors at one institute and 20.7 % at another versus 7.7 % and 1.8 %, respectively, of the controls). Although the Department of Defense presumes cancer survivors to be unfit for military service, it considers waivers on a case-by-case basis for childhood survivors of acute lymphoblastic leukemia who have not had a recurrence and for other survivors who have been out of treatment and cancer-free for 5 years

(2 years for Wilms' tumor, large-cell lymphoma, and germ cell tumors of the testes).

But with the passage of the Americans with Disabilities Act in 1990 and comparable state laws, as well as a sea change in perceptions about living with and beyond cancer, survivors have reported decreasing incidences of work problems attributable to their cancer [5].

A 2006 national survey of cancer survivors found that most employers appear to be highly sensitive and accommodating to the needs of employees who have cancer and to employees who are caregivers for cancer survivors [5]. Three out of five survivors reported receiving coworker support, such as help with work or random acts of kindness. Survivors and caregivers reported very low incidences of negative reactions from their employers and coworkers. The most common negative reaction, reported by one in five survivors, was that an employer gave a survivor less work after diagnosis. Other consequences, such as being fired or laid off (6 %), denied a raise or promotion (7 %), and denied health insurance benefits (4 %), were far less common.

A 2010 study that compared 410 childhood cancer survivors with almost 300,000 controls found that although most childhood cancer survivors were employed as adults, they had lower employment rates than controls.

Employment rates of childhood cancer survivors and controls [15].

|  | Childhood cancer survivors | Controls |
| --- | --- | --- |
| % who held a job in past 12 months | 67.8 | 73.9 |
| % unable to work due to health problems | 20.9 | 6.3 |
| % limited in amount/kind of work because of health problems | 30.9 | 10.6 |

Although incidences of cancer-based employment discrimination have decreased, some survivors still face disparate treatment and seek legal redress. Between 1997 and 2011, 2.3–3.9 % of claims brought under Title I of the ADA alleged "cancer" as a disability [16].

## 21.3  Laws Governing Cancer-Based Discrimination

### 21.3.1  When Cancer-Based Discrimination Is Illegal

Under federal law and most state laws, an employer cannot treat a survivor differently from other workers in job-related activities because of his or her cancer history, provided the survivor is qualified for the job. Individuals are protected by these laws only if:

1. They can do the major duties of the job in question.
2. Their employer treated them differently from other workers in job-related activities because of their cancer history.

#### 21.3.1.1 Americans with Disabilities Act

The Americans with Disabilities Act (ADA) prohibits some types of job discrimination by employers, employment agencies, and labor unions against people who have or had cancer. All private employers with 15 or more employees, state and local governments, the legislative branch of the federal government, employment agencies, and labor unions are covered by the ADA.

A "qualified individual with a disability" is protected by the ADA if he or she can perform the "essential functions" of the job. The ADA prohibits employment discrimination against individuals with a "disability," with a "record" of a "disability," or who are "regarded" as having a "disability." A "disability" is a major health "impairment" that substantially limits the ability to do everyday activities, such as caring for oneself, walking, breathing, or working.

Cancer is an "impairment" as defined by law. In most circumstances, cancer survivors, regardless of whether they are in treatment, in remission, or cured, are protected as persons with a disability because their cancer substantially limited a major life activity. Indeed, the Equal Employment Opportunities Commission (EEOC)

regulations that interpret the ADA consider cancer under most circumstances to be a disability under the ADA. Whether a cancer survivor is covered by the ADA is determined, however, on a case-by-case basis.

The ADA prohibits discrimination in most job-related activities such as hiring, dismissal, and benefits. In most cases, a prospective employer may not ask applicants if they have ever had cancer. An employer has the right to know only if an applicant is able to perform the essential functions of the job. A job offer may be contingent upon passing a relevant medical exam, provided that all prospective employees are subject to the same exam. An employer may ask detailed questions about health only after making a job offer.

Cancer survivors who need extra time or help to work are entitled to a "reasonable accommodation." Common accommodations for survivors include changes in work hours or duties to accommodate medical appointments and treatment side effects. An employer does not have to make changes that would impose an "undue hardship" on the business or other workers. "Undue hardship" refers to any accommodation that would be unduly costly, extensive, substantial, or disruptive or that would fundamentally alter the nature or operation of the business. For example, an employer may replace a survivor who misses 6 months of work that cannot be performed by a temporary employee.

The ADA does not prohibit an employer from ever dismissing or refusing to hire a cancer survivor. Because the law requires employers to treat all employees similarly, regardless of disability, an employer may fire a cancer survivor who would have been dismissed even if he or she were not a survivor.

Most employment discrimination laws protect only the employee. The ADA offers protection more responsive to survivors' needs because it prohibits discrimination against family members, too. Employers may not discriminate against workers because of their relationship or association with a "disabled" person. Employers may not assume that an employee's job performance will be affected by the need to care for a family member who has cancer.

### 21.3.1.2 Family and Medical Leave Act

The Family and Medical Leave Act (FMLA) requires employers with at least 50 workers to provide employees up to 12 weeks of unpaid leave for serious medical illness, including cancer, to care for themselves or dependents. The FMLA provides a number of benefits to people with cancer:

- Requires employers to continue to provide benefits, including health insurance coverage, during the leave period.
- Provides 12 weeks of unpaid leave during any 12-month period.
- Requires employers to restore employees to the same or equivalent position at the end of the leave period.
- Allows leave to care for a spouse, child, or parent who has a serious health condition such as cancer.
- Allows leave because a serious health condition renders the employee unable to perform the functions of the position.
- Allows an intermittent or reduced work schedule when medically necessary. Under some circumstances, an employer may transfer the employee to a position with equivalent pay and benefits to accommodate the new work schedule.
- Allows employees to stack leave under the FMLA with leave allowable under the state medical leave law.

The FMLA reasonably balances the needs of the employer and employee because it:

- Requires employees to make reasonable efforts to schedule foreseeable medical care to minimize workplace disruption
- Requires employees to give employers 30 days' notice of foreseeable medical leave or as much notice as is practicable
- Allows employers to require employees to provide certification of medical needs and allows employers to seek a second opinion, at the employer's expense, to corroborate medical need
- Permits employers to provide leave provisions more generous than those required by the FMLA

### 21.3.1.3 Employee Retirement and Income Security Act

The Employee Retirement and Income Security Act (ERISA) may provide a remedy to an employee who has been denied full participation in an employee benefit plan because of a cancer history. ERISA prohibits an employer from discriminating against an employee for the purpose of preventing him or her from collecting benefits under an employee benefit plan. For example, some employers fear that the participation of a cancer survivor in a group medical plan will increase the employer's insurance costs. An employer may violate ERISA if, upon learning of a worker's cancer history, it dismisses that worker for the purpose of excluding him or her from a group health plan.

### 21.3.1.4 Genetic Information

With the growth of genetic testing, many cancer survivors are concerned that employers will use genetic information as a basis for discrimination. The Genetic Information Nondiscrimination Act (GINA) prohibits an employer, employment agency, labor organization, or training program from using genetic information to make decisions regarding hiring, promotion, terms or conditions, privileges of employment, compensation, or termination. GINA protects employees from discrimination based on the result of a genetic test and information about a family history of a disease. It does not, however, protect employees from discrimination because of a manifested disease or condition. GINA covers the same employers that are covered under the ADA (those with at least 15 employees). An employee who has a genetic predisposition to a disease or condition may still qualify for family or medical leave and may participate in an employer-sponsored wellness program or other genetic services—such as tests, counseling, and education—offered by an employer. The employment provisions of GINA do not interfere with an employee's right to protection under state genetic discrimination laws.

### 21.3.1.5 State Employment Rights Laws

Every state has a law that regulates, to some extent, disability-based employment discrimination.

Some laws clearly prohibit cancer-based discrimination, while others have never been applied to cancer-based discrimination. State laws also vary as to which employers—public or private, large or small—must obey the law.

Several states, such as New Jersey, cover all employers regardless of the number of employees. The laws in most states, however, cover only employers with a minimum number of employees. A small number of states, such as California, Florida, Vermont, and West Virginia, expressly prohibit discrimination based on cancer history. Many state laws protect individuals with real or perceived disabilities and, therefore, cover most cases of cancer-based discrimination. The rights of cancer survivors who are not impaired are unclear in those states where courts have not addressed the issue and where one must have a physical or mental impairment to bring a claim.

Many states have leave laws similar to the federal Family and Medical Leave Act in that they guarantee employees in the private sector unpaid leave for pregnancy, childbirth, and the adoption of a child. Some state laws provide employees with medical leave to address a serious illness, such as cancer. Several states provide coverage more extensive than the federal law.

State medical leave laws vary widely as to:

- How long an employee may take leave
- Which employees may take leave (most states require an employee to have worked for a minimum period of time)
- Which employers must provide leave (a few states have leave laws that apply to employers of fewer than 50 employees)
- The definition of "family member" for whose illness an employee may take family medical leave
- The type of illness that entitles an employee to medical leave
- How much notice an employee must give prior to taking leave
- Whether an employee continues to receive benefits while on leave and who pays for them
- How the law is enforced (by state agency or through private lawsuit)

## 21.4 How to Address Cancer-Based Discrimination

### 21.4.1 How to Avoid Becoming a Victim of Discrimination

Lawsuits are neither the only nor the best way to fight employment discrimination against cancer survivors. State and federal antidiscrimination laws help cancer survivors in two ways. First, they discourage discrimination. Second, they offer remedies when discrimination does occur. These laws, however, should be used as a last resort because lawsuits are costly and time-consuming and may not necessarily result in a fair solution. The first step is to try to avoid discrimination. If that fails, the next step is to attempt a reasonable settlement with the employer. If informal efforts fail, however, a lawsuit may be the most effective next step.

When seeking employment, survivors can lessen the chance they will face cancer-based discrimination by considering the following suggestions:

- Do not volunteer that you have or have had cancer, unless it directly affects your qualifications for the job. An employer has the right—under accepted business practices and most state and federal laws—to know only if you can perform the major duties of the job.
- Do not lie on a job or insurance application. If you are hired and your employer later learns that you lied, you may be fired for your dishonesty. Insurance companies may refuse to pay benefits or may cancel your coverage.
- Apply only for jobs that you are able to do. It is not illegal for an employer to reject you for a job if you are not qualified for it, regardless of your medical history.
- If you have to explain an educational gap or a long period of unemployment during cancer treatment, if possible, explain it in a way that shows you are currently in good health and expected to remain healthy. One way to de-emphasize a gap in your school or work history because of cancer treatment is to organize your resume by experience and skills, instead of by date.

- Offer your employer a letter from your doctor that explains your current health status, prognosis, and ability to work. Be prepared to educate the interviewer about your cancer and why cancer often does not result in death or disability.
- Seek help from a job counselor with resume preparation and job interviewing skills. Practice answers to expected questions such as "why did you miss a year of school?" or "why did you leave your last job?" Answers to these questions must be honest but should stress your current qualifications for the job and not past problems, if any, resulting from your cancer experience.
- If you are interviewing for a job, do not ask about health insurance until after you have been given a job offer. Then ask to see the "benefits package." Prior to accepting the job, review it to make sure it meets your needs.
- If possible, look for jobs with large employers because they are less likely to discriminate.
- Do not discriminate against yourself by assuming you are unable to work at all. Although cancer treatment leaves some survivors with real physical or mental disabilities, most survivors are capable of performing the same duties and activities as they did prior to diagnosis or of adjusting to new job duties. With the help of your medical team, make an honest assessment of your abilities in relation to the mental and physical demands of the job.

## 21.4.2 Fighting Back Against Discrimination

Survivors who suspect that they are being treated differently at work because of their cancer history should consider an informal solution before filing a lawsuit. Survivors who face discrimination may consider the following suggestions:

- Consider using your employer's policies and procedures for resolving employment issues informally. Tell your employer that you know your legal rights and would rather resolve the issues openly and honestly than file a lawsuit.

Be careful of what you say during discussions to avoid saying something that could be used to hurt your claim should your discussions fail to resolve the problem.

- If you need an accommodation to help you work, such as flexible working hours to accommodate doctors' appointments for follow-up or late effects treatment, suggest several alternatives to your employer. If your employer offers you accommodations, do not turn them down lightly. Such an offer may benefit the employer if the case ends up before a court. The Job Accommodation Network, a free service of the United States Department of Labor, helps employers fashion accommodations for disabled employees. Call 1.800.526.7234 or go to www.askjan.org for more information.
- Educate employers and coworkers who might believe that people cannot survive cancer and remain productive workers. For example, you could give your employer a letter from your doctor explaining your cancer history and why you are able to work.
- Ask a member of your health-care team to write or call your supervisor to offer to mediate the conflict and suggest accommodations.
- Consider seeking support from your coworkers. They have an interest in protecting themselves from future discrimination.

Survivors who are considering a lawsuit should take several precautions to protect their rights:

- *Keep carefully written records of all job actions*, *both good and bad*. Good actions, such as positive performance evaluations, may help to show that you were qualified for the job. Bad actions, such as being moved from a job that has much public interaction to a job that has little interaction with the public after your cancer history is disclosed, may be used against your employer to show illegal acts. Keep complete notes of telephone calls and meetings (including dates, times, and attendees), letters, and the names and addresses of witnesses. Make written notes as events occur instead of trying to recall the events weeks or months later.

- *Pause before you sue.* Carefully evaluate your goals. For example, do you want your job back, a change in working conditions, certain benefits, a written apology, or something else? Consider the positive and negative aspects of a lawsuit. Potential positive aspects include getting a job and monetary damages, protecting your rights, and tearing down barriers for other survivors. Potential negative aspects include long court battles with no guarantee of victory, legal fees and expenses, stress, and a hostile relationship between you and the people you sue.
- *Consider an informal settlement of your complaint.* A union representative, human resources employee, or social worker may be able to assist as a mediator. Your state or federal representative or local media may help persuade your employer to treat you fairly. Keep in mind that the first step most government agencies and companies take when they receive a complaint is to try to resolve the dispute without a costly lawsuit.
- *Be aware of filing deadlines so you do not lose your option to file a complaint under state or federal law.* You have 180 days from the date of the action against you to file a complaint with a federal agency. If you work for the federal government, you have only 45 days to begin counseling with an equal employment opportunity counselor. In most states, you have 180 days to file a complaint with the state agency. If you file a complaint and later change your mind, you can drop the lawsuit at any time.

If an informal solution does not work, a lawsuit may be the most appropriate next step for some survivors. To enforce a complaint under the Americans with Disabilities Act, the survivor must file a complaint with the Equal Employment Opportunities Commission (EEOC). The EEOC will attempt to settle the dispute. If no settlement is reached, the EEOC may appoint an investigator to evaluate the claim. If the EEOC determines that your rights may have been violated, the EEOC may sue on your behalf or may grant you the right to file a lawsuit in federal court.

Contact the EEOC at:

- 800.669.4000 to find your local EEOC office
- 800.669.EEOC or 800.669.3362 for more information about the ADA
- www.eeoc.gov

If you can prove that you are qualified for a job but were treated differently because of your cancer history, you may be entitled to:

- Back pay and benefits
- Injunctive relief such as reinstatement
- Monetary damages (e.g., for attorney's fees)

The Americans with Disabilities Act allows an award for compensatory or punitive damages up to $300,000 for intentional discrimination. Intentional discrimination, however, is difficult to prove, and these damages are not available against state or local governments or against a private employer who made a "good faith" effort to accommodate you.

Under the Federal Rehabilitation Act, employees or recipients of federal financial assistance have up to 180 days from the action against them to file a complaint with the federal government. Employees of the federal government, however, have only 30 days.

Survivors must file a complaint with the federal agency that provided federal funds to their employer. For more information, contact:

If your employer receives federal contracts:
United States Department of Labor
Office of Federal Compliance Programs
800.397.6251
www.dol.gov/esa/ofccp
If your employer receives federal financial assistance:
United States Department of Justice
Civil Rights Division, Disability Rights Section
800.514.0301
www.justice.gov/crt/about/drs

Under the Family and Medical Leave Act, you may choose between filing a lawsuit in court or filing a complaint with:
United States Department of Labor
Employment Standards Administration, Wage and Hour
866.487.9243
www.dol.gov/esa/whd/fmla

Most states have a state agency that enforces the law. Some states permit individuals to file a lawsuit in state court to enforce their rights. Under most state laws, employees have up to 180 days from the action against them to file a complaint with the state enforcement agency.

For more information about the laws in your state, contact your state commission on civil or human rights or contact an attorney who is experienced in job discrimination cases. The EEOC Public Information System at 1.800.669.4000 can help you locate the appropriate state enforcement agency.

In some situations, a single act may support a claim of discrimination under more than one law. For example, a cancer survivor who is denied a job by an employer in New York City may have a claim under the New York Human Rights Law (state), the New York City Law on Human Rights (city), and the Americans with Disabilities Act (federal).

Survivors who have a choice of remedies may file a complaint with each relevant enforcement agency. One agency may "stay" (not act on) the claim until another agency issues a decision. A survivor may always drop a complaint at any time once he or she determines which agency is most responsive. Factors to consider when choosing a resource include the types of remedies available, how quickly the agency responds to complaints (ask them how long the process usually takes), and which office is most convenient.

Survivors do not have to have a lawyer to represent them before an enforcement agency or court. However, someone who is represented by a lawyer experienced in job discrimination is more likely to succeed.

## 21.5 Health Insurance

### 21.5.1 The Impact of Cancer on Health Insurance

Because most individuals obtain health insurance through their own, their parents', or their spouse's employment, many insurance problems are related to loss of employment and employment discrimination. Those who are not covered by group policies are the most vulnerable to insurance problems.

Historically, survivors reported a variety of barriers to insurance, including refusal of new applications, policy cancellations or reductions, higher premiums, waived or excluded preexisting conditions, and extended waiting periods [14, 15, 17]. Survivors of childhood cancer also experienced problems obtaining health insurance. Like adult cancer survivors, the more years that had passed since treatment, the better the chances that childhood cancer survivors would obtain health insurance on the same terms as non-survivors [14, 18].

Barriers to adequate health insurance can have a detrimental impact on survivors' physical, emotional, financial, social, and occupational health [19]. Survivors who have private health insurance and higher income experience better cancer screening, treatment, and access to medical care [19]. This discrepancy is so great that survivors who have no or inadequate health insurance experience poorer health and higher mortality risks [19]. With the growth of managed care, survivors are increasingly forced to make decisions regarding their choice of type of treatment, treatment site, and provider, based on whether their insurance plan will cover treatment, rather than on whether their choices satisfy their medical and personal needs [19].

### 21.5.2 Cancer Patients' Health Insurance Rights

Cancer survivors who have health insurance are entitled to all of the rights described in their policies. Insurers who fail to pay for treatment in accordance with the terms of the policies may be sued for violating the contract between the survivor and the insurer.

### 21.5.2.1 Federal Health Insurance Laws

Several federal laws help cancer survivors obtain new health insurance, as well as help them retain insurance. Although they are briefly described below, more information about these laws is available at www.healthcare.gov. The United States Department of Health and Human Services also provides consumer information on health insurance options for children and links to state resources at www.insurekidsnow.gov and 877.543.7669.

### Affordable Care Act

The Affordable Care Act (ACA) significantly expands young adult survivors' access to health insurance. The ACA requires parents' individual and employer-provided health plans to cover their young adult children until the age of 26. This mandate covers married and unmarried young adults and applies to existing employer plans unless the adult child has another offer of employer-based coverage (such as through his or her job). Beginning in 2014, children up to age 26 can stay on their parent's employer plan even if they have another offer of coverage through an employer.

Employers with more than 50 employees must offer health benefits by January 1, 2015, or pay a tax. Employees who do not receive health insurance through work will be able to purchase new health insurance in state-run marketplaces called "exchanges," where they can compare health insurance policies. Families who make between 100 % and 400 % of the federal poverty level will be eligible for tax credits to purchase insurance. Individuals under the age of 65 who earn income up to 133 % of the federal poverty level will be covered by Medicaid.

The ACA prohibits insurers from discriminating against individuals based on preexisting conditions such as a cancer history.

### Americans with Disabilities Act

The ADA prohibits employers from denying health insurance to cancer patients if other employees with similar jobs receive insurance. Because the ADA protects employees from discrimination based on their association with a person with a disability, an employer may not refuse to provide a family health policy solely because one of the employee's dependents has cancer.

### Children's Health Insurance Program

Many low-income children receive health benefits through Medicaid. The Children's Health Insurance Program (CHIP) provides health insurance to children in families with incomes too high to qualify for Medicaid. CHIP is administered by states through state and federal funding. CHIP offers health insurance coverage to low-income, uninsured children under the age of 19. Because each state can design its own CHIP plan, the eligibility requirements vary from state to state. For information about a specific state CHIP, contact your state public welfare or social services department or visit www.healthcare.gov.

### Comprehensive Omnibus Budget Reconciliation Act

The Comprehensive Omnibus Budget Reconciliation Act (COBRA) requires employers to offer group medical coverage to employees and their dependents who otherwise would have lost their group coverage due to individual circumstances. Public and private employers with more than 20 employees are required to make continued insurance coverage available to employees who quit, are terminated, or work reduced hours. Coverage must extend to surviving, divorced, or separated spouses and to dependent children.

By allowing survivors to keep group insurance coverage for a limited time, COBRA provides valuable time to shop for long-term coverage. Although the survivor, and not the former employer, must pay for the continued coverage, the rate may not exceed more than 2 % the rate set for the former coworkers.

Eligibility for the employee, spouse, and dependent child varies under COBRA. The employee becomes eligible if he or she loses group health coverage because of a reduction in hours or because of termination due to reasons other than gross employee misconduct. The spouse of an employee becomes eligible for any of four reasons:

1. Death of spouse.
2. Termination of spouse's employment (for reasons other than gross misconduct) or reduction in spouse's hours of employment.
3. Divorce or legal separation from spouse.
4. Spouse becomes eligible for Medicare.

The dependent child of an employee becomes eligible for any of the five reasons:

1. Death of parent.
2. Termination of parent's employment or reduction in parent's hours.
3. Parent's divorce or legal separation.
4. Parent becomes eligible for Medicare.
5. Dependent ceases to be a dependent child under a specific group plan.

The continued coverage under COBRA must be identical to that offered to the families of the employee's former coworkers. If employment is terminated for any reason other than gross misconduct, the employee and his or her dependents can continue receiving coverage for up to 18 months. A qualified beneficiary who is determined to be disabled for Social Security purposes at the time of the termination of employment or reduction in employment hours can continue COBRA coverage for a total of 29 months. Dependents can continue coverage for up to 36 months if their previous coverage will end because of any of the above reasons.

Continued coverage may be cut short if:

1. The employer no longer provides group health insurance to any of its employees.
2. The continuation coverage premium is not paid.
3. The survivor becomes covered under another group health plan.
4. The survivor becomes eligible for Medicare.

The Employee Benefits Security Administration of the United States Department of Labor enforces COBRA for most employers in the private sector. The Centers for Medicare and Medicaid Services of the United States Department of Health and Human Services regulates COBRA compliance by state and local government employers.

### Health Insurance Portability and Accountability Act (HIPAA)

HIPAA restricts how health information can be used by a health-care provider, health plan, and other related organizations. Health-care providers and employers may not use health information for employment reasons. Information about an individual's health can be used only for reasons related to treatment, payment, and health-care operations. The United States Department of Health and Human Services, Office of Civil Rights, provides information about privacy rights and medical care at http://www.hhs.gov/ocr/hipaa/ and 866.627.7748.

#### 21.5.2.2 State Insurance Laws

Every state regulates policies sold by insurance companies in the state. These laws vary significantly. Some states require insurance policies to cover off-label chemotherapy, minimum hospital stays for cancer surgery, and benefits for certain types of cancer treatment and screening. Most states provide the right to convert a group health insurance policy to an individual policy. The specific rules of open enrollment periods vary from state to state. Additionally, some states provide stronger privacy protections than those provided by HIPAA. Contact your state insurance department for more information.

### 21.5.3 How to Challenge a Denied Claim

Cancer treatment often involves numerous bills from different parties: hospital, physicians (surgeon, anesthesiologist, oncologist, radiologist, etc.), support services (nurse, social worker, nutritionist, therapist, etc.), radiology group, pharmacy (drugs and medical supplies), and consumer businesses (wigs, breast inserts, special clothing, etc.). Insurance companies will pay some of these parties directly, in part or in whole. The survivor must pay other bills and submit copies to the company for reimbursement.

Keeping track of expenses, often amounting to tens of thousands of dollars, can be confusing and exhausting. The key to collecting the maximum benefits covered by the insurance policy is to keep accurate records of all medical expenses by:

- Making photocopies of everything you send to your insurance company, including letters, claim forms, and bills
- Keeping all correspondence you receive from your insurance company
- Submitting a bill, even if you are unsure whether a particular expense is covered by your policy
- Keeping accurate records of your expenses, claim submissions, and payment vouchers

A policyholder has a right to appeal a claim that is denied by a public or private insurer. Because claims are frequently delayed or rejected in part or in full because of errors in filling out the claims forms, carefully provide all the information requested by the insurance company. The following steps could help survivors who are having trouble collecting on their claims:

- Contact your insurance company in writing and insist that they reply in writing. Send copies of all documents and keep the originals for your files.
- Keep a record of your contacts with the insurance company (copies of all letters you send and notes from every telephone call). Write down everything you do, the names of people you talk to, dates, and other facts.
- Contact the state or federal agency that regulates your insurance provider if you do not receive a satisfactory and timely answer from your insurer. Most state insurance departments or commissions help consumers with complaints.
- Contact cancer support organizations in your community. Some offer ombudsman programs to help survivors and their families maximize insurance reimbursement.

- If your claim is still not settled, consider filing a complaint in small claims court or hiring a lawyer to sue your insurance company.

## 21.6 Right to Education

Some survivors of childhood cancer grow up with long-term and late effects of treatment that affect their ability to receive an education and obtain gainful employment. Late effects of radiation, chemotherapy, and surgery can include physical and mental limitations, such as neurocognitive deficits, growth retardation, cardiac dysfunction, second malignancies, and fatigue. Two federal laws protect survivors who have such disabilities from barriers to education, which in turn help expand their employment opportunities.

### 21.6.1 Individuals with Disabilities Education Act

The Individuals with Disabilities Education Act (IDEA) requires states to provide children with disabilities with a free appropriate public education from the age of 3–21. A child with a disability includes a child with developmental disabilities; a hearing, speech, visual, or orthopedic impairment; a serious emotional disturbance; brain injury; autism; learning disability; or other similar health impairment.

The purpose of the IDEA is to ensure that children with disabilities receive a public education that emphasizes special education and related services designed to address their individual needs. Thus, every child is entitled to an individualized education plan (IEP), which is crafted by a team of professionals who are familiar with the child's specific limitations, needs, and abilities. Where possible, school districts are required to provide children with disabilities an education in the regular classroom setting. Schools must provide services that are necessary to help a child benefit from his or her education. These services may include a special education teacher, voice or sign language interpreter, large-print texts, placement in private school, testing accommodations, tutor, special transportation, occupational therapy, physical therapy, speech therapy, or psychotherapy. Although schools are not required to provide all medical services, they must provide certain medical services that are necessary to implement the IEP. For example, a child who uses a catheter is entitled to the services of a school nurse or other trained professional to help keep the catheter clean and functioning during the school day.

## 21.6.2 Americans with Disabilities Act

Students in higher education are covered by the Americans with Disabilities Act. The ADA mandates that no individual with a disability shall be excluded from participation in public services or programs, such as higher education. Educational institutions are required to provide disabled students who can meet the academic standards of the school with reasonable accommodations. For example, a university may be required to provide a sign language interpreter and/or note taker for a cancer survivor who has a hearing loss as a result of treatment. Additionally, the institution may not discriminate on the basis of the student's disability. For example, a survivor who has respiratory fibrosis may not be required to complete the same physical educational standards required of other students.

---

**Conclusion**

Survivors of childhood cancer diagnosed in the twenty-first century can expect fewer legal and economic barriers than those encountered by survivors in the past. Although some barriers to affordable health care remain, the majority of childhood cancer survivors today will enter schools and the job market with a decreasing chance of facing discrimination and an increasing array of legal rights and remedies.

## 21.7 Appendix

Tables 21.1, 21.2, 21.3, and 21.4 give details of some useful resources, outline the main provisions of the Americans with Disabilities Act and the Family and Medical Leave Act, and summarize advice on avoidance and handling of workplace discrimination.

**Table 21.1** Resources

| **National Coalition for Cancer Survivorship** |
|---|
| Provides publications, answers to questions about employment rights, and assistance locating legal resources |
| 877.NCCS.YES or 877.622.7937 |
| www.canceradvocacy.org |
| **National Cancer Legal Services Network** |
| Provides a searchable database of organizations that provide legal services to cancer survivors. The National Cancer Legal Services Network (NCLSN) is a coalition of attorneys, legal service programs, cancer support organizations, and health-care providers |
| www.nclsn.org |
| **Cancer Legal Resource Center** |
| Provides information and education on cancer-related legal issues, including health insurance, employment, government benefits, estate planning, advance health-care directives, family law, and financial assistance. The Cancer Legal Resource Center (CLRC) is a community-based joint program of the Disability Rights Legal Center and Loyola Law School (California) |
| 866.843.2572 |
| www.disabilityrightslegalcenter.org/ |
| **Cancer and Careers** |
| Provides free publications, career coaching, and a series of support groups and educational seminars for employees with cancer and their health-care providers and coworkers |
| www.cancerandcareers.org |
| **Cancer Care, Inc**. |
| Provides assistance by oncology social workers, including answers to questions about employment rights and assistance locating legal resources |
| 800.813.HOPE or 800.813.4673 |
| www.cancercare.org |
| **American Cancer Society** |
| Services vary widely from county to county. Some ACS units may be able to help you find a lawyer in some areas |
| 800.ACS.2345 or 800.227.2345 |
| www.cancer.org |

(continued)

**Table 21.1** (continued)

**Patient Advocate Foundation**

Provides patients with arbitration, mediation, and negotiation to settle issues with access to care, medical debt, and job retention related to their illness

800.532.5274

www.patientadvocate.org/

**The Childhood Cancer Ombudsman Program,** a service provided by the Childhood Brain Tumor Foundation, facilitates problem solving for families, patients, and adult survivors. Services include analysis of cases involving access and discrimination issues in health care, insurance, employment, and education by ombudsman volunteers from medicine, genetics, rehabilitation, ethics, education, psychology, social work, and the law

877.217.4166

www.childhoodbraintumor.org

**Table 21.2** Americans with Disabilities Act

| What the ADA prohibits |
| --- |
| Discrimination based on actual disability, perceived disability, or history of disability |
| Which employers are covered by the ADA |
| Employers with at least 15 employees |
| What the ADA requires |
| Reasonable accommodations |
| Employer may ask only job-related medical questions |
| Employer may not discriminate because a family member is ill |
| How the ADA is enforced |
| Enforced by the EEOC: 800.669.4000 (local EEOC office); 800.669.EEOC (enforcement information) |

**Table 21.3** Family and Medical Leave Act

| Applies to employers with 50+ employees |
| --- |
| Provides 12 weeks of unpaid leave during any 12-month period to care for seriously ill self, spouse, child, or parent |
| Requires employer to continue to provide benefits—including health insurance—during the leave period |
| Requires employer to restore employee to the same or equivalent position at the end of the leave period |
| Requires employee to make reasonable efforts to schedule foreseeable medical care so as not to disrupt the workplace |
| Enforced by private lawsuit |

**Table 21.4** Discrimination

| How to avoid employment discrimination |
| --- |
| Do not volunteer cancer history |
| Do not lie about medical history |
| Keep focus on current health and ability |
| Be prepared with letter from physician |
| Seek employment with large employers |
| Do not ask about health benefits prior to job offer |
| Steps to take if confronted with discrimination |
| Consider resolving problem informally |
| Suggest accommodations |
| Seek support from health-care providers, coworkers, legal resources, and other survivors |
| Keep written records of actions |
| Be aware of filing deadlines |
| Carefully evaluate goals |

# References

1. The 2009 SEER data indicates that 83% of children ages 0 to 19 will be alive five years after their cancer diagnosis. http://seer.cancer.gov/csr/1975_2009_pops09/browse_csr.php?section=28&page=sect_28_table.08.html

2. Bleyer WA (1990) The impact of childhood cancer on the United States and the world. CA Cancer J Clin 40:355–367

3. Meadows A, Green D, Oeffinger K (2003) Pediatric cancer survivors: past history and future challenges. Curr Probl Cancer 27:105–168

4. Siegel R et al (2012) Cancer treatment survivorship and statistic. CA A Cancer J Clin 62(4):220–241

5. Hoffman B (2010) Protecting your patients from job discrimination. Oncol Nurse Ed 24:4, 15

6. Feuerstein M et al (2010) Work in cancer survivors: a model for practice and research. J Cancer Surviv 4:415–416

7. Spelten E (2002) Factors reported to influence the return to work of cancer survivors: a literature review. Psychooncology 11:124–131

8. Short P et al (2005) Employment pathways in a large cohort of adult cancer survivors. Cancer 103(6): 1292–1301

9. Bradley C, Bednarek H (2002) Employment patterns of long-term cancer survivors. Psychooncology 11:188–198

10. Zebrack B (2010) Cancer and job loss. Oncol Nurse Ed 24:4–19

11. Fobair P, Hoppe RT, Bloom J, Cox J, Varghese A, Spiegel D (1986) Psychosocial problems among survivors of Hodgkin's disease. J Clin Oncol 4:805–814

12. Koocher GP, O'Malley JE (1982) The Damocles syndrome: psychosocial consequences of surviving childhood cancer. McGraw-Hill, New York

13. Teta MJ, del Po MC, Kasl SV, Meigs JW, Myers MH, Mulvihill JJ (1986) Psychosocial consequences of childhood and adolescent cancer survival. J Chronic Dis 39:751–759

14. Hays DM et al (1992) Educational, occupational, and insurance status of childhood cancer survivors in their fourth and fifth decades of life. J Clin Oncol 10:1397–1406

15. Dowling E et al (2010) Burden of illness in adult survivors of childhood cancers: findings from a population-based national sample. Cancer 116(15):3712–3721

16. Equal Employment Opportunity Commission, ADA charge data by impairment/bases—receipts, www.eeoc.gov/eeoc/statistics/enforcement/ada-receipts.cfm. Last visited 14 Jun 2012

17. Kornblith AB et al (1998) Comparison of psychosocial adaptation of advanced stage Hodgkin's disease and acute leukemia survivors. Ann Oncol 9: 297–306

18. Vann JC et al (1995) Health insurance access to young adult survivors of childhood cancer in North Carolina. Med Pediatr Oncol 25:389–395

19. Glajchen M (1994) Psychosocial consequences of inadequate health insurance for patients with cancer. Cancer Pract 2:115–120

# Methodology Considerations in the Study of Survivors of Childhood Cancer

**22**

Ann C. Mertens, Wendy Leisenring,
and Yutaka Yasui

## Contents

W. Leisenring, PhD
Cancer Prevention Program, Fred Hutchinson Cancer
Research Center, Seattle, WA

Y. Yasui, PhD
School of Public Health, University of Alberta,
Edmonton, AB, Canada

A.C. Mertens, PhD, MS (✉)
Department of Hematology/Oncology, Children's
Healthcare of Atlanta-Egleston,
2015 Uppergate Drive, Atlanta, GA, 30322, USA
e-mail: ann.mertens@choa.orgit

## 22.1 Introduction

Numerous reports and reviews have been published about the late effects of cancer and its treatment among childhood cancer survivors [17, 19, 22, 27]. This literature describes the sequelae present at, or shortly following, the end of therapy, as well as the occurrence of selected late complications. Most studies of late sequelae focus on medical outcomes, although psychosocial and economic outcomes among survivors have a growing literature. These studies have shown that the type and intensity of therapy, as well as the age of the patient at therapy, are important factors influencing both overall survival and the occurrence of late effects. Children who are younger at diagnosis and treatment are more severely affected than older children, particularly if treatment is administered at a time of significant development and growth. However, specific treatment exposures and outcomes remain to be investigated in depth. Well-designed epidemiologic investigations of these subjects can provide strong and reliable evidence on which to base both clinical practice and health policy. The objectives of this chapter are to present an overview of methodological issues important in the proper conduct and analysis of late-effect studies, to outline briefly several types of study design that are useful, and next steps in the research of childhood cancer survivorship research.

© Springer International Publishing 2015
C.L. Schwartz et al. (eds.), *Survivors of Childhood and Adolescent Cancer:*
*A Multidisciplinary Approach*, Pediatric Oncology, DOI 10.1007/978-3-319-16435-9_22

## 22.2 Methodological Issues Relevant to Survivor Studies

### 22.2.1 Selection of Study Subjects

Studies of late effects begin with the conjecture that a particular factor or exposure may influence the occurrence of a disease or outcome. A study is then designed to test the conjecture or hypothesis. The first, and perhaps the most important, task in the study design is the definition and selection of the population to be tested and the definition and selection of the comparison group, i.e., the group that will appropriately determine whether a statistical association exists between the factor or exposure of interest and the outcome or disease of interest. The study population must be defined in such a way that it is as representative as possible of the wider population of interest (i.e., the entire population of childhood cancer survivors). Care must be exercised in selecting survivors and a non-survivor comparison population to minimize the possibility of differential selection on the basis of exposure. The first step in the survivor case selection is to define the disease/outcome of interest and to establish strict diagnostic criteria to keep the disease entity well defined. Subjects can be obtained from a population-based source, such as a disease registry, from hospital or clinic records over a specified period of time, or they can be members of a defined study cohort assembled from a single institution or a consortium of treating institutions. Each source from which potential study subjects can be drawn will present both drawbacks and benefits. Studies that recruit their subjects from single institutions generally suffer from small sample sizes and findings may be less generalizable. There are advantages to single institution studies, particularly if outcomes of interest require clinic follow-up or testing. Clinical trial consortiums, such as the Children's Oncology Group, have the advantage of being able to evaluate protocol-defined patient cohorts who receive uniform therapies. A drawback, however, is that cases enrolled in the study are not necessarily representative of the full spectrum of a disease or diseases. To define a study cohort based on protocol-defined disease or diseases among such a consortia of institutions allows for complete case ascertainment from each participating institution but can also suffer from low participation rates or from subjects being lost to follow-up.

An important rule of thumb for the selection of the non-survivor comparison group is that it should represent a population with the potential to develop the disease or condition being studied. The use of siblings of survivors as the study's comparison group is appropriate, on the assumption that these individuals share many of the same genetic and environmental factors, with the exception of treatment exposures, and, as a result, that their risk for developing diseases/conditions was comparable to that of their sibling who had had cancer. A significant drawback to using siblings, however, is if the outcomes of interest are factors for which they will be over-matched, such as genetics or other familial factors. There are also limitations if analyses are restricted to complete sibling pairs, such that patients without involved siblings are not represented. The usual alternative is to include all survivors plus any siblings that agree to participate, with care taken to evaluate the degree to which the siblings (or their survivor pair) who participate are representative of those who do not. If they are not representative, then bias may also be introduced in this setting. For all research involving human subjects, it is critical that the study protocol is reviewed and approved by their Institutional Review Board, all potential subjects are properly informed of their risk in participation, and consent is received before subjects are enrolled in research.

### 22.2.2 Bias, Confounding, Matching

Once a well-defined study population has been assembled, it is then necessary to assess the study hypothesis with considerations of possible alternative explanations and whether the statistical association under investigation represents a cause-effect relationship between exposure and disease.

To determine whether a statistical association is valid, possible sources of bias must be considered and, if possible, eliminated. Bias refers to any element of the study design, data collection, or data analysis that introduces a systematic error into the results. It can occur when individuals are selected into a study or through the manner in which information is obtained or reported. Bias is minimized by ensuring that subject selection, exposure assessment, and methods of collecting information are all identical between the two groups being compared.

Confounding is an alternative explanation for an observed association between an outcome and an exposure. Confounding occurs when unmeasured or uncontrolled factors associated both with the exposure and with the outcome explain the observed association. A confounder variable cannot be a step in the causal pathway between the exposure and the outcome. One can control for known confounders either in the study design or analysis phase. To address confounding in the study design, matching can be performed. Matching is the selection of a comparison group that is identical to the group of interest with respect to the distribution of one or more confounders. Often, one matches on known major risk factors, such as age for chronic diseases, in order to remove their effect so that the effect of exposure variables under study can be more clearly discerned. If sufficient numbers of subjects with a full range of confounding covariate values are present in the cohort, then adjusted comparisons can be made using regression techniques for analyses.

## 22.2.3 Exposure Assessment

In assessing the risk of late effects by therapeutic exposure, one must obtain accurate and detailed information on all cancer therapies received by the patients. The assessment process must be unbiased with respect to patients' characteristics, including the types of cancer, the treating institution, whether the patient has experienced any late effects, and the length of follow-up. Specifically, the information must be equally available and of equal quality across all institutions participating in the study. Furthermore, it should include all relevant exposures prior to development of the condition under investigation, including treatment for any recurrence of the individual's original diagnosis and for any subsequent primary cancer. A potential obstacle to the accurate assessment of therapeutic exposures is either incomplete or lost medical records. To ensure accuracy and minimize bias, a detailed, clear protocol for therapeutic exposure assessment must be prepared and followed. Such a protocol includes the development of a structured, medical record abstraction form, as well as consistent training of personnel to abstract the medical records. Alternatively, the late effects resulting from a phase III randomized clinical therapeutic protocol can be evaluated without such an in-depth record review by comparing outcomes based on assigned treatment regimen.

## 22.2.4 Outcome Assessment

While medical records can be used to ascertain outcome data, such records have significant limitations in the study of long-term outcomes in childhood cancer survivors. As survivors grow into adults, the medical facilities at which they receive care will likely shift from the institutions where they were treated for their primary diagnosis to adult care facilities. Because of the large number of adult care facilities involved, requesting copies of records can be costly, as well as inefficient. Direct communication with study subjects – in person, by telephone, or by mail – using standardized interview protocols or questionnaires, is a more practical method of preliminary outcome ascertainment in late-effect research. Data on outcomes for which self-reporting is unreliable can then be supplemented/validated by a focused collection of medical records, potentially using electronic medical records to facilitate these efforts.

A well-constructed survey instrument capable of eliciting reliable and valid medical information from study subjects is crucial to success in late-effect research. Questions must be phrased in such a way as to obtain the most accurate information possible while encouraging high response rates. Both closed and open-ended questions can be useful in late-effect studies. Closed questions require subjects to respond with a limited number of set responses (e.g., a list of drugs); open-ended questions require respondents to recall information and give explanations of events. All questionnaires and other data capture forms must be piloted before first use to determine whether questions are properly phrased, unambiguous, and at an acceptable reading level and to ensure that the contents of the questionnaire and the length of time required to complete it are acceptable to respondents. Determination of these properties of the questionnaire is best performed with individuals who are similar to those to be enrolled in the study (i.e., similar age group, parents of children in hospital with other health conditions), but not be a potential study subject.

### 22.2.4.1 Confirmation of Key Medical Events

Data on key medical events collected by interview or questionnaire can be validated by medical records, particularly for well-known medical events that have clear diagnostic criteria, and where the participant has good recollection of where they were seen for the condition [15]. For example, information about hospitalizations for recurrent or new primary neoplasms can be validated by obtaining the pathology report from the diagnosing hospital. Review of the pathology report can then confirm the diagnosis reported on the questionnaire.

For validation of other medical outcomes, careful consideration has to be made as to which outcomes of interest warrant additional personnel effort and cost. First, outcomes that are self-reported on a study questionnaire can be followed-up with a telephone script to elucidate whether and where the participant received treatment for the reported outcomes. Second, using a signed HIPAA release form, a request for the subject's medical records for the time period of the diagnosis of the selected outcome can then be made to the appropriate institution. Key late effects that can be validated in this fashion, if the medical records can be obtained, include congestive heart failure, myocardial infarction, stroke, and lung fibrosis.

Medical records are useful for identifying false-positive, self-reported outcomes; however, it is difficult to identify false-negative outcome events that are not reported by the respondent. To remedy this, a fraction of the study subjects who do not self-report a selected outcome can be chosen randomly for assessment by medical records. For the analysis of potentially misclassified outcome data with a validation subset such as this, see references [23, 24].

Key medical events can also be validated during a clinical assessment. For example, risk-based health evaluations, as recommended by the Children's Oncology Group for childhood cancer survivors, can be used to document key medical events during a cancer survivor clinic visit [5]. Alternatively, specific physical evaluations could be requested through one of the medical research institutions designated within the Clinical and Translational Science Award (CTSA) program, which is supported by the National Institute of Health [6]. The CTSA Consortium consists of approximately 60 medical research institutions located throughout the United States and provides researchers the use of inpatient and/or outpatient nursing units and/or use of laboratory resources for NIH grant funded projects [9].

## 22.2.5 Need for External Comparisons

A comparison group outside of the survivor population of interest is needed to evaluate the extent of the excess risk of a selected outcome experienced by survivors. For example, it is expected that chronic disease frequencies increase as survivor's age: the question is whether, and to what extent, survivors are experiencing excess risk beyond that seen in the general population. An external control cohort, whose members have not been exposed to the therapy-related risk factors under investigation, such as survivors' close-age siblings or friends, can provide a convenient comparison group. To avoid potential bias, assessments of exposures and outcomes in such an external comparison cohort must be done in an equal manner as in the survivor cohort. Survivor cohorts can also be compared to available population data, such as mortality from vital statistics, cancer incidence from the US surveillance, epidemiology, and end results (SEER) program, or health behaviors reported in the National Health Interview Survey (NHIS). To assure comparability of study data with external population data, it is necessary to use the same definitions of outcomes (e.g., specific types of cancer as defined by SEER) and the same questionnaire items (e.g., smoking question items used in the NHIS) as those used by the population registry or survey to which study participants are being compared.

### 22.2.6 Importance of Thorough Recruitment and Follow-Up

Significant loss of eligible cases in any study can compromise the validity of study findings, since it will be difficult to determine if exposures or outcomes of interest are in some way related to the loss. Non-participation in case-control studies can cause bias if response rates differ between cases and controls and are somehow related to exposure. Loss to follow-up from either cases not found at the initiation of the study or those lost after entry into the cohort introduces another potential source of bias. For example, individuals who remain in the study might be healthier than those who drop out or those who participate may not be truly representative of the population in terms of rates of disease or risk factors.

#### 22.2.6.1 Tracing Techniques

In late-effect research, it is particularly important to achieve maximum ascertainment, enrollment, and follow-up of the eligible study population in order to minimize the potential introduction of bias. One challenge is to locate subjects who may have moved since they became eligible for membership in the cohort [18, 21]. Hospital records are commonly used for assembling a cohort. Because most of the information contained in such records is not collected with the objective of long-term follow-up, key pieces of information that would facilitate tracing and successful location of eligible subjects are often missing.

Moreover, subjects who have ongoing medical conditions, which might include the research outcomes of interest, may be more likely to have been seen in follow-up visits and to have had their addresses updated in their medical records. This increases the potential for enrolling a selected and possibly biased study population.

In attempting to contact a cohort by mail, correspondence can be sent to subjects (or their parents) at the last known address per medical records, via envelopes marked "Address Service Requested." Common tracing techniques for nonrespondents include directory assistance and Internet searches (peoplefinder websites). If these methods fail, commercial survey research firms can be employed for more intensive tracing. The sources such firms might pursue can include telephone directory assistance, reverse telephone directories, Polk's directories, voter registration records, post offices, Department of Motor Vehicles, and commercial credit bureaus. Study subjects who are not successfully traced by these methods can be processed through the National Death Index (NDI) to determine vital status.

With the rapid change of technology over the past decade, however, these traditional methods of patient recruitment need to be reconsidered. Both parents of pediatric patients and those pediatric cancer survivors who are now 18 years of age or older are highly mobile populations. In addition, these two demographic groups are not as available or as responsive to contact by traditional mail mechanisms and are less likely to have a traditional landline telephone. Therefore, successful recruitment of these populations will require capturing relevant contact information through hospital records, such as cell phone numbers and reliable email addresses, and strategies for innovative use of electronic recruitment methods, such as use of various web-based modalities.

### 22.2.7 Use of Molecular Tools

While an increased risk of late effects is often associated with treatment-related factors, individual susceptibility to a particular outcome is clearly variable, with the majority of patients treated for cancer not affected. A possible explanation for unequal susceptibility is variability in the genetic make-up of survivors; differences in drug metabolism may modify the exposure itself, while genetic risk of toxicity affects the outcome of the exposure. Biologic specimens can be collected to evaluate genetic influence on the risk of late effects. Collection of genomic DNA samples, however, is a challenge in a survivor study population that is large, highly mobile, and geographically dispersed.

Several studies have reported success in collecting buccal cell samples by mailing mouthwash to participants and requesting return by mail [8, 14, 20]. Other materials that can be collected for use in genetic or proteomic research are tumor tissue from subsequent cancers and blood specimens. A limitation on the collection of tumor specimens is that many community hospitals store tumor tissues only for a limited time after surgery. Blood specimens can be requested and collected during a participant's regularly scheduled doctor's appointment, although this can be expensive and logistically complex. Another possibility is to contract with a company, such as those that perform insurance physicals, to arrange for a phlebotomist to visit the participant's home or office (or other convenient location) to take the blood specimen. Or, collection of genomic DNA might best be accomplished at diagnosis.

In addition to genetic susceptibility analyses, the biologic specimens can potentially be used for other research purposes, such as the identification of high-risk groups and for genetic/proteomic screening for late effects.

## 22.3	Types of Epidemiologic Study Designs

Two basic types of study design are employed in epidemiologic research of late effects: descriptive studies and analytic studies. Features of both the exposure (usually treatment-related) and the outcome will influence the choice of study design, as will the amount of time needed to collect the data and the resources available to

conduct the study. Results of previous research and gaps in knowledge that remain to be filled must also be taken into account. A given hypothesis can be, and often is, the subject of a progression of different types of studies, each building on a previous study, as researchers attempt to gain increasing precision in their understanding of particular late effects.

### 22.3.1	Descriptive Studies

Descriptive studies are essentially concerned with the distribution of the late effect or disease outcome of interest. These types of studies are primarily used to generate hypotheses. They generally use existing data and are, therefore, relatively inexpensive to conduct. However, they cannot ascertain cause-and-effect relationships between exposure and outcome. The three principal types of descriptive study are case reports, case series, and cross-sectional studies.

Case reports and case series describe the characteristics of one or more subjects with a given disease. Typically, these studies have a relatively small number of subjects. These types of reports can lead to the formulation of hypotheses for testing in analytic studies. An example of a case series report is an early review of retinoblastoma patients treated with radiation who subsequently presented with osteogenic sarcoma as a second primary diagnosis [28]. Because these tumors occurred in the radiation field at sites that were uncharacteristic of spontaneously occurring sarcomas, the investigators suggested a strong role for radiation in their etiology. The link between retinoblastoma and subsequent sarcomas has been confirmed in several follow-up studies.

Cross-sectional studies, also referred to as prevalence studies, are descriptive studies used to assess the presence (or absence) of both exposure and disease at the same point in time. Results from these studies are useful in generating hypotheses regarding possible associations between exposure and disease. As with other descriptive studies, they represent a feasible and affordable strategy for developing etiologic hypotheses. There are many examples of cross-sectional studies in the late-effect literature that have led to further research. For example, Sklar et al. conducted a study of final adult height attainment in long-term survivors of acute lymphoblastic leukemia [30]. This was one of the first studies to track changes in height through adulthood and to associate these findings with different treatment regimens (no cranial radiation, 1,800 cGY cranial radiation, 2,400 cGY cranial radiation). It led to subsequent studies that have confirmed the significance of the association between cranial radiation dosage and final height attainment.

## 22.3.2 Analytic Studies

Analytic studies focus on determinants of a disease and are often set up to test hypotheses generated from previous descriptive studies. Analytic studies are designed to determine whether certain exposures cause (or prevent) a disease of interest. The general approach for analytic studies is first to define the outcome (disease) of interest, then to identify the exposed and unexposed groups. The choice of analytic design depends on the features of the exposure and the disease, the current state of knowledge regarding the hypothesis of interest, and, finally, the available time and financial resources. The methodological issues discussed in the first section of this chapter pertain to the design and conduct of all types of analytic studies of the late effects discussed below.

### 22.3.2.1 Case-Control Study

The case-control study is the most common type of epidemiologic study design. It is often used to determine preliminary information about the etiology of a disease. In this type of study, cases and controls are selected on the basis of the outcome status of interest, and the frequency and/or dosage of the exposure in question is compared between the groups. In late-effect studies, the case-control design is somewhat uncommon because the exposure of interest (specific cancer treatment) is already known. However, case-control studies nested within cohort studies are often employed in late-effect research (see description of nested case-control studies, below).

### 22.3.2.2 Cohort Study

The cohort study is perhaps the most effective study design for late-effect research. A cohort study compares a group of subjects who share a common characteristic (such as being treated for childhood cancer) within a defined time period. Subjects within the cohort are categorized according to exposures of interest. The groups are followed over time and their outcomes are compared. Cohort studies typically enroll large numbers of individuals and follow them for many years. Because of the study population selected, cohort studies allow the assessment of rare exposures (e.g., cranial radiation). They also allow the assessment of multiple outcomes from a single exposure (e.g., development of subsequent CNS tumors, neurocognitive problems). Cohort studies are very expensive to mount. They are also subject to certain types of bias, notably attrition bias resulting from either dropout or loss to follow-up.

A principal benefit of cohort studies is that they make possible the calculation of both the absolute risk and the relative risk of an outcome of interest. Absolute risk is a measure of the occurrence of a disease in a population, divided by the number at risk for the disease. Relative risk is defined as the ratio of the incidence of disease in those exposed, divided by the incidence of disease in those not exposed. It estimates the magnitude of the risk in the exposed group relative to that in the unexposed group.

Many long-term survivor studies have used the cohort design. In the Five-Center Study, for instance, Byrne et al. studied effects of treatment on fertility in 2,283 childhood/adolescent cancer survivors, compared with 3,270 subjects selected from the survivors' siblings [4]. They found that chemotherapy with alkylating agents was associated with a fertility deficit in men, while in women, alkylating agents were associated with only a moderate fertility deficit when administered with radiation below the diaphragm. An example of a larger-scale investigation is the cohort study by Boivin et al., who examined the risk of second cancers by treatment modalities in 10,472 long-term survivors of Hodgkin disease [3].

The largest North American cohort study to date is the Childhood Cancer Survivor Study (CCSS), a multi-institutional collaboration established in 1994, to assess late, adverse events following treatment for childhood or adolescent cancer. Each participating institution identified patients who fulfilled the following eligibility criteria: (a) diagnosis of leukemia, CNS tumors (all histologies), Hodgkin disease, non-Hodgkin lymphoma, malignant kidney tumor (Wilms), neuroblastoma, soft tissue sarcoma, or bone tumor (list of eligible ICD-O codes can be found at www.stjude.org/ccss); (b) diagnosis and initial treatment at 1 of the 26 collaborating CCSS institutions; (c) diagnosis date between January 1, 1970, and December 31, 1986; (d) age less than 21 years at diagnosis; and (e) survival 5 years from diagnosis.

Information on the characteristics of the original cancer diagnosis and treatment was obtained for 20,276 eligible cases from the treating institution [26]. Baseline data were collected for members of the study cohort using a 24-page, self-administered questionnaire; four follow-up surveys have been conducted after the collection of the baseline data from the study cohort. Detailed treatment information was obtained for participants who gave permission to abstract information from their medical records. The data collection surveys are available for review at www.stjude.org/ccss.

### 22.3.2.3 Nested Case-Control Design

Large, well-defined survivor cohorts can provide an ideal setting for smaller analytic studies focusing on rare outcomes. A nested case-control study [16] is a case-control study conducted within a defined cohort. The advantage of a nested case-control study is that it avoids the potential selection bias inherent in standard case-control designs. Nested case-control designs are useful especially when the assessment of exposure is resource-intensive (e.g., radiation dosimetry, genetic studies). Cases are those cohort members who have developed the disease/outcome of interest. Potential controls are all other cohort members who are at risk but have not yet developed the disease. Controls are selected by matching them to cases on potential confounding variables that may be associated with both exposure and outcome, such as age at cancer diagnosis and sex. This technique ensures that potential confounders are distributed in an identical manner among cases and controls. For example, the risk of secondary breast cancer is strongly associated with age at follow-up. Without a proper adjustment for age at follow-up, the risk may appear elevated for those diagnosed with childhood cancer at an older age [33].

After controls have been matched to cases according to potential confounding variables, cases are compared to controls with respect to the exposure of interest. The sources and quality of exposure information (e.g., medical records or biologic specimen) should not differ by case/control status, and it is preferable to have the abstraction of exposure information done with the case/control status blinded. This study design leads to resource savings because the exposure assessment is required only for those cases and sampled controls selected and not for the entire cohort.

A major disadvantage of this type of design is the retrospective assessment of prior exposures. If the exposure assessment relies on self-report, for example, a survivor's recall of exposures may be biased by knowledge of his or her outcome status, or it may be difficult for the subject to assess exposure retrospectively. Also, since the real frequency/rate of outcome in the full study population is not reflected in the case-control sets, one cannot determine the absolute risk of the outcome; only the odds ratio (an estimate) can be determined.

A nested case-control design was used in a long-term cancer-survivor study by Hawkins et al. to investigate second primary bone cancer after childhood cancer [10]. Based on a cohort of 13,175 3-year survivors of childhood cancer in Britain, the analysis comprised 59 cases of second primary bone cancer and 220 controls. The use of the nested case-control design permitted the collection of detailed exposure measurements, such as the site-specific radiation dose and cumulative dose of alkylating agents. The resources needed to collect these measurements would have been about 50 times greater if the study had used a cohort design employing all 13,175 survivors.

### 22.3.2.4 Case-Cohort Design

The case-cohort study [25] proposed in 1986 is a study design that is similar to the nested case-control design, except that the selection of controls is performed without any reference to the specific time of the occurrence of each case's outcome of interest. Case-cohort studies share many of the advantages and disadvantages of nested case-control studies. A key additional advantage of the case-cohort design, compared with the nested case-control design, is the ability to use the same controls for multiple outcomes of interest [13, 30]. This can be particularly relevant to long-term survivor studies, since there may be multiple outcomes of interest, such as mortality from different causes and second cancers at different sites or of different types. External comparisons of the study cohort with a general/reference population are simple with the case-cohort design, and standardized mortality or morbidity ratios, a familiar tool in epidemiology, can be computed [31].

The use of the case-cohort design (although it was not explicitly identified as such) in cancer-survivor studies goes back to Hutchison who studied long-term leukemia risk following radiotherapy for cervical cancer [11]. Boice and Hutchison later discussed the incompleteness of the follow-up in Hutchison's earlier analysis and re-analyzed the data with a greatly extended follow-up of the same cohort [2]. They conducted external comparisons by computing the expected number of leukemia cases in the cohort, based on rates from population cancer registries. In the computation of the expected number, only a 10 % random sample of all patients was used to estimate total person-years in the entire cohort. This greatly minimized the time required for detailed record abstraction and computer analysis.

### 22.3.2.5 Intervention Studies

In contradistinction to the above-described *observational* analytic studies, which test etiologic hypotheses, the purpose of *intervention* studies (also referred to as *randomized controlled trials* or *clinical trials*) is to test the efficacy of a preventive or therapeutic measure, while assessing its potential negative effects (i.e., side effects). In this type of study, investigators have control over the scheme for assigning individuals to groups with different "exposures" of interest (i.e., intervention and control groups). These types of studies are generally considered the strongest design for establishing causal relationships. Therapeutic trials and chemoprevention trials are examples of intervention studies.

Therapeutic trials are conducted on individuals with a disease to determine whether a drug or modified condition of therapy is efficacious as a treatment of the disease without serious toxicity. For example, the therapeutic trials often used in the Children's Oncology Group are designed to test whether modifications in treatment will increase disease-free survival and minimize the occurrence of late effects.

Chemoprevention trials are designed to evaluate whether an agent or procedure can reduce the risk of developing a disease in individuals free of the condition at enrollment. An example of such a trial in late-effect research is a randomized clinical trial of the cardioprotective agent ICRF-187 in pediatric sarcoma patients treated with doxorubicin [32].

Other randomized intervention trials endeavor to modify behavior and minimize late effects. An example is the smoking cessation trial performed within the CCSS, using peer counseling to increase smoking cessation [7].

The advantage of intervention studies is that investigators can create exposure groups with a high degree of comparability (the groups differ only with respect to the interventions of interest) and follow them for differential risk of outcomes, thereby minimizing confounding and increasing the validity of causal inferences. Major drawbacks to intervention studies are the extensive resource requirements, the length of follow-up needed to ascertain outcomes, and lastly, the inability to achieve high compliance to protocols. Other, equally important, drawbacks are possible contaminations across experimental arms and loss to follow-up.

## 22.4 Future Direction: Are There Opportunities Through Comparative Effectiveness Research?

Current knowledge regarding late effects in childhood cancer survivors can be attributed to the diligence of investigators who performed the initial studies and to the wisdom of succeeding researchers who built on previously completed work. The establishment of large, well-characterized cohorts of long-term survivors, such as the CCSS and others (including the British Childhood Cancer Survivor Study, the National Wilms Tumor Study, and the Late Effects Study Group), has created a framework that allows for both the continued surveillance of childhood cancer-survivor populations as they age and the dissemination of the information gained to survivors and clinicians. In addition, the Children's Oncology Group (COG), a National Cancer Institute-supported clinical trials group, is a very good source of information on patient and tumor characteristics, treatments being used, treatment compliance, and morbidities of treatments including long-term complications.

With these excellent resources, we now have the opportunity to consider next steps to unraveling clues in pediatric cancer survivorship. Comparative effectiveness research (CER) is designed to inform health-care decisions by providing evidence on the effectiveness, benefits, and harms of different treatment options and provides an opportunity to improve the quality and outcomes of health care [1, 12]. The question for consideration is, what is the role of CER in survivorship? CER encompasses a wide spectrum of research activities, from primary research, systematic review, and evidence synthesis to the application of evidence in guideline development and decision support [1]. Although most of CER methodology is not new, the available methods when properly used can contribute to informing medical decisions.

Resources within the pediatric cancer-survivor research initiative, such as the Childhood Cancer Survivor Study and the Children's Oncology Group, could support several CER opportunities:

First, CER has described a need for well-designed cohort studies that link clinical information to molecular and genomic data to address outcomes in relevant subgroups. Within our available resources, the biospecimens collected as part of these initiatives may enable studies that can provide insights into which subgroup of patients will benefit from a particular therapy based on expression of a number of putative predictive biomarkers and which patients may experience severe toxicities or poor outcomes.

Second, CER supports high-quality clinical practice guidelines to summarize and apprise the body of evidence and inform recommendations. The Children's Oncology Group Long-Term Follow-Up (COG-LTFU) Guidelines use a mixture of consensus and evidence-based recommendations for exposure-driven, risk-based screening for early detection of long-term complications in childhood cancer survivors. These clinical practice guidelines are well positioned to evaluate improvements in quality of care and system performance and to undertake economic analysis of health-care policy issues.

Lastly, prospective randomized control trials are considered the gold standard of CER. Future steps in late-effect research should also include the conduct of prospective randomized intervention trials that will provide investigators with a platform to prospectively study patient-reported outcomes and quality of life, as well as the most effective methods for modifying behaviors to maximize survivors' future health.

## References

1. Agency for Healthcare, Research and Quality (2012) Effective Health Care Program: what is comparative effectiveness research? Accessed at http://www.effectivehealthcare.ahrq.gov/index.cfm/what-is-comparative-effectiveness-research1/
2. Boice JD, Hutchison GB (1980) Leukemia in women following radiotherapy for cervical cancer: ten-year follow-up of an international study. J Natl Cancer Inst 65:115–129

3. Boivin JF, Hutchison GB, Zauber AG, Bernstein L, Davis FG, Michel RP, Zanke B, Tan CTC, Fuller LM, Mauch P, Ultmann JE (1995) Incidence of second cancers in patients treated for Hodgkin's disease. J Natl Cancer Inst 87:732–741

4. Byrne J, Mulvihill JJ, Myers MH, Connelly RR, Naughton MD, Krauss MR, Steinhorn SC, Hassinger DD, Austin DF, Bragg K, Holmes GF, Holmes FF, Latourette HB, Weyer PJ, Meigs JW, Teta MJ, Cook JW, Strong LC (1987) Effects of treatment of fertility in long-term survivors of childhood or adolescent cancer. N Engl J Med 317:1315–1321

5. Children's Oncology Group (2009) Long-term follow-up guidelines for survivors of childhood, adolescent, and young adult cancers. Accessed at http://www.survivorshipguidelines.org/pdf/LTFUGuidelines.pdf

6. Clinical and Translational Science Award (CTSA) program, support from the National Institute of Health, 2012. Accessed at https://www.ctsacentral.org/

7. Emmons K, Butterfield RM, Puleo E, Park ER, Mertens A, Gritz ER, Lahti M, Li F (2003) Smoking among participants in the childhood cancer survivors cohort: the partnership for health study. J Clin Oncol 21:189–196

8. Feigelson HS, Rodrigeuz C, Robertson AS, Jacobs EJ, Calle EE, Reid YA, Thun MJ (2001) Determinants of DNA yield and quality from buccal cell samples collected with mouthwash. Cancer Epidemiol Biomarkers Prev 10:1005–1008

9. Gurney JG, Ness KK, Sibley SD, O'Leary M, Dengel DR, Lee JM, Youngren NM, Glasser SP, Baker KS (2006) Metabolic syndrome and growth hormone deficiency in adult survivors of childhood acute lymphoblastic leukemia. Cancer 107(6):1303–1312

10. Hawkins MM, Wilson LM, Burton HS, Potok MH, Winter DL, Marsden HB, Stovall MA (1996) Radiotherapy, alkylating agents, and risk of bone cancer after childhood cancer. J Natl Cancer Inst 88:270–278

11. Hutchison GB (1968) Leukemia in patients with cancer of the cervix uteri treated with radiation. A report covering the first 5 years of an international study. J Natl Cancer Inst 40:951–982

12. IOM (Institute of Medicine) (2009) Initial priorities for comparative effectiveness research. The National Academies Press, Washington, DC

13. Langholz B, Thomas DC (1990) Nested case-control and case-cohort methods of sampling from a cohort: a critical comparison. Am J Epidemiol 131:169–176

14. Le Marchand L, Lum-Jones A, Saltzman B, Visaya V, Normua AM, Kolonel LN (2001) Feasibility of collecting buccal cell DNA by mail in a cohort study. Cancer Epidemiol Biomarkers Prev 10:701–703

15. Leisenring WM, Mertens AC, Armstrong GT, Stovall MA, Neglia JP, Lanctot JQ, Boice JD Jr, Whitton JA, Yasui Y (2009) Pediatric cancer survivorship research: experience of the Childhood Cancer Survivor Study. J Clin Oncol 27(14):2319–2327

16. Liddell FDK, McDonald JC, Thomas DC (1977) Methods of cohort analysis: appraisal by application to asbestos mining. J R Stat Soc A 140:469–491

17. Marina N (1997) Long-term survivors of childhood cancer. Pediatr Clin N Am 44:1021–1042

18. McCormick MC, Baker J, Brooks-Gunn J et al (1991) Cohort reconstruction: which infants can be restudied at school age? Paediatr Perinat Epidemiol 5:410–422

19. Meadows AT, Hobbie WL (1986) The medical consequences of cure. Cancer 58:524–528

20. Mertens AC, Mitby PA, Perentesis JP, Radloff G, Kiffmeyer WR, Neglia JP, Meadows A, Jones I, Potter JD, Friedman D, Yasui Y, Robison LL, Davies SM (2004) XRCC1 and glutathione S-transferase polymorphism and susceptibility to therapy-related cancer in Hodgkin's disease survivors: a report from the Childhood Cancer Survivor Study. Cancer 101:1463–1472

21. Mertens AC, Potter JD, Neglia JP, Robison LL (1997) Methods for tracing, contacting, and recruiting a cohort of survivors of childhood cancer. J Pediatr Hematol Oncol 19:212–219

22. Neglia JP (1994) Childhood cancer survivors: past, present, and future. Cancer 73:2883–2885

23. Pepe MS (1992) Inference using surrogate outcome data and a validation sample. Biometrika 79:355–365

24. Pepe MS, Reilly M, Fleming TR (1994) Auxiliary outcome data and the mean score method. J Stat Plan Infer 42:137–160

25. Prentice L (1986) A case-cohort design for epidemiologic cohort studies and disease prevention trials. Biometrika 73:1–11

26. Robison LL, Mertens AC, Boice JD, Breslow NE, Donaldson SE, Green DM, Li FP, Meadows AT, Mulvihill JJ, Neglia JP, Nesbit NE, Packer RJ, Potter JD, Sklar CA, Smith MA, Stovall M, Strong LC, Yasui Y, Zeltzer LK (2002) Study design and cohort characteristics of the Childhood Cancer Survivor Study: a multi-institutional collaborative project. Med Pediatr Oncol 38:229–239

27. Schwartz CL (1995) Late effects of treatment in long-term survivors of cancer. Cancer Treat Rev 21:355–366

28. Schwarz MB, Burgess LP, Fee WE, Donaldson SS (1988) Postirradiation sarcoma in retinoblastoma, induction or predisposition? Arch Otolaryngol Head Neck Surg 114:640–644

29. Sklar C, Mertens A, Walter A, Mitchell D, Nesbit M, O'Leary M, Hutchinson R, Meadows A, Robison L (1993) Final height after treatment for childhood acute lymphoblastic leukemia: comparison of no cranial irradiation with 1800 and 2400 centigrays of cranial irradiation. J Pediatr 123:59–64

30. Wacholder S (1991) Practical considerations in choosing between the case-cohort and nested case-control designs. Epidemiology 2:155–158

31. Wacholder S, Boivin JF (1987) External comparisons with the case-cohort design. Am J Epidemiol 126:1198–1209

32. Wexler LH, Andrich MP, Venzon D, Berg SL, Weaver-McClure L, Chen CC, Dilsizian V, Avila N, Jarosinski P, Balis FM, Poplack DG, Horowitz ME (1996) Randomized trial of the cardioprotective agent ICRF-187 in pediatric sarcoma patients treated with doxorubicin. J Clin Oncol 14:362–372

33. Yasui Y, Liu Y, Neglia J, Friedman D, Bhatia S, Meadows A, Diller L, Mertens A, Whitton J, Robison LL (2003) A methodological issue in the analysis of second cancer incidence in long-term survivors of childhood cancers. Am J Epidemiol 158:1108–1113

# Survivorship Transitions Following Childhood and Adolescent Cancer

**23**

David R. Freyer, Rajkumar Venkatramani, and Debra Eshelman-Kent

## Contents

D.R. Freyer, DO, MS (✉)
Hematology, Oncology and Blood and Marrow
Transplantation, Children's Hospital Los Angeles,
Keck School of Medicine, University of Southern
California, Los Angeles, CA, USA
e-mail: dfreyer@chla.usc.edu

R. Venkatramani, MD
Department of Hematology-Oncology, Texas
Children's Hospital, Baylor College of Medicine,
Houston, TX, USA

D. Eshelman-Kent, MSN, APRN, CPNP
Department of Oncology, Cincinnati Children's
Hospital, Cincinnati, OH, USA

## 23.1     Introduction

For children, adolescents, and their families, the cancer experience is characterized by a series of transitions that begins at diagnosis and, for most patients, ends with entry into long-term survivorship care. Each of these transitions has specific implications for medical care provided during those phases. In pediatric and adolescent oncology, these cancer-related transitions do not occur in isolation but in the context of normal physical, emotional, and social development. Therefore, the successive phases of developmental maturation that begin in infancy and continue through older adolescence not only influence each patient's response to cancer-related transitions but also require support during the cancer experience in order for healthy adulthood to be achieved.

For childhood cancer survivors, the transition from older adolescence to young adulthood is particularly important in that it uniquely encompasses the overlapping complexities of established late effects, emerging risks and need for continued medical surveillance, change from pediatric to adult-focused health-care services, threats to maintaining health insurance, completion of formal education, career planning and entrance to the workforce, attainment of personal independence, and redefinition of familial and societal roles. With more childhood cancer survivors entering young adulthood than ever before,

© Springer International Publishing 2015
C.L. Schwartz et al. (eds.), *Survivors of Childhood and Adolescent Cancer:
A Multidisciplinary Approach*, Pediatric Oncology, DOI 10.1007/978-3-319-16435-9_23

there is a pressing need for effective approaches to health-care transition.

The purpose of this chapter is to discuss key issues in health-care transition for long-term survivors of childhood and adolescent cancer, focusing on the transitions from initial to long-term follow-up and from child-oriented to adult-focused care. Relevant aspects of normal childhood and adolescent development are discussed.

## 23.2 Developmental Aspects of Transition

The cancer experience commonly affects growth and development, both directly and through altered parent/family and peer experiences. An understanding of major developmental tasks of childhood and adolescence is essential for normalizing the cancer experience and interpreting the survivor's response to cancer [1, 2]. As summarized in Table 23.1, survivorship-associated transitions are focused chiefly on maximizing health-related knowledge of the patient and family and facilitating their adaptation to existing late effects and/or future risks resulting from cancer treatment. Over time, explanations should become more detailed commensurate with the increasing cognitive capacity of the maturing young person, and her participation in medical decisions should similarly increase. In pediatric oncology, clinicians need to address the phenomenon of older long-term survivors who were treated as young children but subsequently lack an age-appropriate understanding of their medical histories. As these survivors mature into adolescence, it is essential that they receive sufficient information about their cancer, its treatment, and resulting health implications in order to prepare them properly for health-care transition. It is better for clinicians and parents alike to remember that health-care transition is but a special case of the more general and normative transition to responsible, independent adulthood. Many "teachable moments" present themselves in family life for the maturing teen to assume greater responsibility and accountability in both personal and health-related matters.

## 23.3 The Transition to Long-Term Follow-Up Care

The transition from an initial period of disease-directed to long-term follow-up commonly begins approximately 2 years post-cessation of treatment. For most patients, this phase is open-ended in the sense that lifelong surveillance is recommended for most childhood cancer survivors [3]. The demarcation between the initial and subsequent periods of follow-up care is not uniformly distinct, as the risk for late relapse differs by cancer diagnosis. Cancer survivorship and disease-directed follow-up need not be "either/or" services. At institutions where survivorship referral occurs relatively early, long-term follow-up services may overlap and should continue in parallel with disease-directed surveillance until released by the treating oncologist. The primary focus of this survivorship transition is to establish risk-based monitoring and to provide health-related education to the survivor and family. Whereas relapse is the principal risk during initial posttreatment follow-up, a major subsequent challenge becomes the survivor's potential disengagement from and failure to remain in structured follow-up.

### 23.3.1 Late Effects and the Need for Survivorship Care

Due to the significantly increased risk for late effects, impaired health status, and premature death [4–6], there is expert consensus that most childhood cancer survivors should remain in structured, lifelong follow-up to facilitate risk-based monitoring and health promotion [3]. To assist in this task, the Children's Oncology Group (COG) has developed risk-adapted clinical practice guidelines for late effects surveillance [7]. The guidelines are intended to increase awareness about potential late effects and to standardize the follow-up care of survivors provided by pediatric oncology, subspecialty, and primary care clinicians. Individual guidelines are updated regularly and, along with corresponding patient/family educational materials, may be downloaded

**Table 23.1** Developmental stages and their implications for survivorship transition care

| Developmental stage | Key developmental features [3] | Implications for survivorship transition care |
|---|---|---|
| Preschool (2–5 years) | Acquisition of language and motor skills | Direct anticipatory guidance about late effects toward the parents |
| | Formation of simple concepts of reality | Mention to parents that eventual transition to adult-focused providers will occur |
| | Emotional connection with other people | |
| | Cognitive features of magical thinking, egocentrism, and dominance of perception | |
| Middle childhood (6–12 years) | Expansion of child's world outside the home | Provide simple explanation to child relating prior illness to the need for continued follow-up |
| | Ability to get along with other children | Continue to educate parents on late effects, health, and wellness |
| | Development of concrete operational thinking | Revisit eventual planned transition to adult-focused providers |
| | Acquisition of adult concepts and communication (writing, reading, calculating) | Advise parents against overprotectiveness and encourage normal discipline |
| | | Encourage parents to allow children to have increasing responsibilities at home and an increasing role in personal and medical decisions |
| Early adolescence (10–13 years) | Development of formal logical operations | Provide straightforward but more detailed explanations to survivor about follow-up care |
| | Awareness of changing body and interest in opposite sex | Encourage increased participation in medical decision making and personal health choices |
| | Reduced interest in family-centric activities | Initiate discussions with survivor about eventual transition to adult providers |
| | Increasing peer identification | |
| Middle adolescence (14–16 years) | Importance of physical attractiveness, popularity, and self-esteem | Direct the conversation toward the adolescent with active involvement in decision making |
| | New understanding of abstract concepts and consequences | Reserve "alone time" with teen for a portion of each clinic visit |
| | Reorientation of primary relationships from family to peer groups | Discuss prevention of high-risk behaviors (smoking, alcohol, drug use, unprotected sex) |
| | Start of dating | Discuss targets for transition readiness and provide rationale for transition to adult-focused providers |
| Late adolescence and young adulthood (17–20 years and beyond) | Development of personal independence, core values, ethical principles, and philosophy of life | Encourage a primary role for older adolescent during clinic visits |
| | Attainment of emotional independence | Provide information related to reproductive health and sexuality |
| | Development of intimate relationships | Continue education about importance and rationale for lifelong follow-up |
| | Emerging importance of career decisions as related to self-concept and emerging societal role | Encourage pursuit of higher education and provide information on survivor-focused scholarships and resources (as appropriate) |
| | Preparation for occupation | Emphasize importance of preparing for employment with insurance benefits to cover continued follow-up care (see Fig. 23.2, the "Golden Triangle" of survivorship) |
| | | Help them understand insurance options available for cancer survivors |
| | | Assess transition readiness (see Fig. 23.1) and coordinate transition to adult setting |

Adapted from Venkatramani and Freyer [46]

from the COG website [8]. Research is underway to validate these guidelines and determine their clinical utility [9]. Similar guidelines have been developed by other international cooperative pediatric oncology groups [10–12].

## 23.3.2 Role of the Cancer Survivorship Clinic

The American Academy of Pediatrics has recommended that pediatric cancer treatment centers offer a mechanism for long-term follow-up of successfully treated patients, either at the original treatment center or through referral to a dedicated childhood cancer survivorship program [13]. The main services of cancer survivorship clinic are to provide surveillance for late effects, identify and address medical and psychosocial issues, provide health education and health promotion interventions to modify risk, and conduct longitudinal research in this population (Table 23.2). Various effective models exist for delivering such care [14]. Most cancer survivorship clinics are staffed by physicians, nurse practitioners, and social workers with expertise in childhood cancer survivorship. Referral access should also be available to other specialists such as psychologists, nutritionists, genetic counselors, cardiologists, endocrinologists, fertility specialists, and orthopedic surgeons. However, given that a recent survey of COG centers found that only 59 % have dedicated cancer survivorship clinics, many institutions provide long-term follow-up care by the treating oncologist [15]. Comprehensive survivorship evaluation is resource intensive, beginning with generating a detailed cancer treatment history, performing a complete physical assessment, preparing a treatment summary and survivorship care plan, and educating the survivor and family to improve health-related knowledge, attitudes, and behaviors.

Referral to cancer survivorship clinic generally represents the "official" transition to long-term follow-up care. When this should be initiated is a matter of varying practice and some debate. A survey of 24 comprehensive pediatric survivorship programs found that most patients were

**Table 23.2** Components and tasks of survivorship care

| Components of ideal system of survivorship care |
|---|
| 1. Provide a range of direct services to survivors to identify, prevent, treat, and manage late effects |
| 2. Bridge the realms of primary and specialty health care with education and outreach |
| 3. Coordinate medical care with educational and occupational services |
| 4. Conduct research to better understand late effects and their prevention |
| Specific tasks of survivorship program |
| 1. Risk-based monitoring for late complications of cancer treatment |
| 2. Coordinating specialized care for established late complications of cancer treatment |
| 3. Educating and counseling survivors regarding the specific conditions to which they are susceptible and guidance of self-monitoring of late effects |
| 4. Applying preventive approaches known to be effective for the general population, including encouragement of abstinence from tobacco, limited exposure to alcohol, sun protection, physical activity, maintenance of a healthy weight, consumption of fruits and vegetables |
| 5. Providing psychosocial support services to survivors and their families |
| 6. Providing reproductive and sexuality counseling |
| 7. Providing genetic counseling for individuals with a hereditary cancer and their family members |
| 8. Assistance with identifying and meeting financial challenges |

referred to long-term follow-up clinics when they reached 5 years post-diagnosis and 2 years off therapy, whichever was later [16]. The rationale for this relatively late time point is that the risk for relapse is minimal for most pediatric cancers. One concern about such a late time point is that for cancers treated with relatively brief therapy (e.g., Wilms' tumor and Hodgkin's lymphoma), the duration of time between end of treatment and survivorship referral is relatively long and may result in attrition of survivors. Consequently, some programs are experimenting with earlier referral while patients are still in disease-directed follow-up in order to improve sustained engagement of survivors.

Challenges may be encountered in launching this transition. Even well-established pediatric survivorship clinics within large cancer treatment programs at prominent hospitals report capturing only a portion of eligible survivors. The reasons for this have not been studied extensively, but one survey of survivorship programs suggests that factors related to both the institution (such as inadequate resources, low institutional commitment, and lack of capacity to care for the growing population of survivors) and the survivor (including lack of awareness of health risks) may contribute [16]. Patients/families may be reluctant to relinquish their trusted treating oncologist in order to see the survivorship team. Treating oncologists may need to confront their own reluctance to "let go" of established patients. Some patients may find it difficult to come to the same clinic where they experienced the trauma of cancer treatment; thus, it is ideal, though not always feasible, to hold survivorship clinic in a separate setting. Survivors and their families may lack financial resources or face geographical barriers in traveling to the treatment center. Lack of health insurance coverage for surveillance tests may be an issue, although most states in the United States (US) provide catastrophic health insurance programs that cover follow-up services up to 21 years of age. The Patient Protection and Affordable Care Act, passed in 2010 by the US Congress, now allows young adults to continue receiving health insurance coverage through their parents' policy until 26 years of age and prohibit exclusions based on prior health conditions [17, 18]. All of these provisions benefit young adult survivors of childhood and adolescent cancer.

## 23.4 The Transition from Child-Oriented to Adult-Focused Care

As developed by the Society for Adolescent Medicine, the now-classic definition of health-care transition is the planned movement of adolescents and young adults with chronic physical and medical conditions from child-centered to adult-oriented health-care systems [19]. Its overarching purpose is to provide continuous, well-coordinated care that is both medically and developmentally appropriate. As mentioned previously, continuing needs for late effects surveil-

lance, health promotion, and personal advocacy/empowerment provide the medical rationale for health-care transition of childhood cancer survivors. While health-care transition is a concept now being applied broadly across most chronic diseases or conditions originating in childhood [20–22], cancer survivorship is different in that patients are considered cured but remain at risk for developing late effects. Most are asymptomatic, leading many survivors to question why continued medical care is necessary. In order to ensure a successful transition, adolescents and young adults should be encouraged to take responsibility for their wellness. Communication should be directed toward the adolescent/young adult rather than the parent in order to address important issues such as sexuality, reproductive health, substance abuse, and other risk-taking behaviors [19]. Most adolescent cancer survivors undergo the same developmentally appropriate shifts as their peers, including educational advancement, change in residence, reorientation of primary relationships, need for employment and health insurance, and switching to an adult-focused health-care provider [23]. It is important for health-care transition to address these needs in a way that is relevant for childhood cancer survivors. In particular, adolescent survivors need to understand the interrelationship of education, employment, and health insurance—the "Golden Triangle" of childhood cancer survivorship (Fig. 23.1). In the United States, most health insurance for adults is provided through an employer-based benefits package. Thus, securing health insurance requires having a job with benefits, which is facilitated, in turn, by completing formal education and career planning. According to the US Department of Labor, among Americans aged 25 years and older in November 2012, unemployment rates by educational level, categorized as some high school, high school graduate, some college/associate's degree, and bachelor's degree or beyond, were 12.2 %, 8.1 %, 6.5 %, and 3.8 %, respectively [24]. Given that young adult cancer survivors already exhibit higher levels of nonemployment than their siblings [25] coupled with their need for health insurance, it becomes especially important to

**Fig. 23.1** The "Golden Triangle" of childhood cancer survivorship indicating the interrelationship of the survivor's formal education, employment, and obtaining of health insurance. The rationales for each point of the triangle as explained to the survivor are shown

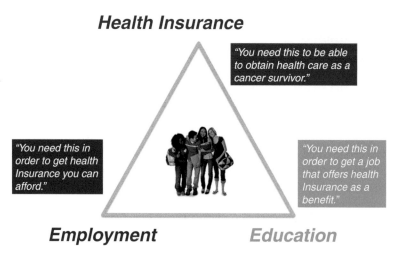

### Health Insurance

*"You need this to be able to obtain health care as a cancer survivor."*

*"You need this in order to get health Insurance you can afford."*

*"You need this in order to get a job that offers health Insurance as a benefit."*

### Employment                    Education

encourage postsecondary education leading to employable careers for adolescent and young adult survivors who have the potential to succeed.

Health-care transition generally occurs in the age range of 18–21 years. This is also the age when most pediatric hospitals are less able to serve the needs of adult patients, due to child-oriented facilities and lack of convenient access to adult-focused specialists. Recent studies have found there is considerable variation in timing of transition among pediatric oncology centers. In a recent survey of 220 COG institutions, 35 % of respondents reported having no formal transitional care mechanism, 31 % reported transition is carried out when the patient is deemed ready, and the remainder carries out transition at varying points between 18 and 30 years of age [15]. In a survey of 12 academic centers in New England, only 4 of the 11 with established survivorship clinics reported having an age-specific policy for transition, with their median age of transition being 32 years (range, 21–40) [26]. In a survey of Canadian pediatric oncology centers, 8 of 15 reported having formal programs for adult survivors, with 2 more in development; although age at transition was not reported, only 4 of these 10 centers estimated that 50 % or more of their adult survivors were being followed [27]. Some have drawn support for delaying transition until the mid- to late-twenties from recent evidence that neurobiological maturation

in brain regions responsible for risk assessment, motivation, and choice is not complete until that time [28].

Relatively little is known about what factors contribute to successful health-care transition, particularly for childhood cancer survivors. Through focus group interviews of adolescents with special health-care needs, their parents, and providers, Reiss and Gibson identified the following factors as important: (1) having a future-focused orientation throughout care, (2) viewing transition positively as a normal milestone of late adolescence, (3) starting the transition process early, (4) fostering personal and medical independence by promoting early involvement of the child in medical decision making, and (5) maintaining continuous, uninterrupted health-care insurance if possible [29]. Inasmuch as the majority of childhood cancer patients become long-term survivors, it is appropriate to make first mention of health-care transition even as early as the initial family conference at diagnosis and to revisit the topic at the end of therapy and upon referral to survivorship clinic. In their model of transition for adolescent childhood cancer survivors, Schwartz and colleagues have described a "window of modifiability" between end of treatment and engagement in adult care during which transition readiness increases through the application of interventions targeted at variables including knowledge, skills/efficacy, beliefs/expectations, goals, relationships, and psychosocial functioning [30].

The transitional care visit itself should accomplish the following four tasks: (1) assessment of readiness for transition; (2) education of the survivor/family on essential skills needed in the adult health-care system; (3) preparation of an updated health-care summary, including past cancer treatment, current and potential health problems, and recommended late effects surveillance (survivorship care plan); and (4) communication with the new adult-focused provider(s) including a clear transfer of responsibility for follow-up.

## 23.4.1 Transitional Care Models for Young Adult Survivors

A variety of models are in use for care of young adult survivors. No single care model is optimal for all settings, and more research is needed to define "best practices" in this area. In general, existing programs fall into the three broad categories of cancer center-based, community-based, or hybrid models [14].

### 23.4.1.1 Cancer Center-Based Model

In this model, adult-focused care continues to be provided to all survivors within the same cancer center or health system where treatment was given. This model is more prevalent in institutions where both children and adults are treated and in a recent survey of COG institutions was the most common model used for care of adult survivors [15]. In this model, the post-transition team includes an adult-focused primary care provider (internist, family medicine, medicine/pediatrics) and/or medical oncologist, plus pediatric survivorship specialists. This model involves transition to adult services but not transfer of care from the institution. An advantage of this model is continuity of providers and medical records. Disadvantages are that survivors may be required to travel long distances and not all may need this degree of resource intensity.

### 23.4.1.2 Community-Based Model

In this model, survivorship care is provided to all survivors by a community-based primary care provider [14]. Here, there is both transition and transfer of care. In this model, the treatment center provides the identified primary care provider with a formal survivorship care plan (as described above). Advantages of this model include geographic convenience, an emphasis on wellness/prevention that characterizes primary care, and integration of cancer survivorship into routine health care. The chief disadvantage may be a relative lack of familiarity with late effects on the part of the primary care provider.

### 23.4.1.3 Hybrid and Risk-Stratified Models

In the hybrid model, a combined approach is used that involves both the community-based primary care provider and the cancer treatment center. Survivors undergo transition and transfer of care, but in this case, an active linkage is maintained between the pediatric survivorship center and the primary care provider. A formal survivorship care plan is provided to the primary care provider, but regular communication with the survivorship center permits updates on the survivor's status and evolving long-term follow-up monitoring guidelines. In theory, the hybrid model offers the advantages of both the cancer center-based and community-based models but offsets the disadvantages of each. Delivery of survivorship care by the primary care provider is appealing because CCSS data have shown better utilization of general medical care than cancer center care among young adult survivors [31]. A recent study from the Netherlands showed that a coordinated program involving the childhood cancer treatment center and family physicians resulted in good outcomes and provider satisfaction [32]. A Web-based initiative was reported recently that involves primary care providers in shared care of pediatric cancer survivors through concise summaries of late effects and continuing education modules that are available online [33].

A variant of the hybrid model, called the risk-stratified model, is utilized in some survivorship programs, including the LIFE Cancer Survivorship and Transition Program at Children's Hospital Los Angeles (CHLA). In this model, the locus of post-transitional survivorship care is determined by the classification

**Fig. 23.2** The risk-stratified model for post-transitional care as utilized by the LIFE Cancer Survivorship and Transition Program at Children's Hospital Los Angeles. Modified from Venkatramani and Freyer [46]

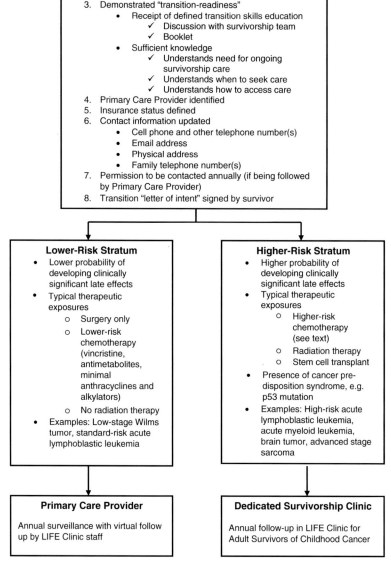

**Criteria for Undergoing Survivorship Transition**

1. Current age ≥21 years
2. Stable medical and emotional status
3. Demonstrated "transition-readiness"
   - Receipt of defined transition skills education
     - ✓ Discussion with survivorship team
     - ✓ Booklet
   - Sufficient knowledge
     - ✓ Understands need for ongoing survivorship care
     - ✓ Understands when to seek care
     - ✓ Understands how to access care
4. Primary Care Provider identified
5. Insurance status defined
6. Contact information updated
   - Cell phone and other telephone number(s)
   - Email address
   - Physical address
   - Family telephone number(s)
7. Permission to be contacted annually (if being followed by Primary Care Provider)
8. Transition "letter of intent" signed by survivor

**Lower-Risk Stratum**
- Lower probability of developing clinically significant late effects
- Typical therapeutic exposures
  - Surgery only
  - Lower-risk chemotherapy (vincristine, antimetabolites, minimal anthracyclines and alkylators)
  - No radiation therapy
- Examples: Low-stage Wilms tumor, standard-risk acute lymphoblastic leukemia

**Higher-Risk Stratum**
- Higher probability of developing clinically significant late effects
- Typical therapeutic exposures
  - Higher-risk chemotherapy (see text)
  - Radiation therapy
  - Stem cell transplant
- Presence of cancer pre-disposition syndrome, e.g. p53 mutation
- Examples: High-risk acute lymphoblastic leukemia, acute myeloid leukemia, brain tumor, advanced stage sarcoma

**Primary Care Provider**

Annual surveillance with virtual follow up by LIFE Clinic staff

**Dedicated Survivorship Clinic**

Annual follow-up in LIFE Clinic for Adult Survivors of Childhood Cancer

of survivors according to risk for developing clinically significant late effects. As shown in Fig. 23.2, transition-ready survivors are classified as either lower or higher risk using an adaption of validated criteria for survivorship risk assignment [34, 35]. At 21 years of age, lower-risk survivors undergo transition to their primary care providers to continue lifelong follow-up as specified in their survivorship care plan. Following transition, lower-risk survivors are contacted annually by the LIFE Program to ascertain current health status and adherence to recommended surveillance ("virtual follow-up"). Those deemed to be higher risk return annually to the LIFE Clinic for Adult Survivors of Childhood Cancer, a collaborative clinic involving adult-focused providers at the University of Southern California (USC) Norris Comprehensive Cancer Center. Chemotherapy criteria currently used to identify higher risk transition status are based on the COG Long-Term

Follow-Up Guidelines [8], namely cumulative anthracycline dose meriting echocardiogram every 1–2 years or cumulative alkylator doses that are deemed therein as high risk. In this overall LIFE Clinic model, all survivors undergo transition, but full transfer of care occurs only for those classified as lower risk. Transition-related outcomes data are now being collected to evaluate efficacy and satisfaction with this model. One anticipated benefit is more rational, risk-based utilization of valuable survivorship resources. However, this and the extent to which risk stratification is used in transitional survivorship care need to be documented through health services research efforts.

## 23.4.2 Barriers to Transition of Young Adult Survivors

Significant barriers to successful health-care transition may be encountered at the level of the survivor, health-care provider, and medical systems (Table 23.3). While some have been the subject of research, others remain clinical observations and anecdotal impressions.

### 23.4.2.1 Barriers Related to the Survivor

Certain negative perceptions and lack of relevant health-related knowledge may interfere with follow-up. These factors include a lack of awareness about long-term risks and need for continued monitoring [36, 37], reluctance to terminate long-standing relationships with their pediatric providers, and the challenge of building relationships in new health-care settings [29]. The perceived stigma of a cancer history and emotional difficulty of discussing the cancer experience may contribute, especially for Latino adolescent/young adult survivors [38]. Deficits in survivor knowledge regarding medical indications for continued follow-up have been documented [39], and there is some evidence to suggest that targeted educational interventions might result in improved adherence to recommended late effects screening. Seventy-two survivors of Hodgkin's lymphoma who were at increased risk of breast cancer or cardiomyopathy but had not undergone

**Table 23.3** Summary of barriers to survivorship transition

| Survivor related | Complex cancer treatment history |
| | Multiple long-term health risks |
| | Failure or inability to assume personal responsibility for health |
| | Lack of personal support systems |
| | Lack of trust in new health-care provider |
| Survivor/family related | Overprotectiveness |
| | Fear of loss of control |
| | Emotional dependency on child survivor |
| | Lack of trust in new health-care provider |
| Adult-focused provider related | Lack of knowledge or experience in post-transitional care and survivor's underlying medical condition and health risks |
| | No preexisting emotional bond with survivor/family |
| | Burden of assuming care for unfamiliar, occasionally complex survivors |
| Health system related | Lack of seamless referral networks linking pediatric and adult-oriented providers |
| | Lack of systemic training of health-care professionals in posttranslational health care |
| | Loss of health insurance needed for continuation of survivorship care in young adulthood and beyond |

Adapted from Freyer [23]

recommended screening during the previous 2 years were mailed a 1-page survivorship care plan containing applicable surveillance recommendations [40]. Their primary physicians were given patient-specific information. Within 6 months, 41 % of survivors completed the recommended mammogram and 20 % completed the echocardiogram. However, providing written directives may not be enough, as they can be easily misplaced or lost [39]. Electronic health records accessible by survivors or their care providers through secure Internet portals, such as the

Passport for Care initiative [41], may address some of these issues.

### 23.4.2.2 Barriers Related to the Health-Care Provider

Barriers related to the health-care provider involve both the pediatric cancer specialist and the adult-focused physician. Among both pediatric oncology clinicians and survivors, there are concerns that adult-focused primary care providers lack survivorship expertise [15, 36, 37]. A factor likely contributing to this is the current paucity of survivorship-related content in medical school curricula, primary care residency training, and family nurse practitioner or physician assistant training, in comparison with pediatric oncology fellowships where survivorship training is improving [42]. However, even with such exposure during training, the relative rarity of childhood cancer makes it difficult for the typical primary care provider to accumulate significant experience and maintain knowledge in this area.

This lack of survivorship expertise might be addressed in several ways. Fundamentally, clinical survivorship and health-care transition must be addressed at multiple levels of education for health-care professionals, particularly during the training of primary care providers, including physicians in family medicine, internal medicine, and medicine/pediatrics, as well as family nurse practitioners and physician assistants. It also needs to be included as a topic in continuing medical education conferences and online courses, such as the "Focus Under Forty" series offered by the American Society of Clinical Oncology [41]. As discussed earlier, risk stratification at survivorship transition could be used to direct only the lowest risk patients to primary care providers. Models of shared care between survivorship centers and primary care providers show encouraging preliminary experience [32, 33]. Another strategy is to make patient-specific treatment information and monitoring recommendations available to both survivors and their primary care providers through a secure, interactive online resource that can be accessed in real time at the point of care, the prototype for this being

Passport for Care [41]. Passport for Care could prove helpful even for some pediatric oncologists, as a recent survey documented suboptimal screening guideline knowledge when they were given a clinical vignette describing a young woman previously treated for Hodgkin's lymphoma with chest irradiation and anthracycline chemotherapy [43].

### 23.4.2.3 Barriers Related to Systems of Care

Two important system-based issues serve as barriers to effective survivorship care. The first is a lack of survivorship care networks linking pediatric and adult-focused providers. A key element for facilitating this is a shared electronic medical record (EMR) containing relevant clinical detail for each patient. Currently, very few institutional EMR systems are capable of interfacing with outside providers, which severely hampers their utility in survivorship care. In the interim, it is especially important for transition-related medical information to be transmitted from the pediatric treatment center to the adult service by other means. The Web-based Passport for Care initiative represents another emerging option [41].

The second issue, particularly pertinent in the United States, is the lack of continuous health insurance coverage over the transitional age period. Data from the CCSS have documented that, compared with siblings, young adult survivors have less health insurance coverage and encounter greater difficulty obtaining it [44]. In the United States, young adults in general are the most underinsured segment of the population [45]. Typically, children with cancer are covered by Medicaid-funded state programs for catastrophic illness, but this coverage usually ends at 21 years of age, resulting in the "aging out" phenomenon commonly mentioned in US transitional care literature. For young adult survivors fortunate enough to qualify for coverage on their parents' private health insurance policy, a provision of the Patient Protection and Affordable Care Act passed in 2010 by the US Congress permits them to remain covered until 26 years of age and to be exempt from exclusion for prior conditions [18].

## Conclusions

The transition to long-term cancer survivorship care takes place against a backdrop of each patient's normal physical and psychosocial development. Understanding the major developmental tasks of childhood and adolescence is essential for normalizing the cancer survivorship experience and for taking advantage of opportunities to prepare maturing teens for medical decision making and other health-related responsibilities of adulthood. Many survivors remain at increased lifelong risk for clinically significant complications of their cancer therapy. The major objectives of long-term follow-up care are risk-based monitoring for late effects and provision of health information to the survivor and family. Successful transition of young adult survivors from the pediatric to adult-focused setting must overcome barriers at the level of survivors, providers, and health-care systems but is essential nonetheless for continuing medically and developmentally appropriate survivorship care over the lifespan.

## References

1. Hobbie WL (1986) The role of the pediatric oncology nurse specialist in a follow-up clinic for long-term survivors of childhood cancer. J Assoc Pediatr Oncol Nurses 3:9–12, 24
2. Needlman RD (2004) Growth and development. In: Behrman R, Kliegman R, Jenson H (eds) Nelson textbook of pediatrics, 17th edn. W.B. Saunders, Philadelphia
3. Hewitt M, Weiner S, Simone J (2003) Childhood cancer survivorship: improving care and quality of life. National Academies Press, Washington, DC
4. Hudson MM, Mulrooney DA, Bowers DC et al (2009) High-risk populations identified in Childhood Cancer Survivor Study investigations: implications for risk-based surveillance. J Clin Oncol 27:2405–2414
5. Mertens AC, Liu Q, Neglia JP et al (2008) Cause-specific late mortality among 5-year survivors of childhood cancer: the Childhood Cancer Survivor Study. J Natl Cancer Inst 100:1368–1379
6. Oeffinger KC, Mertens AC, Sklar CA et al (2006) Chronic health conditions in adult survivors of childhood cancer. N Engl J Med 355:1572–1582
7. Landier W, Bhatia S, Eshelman DA et al (2004) Development of risk-based guidelines for pediatric cancer survivors: the Children's Oncology Group Long-Term Follow-Up Guidelines from the Children's Oncology Group Late Effects Committee and Nursing Discipline. J Clin Oncol 22:4979–4990
8. Children's Oncology Group [Internet] (cited 21 May 2012). Available from: http://www.survivorshipguidelines.org/
9. Landier W, Armenian SH, Lee J et al (2012) Yield of screening for long-term complications using the Children's Oncology Group Long-Term Follow-Up Guidelines. J Clin Oncol 30:4401–4408
10. CCLG – therapy based long term follow up, 2nd edn. [Internet] (cited 28 Sep 2011). Available from: http://www.cclg.org.uk/researchandtreatment/content.php?3id=29&2id=19
11. Jaspers MWM, Van den Bos C, Heinen RC et al (2007) Development of a national protocol to screen Dutch cancer survivors on late cancer treatment effects. Int J Med Inform 76:297–305
12. Long term follow up care or survivors of childhood cancer [Internet] (cited 28 Sep 2011). Available from: http://www.sign.ac.uk/guidelines/fulltext/76/
13. American Academy of Pediatrics Section Statement Section on Hematology/Oncology (1997) Guidelines for the pediatric cancer center and role of such centers in diagnosis and treatment. Pediatrics 99:139–141
14. Friedman DL, Freyer DR, Levitt GA (2006) Models of care for survivors of childhood cancer. Pediatr Blood Cancer 46:159–168
15. Eshelman-Kent D, Kinahan KE, Hobbie W et al (2011) Cancer survivorship practices, services, and delivery: a report from the Children's Oncology Group (COG) nursing discipline, adolescent/young adult, and late effects committees. J Cancer Surviv 5:345–357
16. Aziz NM, Oeffinger KC, Brooks S et al (2006) Comprehensive long-term follow-up programs for pediatric cancer survivors. Cancer 107:841–848
17. McCabe MS, Bhatia S, Oeffinger KC et al (2013) American Society of Clinical Oncology statement: achieving high-quality cancer survivorship care. J Clin Oncol 31:631–640
18. Wolfson J, Ruccione K, Reaman GH (2010) Health care reform 2010: expected favorable impact on childhood cancer patients and survivors. Cancer J 16:554–562
19. Blum RW, Garell D, Hodgman CH et al (1993) Transition from child-centered to adult health-care systems for adolescents with chronic conditions: a position paper of the Society for Adolescent Medicine. J Adolesc Health 14:570–576
20. Cameron JS (2001) The continued care of children with renal disease into adult life. Pediatr Nephrol 16:680–685
21. Knauth A, Verstappen A, Reiss J et al (2006) Transition and transfer from pediatric to adult care of the young adult with complex congenital heart disease. Cardiol Clin 24:619–629
22. McDonagh JE (2007) Transition of care from paediatric to adult rheumatology. Arch Dis Child 92:802–807

23. Freyer DR (2010) Transition of care for young adult survivors of childhood and adolescent cancer: rationale and approaches. J Clin Oncol 28:4810–4818

24. Table A-4. Employment status of the civilian population 25 years and over by educational attainment [Internet] (cited 16 Dec 2012). Available from: http://www.bls.gov/news.release/empsit.t04.htm

25. Kirchhoff AC, Leisenring W, Krull KR et al (2010) Unemployment among adult survivors of childhood cancer: a report from the childhood cancer survivor study. Med Care 48:1015–1025

26. Kenney LB, Bradeen H, Kadan-Lottick NS et al (2011) The current status of follow-up services for childhood cancer survivors, are we meeting goals and expectations: a report from the Consortium for New England Childhood Cancer Survivors. Pediatr Blood Cancer 57:1062–1066

27. Guilcher GMT, Fitzgerald C, Pritchard S (2009) A questionnaire based review of long-term follow-up programs for survivors of childhood cancer in Canada. Pediatr Blood Cancer 52:113–115

28. Sturman DA, Moghaddam B (2011) The neurobiology of adolescence: changes in brain architecture, functional dynamics, and behavioral tendencies. Neurosci Biobehav Rev 35:1704–1712

29. Reiss J, Gibson R (2002) Health care transition: destinations unknown. Pediatrics 110:1307–1314

30. Schwartz LA, Tuchman LK, Hobbie WL et al (2011) A social-ecological model of readiness for transition to adult-oriented care for adolescents and young adults with chronic health conditions. Child Care Health Dev 37:883–895

31. Oeffinger KC, Mertens AC, Hudson MM et al (2004) Health care of young adult survivors of childhood cancer: a report from the Childhood Cancer Survivor Study. Ann Fam Med 2:61–70

32. Blaauwbroek R, Tuinier W, Meyboom-de Jong B et al (2008) Shared care by paediatric oncologists and family doctors for long-term follow-up of adult childhood cancer survivors: a pilot study. Lancet Oncol 9:232–238

33. Meacham LR, Edwards PJ, Cherven BO et al (2012) Primary care providers as partners in long-term follow-up of pediatric cancer survivors. J Cancer Surviv 6:270–277

34. Eiser C, Absolom K, Greenfield D et al (2006) Follow-up after childhood cancer: evaluation of a three-level model. Eur J Cancer 42:3186–3190

35. Wallace WHB, Blacklay A, Eiser C et al (2001) Developing strategies for long term follow up of survivors of childhood cancer. BMJ 323:271–274

36. Mertens AC, Cotter KL, Foster BM et al (2004) Improving health care for adult survivors of childhood cancer: recommendations from a delphi panel of health policy experts. Health Policy 69:169–178

37. Zebrack BJ, Eshelman DA, Hudson MM et al (2004) Health care for childhood cancer survivors. Cancer 100:843–850

38. Casillas J, Kahn KL, Doose M et al (2010) Transitioning childhood cancer survivors to adult-centered healthcare: insights from parents, adolescent, and young adult survivors. Psychooncology 19:982–990

39. Kadan-Lottick NS, Robison LL, Gurney JG et al (2002) Childhood cancer survivors' knowledge about their past diagnosis and treatment. JAMA J Am Med Assoc 287:1832–1839

40. Oeffinger KC, Hudson MM, Mertens AC et al (2011) Increasing rates of breast cancer and cardiac surveillance among high-risk survivors of childhood Hodgkin lymphoma following a mailed, one-page survivorship care plan. Pediatr Blood Cancer 56:818–824

41. Horowitz ME, Fordis M, Krause S, McKellar J, Poplack DG. J Oncol Pract 2009; 5(3):110–112. doi:10.1200/JOP.0934405

42. Nathan PC, Schiffman JD, Huang S et al (2011) Childhood cancer survivorship educational resources in North American pediatric hematology/oncology fellowship training programs: a survey study. Pediatr Blood Cancer 57:1186–1190

43. Henderson TO, Hlubocky FJ, Wroblewski KE et al (2010) Physician preferences and knowledge gaps regarding the care of childhood cancer survivors: a mailed survey of pediatric oncologists. J Clin Oncol 28:878–883

44. Park ER, Li FP, Liu Y et al (2005) Health insurance coverage in survivors of childhood cancer: the Childhood Cancer Survivor Study. J Clin Oncol 23:9187–9197

45. Nicholson J, Collins S, Mahato B et al (2009) Rite of passage? Why young adults become uninsured and how new policies can help, 2009 update. Commonw Fund 64:1–20

46. Venkatramani R, Freyer DR (2012) Transitional phases from acute care to long term follow up and adult survivorship. In: Mucci GA, Torno L et al (eds) Handbook of long term care of the childhood cancer survivor. Springer, New York

# Health Promotion

24

Holly DeLuca and Karim Thomas Sadak

## Contents

H. DeLuca (✉)
Division of Pediatric Hematology/Oncology,
University of Maryland Medical Center
Children's Hospital, Baltimore, MD, USA
e-mail: hdeluca@umm.edu

K.T. Sadak
Division of Pediatric Hematology/Oncology,
University of Minnesota Masonic Children's Hospital,
Minneapolis, MN, USA

## 24.1   Introduction

Long-term follow-up care for the childhood cancer survivor has evolved from describing late effects to evaluating interventions that might prevent or reduce the severity of long-term complications from previous life-saving treatments. This progression has led to an emphasis on disease prevention through health promotion. Guidance for health promotion has traditionally been provided to patients by a primary care provider. Due to the potential for adverse health outcomes in childhood cancer survivors, health-care providers must be aware of routine health promotion guidelines as well as those that are specifically relevant for the survivor. This chapter includes information on appropriate diet and physical activity, health-risk behaviors, complementary and alternative medicine, and general cancer screening that can be used by health-care providers counseling survivors about health promotion.

## 24.2   Diet and Physical Activity

The Childhood Cancer Survivor Study (CCSS) reports that 62.3 % of survivors have at least one chronic health condition compared to 36.8 % of sibling controls. The most common chronic conditions reported in the CCSS cohort are cardiovascular disease, kidney dysfunction, musculoskeletal problems, endocrinopathies, and

© Springer International Publishing 2015
C.L. Schwartz et al. (eds.), *Survivors of Childhood and Adolescent Cancer:*
*A Multidisciplinary Approach*, Pediatric Oncology, DOI 10.1007/978-3-319-16435-9_24

second cancers [1]. Survivors in the CCSS cohort are almost twice as likely as siblings to take medications for hypertension. Anthracycline exposure and abdomen or chest radiation increased the risk for hypertension [2]. An increased prevalence of hypertension has also been reported in survivors of childhood acute lymphoblastic leukemia [3].

Corticosteroids, methotrexate, and radiation to weight-bearing bones as well as growth hormone, testosterone, and/or estrogen deficiency enhance risk for low bone mineral density (BMD) with subsequent risk of fracture [4–6]. More severe sequelae such as osteonecrosis (ON) or avascular necrosis may also be associated with cancer treatment.

Childhood cancer survivors are at increased risk for obesity compared to US normative data [7]. Hypothalamic/pituitary injury may lead to hypothalamic obesity syndrome including fatigue, decreased physical activity, insulin and leptin resistance, uncontrolled appetite, and morbid obesity [8–10]. The incidence of severe obesity in children and adolescents who have undergone surgical resection of a craniopharyngioma is 22–62 % [8–10]. Risk factors for obesity include cancer diagnosed at 5–9 years of age, female sex, abnormal physical function, cranial radiation doses of 20–30 Gy, and exposure to high levels of corticosteroids [7, 11].

Physical inactivity and poor diet are believed to enhance risk or severity of late effects of treatment [6, 12–15]. Several studies indicate that less than 50 % of survivors meet the recommended guidelines for physical activity [13, 16–19]. In addition, childhood cancer survivors have been shown to have poor dietary habits, consume excessive calories, and not follow dietary guidelines in two reports [20, 21]. Conversely, a significant proportion of adult survivors of childhood cancer are underweight. In the CCSS cohort, these underweight survivors were most likely to report adverse health outcomes and major medical conditions [7]. It is unclear what impact this may have on future health outcomes or whether this is a consequence of active medical conditions.

The following will review the recommended physical activity and dietary guidelines most relevant to childhood cancer survivors.

## 24.2.1 Physical Activity

In 2008, the US Department of Health and Human Services Centers for Disease Control and Prevention (CDC) published physical activity guidelines: *2008 Physical Activity Guidelines for Americans* [22]. These guidelines provide evidence-based recommendations to help all Americans improve their health through physical activity. They are especially important for childhood cancer survivors. Maintaining a physically active lifestyle provides health benefits to individuals of all ages by reducing the risk of chronic illness that may lead to disability and/or premature death. These include coronary heart disease, stroke, osteoporosis, depression, type 2 diabetes, and some cancers.

According to the *2008 Physical Activity Guidelines for Americans*, aerobic activity, muscle strengthening activity, and bone strengthening activity are necessary to achieve the health benefits listed in Table 24.1. Intensity, frequency, and duration/repetition are important components of all of these. However, the total amount of physical activity is more important for achieving health

**Table 24.1** Health benefits associated with regular physical activity

| Children and adolescents |
| --- |
| Improved cardiopulmonary and muscular fitness |
| Improved bone health |
| Improved cardiovascular and metabolic health biomarkers |
| Reduced symptoms of depression |
| Adults |
| Lower risk of early death |
| Lower risk of coronary artery disease |
| Lower risk of stroke |
| Lower risk of hypertension |
| Lower risk of type 2 diabetes |
| Lower risk of metabolic syndrome |
| Lower risk of colon and breast cancer |
| Improved cardiopulmonary and muscular fitness |
| Improved bone density |
| Improved blood lipid profile |
| Weight loss and prevention of weight gain |
| Reduced symptoms of depression |

Adapted from *2008 Physical Activity Guidelines for Americans*

**Table 24.2**  Minimum physical activity requirements to achieve health benefits

| Level of intensity | Adults | Children and adolescents |
|---|---|---|
| *Moderate intensity* Individual participating in the activity can talk but not sing during the activity | 150 min moderate-intensity aerobic activity each week OR 75 min vigorous-intensity aerobic activity each week | 60 min or more daily moderate to vigorous-intensity aerobic activity Activities should be age appropriate, varied, and enjoyable |
| Energy expenditure is 3–5.9 times the amount of energy expended at rest | At least 10 min intervals of activity spread throughout the week | |
| *Vigorous intensity* Individual participating in the activity cannot say more than a few words without pausing for a breath Energy expenditure is 6 or more times the amount of energy expended at rest | Muscle strengthening activities 2 or more days each week. Work all major muscle groups (legs, hips, back, abdomen, chest, shoulders, and arms) in sets of 8–12 repetitions | Muscle strengthening and weight-bearing activities that produce force on the bones at least 3 days each week as part of the 60 min per day of physical activity Work all the major muscle groups of the body |

Adapted from *2008 Physical Activity Guidelines for Americans*

benefits than is any one component or specific combination of activities. The minimum physical activity requirements recommended by the CDC to obtain substantial health benefits are detailed in Table 24.2.

Health-care providers should encourage survivors to participate in physical activity as recommended by the CDC guidelines. The risk of developing many of the late effects of childhood cancer therapy can be decreased through regular exercise including cardiovascular disease, diabetes, obesity, stroke, decreased bone mineral density, and some second malignant neoplasms. Existing late effects may also be ameliorated through participation in adequate physical activity. Bone strengthening activities are especially important for child and adolescent survivors at risk for low BMD since the greatest increase in bone mass occurs just before and during puberty and peak bone mass is obtained by the end of adolescence [23]. Participation in regular weight-bearing exercise during adolescent growth can significantly increase bone mineral content [24, 25].

### 24.2.1.1 Physical Activity: Special Considerations

The Children's Oncology Group (COG) Long-Term Follow-Up Guidelines recommend that survivors who received anthracycline chemotherapy and/or chest radiation should be coun-

seled to avoid intense isometric exercise as this has been reported to precipitate cardiac events in survivors. Aerobic exercise and high repetition lifting of light weights are generally thought to be safe in this population, although this has not been studied prospectively due to obvious difficulties with study design. Survivors who choose to participate in strenuous activity or competitive sports should discuss their personal risk with a health-care provider and receive ongoing monitoring by a cardiologist [26].

Survivors who had limb-sparing surgery should discuss limitations on physical activity with their orthopedic surgeon. High levels of physical activity may damage the endoprosthesis [26]. However, regular participation in approved exercise should be encouraged to prevent functional limitation and decreased bone mineral density [4].

Survivors who have undergone nephrectomy should protect their single kidney during physical activity by staying well hydrated [26]. Survivors with a single kidney should be encouraged to discuss their kidney status with a health-care provider before participation in contact sports or recreational activities. Caution should be taken to avoid bicycle handlebar injuries. A kidney guard may be worn during activities with an increased risk for renal injury. Survivors should wear a medical alert bracelet or carry a card in their wallet indicating that they have a single kidney.

The CDC recommends all individuals to wear a helmet when participating in sports that carry a risk of traumatic brain injury. Survivors should be counseled to wear a fitted and well-maintained helmet when riding a bike, skateboard, or scooter; playing a contact sport such as football or hockey; using in-line skates; horseback riding; skiing or snowboarding; and batting/running bases in baseball or softball [27].

## 24.2.2 Diet

A healthy diet can reduce the risk of major chronic health conditions such as heart disease, diabetes, osteoporosis, and cancer. The US Department of Health and Human Services (HHS) and the US Department of Agriculture (USDA) jointly publish Dietary Guidelines every 5 years, including the most recent edition: *Dietary Guidelines for Americans, 2010* [28]. While these goals are intended for the general population, they are especially relevant for childhood cancer survivors.

### 24.2.2.1 Diet: Weight Management

Weight management is a well-documented challenge for survivors of childhood cancer. This includes both being underweight and being obese. *Dietary Guidelines for Americans, 2010* provides basic information readily available to all that can serve as a foundation for dietary health promotion. When available, individualized dietary recommendations from a registered dietician can help minimize the many risk factors associated with obesity or being underweight in the childhood cancer survivor.

*Dietary Guidelines for Americans, 2010* has three major goals that can assist in preventing and/or treating obesity:

1. Balance calories with physical activity to manage weight
2. Consume more of certain foods and nutrients such as fruits, vegetables, whole grains, fat-free and low-fat dairy products, and seafood
3. Consume fewer foods with sodium (salt), saturated fats, trans fats, cholesterol, added sugars, and refined grains

The USDA recommends using a Daily Food Plan to optimize food consumption and caloric intake that promotes a healthy weight. A Daily Food Plan summarizes what and how much to eat within a specific calorie allowance that is based on age, sex, height, weight, and physical activity level [29]. The five recommended food groups are fruit, vegetables, grains, protein, and dairy. For the 2,000 calorie per day level, recommended intakes include 2 cups fruit, 2.5 cups vegetables, 6 oz grains, 5.5 oz protein foods, and 3 cups dairy [30]. Just as an exercise scientist or physical therapist can create a personalized exercise regimen or physical activity plan, a registered dietician can create a personalized nutrition plan that can best help the survivor manage their weight.

### 24.2.2.2 Diet: Hypertension

Like obesity, hypertension is a significant risk factor for heart disease, but can be modified with dietary changes. The Seventh Report of the Joint National Committee on Prevention, Detection, Evaluation, and Treatment of High Blood Pressure (JNC 7) calls for an aggressive approach to treating hypertension including lifestyle modifications with an emphasis on dietary changes before the initiation of drug therapy. The JNC 7 recommends adopting an eating plan that is rich in fruits, vegetables, and low-fat dairy products with reduced content of saturated and total fat [31]. These dietary modifications have been shown to reduce systolic blood pressure by 8–14 mmHg [32, 33]. Blood pressure classifications are summarized in Table 24.3.

An appropriate dietary plan should serve as the mainstay of heart health promotion, along with weight loss and physical activity.

Table 24.3 Classification of blood pressure (BP) ranges for adults

| BP classification | Systolic BP (mmHg) | Diastolic BP (mmHg) |
|---|---|---|
| Normal | <120 | and <80 |
| Prehypertension | 120–139 | or 80–89 |
| Stage 1 hypertension | 140–159 | or 90–99 |
| Stage 2 hypertension | ≥160 | or ≥100 |

Adapted from *JNC 7 Express: The Seventh Report of the Joint National Committee on Prevention, Detection, Evaluation, and Treatment of High Blood Pressure*, 2003

### 24.2.2.3 Diet: Bone Health

Appropriate amounts of dietary calcium and vitamin D are necessary to maintain proper levels of calcium and bone mass. Physiological vitamin D also comes from synthesis in the skin through sunlight exposure. In 2010, the Institute of Medicine (IOM) was commissioned to assess the current data on health outcomes associated with calcium and vitamin D [4]. Their exhaustive review of the evidence determined that calcium and vitamin D have a role in bone health but not in other health conditions. It was concluded that Americans are receiving adequate amounts of both calcium and vitamin D. Additionally, the IOM report indicated that too much of these nutrients may be harmful. The recommended amounts of intake for the general population were based on age and assumed minimal sun exposure. Recommended dietary intake for calcium and vitamin D are summarized in Table 24.4.

It has been hypothesized that in addition to treatment-related risk factors, sedentary lifestyle and inflammation may play a role in bone deficits in childhood cancer survivors [6]. While lifestyle changes are possible, appropriate dietary guidelines should be followed for calcium and vitamin D supplementation to optimize bone health.

Evidence-based guidelines now exist for calcium and vitamin D supplementation. Given the concern for low BMD in both child and adult survivors of childhood cancer, it is prudent to use the IOM recommendations (see Table 24.4 above) regarding calcium and vitamin D as a foundation for supplementation therapy. It is advisable to consult with a registered dietician or endocrinologist for the optimal calcium and vitamin D doses needed by the childhood cancer survivor based on the individual risk for poor bone health.

Table 24.4 Recommended dietary allowance (RDA) for calcium and vitamin D

| Age (years) | Calcium RDA (mg) | Vitamin D (IU) |
| --- | --- | --- |
| 1–3 | 700 | 600 |
| 4–8 | 1,000 | 600 |
| 9–18 | 1,300 | 600 |
| 19–30 | 1,000 | 600 |

Adapted from *Dietary Reference Intakes for Calcium and Vitamin D*, Institute of Medicine, 2010

Special attention must be paid to women on hormonal therapy as that also can affect bone health. In conjunction with the appropriate physical activity regimen, such supplementation can maintain optimal bone health and help prevent low BMD and its serious sequelae such as ON.

## 24.3 Health-Risk Behaviors

A key component of survivor health promotion is minimizing health-risk behaviors. Research indicates that childhood cancer survivors participate in health-risk behaviors at rates similar to their healthy peers. These include tobacco and alcohol use, substance abuse, inadequate sun protection, unsafe sexual practices, poor adherence to general recommendations for diet/exercise, and injury prevention [34–41]. This may not provide survivors with adequate risk reduction given their increased likelihood of chronic health conditions and adverse health outcomes [1]. Some survivors have reported a perception of being more vulnerable to health problems and needing to protect their health [34–42]. Providers must leverage this sentiment to empower survivors with the education and medical assistance needed to promote health-protective behaviors. Behavioral change is a challenge, as factors other than health perceptions are involved, but survivor behaviors can directly determine several health outcomes that must be addressed as part of comprehensive survivorship care [35–43].

### 24.3.1 Tobacco

Tobacco use is the leading cause of preventable illness and death in the United States [36–44]. More than 600,000 middle school students and three million high school students smoke cigarettes [37–45]. In the CCSS, 28 % reported ever smoking with 17 % being current smokers [40]. Adolescent survivors had rates of tobacco use similar to their cancer-free siblings [35, 38–45]. This is still concerning as survivors used tobacco at higher rates than expected given their increased risk of cardiac and pulmonary complications [35, 39–46]. When compared to the general population, survivors of childhood cancer were, in fact, more likely to report being a current smoker than their noncancer peer controls [35, 40–47]. In countries outside the United States, tobacco use among survivors has varied. For example, in Great Britain, the prevalence of smoking among adult survivors of childhood cancer is substantially less overall than that in the general population [35, 40, 42–48]. Given the multiple risks associated with tobacco use, survivorship care should routinely screen for its use and have accessible smoking cessation resources readily available [35, 40, 43–49]. Multiple options exist for smoking cessation, but interventions designed to build self-efficacy may be specifically beneficial for this population [35, 40, 44–50]. Data from the CCSS showed that >69 % of survivors studied engaged in two or more other health-risk behaviors [51]. Reducing other risk behaviors might also encourage survivors to quit smoking [51].

## 24.3.2 Substance Abuse

According to the Centers for Disease Control and Prevention's (CDC) 2011 Youth Risk Behavior Surveillance System (YRBSS), 38.7 % of US high school students had at least one alcoholic drink in the 30 days prior to being surveyed, and 39.9 % had used marijuana one or more times during their life [52]. Varying reports exist on the prevalence of alcohol and drug use by survivors of childhood cancer. Some reports have found no significant difference between survivors and their peers in regard to alcohol use [47]. There is still great concern, however, as the rate of alcohol use in long-term survivors was higher than expected given the increased risk of cardiac and pulmonary sequelae [46]. Another study reported that adult survivors of childhood cancer have decreased alcohol consumption compared to their peers [53]. This trend was also seen in a British cohort of childhood cancer survivors [42]. Illicit drugs that have a stimulatory effect on the cardiovascular system may also pose significant health risks. Therefore, survivors at risk for cardiac long-term complications should be specifically counseled regarding the dangers of any

drug use that may be associated with cardiac side effects, such as cocaine use or methamphetamine abuse and smoking risk factors with marijuana.

Evidence-based interventions are needed to address substance abuse among survivors. The multiorgan damage associated with excessive alcohol consumption can quickly compound the risks of potential cardiac, pulmonary, hepatic, and endocrine complications for the childhood cancer survivor. Interventions specific to the childhood cancer survivor are currently under investigation and many show promise [54, 55]. If substance abuse is suspected by a survivorship provider, a quick and definitive referral to an addiction specialist is necessary for further evaluation and treatment.

## 24.3.3 Sun Safety

Inadequate sun protection is a health-risk behavior that can have serious consequences for the cancer survivor. The risk of skin cancer as a second malignant neoplasm is especially relevant for those who received radiation therapy for their primary malignancy. The CDC recommends that all people take precautions against sun exposure every day of the year, especially during midday hours. This is the time period when ultraviolet (UV) rays are strongest and can do the most damage. UV rays are not blocked by clouds and can damage unprotected skin in as little as 15 min [56]. The CDC recommends the following sun protection (Table 24.5).

In a study of 75 adolescent survivors of childhood cancer, nonadherence to sun protection was the single most common health-risk behavior reported [57]. An educational intervention

Table 24.5 CDC recommendations for sun protection [56]

| | |
|---|---|
| Seek shade, especially during midday hours | Avoid tanning beds and sunlamps |
| Cover up with clothing to protect exposed skin | Use UVA and UVB sunscreen |
| Wear a hat with a wide brim to shade the face, head, ears, and neck | Use sunscreen with protective factor (SPF) 15 or higher |

for these survivors was found to be efficacious in improving short-term self-reported sun safety practices [58]. Nevertheless, sun protection behaviors are difficult to instill in survivors, as in the general population. Even in a group of primary melanoma survivors, the rates of sun protection were no higher than the estimates for the general population [59]. Survivors should also be cautioned about the use of tanning beds which also increases the risk of skin cancer.

### 24.3.4 Injury Prevention

Single kidney health guidelines have been reviewed in the *Physical Activity: Special Considerations* section of this chapter. The use of a helmet when engaging in physical activities that involve movement at high speeds may prevent head injury. The CDC YBRSS found that 87.5 % of youth who had ridden a bicycle in the last year prior to the survey reported not wearing a helmet [52]. As with the general population, age-appropriate preventive medicine and anticipatory guidance should be communicated to all childhood cancer survivors. This involves reviewing seat belt guidelines, especially when survivors approach the legal driving age. Seat belt laws vary, but most states mandate the use of seat belts for drivers and front seat passengers, while many require that all passengers wear seat belts when riding in a passenger vehicle. This anticipatory guidance is critical as 7.7 % of youth surveyed for the YBRSS rarely or never wore a seat belt when riding in a car driven by someone else [52]. Distracted driving should also be included as a risk-taking behavior that should be avoided by survivors. It is now estimated that 33 % of youth text or email while driving a car [52].

### 24.3.5 STI Prevention

It is imperative that all survivors understand their risks for sexually transmitted infections (STIs). Young people in the United States account for nearly half of all new STIs, yet they represent only 25 % of the sexually active population [60].

Consequently, a sexual history should be obtained on all adolescent and young adult survivors of childhood cancer as part of routine survivorship health promotion. In the CCSS cohort, survivors were more likely than their siblings to report being tested for human immunodeficiency virus (HIV) [47]. Furthermore, providers must dispel any survivor misconception that infertility is protective against contracting STIs. Another opportunity for survivor health promotion includes anticipatory guidance regarding human papillomavirus (HPV) infections [61]. A recent study found that the rate of HPV vaccination among female pediatric cancer survivors was not appreciably different than that seen in the general population [62]. Unsafe sexual practices and their associated significant health risks must be addressed as part of childhood cancer survivor health promotion.

## 24.4 Complementary and Alternative Medicine

Complementary and alternative medicine (CAM) is defined by the National Center for Complementary and Alternative Medicine as "a group of diverse medical and healthcare systems, practices, and products that are not presently considered to be a part of conventional medicine" [63]. It includes both biological and nonbiological agents. Some CAM practices fit into more than one category (Table 24.6).

In the general pediatric population, CAM usage rates have been reported to be between 20 % and 40 % [64]. In surveys of children with malignancies, usage rates ranged from 59 % to 84 % [65, 66]. The CCSS reports 39.4 % of adult survivors of childhood cancer used some form of CAM [67]. Another study of 119 childhood cancer survivors ages 7–19 years, who were at least 3 months post completion of therapy, revealed that 82.3 % used at least one form of CAM and 58.9 % used more than one CAM modality. The survivors in this study reported using CAM to reduce the risk of relapse, cope with long-term effects of cancer treatment, or reduce their risk of developing a late effect [68].

**Table 24.6** Types of complementary and alternative medicine

| Whole medical systems | Homeopathic medicine | Small doses of diluted substances that in larger doses would produce illness |
|---|---|---|
| | Naturopathic medicine | Dietary and lifestyle changes with herbs, massage and joint manipulation aiming to support the body's own healing |
| | Traditional Chinese medicine | Combination of herbs, meditation, massages, and acupuncture that aims to aid healing |
| | Ayurveda | Combination of herbs, massage, and yoga aiming to integrate the body, mind, and spirit to prevent and treat disease |
| Mind-body medicine | Mental control and meditation | Hypnosis, hypnotherapy, meditation, faith healers, imagery |
| | Creative outlets | Art, music, or dance |
| Biologically based therapies | Herbal products | For example: curcumin, mistletoe, ginseng, mushrooms, milk thistle, echinacea, saw palmetto, essiac, selenium, ginkgo biloba, valerian, green tea |
| | Dietary supplements | Vitamins, minerals, fatty acids, amino acids, garlic |
| Manipulative and body-based practices | Osteopathic manipulation | Spinal manipulation to relieve pain and improve physical function |
| | Massage | Manipulation of the muscles and soft tissues of the body to relieve pain, reduce stress, increase relaxation, treat anxiety/depression, and aid in general well-being |
| Energy medicine | Bio-field therapies | Acupuncture, acupressure, Reiki, qi gong, therapeutic touch |
| | Bio-electromagnetic-based therapies | Use of electromagnetic fields, such as pulsed fields, magnetic fields, or alternating-current or direct-current fields |

Adapted from http://nccam.nih.gov/health/whatiscam

Despite the popularity of CAM in pediatrics, there is little research on the effectiveness of most CAM in children. In addition, many patients and parents do not disclose CAM use to their health-care providers, and most pediatric oncologists do not ask about CAM use [66, 68, 69]. The discrepancy between patient use and disclosure to health-care providers is potentially dangerous for patients.

The use of CAM as part of a healthy lifestyle may provide support to survivors coping with late effects of their disease and cancer treatment. For example, yoga and meditation may reduce anxiety, improve physical function in balance or gait, and assist with maintaining a healthy weight. Acupuncture may relieve chronic fatigue and pain. Some providers feel that the use of dietary supplements may help optimize bone density and support psychological well-being [70].

Health-care providers should routinely discuss CAM usage with their patients. All uses and effects of CAM therapies should be documented in the medical record. For childhood cancer survivors, the emphasis should be on using CAM therapies to promote overall wellness. This will support health promotion and late effects symptom management and prevention.

## 24.5 Cancer Screening

Comprehensive survivorship care includes routine health maintenance such as age-appropriate cancer screening. For the pediatric provider, this can represent a significant knowledge void as most screening tests begin later in adulthood. Breast cancer screening and guidelines for the cancer survivor have been described previously.

All women are at risk for cervical cancer, with approximately 12,000 women affected in the United States each year [71]. However, early detection and intervention are associated with good long-term survival and quality of life. The American College of Obstetricians and Gynecologists (ACOG) published cervical cancer screening guidelines for average-risk women in 2009. ACOG recommends screening with a Papanicolaou (Pap) test every 2 years starting at age 21 regardless of the age of onset of sexual activity. This interval may be extended to every 3 years at age 30 years with a history of three consecutive negative tests [72]. In a CCSS cohort of 3,392 average-risk female survivors, 80.9 % reported having a Pap smear within the recommended time frame [73]. In order to promote optimal health, female cancer survivors age 21 years and older should be advised to undergo screening for cervical cancer according to the ACOG guidelines. Survivors who are immunocompromised, are HIV positive, have a history of cervical cancer, have human papillomavirus, or have a high-grade pre-cancerous cervical lesion and those who were exposed in utero to diethylstilbestrol are at higher risk for cervical cancer and should seek further advice from a gynecologist for personalized screening recommendations [72].

Colon cancer screening guidelines have also been adapted for the at-risk childhood cancer survivor. Survivors who have received >30 Gy of radiation therapy to any region of the body that may have affected the intestinal tract are at greatest risk for secondary colorectal cancers. Colorectal cancer screening includes colonoscopies every 5 years, starting 10 years after the radiation therapy or at age 35 years (whichever comes last). The highest-risk groups include survivors with concurrent conditions that separately increase the risk of colorectal cancer, such as familial adenomatous polyposis or inflammatory bowel disease. In these cases, colonoscopies should be obtained more frequently [26].

Currently, there is insufficient evidence to suggest that self-testicular exams decrease mortality from testicular cancer. However, many providers instruct patients to perform monthly self-examinations to develop awareness of testicular contour that will increase the chances of identifying testicular irregularities in the future. The optimal time to perform a self-testicular exam is during or after a warm bath or shower, when the skin of the scrotum is most relaxed. The American Cancer Society gives the following instructions for self-exams:

1. Hold the penis out of the way and check one testicle at a time.
2. Hold the testicle between the thumbs and fingers of both hands and roll it gently between all fingers.
3. Look and feel for any hard lumps or smooth rounded bumps or any change in the size, shape, or consistency of the testes [74].

A history of testicular cancer or leukemia is a significant risk factor for testicular disease that warrants survivor self-examinations. Survivors should be educated on how to perform self-examinations and counseled to do so monthly.

Self breast examinations recommendations are covered in the breast chapter, which vary based on the treatment received during cancer therapy.

## Conclusion

Health-care providers in childhood cancer survivorship care need to be aware of age-appropriate recommendations for disease prevention in order to deliver appropriate counseling for health promotion. This knowledge, combined with their expertise in long-term effects of pediatric cancer treatment, will facilitate the adaptation of national health promotion guidelines to meet the needs of each survivor based on his or her individual risk. Table 24.7 includes a list of materials/websites that can be used in patient education regarding health promotion.

**Table 24.7** Resources for patient/family health promotion education

| | |
|---|---|
| *2008 Physical Activity Guidelines for Americans*, US Department of Health and Humans Services | http://www.health.gov/paguidelines/ |
| Cancer Survivors' Network – American Cancer Society | www.cancersurvivorsnetwork.org |
| *Childhood Cancer Survivors: A Practical Guide to Your Future, Third Edition* (includes chapter on staying healthy) | Nancy Keene, Wendy Hobbie, ad Kathy Ruccione. O'Reilly, 2012 |
| Children's Oncology Group Long-Term Follow-Up Guidelines and Health Links (printable patient/family handouts) | www.survivorshipguidelines.org |
| *Dietary Guidelines for Americans 2010* (Updated every 5 years by the US Departments of Agriculture and Health and Human Services) | http://www.cnpp.usda.gov/dietaryguidelines.htm |
| *Eating Well Through Cancer: Easy Recipes & Recommendations During & After Treatment* | Holly Clegg and Gerald Miletello. Favorite Recipes Press, 2006 |
| National Center for Complementary and Alternative Medicine (NCCAM) | http://nccam.nih.gov/health/providers/forpatients.htm |
| National Children's Cancer Society: Beyond the Cure | www.beyoundthecure.org |
| OncoLink | www.oncolink.org |
| Smokefree.gov (information and professional guidance from the National Cancer Institute to help smokers quit) | www.smokefree.gov |

# References

1. Oeffinger KC, Mertens AC, Sklar CA et al (2006) Chronic health conditions in adult survivors of childhood cancer. N Engl J Med 355:1572–1582
2. Meacham LR, Chow EJ, Ness KK et al (2010) Cardiovascular risk factors in adult survivors of pediatric cancer – a report from the childhood cancer survivor study. Cancer Epidemiol Biomarkers Prev 19(1):170–181
3. Chow EJ, Pihoker C, Hunt K, Wilkinson K, Friedman DL (2007) Obesity and hypertension among children after treatment for acute lymphoblastic leukemia. Cancer 110(10):2313–2320
4. Thomas IJ, Donohue JE, Ness KK, Dengel DR, Baker KS, Gurney JG (2008) Bone mineral density in young adult survivors of acute lymphoblastic leukemia. Cancer 113(11):3248–3256
5. LeMeignen M, Auquier P, Barlogis V et al (2011) Bone mineral density in adult survivors of childhood acute leukemia: impact of hematopoietic stem cell transplantation and other treatment modalities. Blood 118(6):1481–1489
6. Polgreen LE, Petryk A, Dietz AC et al (2012) Modifiable risk factors associated with bone deficits in childhood cancer survivors. BMC Pediatr 12(1):40
7. Meacham LR, Gurney JG, Mertens AC et al (2005) Body mass index in long-term adult survivors of childhood cancer: a report of the Childhood Cancer Survivor Study. Cancer 103:1730–1739
8. Roth C (2011) Hypothalamic obesity in patients with craniopharyngioma: profound changes of several weight regulatory circuits. Front Endocrinol 2(49):1–6
9. Muller HL (2008) Childhood craniopharyngioma. Recent advances in diagnosis, treatment, and follow-up. Horm Res 69:193–202
10. Shwartz MW, Woods SC, Porte D et al (2000) Central nervous system control of food intake. Nature 404:661–667
11. Green DM, Cox CL, Zhu L, Krull KR, Srivastava DK, Stovall M et al (2012) Risk factors for obesity in adult survivors of childhood cancer: a report from the Childhood Cancer Survivor Study. J Clin Oncol 30(3):246–255
12. Hoffman KE, Derdak J, Bernstein D et al (2008) Metabolic syndrome traits in long-term survivors of pediatric sarcoma. Pediatr Blood Cancer 50:341–346
13. Florin TA, Fryer GE, Miyoshi T et al (2007) Physical inactivity in adult survivors of childhood acute lymphoblastic leukemia: a report from the childhood cancer survivorship study. Cancer Epidemiol Biomark Prev 16:1356–1363
14. Oeffinger KC (2008) Are survivors of acute lymphoblastic leukemia (all) at increased risk of cardiovascular disease? Pediatr Blood Cancer 50:462–467
15. Oeffinger KC, Nathan PC, Kremer LCM (2008) Challenges after curative treatment for childhood cancer and long-term follow-up of survivors. Pediatr Clin N Am 55:251–273
16. Ness KK, Wendy ML, Sujuan H et al (2009) Predictors of inactive lifestyle among adult survivors of childhood cancer. Cancer 115:1984–1994
17. Keats MR, Culos-Reed SN, Courneya KS et al (2006) An examination of physical activity behaviors in a sample of adolescent cancer survivors. J Pediatr Oncol Nurs 23:135–142
18. Castillino SM, Casillas J, Hudson MM et al (2005) Minority adult survivors of childhood cancer: a

comparison of long-term outcomes, health care utilization, and health-related behaviors from the childhood cancer survivor study. J Am Soc Clin Oncol 23:6499–6507

19. Hocking MC, Schwartz LA, Hobbie WL et al (2012) Prospectively examining physical activity in young adult survivors of childhood cancer and healthy controls. Pediatr Blood Cancer. doi:10.1002/pbc

20. Cohen J, Wakefield CE, Fleming CA, Gawthorne R, Tapsell LC, Cohn RJ (2012) Dietary intake after treatment in child cancer survivors. Pediatr Blood Cancer 58(5):752–757

21. Robien K, Ness KK, Klesges LM, Baker KS, Gurney JG (2008) Poor adherence to dietary guidelines among adult survivors of childhood acute lymphoblastic leukemia. J Pediatr Hematol Oncol 30(11):815–822

22. U.S. Department of Health and Human Services (2008) 2008 physical activity guidelines for Americans. Office of Disease Prevention and Health Promotion publication No. U0036

23. Pitukcheewanont P, Punyasavatsut N, Feuille M (2010) Physical activity and bone health in children and adolescents. Pediatr Endocrinol Rev 7(3):275–282

24. Kato T, Yamashita T, Mizutani S et al (2009) Adolescent exercise associated with long-term superior measures of bone geometry: a cross-sectional DXA and MRI study. Br J Sports Med 43(12):932–935

25. Wang Q, Alen M, Nicholson P et al (2007) Weight-bearing, muscle loading and bone mineral accrual in pubertal girls: a 2-year longitudinal study. Bone 40(5):1196–1202

26. The Children's Oncology Group long-term follow-up guidelines for survivors of childhood, adolescent and young adult cancers, version 3.0 – Oct 2008. www.survivorshipguidelines.org

27. Injury prevention and control: traumatic brain injury (May 2012). Center for Disease Control and Prevention, National Center for Injury Prevention and Control. http://www.cdc.gov/traumaticbraininjury/prevention.html Accessed on 24 Jul 2012

28. U.S. Department of Agriculture, U.S. Department of Health and Human Services (2010) Dietary guidelines for Americans, 2010, 7th edn. U.S. Government Printing Office, Washington, DC

29. Super Tracker & Other Tools: Daily Food Plans (2011) In ChooseMyPlate.gov. Retrieved from http://www.choosemyplate.gov/supertracker-tools/daily-food-plans.html

30. FAQs: I. Food and Diet (2011) In ChooseMyPlate.gov. Retrieved from http://www.choosemyplate.gov/faqs.html

31. Chobanian AV, Bakris GL, Black HR et al (2003) Seventh report of the Joint National Committee on prevention, detection, evaluation, and treatment of high blood pressure. Hypertension 42(6):1206–1252

32. Sacks FM, Svetkey LP, Vollmer WM et al (2001) Effects on blood pressure of reduced dietary sodium and the Dietary Approaches to Stop Hypertension (DASH) diet. DASH-Sodium Collaborative Research Group. N Engl J Med 344:3–10

33. Vollmer WM, Sacks FM, Ard J et al (2001) Effects of diet and sodium intake on blood pressure: subgroup analysis of the DASH-sodium trial. Ann Intern Med 135:1019–1028

34. Ford JS, Ostroff JS (2006) Health behaviors of childhood cancer survivors: what we've learned. J Clin Psych Med Set 13(2):151–167

35. Klosky JL, Howell CR, Li Z, Foster RH et al (2012) Risky health behavior among adolescents in the childhood cancer survivor study cohort. J Pediatr Psychol 37(6):634–646

36. Oeffinger KC (2003) Longitudinal risk-based health care for adult survivors of childhood cancer. Curr Probl Cancer 27(3):143–163

37. Cox CL, Rai SN, Rosenthal D, Phipps S, Hudson MM (2008) Subclinical late cardiac toxicity in childhood cancer survivors: impact on self-reported health. Cancer 112(8):1835–1844

38. Carpentier MY, Mullins LL, Elkin TD, Wolfe-Christensen C (2008) Predictors of health-harming and health-protective behaviors in adolescents with cancer. Pediatr Blood Cancer 51(4):525–530

39. Arroyave WD, Clipp EC, Miller PE et al (2008) Childhood cancer survivors' perceived barriers to improving exercise and dietary behaviors. Oncol Nurs Forum 35(1):121–130

40. Emmons K, Li FP, Whitton J et al (2002) Predictors of smoking initiation and cessation among childhood cancer survivors: a report from the childhood cancer survivor study. J Clin Onc 20(6):1608–1616

41. Hollen PJ, Hobbie WL, Donnangelo SF, Shannon S, Erikson J (2007) Substance use risk behaviors and decision-making skills among cancer-surviving adolescents. J Pediatr Oncol Nurs 24(5):264–273

42. Tyc VL, Hadley W, Crockett G (2001) Prediction of health behaviors in pediatric cancer survivors. Med Pediatr Oncol 37:42–46

43. Hudson MM, Findlay S (2006) Health-risk behaviors and health promotion in adolescent and young adult cancer survivors. Cancer 107:1695–1701

44. U.S. Department of Health and Human Services. Center for Disease Control (2004) 2004 surgeon general's report: the health consequences of smoking. Retrieved from http://www.cdc.gov/tobacco/data_statistics/sgr/2004/index.htm

45. U.S. Department of Health and Human Services. Center for Disease Control (2012) Preventing tobacco use among youth and young adults fact sheet. Retrieved from http://www.surgeon-general.gov/library/reports/preventing-youth-tobacco-use/fact-sheet.html

46. Nathan PC, Ford JS, Henderson TO et al (2009) Health behaviors, medical care, and interventions to promote healthy living in the Childhood Cancer Survivor Study cohort. J Clin Oncol 27(14):2363–2373

47. Phillips-Salimi CR, Lommel K, Andrykowski MA (2012) Physical and mental health status and health behaviors of childhood cancer survivors: findings from the 2009 BRFSS survey. Pediatr Blood Cancer 58(6):964–970

48. Frobisher C, Winter DL, Lancashire ER et al (2008) Extent of smoking and age at initiation of smoking among adult survivors of childhood cancer in Britain. J Natl Cancer Inst 100(15):1068–1081

49. de Moor JS, Puleo E, Ford JS et al (2011) Disseminating a smoking cessation intervention to childhood and young adult cancer survivors: baseline characteristics and study design of the partnership for health-2 study. BMC Cancer 11:165

50. Asfar T, Klesges RC, Sanford SD et al (2010) Trial design: the St. Jude Children's Research Hospital cancer survivors tobacco quit line study. Contemp Clin Trials 31(1):82–91

51. Butterfield RM, Park ER, Puleo E et al (2004) Multiple risk behaviors among smokers in the childhood cancer survivors study cohort. Psychooncology 13(9):619–629

52. The Centers for Disease Control and Prevention (2012) Morbidity and mortality weekly report. Youth risk behavior surveillance—United States 2011. Retrieved from http://www.cdc.gov/mmwr/pdf/ss/ss6104.pdf

53. Lown EA, Goldsby R, Mertens AC et al (2008) Alcohol consumption patterns and risk factors among childhood cancer survivors compared to siblings and general population peers. Addiction 103(7):1139–1148

54. Hollen PJ, Hobbie WL, Finley SM (1999) Testing the effects of a decision-making and risk-reduction program for cancer-surviving adolescents. Oncol Nurs Forum 26(9):1475–1486

55. Bauld C, Toumbourou JW, Anderson V et al (2005) Health-risk behaviours among adolescent survivors of childhood cancer. Pediatr Blood Cancer 45(5):706–715

56. The Centers for Disease Control and Prevention (2012) Skin cancer awareness: protect your skin. Retrieved from http://www.cdc.gov/Features/SkinCancer/

57. Tercyak KP, Donze JR, Prahlad S et al (2006) Multiple behavioral risk factors among adolescent survivors of childhood cancer in the Survivor Health and Resilience Education (SHARE) program. Pediatr Blood Cancer 47(6):825–830

58. Mays D, Black JD, Mosher RB et al (2011) Improving short-term sun safety practices among adolescent survivors of childhood cancer: a randomized controlled efficacy trial. J Cancer Surviv 5(3):247–254

59. Mujumdar UJ, Hay JL, Monroe-Hinds YC et al (2009) Sun protection and skin self-examination in melanoma survivors. Psychooncology 18(10):1106–1115

60. The Centers for Disease Control and Prevention (2010) 2010 sexually transmitted diseases surveillance. STD Trends in the United States: 2010 national data for gonorrhea, chlamydia, and syphilis. Retrieved from http://www.cdc.gov/std/stats10/trends.htm/

61. Klosky JL, Gamble HL, Spunt SL et al (2009) Human papillomavirus vaccination in survivors of childhood cancer. Cancer 115(24):5627–5736

62. Hoffman L, Okcu MF, Dreyer ZE, et al (2012) Human papillomavirus vaccination in female pediatric cancer survivors. J Pediatr Adolesc Gynecol. [Epub ahead of print]

63. NCCAM National Institutes of Health. http://nccam.nih.gov/health/whatiscam. Accessed 10 Jul 2012; 25(5):305–307

64. Highfield ES, McLellan MC, Kemper KJ et al (2005) Integration of complementary and alternative medicine in a major pediatric teaching hospital: an initial overview. J Altern Complement Med 11:373–380

65. Post-White J, Fitzgerald M, Hageness S et al (2009) Complementary and alternative medicine use in children with cancer and general and specialty pediatrics. J Pediatr Oncol Nurs 26:7–15

66. Kelly KM, Jacobson JS, Kennedy DD et al (2000) Use of unconventional therapies by children with cancer at an urban medical center. J Pediatr Hematol Oncol 22:412–416

67. Mertens AC, Sencer S, Myers CD, et al (2008) Complementary and alternative therapy use in adult survivors of childhood cancer: a report from the childhood cancer survivor study. Pediatr Blood Cancer 50(1):90–97

68. Nees S, Ladas EJ, Hughes D et al (2008) Complementary/alternative medical therapies used by survivors of childhood cancer [abstract]. J Soc Integr Oncol 6:178

69. Roth M, Lin J, Kim M et al (2009) Pediatric oncologists' views toward the use of complementary and alternative medicine in children with cancer. J Pediatr Hematol Oncol 31:177–182

70. Kemper KJ, Shannon S (2007) Complementary and alternative medicine therapies to promote healthy mood. Pediatr Clin N Am 54:901–926

71. U.S. Cancer Statistics Working Group (2012) United States Cancer Statistics: 1999–2008 incidence and mortality web-based report. Atlanta: Department of Health and Human Services, Centers for Disease Control and Prevention, and National Cancer Institute. Available at: http://www.cdc.gov/uscs. Accessed 31 Jul 2012

72. ACOG practice bulletin no. 109: Cervical cytology screening (2009). ACOG committee on practice bulletins – gynecology. Obstet Gynecol 114(6):1409–1420.

73. Nathan PC, Ness KK, Mahoney MC et al (2010) Screening and surveillance for second malignant neoplasms in adult survivors of childhood cancer: a report from the childhood cancer survivor study. Ann Intern Med 153(7):442–451

74. The American Cancer Society (2012). Do I have testicular cancer?. Retrieved from http://www.cancer.org/Cancer/TesticularCancer/MoreInformation/DoIHaveTesticularCancer/do-i-have-testicular-cancer-self-exam